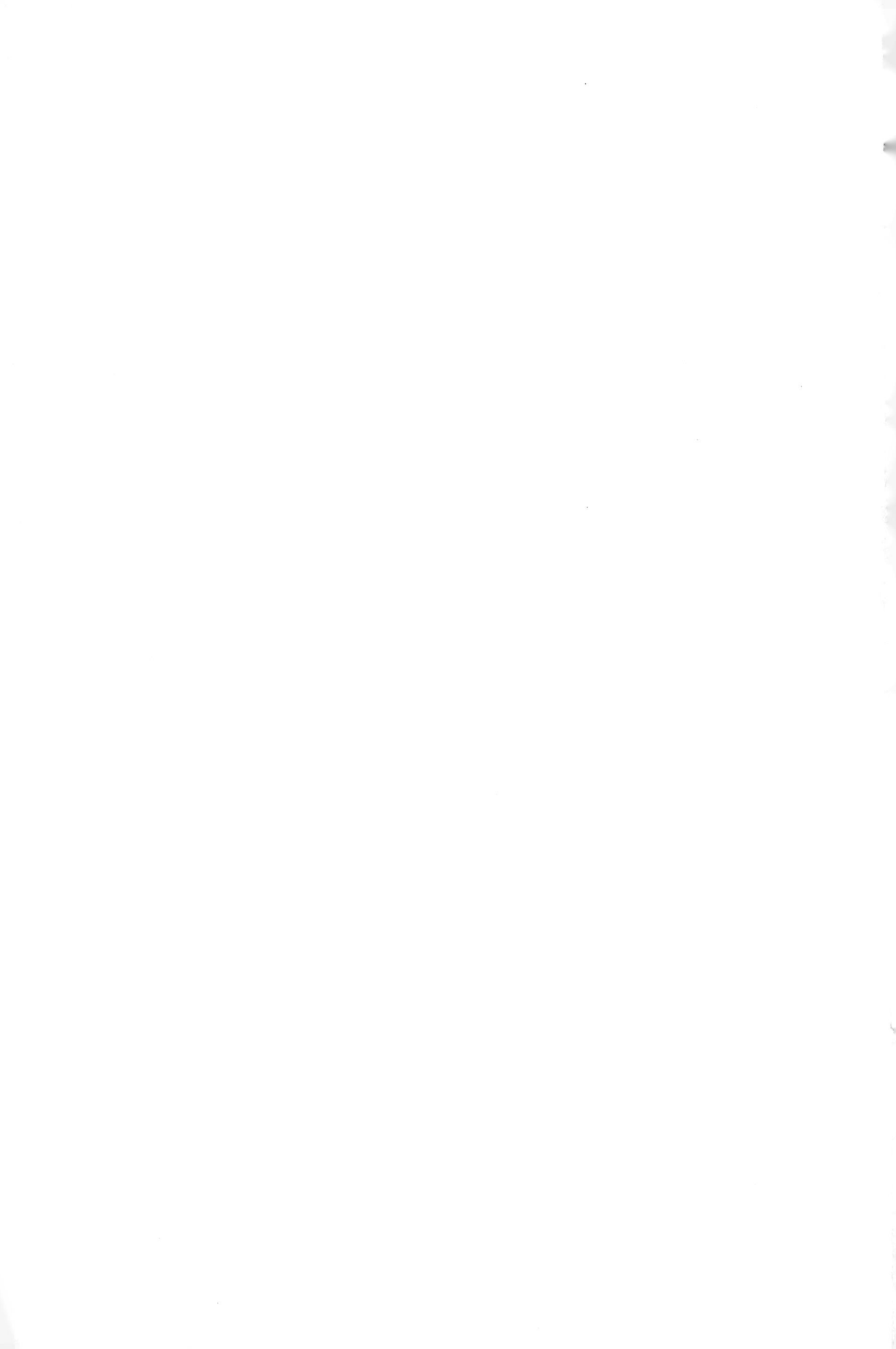

Updates on Breast Cancer

Updates on Breast Cancer

Editors

Enrico Cassano
Filippo Pesapane

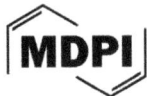 Basel • Beijing • Wuhan • Barcelona • Belgrade • Novi Sad • Cluj • Manchester

Editors

Enrico Cassano
IEO European Institute of
Oncology IRCCS
Milan
Italy

Filippo Pesapane
European Institute of
Oncology (IEO)
Milan
Italy

Editorial Office
MDPI
St. Alban-Anlage 66
4052 Basel, Switzerland

This is a reprint of articles from the Special Issue published online in the open access journal *Cancers* (ISSN 2072-6694) (available at: https://www.mdpi.com/journal/cancers/special_issues/updates_breast_cancer).

For citation purposes, cite each article independently as indicated on the article page online and as indicated below:

Lastname, A.A.; Lastname, B.B. Article Title. *Journal Name* **Year**, *Volume Number*, Page Range.

ISBN 978-3-7258-0389-7 (Hbk)
ISBN 978-3-7258-0390-3 (PDF)
doi.org/10.3390/books978-3-7258-0390-3

© 2024 by the authors. Articles in this book are Open Access and distributed under the Creative Commons Attribution (CC BY) license. The book as a whole is distributed by MDPI under the terms and conditions of the Creative Commons Attribution-NonCommercial-NoDerivs (CC BY-NC-ND) license.

Contents

About the Editors vii

Preface ix

Filippo Pesapane, Luca Nicosia and Enrico Cassano
Updates on Breast Cancer
Reprinted from: *Cancers* 2023, 15, 5392, doi:10.3390/cancers15225392 1

**Bálint Cserni, Darren Kilmartin, Mark O'Loughlin, Xavier Andreu,
Zsuzsanna Bagó-Horváth, Simonetta Bianchi, et al.**
ONEST (Observers Needed to Evaluate Subjective Tests) Analysis of Stromal
Tumour-Infiltrating Lymphocytes (sTILs) in Breast Cancer and Its Limitations
Reprinted from: *Cancers* 2023, 15, 1199, doi:10.3390/cancers15041199 5

Fátima Liliana Monteiro, Lina Stepanauskaite, Cecilia Williams and Luisa A. Helguero
SETD7 Expression Is Associated with Breast Cancer Survival Outcomes for Specific Molecular
Subtypes: A Systematic Analysis of Publicly Available Datasets
Reprinted from: *Cancers* 2022, 14, 6029, doi:10.3390/cancers14246029 16

Liu Yang, Wei Du, Taobo Hu, Miao Liu, Li Cai, Qiang Liu, et al.
Survival in Breast Cancer Patients with Bone Metastasis: A Multicenter Real-World Study on the
Prognostic Impact of Intensive Postoperative Bone Scan after Initial Diagnosis of Breast Cancer
(CSBrS-023)
Reprinted from: *Cancers* 2022, 14, 5835, doi:10.3390/cancers14235835 40

**Olha Kholod, William I. Basket, Jonathan B. Mitchem, Jussuf T. Kaifi, Richard D. Hammer,
Christos N. Papageorgiou, et al.**
Immune-Related Gene Signatures to Predict the Effectiveness of Chemoimmunotherapy in
Triple-Negative Breast Cancer Using Exploratory Subgroup Discovery
Reprinted from: *Cancers* 2022, 14, 5806, doi:10.3390/cancers14235806 54

**Evan N. Cohen, Gitanjali Jayachandran, Richard G. Moore, Massimo Cristofanilli,
Julie E. Lang, Joseph D. Khoury, et al.**
A Multi-Center Clinical Study to Harvest and Characterize Circulating Tumor Cells from
Patients with Metastatic Breast Cancer Using the Parsortix® PC1 System
Reprinted from: *Cancers* 2022, 14, 5238, doi:10.3390/cancers14215238 66

**Francesca Carlino, Anna Diana, Anna Ventriglia, Antonio Piccolo, Carmela Mocerino,
Ferdinando Riccardi, et al.**
HER2-Low Status Does Not Affect Survival Outcomes of Patients with Metastatic Breast Cancer
(MBC) Undergoing First-Line Treatment with Endocrine Therapy plus Palbociclib: Results of a
Multicenter, Retrospective Cohort Study
Reprinted from: *Cancers* 2022, 14, 4981, doi:10.3390/cancers14204981 92

**Alberto Valenzuela-Palomo, Lara Sanoguera-Miralles, Elena Bueno-Martínez,
Ada Esteban-Sánchez, Inés Llinares-Burguet, Alicia García-Álvarez, et al.**
Splicing Analysis of 16 *PALB2* ClinVar Variants by Minigene Assays: Identification of Six Likely
Pathogenic Variants
Reprinted from: *Cancers* 2022, 14, 4541, doi:10.3390/cancers14184541 103

Marine C. N. M. Blackman, Tania Capeloa, Justin D. Rondeau, Luca X. Zampieri,
Zohra Benyahia, Justine A. Van de Velde, et al.
Mitochondrial Protein Cox7b Is a Metabolic Sensor Driving Brain-Specific Metastasis of Human Breast Cancer Cells
Reprinted from: *Cancers* 2022, 14, 4371, doi:10.3390/cancers14184371 121

Mohammad Alkhaleefah, Tan-Hsu Tan, Chuan-Hsun Chang, Tzu-Chuan Wang,
Shang-Chih Ma, Lena Chang, et al.
Connected-SegNets: A Deep Learning Model for Breast Tumor Segmentation from X-ray Images
Reprinted from: *Cancers* 2022, 14, 4030, doi:10.3390/cancers14164030 145

Antonella Petrillo, Roberta Fusco, Elio Di Bernardo, Teresa Petrosino, Maria Luisa Barretta,
Annamaria Porto, et al.
Prediction of Breast Cancer Histological Outcome by Radiomics and Artificial Intelligence Analysis in Contrast-Enhanced Mammography
Reprinted from: *Cancers* 2022, 14, 2132, doi:10.3390/cancers14092132 161

Luca Nicosia, Anna Carla Bozzini, Silvia Penco, Chiara Trentin, Maria Pizzamiglio,
Matteo Lazzeroni, et al.
A Model to Predict Upstaging to Invasive Carcinoma in Patients Preoperatively Diagnosed with Low-Grade Ductal Carcinoma In Situ of the Breast
Reprinted from: *Cancers* 2022, 14, 370, doi:10.3390/cancers14020370 174

Syazalina Zahari, Saiful Effendi Syafruddin and M. Aiman Mohtar
Impact of the Cancer Cell Secretome in Driving Breast Cancer Progression
Reprinted from: *Cancers* 2023, 15, 2653, doi:10.3390/cancers15092653 185

Loïck Galland, Nicolas Roussot, Isabelle Desmoulins, Didier Mayeur, Courèche Kaderbhai,
Silvia Ilie, et al.
Clinical Utility of Genomic Tests Evaluating Homologous Recombination Repair Deficiency (HRD) for Treatment Decisions in Early and Metastatic Breast Cancer
Reprinted from: *Cancers* 2023, 15, 1299, doi:10.3390/cancers15041299 202

Nazia Riaz, Tiffany Jeen, Timothy J. Whelan and Torsten O. Nielsen
Recent Advances in Optimizing Radiation Therapy Decisions in Early Invasive Breast Cancer
Reprinted from: *Cancers* 2023, 15, 1260, doi:10.3390/cancers15041260 228

Huina Zhang and Yan Peng
Current Biological, Pathological and Clinical Landscape of HER2-Low Breast Cancer
Reprinted from: *Cancers* 2023, 15, 126, doi:10.3390/cancers15010126 262

Stephen Safe and Lei Zhang
The Role of the Aryl Hydrocarbon Receptor (AhR) and Its Ligands in Breast Cancer
Reprinted from: *Cancers* 2022, 14, 5574, doi:10.3390/cancers14225574 277

Alexandra Derevianko, Silvia Francesca Maria Pizzoli, Filippo Pesapane, Anna Rotili,
Dario Monzani, Roberto Grasso, et al.
The Use of Artificial Intelligence (AI) in the Radiology Field: What Is the State of Doctor–Patient Communication in Cancer Diagnosis?
Reprinted from: *Cancers* 2023, 15, 470, doi:10.3390/cancers15020470 298

About the Editors

Enrico Cassano

Dr. Enrico Cassano, MD, is a distinguished medical professional with a rich academic background and a profound commitment to breast imaging and oncology. Since the year 2000, Dr. Cassano has held the esteemed position of Director of the Breast Imaging Division at the referral cancer center European Institute of Oncology (IEO) in Milan (Italy). In this role, he has been pivotal in advancing breast imaging practices and patient care. Additionally, he serves as a dedicated tutor for the Postgraduate School of Radiology at the University of Milan and as a lecturer at the Italian School of Senology, where he is also a valued member of its scientific committee. His dedication to improving breast health is further underscored by his role as a member of the Scientific Committee and the Committee for Quality Control of the Mammographic Screening Programme of Milan in 1999 and 2000. Dr. Cassano is an accomplished author and co-author with a portfolio of more than 100 international publications. Beyond his professional accomplishments, Dr. Cassano is deeply committed to humanitarian efforts. He collaborates with various foundations, notably the Fondazione Umberto Veronesi and Fondazione Francesca Rava, where he actively participates in programs that aim to impact humanity positively. Dr. Cassano has received two prestigious international awards for his outstanding contributions to the medical and humanitarian spheres. In 2019, he was honored with the International Standout Woman Award at Palazzo Madama in Rome, where he received the "Standout Man Award." In 2020, he was the recipient of the International Award "Semplicemente Donna Harmony Award" in the category of "Human Rights Figure" during the 8th edition held in Castiglion Fiorentino (Italy). Dr. Enrico Cassano's illustrious career and unwavering commitment to breast health, research, and humanitarian endeavors stand as a testament to his dedication to improving lives and advancing medical science.

Filippo Pesapane

Dr. Filippo Pesapane, MD, is a highly accomplished radiologist with four board certifications, specializing as a breast radiologist at the European Institute of Oncology in Milan (Italy). He also collaborates with the University of Milan as a teacher and tutor for radiology residents. With a profound passion for research, Dr. Pesapane boasts an impressive track record in cancer imaging and has published numerous articles in esteemed peer-reviewed journals. He has undertaken honorary fellowships at renowned institutions, including the University Hospital of Gent in Belgium, the National Institute of Health in Bethesda, USA, and prominent hospitals in London, such as King's College Hospital and the Royal Marsden Hospital in the UK. Dr. Pesapane's primary research focuses on pioneering imaging techniques in breast radiology, reflecting his commitment to innovative research. His dedication has earned him grants and fellowships from prestigious international societies, including the European School of Radiology and the Radiological Society of North America. In recognition of his outstanding contributions, he received the Radiology Rising Star award during the European Conference of Radiology in Vienna, Austria, in 2019. In 2020, Dr. Pesapane obtained the Italian national academic qualification as an associate professor, further solidifying his expertise and commitment to academia. His influence extends to the Editorial realm, as he assumed the role of an Editorial Board Member at European Radiology Experimental in 2021 and an Editorial Advisory Board Member at AuntminnieEurope in 2023. Dr. Filippo Pesapane's career exemplifies his dedication to advancing radiology, particularly in breast imaging. His contributions continue to shape the future of medical research and patient care, making him a prominent figure in the field.

Preface

Welcome to the *Cancers'* Special Issue "Updates on Breast Cancer." This collection of research represents a collaborative effort from distinguished experts in the field of breast cancer, driven by a shared commitment to advancing our understanding and treatment of this complex disease.

Breast cancer remains a global health challenge, affecting countless lives and demanding relentless pursuit of scientific breakthroughs. In this Special Issue, we delve into the multifaceted nature of breast cancer, exploring the latest developments in diagnostics, treatments, and patient care.

The motivation behind this endeavor is rooted in our unwavering dedication to improving the lives of breast cancer patients worldwide. With this collection, we aim to shed light on the remarkable progress that has been achieved through the tireless efforts of researchers, clinicians, and healthcare professionals.

We extend our heartfelt gratitude to all the authors whose contributions have enriched this Special Issue: their expertise and commitment have been instrumental in bringing this body of work to fruition, and we acknowledge their invaluable assistance.

As we embark on this journey through the pages of "Updates on Breast Cancer," we invite the medical community, especially those at the forefront of breast cancer care, to embrace these advancements. Together, we look forward to a future filled with promise and hope in the ongoing battle against breast cancer.

Enrico Cassano and Filippo Pesapane
Editors

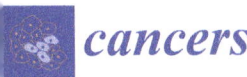

Editorial

Updates on Breast Cancer

Filippo Pesapane *, Luca Nicosia and Enrico Cassano

Breast Imaging Division, IEO European Institute of Oncology IRCCS, 20141 Milan, Italy; luca.nicosia@ieo.it (L.N.); enrico.cassano@ieo.it (E.C.)
* Correspondence: filippo.pesapane@ieo.it; Tel.: +39-02-57489-1

Citation: Pesapane, F.; Nicosia, L.; Cassano, E. Updates on Breast Cancer. *Cancers* **2023**, *15*, 5392. https://doi.org/10.3390/cancers15225392

Received: 20 September 2023
Accepted: 9 November 2023
Published: 13 November 2023

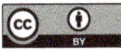

Copyright: © 2023 by the authors. Licensee MDPI, Basel, Switzerland. This article is an open access article distributed under the terms and conditions of the Creative Commons Attribution (CC BY) license (https://creativecommons.org/licenses/by/4.0/).

This collection of 18 articles, comprising 12 original studies, 1 systematic review, and 5 reviews, is a collaborative effort by distinguished experts in breast cancer research, and it has been edited by Dr. Enrico Cassano and Dr. Filippo Pesapane, who both work at an international breast cancer referral center [1].

Breast cancer, a globally prevalent malignancy primarily afflicting women [2], remains a pivotal focus of medical research and innovation. In our Special Issue, titled "Updates on Breast Cancer", we present the latest developments in breast cancer diagnostics, treatments, and patient care, offering an in-depth exploration of the multifaceted nature of breast cancer and the way in which science is transforming this field.

Nowadays, though precision diagnosis and personalized medicine are cornerstones of effective breast cancer management, achieving consistent and reproducible diagnostic assessments remains a challenge. Cserni B. et al. [3] introduce a groundbreaking methodology known as the ONEST (Observers Needed to Evaluate Subjective Tests) analysis. By determining the optimal number of observers required for reliable tumor-infiltrating lymphocyte categorization, ONEST has the potential to revolutionize diagnostic accuracy, providing a more robust and consistent framework for assessing breast cancer pathology.

Precision diagnosis also allows clinicians to understand the molecular intricacies of breast cancer. Monteiro F.L. et al. [4] performed a meticulous analysis that unveils the enigmatic role played by SETD7, a lysine N-methyltransferase, in breast cancer. Among her notable findings is the correlation between high SETD7 expression and worse recurrence-free survival in the basal-like subtype, underscoring this molecule's clinical significance as a potential treatment-predictive marker.

The study of Nicosia L. et al. [5] introduces a novel nomogram aimed at predicting the likelihood of upstaging low-grade ductal carcinoma in situ in patients who have previously undergone vacuum-assisted breast biopsy, followed by surgical excision. This innovative tool leverages radiological and pathological criteria to provide a tailored framework for making treatment decisions. By identifying patients with a low risk of upstaging to infiltrating carcinomas, this nomogram has the potential to reduce overtreatment and improve patient outcomes, once again showing that personalized medicine is increasingly paramount in breast cancer care.

Radiomics and artificial intelligence (AI) are also driving significant advances in precision diagnosis. Petrillo et al. [6] launch a comprehensive investigation, leveraging radiomics features derived from contrast-enhanced mammography to predict various histological outcomes.

Radiomics, the extraction and analysis of quantitative features from medical images, holds promise in terms of providing valuable information beyond what the human eye can perceive [7–9]. The results of Petrillo et al.'s study rested on the analysis of a staggering 837 textural metrics that demonstrate an accuracy of 88.98%, enabling the differentiation of malignant and benign lesions. Beyond this distinction, the study attempted to predict histological grading, the presence of hormone receptors, and the status of human epidermal growth factor receptor 2 (HER2) in breast cancer patients.

As we continue to harness the capabilities of radiomics and AI, we move closer to developing more effective breast cancer management practices, offering hope and improved prospects for afflicted women.

Mohammad Alkhaleefah M. et al. [10] present an innovative deep learning model named Connected-SegNets. This model is engineered for the precise segmentation of breast tumors from X-ray images, incorporating skip connections between layers, thus replacing the conventional loss function with intersection over union to fortify robustness against noise during training.

These findings all highlight the immense potential of radiomics and AI in the realm of breast cancer care [7–9]. However, while the integration of AI into radiology is revolutionizing breast cancer diagnosis, continuing to focus on the patient and preserving the doctor–patient relationship is crucial. Derevianko et al.'s study [11] delves into the impact of AI on doctor–patient communication, particularly within the context of cancer diagnosis. Their systematic review emphasizes the need for transparent and informative communication to establish patient trust in AI-driven diagnostic processes, ultimately improving healthcare interactions. Ad it remains uncertain to what extent and under which conditions the general population will embrace the use of AI [12], this study highlights the need to conduct larger-scale research to better understand women's demands and concerns regarding the potential applications of AI in breast cancer care.

In addition to these improvements in breast cancer diagnosis, advances in postoperative surveillance have significantly contributed to the improved survival rates identified in breast cancer patients. Yang L. et al. [13] present a multicenter real-world study conducted across medical centers in China. Their study investigates the prognostic value of intensive postoperative bone scans for patients with breast cancer and bone metastasis. The findings provide compelling evidence of the benefits of this screening method, showcasing its potential to extend both overall survival and overall survival after bone metastasis.

Despite such improvement, in a breast cancer scenario, triple-negative breast cancer (TNBC) remains a formidable clinical challenge due to its limited therapeutic options. Kholod O. et al. [14] decode the immune-related gene signatures that hold the key to predicting chemoimmunotherapy outcomes in TNBC patients, analyzing a vast dataset encompassing 422 patients across 24 studies. Through an algorithmic approach, they categorize patients into 12 homogenous subgroups based on various parameters, including tumor mutational burden, relapse status, tumor cellularity, menopausal status, and tumor stage.

A comprehensive analysis of the clinical utility of genomic tests in breast cancer care is provided by Galland et al. [15], who explore the clinical utility of genomic tests evaluating homologous recombination repair deficiency in breast cancer treatment decisions. Moreover, Safe S. et al. [16] show the roles played by the aryl hydrocarbon receptor and its ligands in breast cancer progression and the potentialities for homologous recombination repair deficiency in early and metastatic breast cancer. Finally, Valenzuela-Palomo et al. [17] delve into the impacts of these variants on splicing, a crucial step in gene expression regulation. Their use of minigene assays to analyze 16 PALB2 variants at intron/exon boundaries reveals that 12 of these variants disrupt splicing, with 6 variants being classified as likely pathogenic in nature. This study offers essential insights into the clinical management of carrier patients and their families, enabling tailored prevention and therapy protocols.

Our Special Issue exceeds the traditional boundaries of breast cancer research, exploring a diverse array of topics that all enrich our understanding of this complex disease. From the characterization of circulating tumor cells using cutting-edge technology like the Parsortix® PC1 System [18] to investigating the clinical landscape of HER2-Low breast cancer [19], these studies broaden our horizons. With regard to radiation therapy, which is a crucial component of breast cancer treatment, Riaz et al. [20] analyze recent advances in optimizing radiation therapy decisions for early invasive breast cancer. Their exploration of strategies to identify patients who may benefit from tailored radiation therapy regimens shows a commitment to enhancing patient care and outcomes. Lastly, Zahari et al. [21]

provide a review of the role played by the cancer cell secretome in breast cancer progression, explaining how the secretome shapes the tumor microenvironment, influences treatment resistance, and offer insights into potential therapeutic strategies targeting its components.

In conclusion, our Special Issue, titled "Updates on Breast Cancer," shows the remarkable progress taking place within the field of breast cancer research. Technological innovations like radiomics and AI, together with the collective efforts of dedicated researchers, have paved the way for precision diagnosis, enhanced treatment strategies, and more personalized patient care. As we journey through this compendium of research, we are reminded that the pursuit of knowledge and innovation is limitless. The future of breast cancer care is being shaped right now, guided by the dedication and unwavering commitment of the scientific community. We invite our readers to help us to embrace these advancements, as we look forward to a brighter and more promising future in the battle against breast cancer.

Conflicts of Interest: The authors declare no conflict of interest.

References

1. Pesapane, F.; Penco, S.; Rotili, A.; Nicosia, L.; Bozzini, A.; Trentin, C.; Dominelli, V.; Priolo, F.; Farina, M.; Marinucci, I.; et al. How we provided appropriate breast imaging practices in the epicentre of the COVID-19 outbreak in Italy. *Br. J. Radiol.* **2020**, *93*, 20200679. [CrossRef] [PubMed]
2. Sung, H.; Ferlay, J.; Siegel, R.L.; Laversanne, M.; Soerjomataram, I.; Jemal, A.; Bray, F. Global cancer statistics 2020: GLOBOCAN estimates of incidence and mortality worldwide for 36 cancers in 185 countries. *CA Cancer J. Clin.* **2021**, *71*, 209–249. [CrossRef]
3. Cserni, B.; Kilmartin, D.; O'Loughlin, M.; Andreu, X.; Bago-Horvath, Z.; Bianchi, S.; Chmielik, E.; Figueiredo, P.; Floris, G.; Foschini, M.P.; et al. ONEST (Observers Needed to Evaluate Subjective Tests) Analysis of Stromal Tumour-Infiltrating Lymphocytes (sTILs) in Breast Cancer and Its Limitations. *Cancers* **2023**, *15*, 1199. [CrossRef] [PubMed]
4. Monteiro, F.L.; Stepanauskaite, L.; Williams, C.; Helguero, L.A. SETD7 Expression Is Associated with Breast Cancer Survival Outcomes for Specific Molecular Subtypes: A Systematic Analysis of Publicly Available Datasets. *Cancers* **2022**, *14*, 6029. [CrossRef] [PubMed]
5. Nicosia, L.; Bozzini, A.C.; Penco, S.; Trentin, C.; Pizzamiglio, M.; Lazzeroni, M.; Lissidini, G.; Veronesi, P.; Farante, G.; Frassoni, S.; et al. A Model to Predict Upstaging to Invasive Carcinoma in Patients Preoperatively Diagnosed with Low-Grade Ductal Carcinoma In Situ of the Breast. *Cancers* **2022**, *14*, 370. [CrossRef] [PubMed]
6. Petrillo, A.; Fusco, R.; Di Bernardo, E.; Petrosino, T.; Barretta, M.L.; Porto, A.; Granata, V.; Di Bonito, M.; Fanizzi, A.; Massafra, R.; et al. Prediction of Breast Cancer Histological Outcome by Radiomics and Artificial Intelligence Analysis in Contrast-Enhanced Mammography. *Cancers* **2022**, *14*, 2132. [CrossRef]
7. Pesapane, F.; De Marco, P.; Rapino, A.; Lombardo, E.; Nicosia, L.; Tantrige, P.; Rotili, A.; Bozzini, A.C.; Penco, S.; Dominelli, V.; et al. How Radiomics Can Improve Breast Cancer Diagnosis and Treatment. *J. Clin. Med.* **2023**, *12*, 1372. [CrossRef]
8. Pesapane, F.; Rotili, A.; Agazzi, G.M.; Botta, F.; Raimondi, S.; Penco, S.; Dominelli, V.; Cremonesi, M.; Jereczek-Fossa, B.A.; Carrafiello, G.; et al. Recent Radiomics Advancements in Breast Cancer: Lessons and Pitfalls for the Next Future. *Curr. Oncol.* **2021**, *28*, 2351–2372. [CrossRef]
9. Pesapane, F.; Suter, M.B.; Rotili, A.; Penco, S.; Nigro, O.; Cremonesi, M.; Bellomi, M.; Jereczek-Fossa, B.A.; Pinotti, G.; Cassano, E. Will traditional biopsy be substituted by radiomics and liquid biopsy for breast cancer diagnosis and characterisation? *Med. Oncol.* **2020**, *37*, 29. [CrossRef]
10. Alkhaleefah, M.; Tan, T.H.; Chang, C.H.; Wang, T.C.; Ma, S.C.; Chang, L.; Chang, Y.L. Connected-SegNets: A Deep Learning Model for Breast Tumor Segmentation from X-ray Images. *Cancers* **2022**, *14*, 4030, Correction in *Cancers* **2023**, *15*, 2237. [CrossRef]
11. Derevianko, A.; Pizzoli, S.F.M.; Pesapane, F.; Rotili, A.; Monzani, D.; Grasso, R.; Cassano, E.; Pravettoni, G. The Use of Artificial Intelligence (AI) in the Radiology Field: What Is the State of Doctor-Patient Communication in Cancer Diagnosis? *Cancers* **2023**, *15*, 470. [CrossRef] [PubMed]
12. Pesapane, F.; Rotili, A.; Valconi, E.; Agazzi, G.M.; Montesano, M.; Penco, S.; Nicosia, L.; Bozzini, A.; Meneghetti, L.; Latronico, A.; et al. Women's perceptions and attitudes to the use of AI in breast cancer screening: A survey in a cancer referral centre. *Br. J. Radiol.* **2023**, *96*, 20220569. [CrossRef] [PubMed]
13. Yang, L.; Du, W.; Hu, T.; Liu, H.; Cai, L.; Liu, Q.; Yu, Z.; Liu, G.; Wang, S. Survival in Breast Cancer Patients with Bone Metastasis: A Multicenter Real-World Study on the Prognostic Impact of Intensive Postoperative Bone Scan after Initial Diagnosis of Breast Cancer (CSBrS-023). *Cancers* **2022**, *14*, 5835. [CrossRef] [PubMed]
14. Kholod, O.; Basket, W.I.; Mitchem, J.B.; Kaifi, J.T.; Hammer, R.D.; Papageorgiou, C.N.; Shyu, C.R. Immune-Related Gene Signatures to Predict the Effectiveness of Chemoimmunotherapy in Triple-Negative Breast Cancer Using Exploratory Subgroup Discovery. *Cancers* **2022**, *14*, 5806. [CrossRef]

15. Galland, L.; Roussot, N.; Desmoulins, I.; Mayeur, D.; Kaderbhai, C.; Ilie, S.; Hennequin, A.; Reda, M.; Albuisson, J.; Arnould, L.; et al. Clinical Utility of Genomic Tests Evaluating Homologous Recombination Repair Deficiency (HRD) for Treatment Decisions in Early and Metastatic Breast Cancer. *Cancers* **2023**, *15*, 1299. [CrossRef]
16. Safe, S.; Zhang, L. The Role of the Aryl Hydrocarbon Receptor (AhR) and Its Ligands in Breast Cancer. *Cancers* **2022**, *14*, 5574. [CrossRef]
17. Valenzuela-Palomo, A.; Sanoguera-Miralles, L.; Bueno-Martinez, E.; Esteban-Sanchez, A.; Llinares-Burguet, I.; Garcia-Alvarez, A.; Perez-Segura, P.; Gomez-Barrero, S.; de la Hoya, M.; Velasco-Sampedro, E.A. Splicing Analysis of 16 PALB2 ClinVar Variants by Minigene Assays: Identification of Six Likely Pathogenic Variants. *Cancers* **2022**, *14*, 4541. [CrossRef]
18. Cohen, E.N.; Jayachandran, G.; Moore, R.G.; Cristofanilli, M.; Lang, J.E.; Khoury, J.D.; Press, M.F.; Kim, K.K.; Khazan, N.; Zhang, Q.; et al. A Multi-Center Clinical Study to Harvest and Characterize Circulating Tumor Cells from Patients with Metastatic Breast Cancer Using the Parsortix® PC1 System. *Cancers* **2022**, *14*, 5328. [CrossRef]
19. Zhang, H.; Peng, Y. Current Biological, Pathological and Clinical Landscape of HER2-Low Breast Cancer. *Cancers* **2022**, *15*, 126. [CrossRef]
20. Riaz, N.; Jeen, T.; Whelan, T.J.; Nielsen, T.O. Recent Advances in Optimizing Radiation Therapy Decisions in Early Invasive Breast Cancer. *Cancers* **2023**, *15*, 1260. [CrossRef]
21. Zahari, S.; Syafruddin, S.E.; Mohtar, M.A. Impact of the Cancer Cell Secretome in Driving Breast Cancer Progression. *Cancers* **2023**, *15*, 2653. [CrossRef] [PubMed]

Disclaimer/Publisher's Note: The statements, opinions and data contained in all publications are solely those of the individual author(s) and contributor(s) and not of MDPI and/or the editor(s). MDPI and/or the editor(s) disclaim responsibility for any injury to people or property resulting from any ideas, methods, instructions or products referred to in the content.

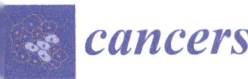

Article

ONEST (Observers Needed to Evaluate Subjective Tests) Analysis of Stromal Tumour-Infiltrating Lymphocytes (sTILs) in Breast Cancer and Its Limitations

Bálint Cserni [1], Darren Kilmartin [2], Mark O'Loughlin [2], Xavier Andreu [3], Zsuzsanna Bagó-Horváth [4], Simonetta Bianchi [5], Ewa Chmielik [6], Paulo Figueiredo [7], Giuseppe Floris [8], Maria Pia Foschini [9], Anikó Kovács [10], Päivi Heikkilä [11], Janina Kulka [12], Anne-Vibeke Laenkholm [13], Inta Liepniece-Karele [14], Caterina Marchiò [15,16], Elena Provenzano [17,18], Peter Regitnig [19], Angelika Reiner [20], Aleš Ryška [21], Anna Sapino [15,16], Elisabeth Specht Stovgaard [22], Cecily Quinn [23,24], Vasiliki Zolota [25], Mark Webber [2], Sharon A. Glynn [2], Rita Bori [26], Erika Csörgő [26], Orsolya Oláh-Németh [27], Tamás Pancsa [27], Anita Sejben [27], István Sejben [26], András Vörös [27], Tamás Zombori [27], Tibor Nyári [28], Grace Callagy [2] and Gábor Cserni [26,27,*]

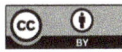

Citation: Cserni, B.; Kilmartin, D.; O'Loughlin, M.; Andreu, X.; Bagó-Horváth, Z.; Bianchi, S.; Chmielik, E.; Figueiredo, P.; Floris, G.; Foschini, M.P.; et al. ONEST (Observers Needed to Evaluate Subjective Tests) Analysis of Stromal Tumour-Infiltrating Lymphocytes (sTILs) in Breast Cancer and Its Limitations. *Cancers* **2023**, *15*, 1199. https://doi.org/10.3390/cancers15041199

Academic Editors: Enrico Cassano and Filippo Pesapane

Received: 20 January 2023
Revised: 4 February 2023
Accepted: 9 February 2023
Published: 14 February 2023

Copyright: © 2023 by the authors. Licensee MDPI, Basel, Switzerland. This article is an open access article distributed under the terms and conditions of the Creative Commons Attribution (CC BY) license (https://creativecommons.org/licenses/by/4.0/).

1. TNG Technology Consulting GmbH, Király u. 26., 1061 Budapest, Hungary
2. Discipline of Pathology, Lambe Institute for Translational Research, School of Medicine, University of Galway, H91 TK33 Galway, Ireland
3. Pathology Department, Atryshealth Co., Ltd., 08039 Barcelona, Spain
4. Department of Pathology, Medical University of Vienna, Währinger Gürtel 18-20, 1090 Vienna, Austria
5. Division of Pathological Anatomy, Department of Health Sciences, University of Florence, 50134 Florence, Italy
6. Tumor Pathology Department, Maria Sklodowska-Curie National Research Institute of Oncology, Gliwice Branch, 44-102 Gliwice, Poland
7. Laboratório de Anatomia Patológica, IPO Coimbra, 3000-075 Coimbra, Portugal
8. Laboratory of Translational Cell & Tissue Research and KU Leuven, Department of Imaging and Pathology, Department of Pathology, University Hospitals Leuven, University of Leuven, Oude Market 13, 3000 Leuven, Belgium
9. Unit of Anatomic Pathology, Department of Biomedical and Neuromotor Sciences, University of Bologna, Bellaria Hospital, 40139 Bologna, Italy
10. Department of Clinical Pathology, Sahlgrenska University Hospital, 41345 Gothenburg, Sweden
11. Department of Pathology, Helsinki University Central Hospital, 00029 Helsinki, Finland
12. Department of Pathology, Forensic and Insurance Medicine, Semmelweis University Budapest, Üllői út 93, 1091 Budapest, Hungary
13. Department of Surgical Pathology, Zealand University Hospital, 4000 Roskilde, Denmark
14. Department of Pathology, Riga Stradins University, Riga East Clinical University Hospital, LV-1038 Riga, Latvia
15. Unit of Pathology, Candiolo Cancer Institute FPO-IRCCS, 10060 Candiolo, Italy
16. Department of Medical Sciences, University of Turin, 10126 Turin, Italy
17. Department of Histopathology, Cambridge University Hospitals National Health Service (NHS) Foundation Trust, Cambridge CB2 0QQ, UK
18. National Institute for Health Research Cambridge Biomedical Research Centre, Cambridge CB2 0QQ, UK
19. Diagnostic and Research Institute of Pathology, Medical University of Graz, 8010 Graz, Austria
20. Department of Pathology, Klinikum Donaustadt, 1090 Vienna, Austria
21. The Fingerland Department of Pathology, Charles University Medical Faculty and University Hospital, 50003 Hradec Kralove, Czech Republic
22. Pathology Department, Herlev University Hospital, DK-2730 Herlev, Denmark
23. Department of Histopathology, Irish National Breast Screening Programme, BreastCheck, St. Vincent's University Hospital and School of Medicine, University College Dublin, D04 T6F4 Dublin, Ireland
24. School of Medicine, University College Dublin, D04 V1W8 Dublin, Ireland
25. Department of Pathology, School of Medicine, University of Patras, 26504 Rion, Greece
26. Department of Pathology, Bács-Kiskun County Teaching Hospital, 6000 Kecskemét, Hungary
27. Department of Pathology, University of Szeged, 6720 Szeged, Hungary
28. Department of Medical Physics and Informatics, University of Szeged, 6720 Szeged, Hungary
* Correspondence: csernig@kmk.hu

Simple Summary: Tumour-infiltrating lymphocytes (TILs) reflect the host's response against tumours. TILs have a strong prognostic effect in the so-called triple-negative (oestrogen receptor, progesterone receptor, and human epidermal growth factor receptor-2 negative) subset of breast cancers and predict a better response when primary systemic (neoadjuvant) treatment is administered. Although they are easy to assess, their quantitative assessment is subject to some inter-observer variation. ONEST (Observers Needed to Evaluate Subjective Tests) is a new way of analysing inter-observer variability and helps in estimating the number of observers required for a more reliable estimation of this phenomenon. This aspect of reproducibility for TILs has not been explored previously. Our analysis suggests that between six and nine pathologists can give a good approximation of inter-observer agreement in TIL assessments.

Abstract: Tumour-infiltrating lymphocytes (TILs) reflect antitumour immunity. Their evaluation of histopathology specimens is influenced by several factors and is subject to issues of reproducibility. ONEST (Observers Needed to Evaluate Subjective Tests) helps in determining the number of observers that would be sufficient for the reliable estimation of inter-observer agreement of TIL categorisation. This has not been explored previously in relation to TILs. ONEST analyses, using an open-source software developed by the first author, were performed on TIL quantification in breast cancers taken from two previous studies. These were one reproducibility study involving 49 breast cancers, 23 in the first circulation and 14 pathologists in the second circulation, and one study involving 100 cases and 9 pathologists. In addition to the estimates of the number of observers required, other factors influencing the results of ONEST were examined. The analyses reveal that between six and nine observers (range 2–11) are most commonly needed to give a robust estimate of reproducibility. In addition, the number and experience of observers, the distribution of values around or away from the extremes, and outliers in the classification also influence the results. Due to the simplicity and the potentially relevant information it may give, we propose ONEST to be a part of new reproducibility analyses.

Keywords: ONEST; observers needed to evaluate subjective tests; TILs; sTILs; tumour-infiltrating lymphocytes; triple-negative; breast cancer; reproducibility; international immuno-oncology biomarker working group; European Working Group for Breast Screening Pathology

1. Introduction

Tumour-infiltrating lymphocytes (TILs) are a reflection of antitumour immunity. Different compartments and populations are recognised; for breast carcinomas, stromal lymphocytes have been accepted as the most practically assessable compartment of TILs, and their quantity correlates with that of intra-epithelial TILs [1]. On the basis of meta-analyses, stromal TILs (sTILs) have been proven to be predictive of the response to neoadjuvant chemotherapy [2] and to be associated with better prognosis after adjuvant treatment of triple-negative breast carcinomas (TNBCs) [3]. TILs have also been linked to the rare phenomenon of spontaneous regression in TNBC [4]. The accumulated data on the value of TILs have matured enough to recommend this biomarker for implementation in daily routine [5].

However, there are a number of other events (e.g., necrosis or previous biopsy) that lead to the accumulation of inflammatory cells, and these have been taken into consideration when defining the rules for quantifying the amount of sTILs relevant for antitumour immunity. This has led to the formulation of guidelines recommending that sTILs should be evaluated as the average proportion of the stromal area occupied by TILs, including both lymphocytes and plasma cells. In the assessment, the total stromal area excludes areas of regressive hyalinisation, necrosis, and previous needle biopsy sites. Mononuclear cells around in situ carcinoma and normal structures should also be excluded, and all estimations should be restricted to the tumour area [6]. A later addendum suggested that the invasive front (1 mm at the edge of the tumour) should also be included [7]. The human brain tries to simplify things; therefore, the rules for quantifying sTILs predispose this biomarker to being poorly reproducible. Nevertheless, good reproducibility was documented by the International Immuno-oncology Biomarker Working Group (IIOBMWG) after the introduction of a direct online feedback software helping in the calibration of sTIL percentages in pre-selected fields of view (FOVs) [8].

Members of the European Working Group for Breast Screening Pathology (EWGBSP) have also assessed the reproducibility of scoring sTILs on digitised needle core biopsy specimens using the same performance-improving online tool that was used for training by Denkert et al. [8,9] and found moderate reproducibility for biopsy specimens (intraclass correlation coefficient, ICC 0.634, 95% CI 0.539–0.735) but good reproducibility for selected triplets of FOVs (ICC 0.798, 95% CI 0.727–0.864) [10]. In the present work, we use the same data to perform an ONEST (Observers Needed to Evaluate Subjective Tests) analysis of sTILs.

ONEST is a recently developed method that complements inter-observer agreement studies by helping to estimate the number of observers required for a reliable estimation of reproducibility [11]. ONEST uses 100 randomly selected permutations of all participating pathologists (observers or raters) and plots the overall percent agreement (OPA) values for an increasing number of observers, looking for the worst (lowest) curve to reach a plateau, beyond which an increasing number of observers does not have a substantial effect on agreement [11–13]. Additionally, ONEST has been recognised to be valuable as a visual complement to demonstrate the degree of reproducibility of subjectively evaluated parameters such as oestrogen receptor (ER) quantification, Ki-67 labelling, or histological grade, as well as the difference between observers and how these compare to the overall percent agreement (OPA) of all observers [12,13]. The aim of this study is to evaluate sTIL quantification using ONEST and to estimate the number of observers needed for a reliable evaluation of its reproducibility. The relatively large number of observers in our previous study [9] allows for a better evaluation of ONEST itself as a method.

2. Materials and Methods

We used anonymised results from the EWGBSP analysis of reproducibility [9]. In that study, 23 pathologists assessed 49 core needle biopsies from TNBCs in circulation 1 (C1), and 14 pathologists, as a subset, assessed both C1 (this subset of C1 denoted as C1s) in addition to 3 pre-selected digital FOVs of the same 49 cases with different labels to prevent comparisons (C2). The corresponding author of this previous study (Grace Callagy) has released the sTIL percentage values reported by the 23 and 14 participants for each case in a tabulated format, with rows representing cases and columns representing one or the other observer, and these values were used for the ONEST analyses of C1 and C2, respectively. There were 2 missing values in all circulations (C1, C1s, and C2) which were replaced by mean sTIL percentages rounded to the closest integer. For the ONEST analysis, as per the introduction of the method and its subsequent uses [11–13], 100 randomly selected permutations were selected for the values of the ONEST plots. Four selected cut-offs were used to define categories: <60% vs. ≥60%, e.g., [14], and <50% vs. ≥50%, e.g., [15,16], to match two different definitions of lymphocyte-predominant breast cancers, which are the likeliest responders to neoadjuvant treatment [6]; <30% vs. ≥30% to match a cut-off proposed for a strong prognostic role in the adjuvant setting [3]; and 0–20%, 21–49%, and ≥50% to match a three-tiered classification used in the IIOBWG ring studies [8].

In a previous study, 9 pathologists assessed the ER, the progesterone receptor (PR) status, Ki67 labelling [12], and histological grade [13] of breast cancers in 50 core needle biopsies and 50 resection specimens represented on a full-face glass slide for each case. While assessing these parameters, the participants were also asked to document sTILs based on the IIOBMWG recommendations [6,7], which are also part of the Hungarian recommendation [17,18]. These results have never been analysed previously and were also used for a separate ONEST analysis as circulation 3 (C3).

A full ONEST plot includes all OPA values per increasing number of observers for the 100 randomly obtained permutations of observers, i.e., it represents 100 OPA curves (OPACs), each representing the OPA values of a given permutation (Figure 1A). We also introduced a simplified ONEST plot, which includes only the maximum OPA values (maximum curve—best scenario), the minimum OPA values (minimum curve—worst scenario), and a median value curve. The maximum and minimum curves do not necessarily represent an OPAC from the 100 randomly selected permutations, but they obviously coincide with an OPAC from all possible permutations. Figure 1A and 1B compare the full and simplified ONEST plots of the same entity studied. The ONEST value is the integer from axis x (the number of pathologists), which reflects the minimum curve OPA value beyond which there is no more relevant decrease in OPA values with further increase in observers. Bandwidth is defined as the difference between the highest and lowest OPA values with 2 pathologists assessing sTILs, i.e., this is the difference in OPA of the maximum and minimum curves with 2 observers. Finally, OPA(n) is the OPA value for all observers, the percentage of cases upon which all assessing observers agree. Good reproducibility implies a high OPA(n), a low ONEST value, and narrow bandwidth, whereas the opposite is true for poor reproducibility. The worst scenario is when OPA(n) = 0, i.e., there are no cases on which all observers agree. This latter scenario is unacceptable for biomarker studies or subjective tests on relevant issues in general and should be remedied by improving reproducibility or dropping the test and substituting it with a better one. An open-source software designed by the first author for randomly selecting 100 permutations from all possible ones and making a basic ONEST analysis is available at github.com (accessed on 12 November 2022) [19].

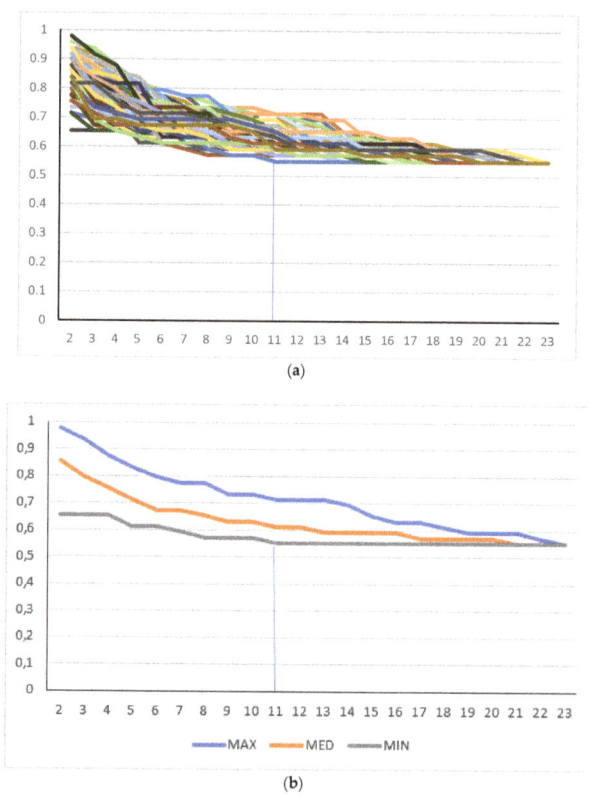

Figure 1. *Cont.*

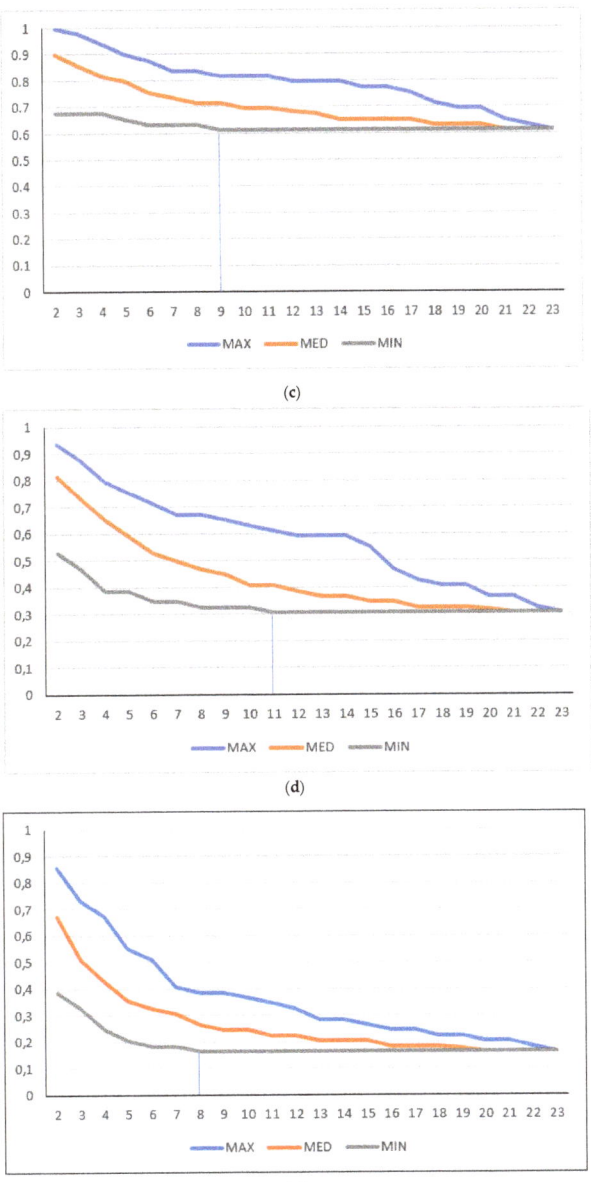

Figure 1. ONEST plots of different cut-off values for 23 pathologists. (**a**) Full and (**b**) simplified ONEST plots for the 49 cases assessed by 23 pathologists for a cut-off of <50% vs. ≥50% sTILs. (**c–e**) Simplified ONEST plots for further cut-off values studied: (**c**) <60% vs. ≥60%; (**d**) <30% vs. ≥30%; and (**e**) <20%, 21–50%, >50%. Readings from the plots are included in Table 1. OPA (n = 23) values are the OPA values at the right side of the plots and reflect the proportion of cases with full agreement. ONEST values correspond to the number of observers on the x-axis, where the minimum curve levels off, and no substantial decrease is noted with further increase in the number of observers (this is highlighted by vertical segments between the x-axis value and the minimum curve). The bandwidth of the ONEST plot is visualised on the left side of the plot as the difference between the maximum and the minimum curves with 2 observers; this is the largest difference in agreement between two observers.

Table 1. ONEST analyses of different circulations and cut-off values of sTILs.

<50% vs. ≥50%	C1	C1 without Divergent Raters 7 and 20	C1s	C2	C2 without Divergent Raters 4 and 13	C3
n	23	21	14	14	12	9
OPA(n)	0.551	0.612	0.571	0.776	0.816	0.89
Bandwidth	0.327	0.245	0.265	0.184	0.143	0.07
ONEST	11	7	8	6	3	6
<60% vs. ≥60%						
n	23	21	14	14	12	9
OPA(n)	0.612	0.796	0.612	0.796	0.837	0.91
Bandwidth	0.327	0.286	0.612	0.163	0.163	0.07
ONEST	9	7	4	6	2	2
<30% vs. ≥30%						
n	23	21	14	14	12	9
OPA(n)	0.306	0.347	0.327	0.551	0.592	0.81
Bandwidth	0.408	0.306	0.306	0.306	0.204	0.09
ONEST	11	8	9	8	7	6
≤20%, 21–49%, ≥50%						
n	23	21	14	14	12	9
OPA(n)	0.163	0.204	0.408	0.408	0.449	0.74
Bandwidth	0.469	0.388	0.143	0.265	0.245	0.12
ONEST	8	7	7	5	6	6

C1: circulation 1 with 23 pathologists and 49 digital slides of core needle biopsy samples; C1s: subset of C1 with the 14 pathologists taking part in C2; C2: circulation 2 with 14 pathologists and 3 preselected fields of view of the 49 cases viewed in C1; C3: circulation 3 is independent from C1 and C2 and involves 9 pathologists assessing 100 cases, half from core needle biopsies and half from excision specimens. For further details, see the Materials and Methods section.

For the analysis with a cut-off value of <50% vs. ≥50% sTILs, ONEST analyses were repeated 3 times (3 random selections of 100 permutations in which the chances of identical permutations are practically nil), and the minimum curves obtained were compared by means of the Kruskal–Wallis test. In the original series, two pathologists (numbers 7 and 20) substantially diverged in their opinions from the rest of the group in C1, whereas two pathologists (numbers 4 and 13) diverged from others in C2. To test the influence of these divergently classifying pathologists, 3 and 3 ONEST plots for the same cut-off values (<50% vs. ≥50%) were also generated after the removal of results by these observers, and the ONEST values were determined from all plots. The ONEST values obtained with or without the deviant classifiers were compared by means of the two sample Wilcoxon rank sum test. Statistical analyses were performed in Excel with the Real Statistics Add-Ins [20] and STATA Software version 17.0 (StataCorp LP, College Station, TX, USA).

3. Results

The results of the C1 were selected to be represented by the ONEST plots in Figure 1. Readings of this and other ONEST analyses from C2 and C3 are represented in Table 1. With different approaches, pathologists, and numbers of pathologists, the ONEST values varied between 2 and 11 (Table 1). There were two pathologists, in both circulations C1 and C2, who substantially deviated from the overall average ratings; separate ONEST analyses were also performed without these participants. Not surprisingly, not only did the OPA(n) values increase, but the bandwidth became smaller, and the ONEST values decreased. With the exception of the C1 (n = 23 pathologists) for the <50% vs. ≥50% and the <30% vs. ≥30% categorisations, the ONEST values were not greater than 9; the number of pathologists involved in the C3 yielded the best OPA(n) values, i.e., the best reproducibility (Table 1).

One of the sTIL categorisations was used to test the ONEST plots. Three random selections of 100 permutations were compared with the Kruskal–Wallis test for the chosen (<50% vs. ≥50%) sTIL categorisation for C1, C1 without the two substantially divergent raters, C1s, C2, and C2 without the two substantially divergent raters. Although sometimes there was a small shift in the ONEST and other values, these permutations were not statistically different with regard to the minimum curves; their p-values were 0.937, 0.271, 0.877, 0.855, and 1, respectively (Figure 2).

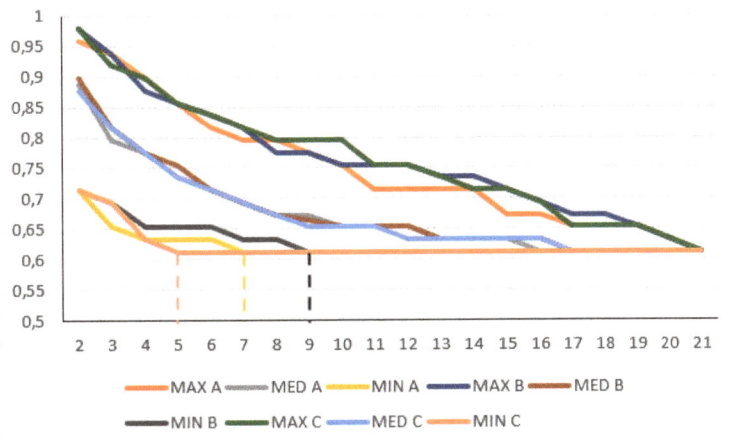

Figure 2. Partly overlapping simplified ONEST plots of 3 randomly selected 100 permutations (A, B, and C) for the <50% sTIL or more classification in C1 circulation without the two divergent classifiers; this example showed the lowest *p*-value in the Kruskal–Wallis test. Note: the *y*-axis only represents values between 0.5 and 1; despite not being statistically significantly different, the 3 randomly selected ONEST plots of 100 permutations yield 3 different ONEST values: 7 (A), 9 (B), and 5 (C) (to ease reading of the values, these are highlighted by vertical dashed segments between the *x*-axis value and the minimum curves), whereas the bandwidth is very similar (0.245 A, 0.265 B and C), and by definition, the OPA(21) value is identical (0.612). MAX: maximum curve; MED: median curve; MIN: minimum curve.

Furthermore, the three random permutations from C1 and C1 without the outlying classifiers; C2 and C2 without the outlying classifiers; and finally, C1 and C2, were also compared with the Wilcoxon rank sum test for the ONEST values that could be derived from them, and this demonstrated significant differences ($p = 0.046$, $p = 0.034$, and $p = 0.043$, respectively) for each of these comparisons.

4. Discussion

ONEST is a recently described additional analysis that can complement reproducibility studies [11–13]. Although it was introduced to estimate the minimum number of observers required to provide a reliable estimate of the reproducibility of a given classification [11], it also gives a visual impression of how much agreement is reached when categorising items into predefined classes and the difference one can expect between two observers. However, as a complementary tool, ONEST is not independent of the studied "population" and the observers.

It is generally accepted that two-tiered classifications are more reproducible than those with more than two categories, e.g., [21]. This also applies to ONEST, as reported for PD-L1 [9] and Ki67 [10], and this is also supported by our analysis of the three-tiered classification in the present study, which demonstrated the worst OPA(n) values in nearly all circulations (Table 1).

Although our attempt to analyse the data without the two observers who substantially deviated from the majority opinion resulted in "improved" results in both C1 and C2 (i.e., greater OPA(n), narrower bandwidth, and lower ONEST values), the analyses without these outliers may not reflect real-life assessments. It is well accepted that populations are generally described with their average values of measurable things, but they also have members that are above and below the average. Therefore, if one wishes to estimate the real-life performance of a classification, all raters, and not only the best raters, should be included in the analysis.

Reproducibility is also dependent on the distribution of the parameter being evaluated in the cases. While assessing three nuclear immunostains for ER, PR, and Ki67 in a different study, we found that using the same cut-off values for all three biomarkers resulted in different reproducibility and ONEST estimations [12]. This was explained by the difference in the number of cases close to or away from the extreme values (0% and 100%). Most values for ER staining were in the 90–100% or 0% range, whereas PR values showed more divergence, Ki67 scores were distributed over a wider range, and ONEST values increased in a respective manner. This phenomenon is likely to be the most important contributor to the surprisingly good results observed for the C3 circulation in the present study (Table 1). Indeed, in C3, there were only 45/900 ratings for sTILs $\geq$ 50% involving 8/100 cases.

The homogeneity versus heterogeneity of the entity being observed also influences reproducibility, and this is substantiated by earlier studies. ER staining is generally more homogeneous than Ki67, as reflected in the lower inter-observer agreement for the latter [12]. On the other hand, sTILs often have a heterogeneous distribution, making it more difficult to assess the overall average distribution. This phenomenon, i.e., heterogenous distribution, was identified as the main contributor to the weaker reproducibility for some cases in our previous study [9] and was also reported by others [22]. Scoring preselected FOVs (C2) eliminates the variability associated with the observers selecting the areas to score in the case of heterogeneously distributed sTILs and results in substantially better reproducibility (ICC for absolute sTILs with preselected FOVs vs. the case when observers had selected their FOVs to be assessed: 0.798 vs. 0.634) [9]. This improved reproducibility was also reflected by key values of ONEST plot analyses: higher OPA(n) values, lower bandwidth, and lower ONEST values in C2 vs. C1 for all categorical classifications.

The number of observers may also influence reproducibility and ONEST plots. For example, C2 versus C1, without the discordant raters (with 12 observers of the former all included in the 21 of the latter), resulted in different OPA(n) values (82% vs. 61% agreement for, e.g., sTILs $\geq$ 50% or fewer). The number of observers also greatly impacts the number of possible permutations, being 2.585×10^{22} for C1 (n = 23), 87,178,291,200 for C2 (n = 14), and "only" 362,880 for C3 (n = 9). In a previous study, also with nine observers [12], we verified that the minimum curve of the 100 randomly selected permutations does not significantly differ from the minimum OPAC of all permutations. In the present analysis, three random ONEST plots were examined for all circulations with one of the cut-offs (<50% vs. the $\geq$50%), and no significant difference was found between their minimum curves. This is also reflected in Figure 2, in which the minimum (and the maximum and median) curves of the three plots substantially overlap with each other. Despite this, there were minor alterations in the bandwidths and ONEST values from the three analyses of the same datasets. This leads us to conclude that even ONEST readings are just estimations and might have a range, but depending on how close the ONEST value is to 2, we can estimate how a reproducibility study with a low number of participants may reflect real-life performance for the test in question. An early study of TILs with 99 cases suggested an 85% (95% CI, 76% to 91%) agreement with no more than a 10% difference in absolute sTIL ratings between two observers [23]. Kojima and colleagues reported an 81% agreement between two observers when classifying sTILs into three categories in 129 cases [24]. A report on 100 cases and >90% mean pairwise agreement on sTILs, by any of six pathologists, with a seventh pathologist serving as the main reviewer for a study, also suggests excellent reproducibility [25]. However, Figure 1A clearly shows that two observers randomly selected from a pool of observers or pairwise comparisons may have minimal discrepancies or no discrepancy at all, but the bandwidth may be much wider than this. Four pathologists also achieved a good agreement scoring sTILs in 121 cases [26] and substantial agreement in 75 cases [27], but Table 1 suggests that this number is still prone to underestimating real-life conditions. Certainly, two observers [23,24,28,29] do not accurately reflect inter-observer agreement [11], and most readings from the ONEST plots (Table 1) with a different number or quality of readers suggest that between 6 and 11 readers are required for a reasonable estimation of inter-observer agreement.

As a limitation, ONEST analyses can only be performed for categorical classifications. Agreement for scoring some markers (e.g., sTILs) as a continuous variable is generally better than the agreement observed using categories defined by given cut-off values [30]. On the other hand, therapeutic decisions are generally made using cut-off values for a biomarker.

Finally, after considering the factors influencing the reproducibility of a subjective test, such as scoring sTILs in breast cancer, it is the case that other variables (e.g., number and experience of observers, distribution of the cases around or away from the extremes, and heterogeneity between fields to assess) also influence ONEST analyses and the ONEST values. Therefore, we can state that two to four observers are certainly not sufficient to reflect the actual inter-observer agreement for evaluating sTILs in breast cancer, but between 6 and 11 observers would be sufficient. The studies by the IIOBMWG largely fulfil this requirement, and their reported values of good reproducibility should be considered reliable [8]. Notwithstanding, the finding that our group, also with a sufficient number of pathologists, was only able to match their high ICC values when scoring sTILs on preselected FOVs, but not when full digital slides were scored, clearly means that factors other than the number of observers contribute to reproducibility [11]. This is also substantiated by another study involving 41 cases of digitised core needle biopsies scored by 40 pathologists, where the ICC values ranged between -0.376 and 0.947, with a mean of 0.659 [31]. In addition to applying methods such as ONEST, the development of tools that can quantify other contributors to lower reproducibility will be useful in the design of reproducibility studies. Due to its simplicity and the data it gives, we also propose that an ONEST analysis could be a part of reproducibility studies to explore the reliability of the results presented or published previously, as not all reports satisfy the suggested minimum number of observers to reach the best possible conclusions. However, the limitations described in the present article must be kept in mind.

5. Conclusions

The reproducibility of sTIL assessments in breast cancer has been examined in several studies. Our results using ONEST indicate that between six and nine observers are expected to give a good estimate of inter-observer variability, and studies involving fewer than these numbers may overestimate agreement between observers. As sTIL evaluation becomes part of daily practice [5], efforts to characterise factors interfering with the reproducibility of scoring are welcome.

Author Contributions: Conceptualisation, B.C. and G.C. (Gábor Cserni); methodology, B.C., G.C. (Gábor Cserni), and T.N.; scoring cases (investigation), X.A., R.B., Z.B.-H., S.B., E.C. (Erika Csörgő), E.C. (Ewa Chmielik), G.C. (Grace Callagy), G.C. (Gábor Cserni), P.F., G.F., M.P.F., A.K., P.H., J.K., A.-V.L., I.L.-K., C.M., O.O.-N., T.P., E.P., P.R., A.R. (Aleš Ryška), A.R. (Angelika Reiner), A.S. (Anna Sapino), A.S. (Anita Sejben), E.S.S., I.S., C.Q., A.V., V.Z. and T.Z.; formal analysis and data curation, B.C., G.C. (Gábor Cserni), T.N.; D.K., M.O. and S.A.G.; digitisation, case distribution, M.W.; writing—original draft preparation, B.C. and G.C. (Gábor Cserni); writing—review and editing, all authors. All authors have read and agreed to the published version of the manuscript.

Funding: This research received no external funding.

Institutional Review Board Statement: This study was conducted according to the guidelines of the Declaration of Helsinki; it involved no patient data, and no ethical approval was deemed necessary.

Informed Consent Statement: Not applicable.

Data Availability Statement: Data are available from the corresponding author and will be released upon reasonable request.

Conflicts of Interest: The authors declare no conflict of interest.

References

1. El Bairi, K.; Haynes, H.R.; Blackley, E.; Fineberg, S.; Shear, J.; Turner, S.; de Freitas, J.R.; Sur, D.; Amendola, L.C.; Gharib, M.; et al. The tale of TILs in breast cancer: A report from The International Immuno-Oncology Biomarker Working Group. *N.P.J. Breast Cancer.* **2021**, *7*, 150. [CrossRef] [PubMed]
2. Denkert, C.; von Minckwitz, G.; Darb-Esfahani, S.; Lederer, B.; Heppner, B.I.; Weber, K.E.; Budczies, J.; Huober, J.; Klauschen, F.; Furlanetto, J.; et al. Tumour-infiltrating lymphocytes and prognosis in different subtypes of breast cancer: A pooled analysis of 3771 patients treated with neoadjuvant therapy. *Lancet Oncol.* **2018**, *19*, 40–50. [CrossRef]
3. Loi, S.; Drubay, D.; Adams, S.; Pruneri, G.; Francis, P.A.; Lacroix-Triki, M.; Joensuu, H.; Dieci, M.V.; Badve, S.; Demaria, S.; et al. Tumor-infiltrating lymphocytes and prognosis: A pooled individual patient analysis of early-stage triple-negative breast cancers. *J. Clin. Oncol.* **2019**, *37*, 559–569. [CrossRef] [PubMed]
4. Cserni, G.; Serfőző, O.; Ambrózay, É.; Markó, L.; Krenács, L. Spontaneous pathological complete regression of a high grade triple negative breast cancer with axillary metastasis–report of a case. *Pol. J. Pathol.* **2019**, *70*, 139–143. [CrossRef] [PubMed]
5. Laenkholm, A.V.; Callagy, G.; Balancin, M.; Bartlett, J.M.S.; Sotiriou, C.; Marchio, C.; Kok, M.; Dos Anjos, C.H.; Salgado, R. Incorporation of TILs in daily breast cancer care: How much evidence can we bear? *Virchows Arch.* **2022**, *480*, 147–162. [CrossRef] [PubMed]
6. Salgado, R.; Denkert, C.; Demaria, S.; Sirtaine, N.; Klauschen, F.; Pruneri, G.; Wienert, S.; Van den Eynden, G.; Baehner, F.L.; Penault-Llorca, F.; et al. The Evaluation of Tumor-Infiltrating Lymphocytes (TILs) in Breast Cancer: Recommendations by an International TILs Working Group 2014. *Ann. Oncol.* **2015**, *26*, 259–271. [CrossRef]
7. Dieci, M.V.; Radosevic-Robin, N.; Fineberg, S.; van den Eynden, G.; Ternes, N.; Penault-Llorca, F.; Pruneri, G.; D'Alfonso, T.M.; Demaria, S.; Castaneda, C.; et al. Update on Tumor-Infiltrating Lymphocytes (TILs) in Breast Cancer, Including Recommendations to Assess TILs in Residual Disease After Neoadjuvant Therapy and in Carcinoma In Situ: A Report of the International Immuno-Oncology Biomarker Working Group on Breast Cancer. *Semin. Cancer Biol.* **2018**, *52*, 16–25. [CrossRef]
8. Denkert, C.; Wienert, S.; Poterie, A.; Loibl, S.; Budczies, J.; Badve, S.; Bago-Horvath, Z.; Bane, A.; Bedri, S.; Brock, J.; et al. Standardized evaluation of tumor-infiltrating lymphocytes in breast cancer: Results of the ring studies of the international immuno-oncology biomarker working group. *Mod. Pathol.* **2016**, *29*, 1155–1164. [CrossRef]
9. Kilmartin, D.; O'Loughlin, M.; Andreu, X.; Bagó-Horváth, Z.; Bianchi, S.; Chmielik, E.; Cserni, G.; Figueiredo, P.; Floris, G.; Foschini, M.P.; et al. Intra-Tumour Heterogeneity Is One of the Main Sources of Inter-Observer Variation in Scoring Stromal Tumour Infiltrating Lymphocytes in Triple Negative Breast Cancer. *Cancers* **2021**, *13*, 4410. [CrossRef]
10. Koo, T.K.; Li, M.Y. A guideline of selecting and reporting intraclass correlation coefficients for reliability research. *J. Chiropr. Med.* **2016**, *15*, 155–163. [CrossRef]
11. Reisenbichler, E.S.; Han, G.; Bellizzi, A.; Bossuyt, V.; Brock, J.; Cole, K.; Fadare, O.; Hameed, O.; Hanley, K.; Harrison, B.T.; et al. Prospective multi-institutional evaluation of pathologist assessment of PD-L1 assays for patient selection in triple negative breast cancer. *Mod. Pathol.* **2020**, *33*, 1746–1752. [CrossRef] [PubMed]
12. Cserni, B.; Bori, R.; Csörgő, E.; Oláh-Németh, O.; Pancsa, T.; Sejben, A.; Sejben, I.; Vörös, A.; Zombori, T.; Nyári, T.; et al. The additional value of ONEST (Observers Needed to Evaluate Subjective Tests) in assessing reproducibility of oestrogen receptor, progesterone receptor and Ki67 classification in breast cancer. *Virchows Arch.* **2021**, *479*, 1101–1109. [CrossRef]
13. Cserni, B.; Bori, R.; Csörgő, E.; Oláh-Németh, O.; Pancsa, T.; Sejben, A.; Sejben, I.; Vörös, A.; Zombori, T.; Nyári, T.; et al. ONEST (Observers Needed to Evaluate Subjective Tests) suggests four or more observers for a reliable assessment of the consistency of histological grading of invasive breast carcinoma—A reproducibility study with a retrospective view on previous studies. *Pathol. Res. Pract.* **2021**, *229*, 153718. [CrossRef]
14. Stanton, S.E.; Disis, M.L. Clinical significance of tumor-infiltrating lymphocytes in breast cancer. *J. Immunother. Cancer* **2016**, *4*, 59. [CrossRef] [PubMed]
15. Loi, S.; Michiels, S.; Salgado, R.; Sirtaine, N.; Jose, V.; Fumagalli, D.; Kellokumpu-Lehtinen, P.L.; Bono, P.; Kataja, V.; Desmedt, C.; et al. Tumor infiltrating lymphocytes are prognostic in triple negative breast cancer and predictive for trastuzumab benefit in early breast cancer: Results from the FinHER trial. *Ann. Oncol.* **2014**, *25*, 1544–1550. [CrossRef]
16. Sasaki, R.; Horimoto, Y.; Yanai, Y.; Kurisaki-Arakawa, A.; Arakawa, A.; Nakai, K.; Saito, M.; Saito, T. Molecular Characteristics of Lymphocyte-predominant Triple-negative Breast Cancer. *Anticancer Res.* **2021**, *41*, 2133–2140. [CrossRef] [PubMed]
17. Cserni, G.; Francz, M.; Járay, B.; Kálmán, E.; Kovács, I.; Krenács, T.; Udvarhelyi, N.; Tóth, E.; Vass, L.; Vörös, A.; et al. Pathological diagnosis, work-up and reporting of breast cancer. Recommendations from the 4th Breast Cancer Consensus Conference. *Magy. Onkol.* **2020**, *64*, 301–328. (In Hungarian) [PubMed]
18. Cserni, G.; Francz, M.; Járay, B.; Kálmán, E.; Kovács, I.; Krenács, T.; Udvarhelyi, N.; Tóth, E.; Vass, L.; Vörös, A.; et al. Pathological Diagnosis, Work-Up and Reporting of Breast Cancer 1st Central-Eastern European Professional Consensus Statement on Breast. *Cancer. Pathol. Oncol. Res.* **2022**, *28*, 1610373. [CrossRef]

19. Cserni, B. ONEST Calculator. Available online: https://github.com/csernib/onest (accessed on 12 November 2022).
20. Zaiontz, C. Real Statistics Resource Pack | Real Statistics Using Excel. Available online: https://real-statistics.com (accessed on 22 September 2022).
21. Tramm, T.; Di Caterino, T.; Jylling, A.-M.B.; Lelkaitis, G.; Lænkholm, A.-V.; Ragó, P.; Tabor, T.P.; Talman, M.-L.M.; Vouza, E.; Scientific Committee of Pathology, Danish Breast Cancer Group (DBCG). Standardized assessment of tumor-infiltrating lymphocytes in breast cancer: An evaluation of inter-observer agreement between pathologists. *Acta. Oncol.* **2018**, *57*, 90–94. [CrossRef]
22. Kos, Z.; Roblin, E.; Kim, R.S.; Michiels, S.; Gallas, B.D.; Chen, W.; van de Vijver, K.K.; Goel, S.; Adams, S.; Demaria, S.; et al. Pitfalls in assessing stromal tumor infiltrating lymphocytes (sTILs) in breast cancer. *N.P.J. Breast Cancer* **2020**, *6*, 17. [CrossRef]
23. Adams, S.; Gray, R.J.; Demaria, S.; Goldstein, L.; Perez, E.A.; Shulman, L.N.; Martino, S.; Wang, M.; Jones, V.E.; Saphner, T.J.; et al. Prognostic value of tumor-infiltrating lymphocytes in triple-negative breast cancers from two phase III randomized adjuvant breast cancer trials: ECOG 2197 and ECOG 1199. *J. Clin. Oncol.* **2014**, *32*, 2959–2966. [CrossRef] [PubMed]
24. Kojima, Y.A.; Wang, X.; Sun, H.; Compton, F.; Covinsky, M.; Zhang, S. Reproducible evaluation of tumor-infiltrating lymphocytes (TILs) using the recommendations of International TILs Working Group 2014. *Ann. Diagn. Pathol.* **2018**, *35*, 77–79. [CrossRef] [PubMed]
25. Kim, R.S.; Song, N.; Gavin, P.G.; Salgado, R.; Bandos, H.; Kos, Z.; Floris, G.; Eynden, G.G.G.M.V.D.; Badve, S.; Demaria, S.; et al. Stromal Tumor-infiltrating Lymphocytes in NRG Oncology/NSABP B-31 Adjuvant Trial for Early-Stage HER2-Positive Breast Cancer. *J. Natl. Cancer Inst.* **2019**, *111*, 867–871. [CrossRef] [PubMed]
26. Buisseret, L.; Desmedt, C.; Garaud, S.; Fornili, M.; Wang, X.; Van den Eyden, G.; de Wind, A.; Duquenne, S.; Boisson, A.; Naveaux, C.; et al. Reliability of tumor-infiltrating lymphocyte and tertiary lymphoid structure assessment in human breast cancer. *Mod. Pathol.* **2017**, *30*, 1204–1212. [CrossRef]
27. Swisher, S.K.; Wu, Y.; Castaneda, C.A.; Lyons, G.R.; Yang, F.; Tapia, C.; Wang, X.; Casavilca, S.A.; Bassett, R.; Castillo, M.; et al. Interobserver Agreement Between Pathologists Assessing Tumor-Infiltrating Lymphocytes (TILs) in Breast Cancer Using Methodology Proposed by the International TILs Working Group. *Ann. Surg. Oncol.* **2016**, *23*, 2242–2248. [CrossRef] [PubMed]
28. Cabuk, F.K.; Aktepe, F.; Kapucuoglu, F.N.; Coban, I.; Sarsenov, D.; Ozmen, V. Interobserver reproducibility of tumor-infiltrating lymphocyte evaluations in breast cancer. *Indian J. Pathol. Microbiol.* **2018**, *61*, 181–186. [CrossRef]
29. Khoury, T.; Peng, X.; Yan, L.; Wang, D.; Nagrale, V. Tumor-Infiltrating Lymphocytes in Breast Cancer: Evaluating Interobserver Variability, Heterogeneity, and Fidelity of Scoring Core Biopsies. *Am. J. Clin. Pathol.* **2018**, *150*, 441–450. [CrossRef]
30. O'Loughlin, M.; Andreu, X.; Bianchi, S.; Chemielik, E.; Cordoba, A.; Cserni, G.; Figueiredo, P.; Floris, G.; Foschini, M.P.; Heikkilä, P.; et al. Reproducibility and predictive value of scoring stromal tumour infiltrating lymphocytes in triple-negative breast cancer: A multi-institutional study. *Breast Cancer Res. Treat.* **2018**, *171*, 1–9. [CrossRef]
31. Van Bockstal, M.R.; François, A.; Altinay, S.; Arnould, L.; Balkenhol, M.; Broeckx, G.; Burguès, O.; Colpaert, C.; Dedeurwaerdere, F.; Dessauvagie, B.; et al. Interobserver variability in the assessment of stromal tumor-infiltrating lymphocytes (sTILs) in triple-negative invasive breast carcinoma influences the association with pathological complete response: The IVITA study. *Mod. Pathol.* **2021**, *34*, 2130–2140. [CrossRef]

Disclaimer/Publisher's Note: The statements, opinions and data contained in all publications are solely those of the individual author(s) and contributor(s) and not of MDPI and/or the editor(s). MDPI and/or the editor(s) disclaim responsibility for any injury to people or property resulting from any ideas, methods, instructions or products referred to in the content.

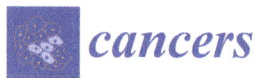

Article

SETD7 Expression Is Associated with Breast Cancer Survival Outcomes for Specific Molecular Subtypes: A Systematic Analysis of Publicly Available Datasets

Fátima Liliana Monteiro [1], Lina Stepanauskaite [2,3], Cecilia Williams [2,3,†] and Luisa A. Helguero [2,*,†]

[1] Department of Medical Sciences, Institute of Biomedicine—iBiMED, University of Aveiro, 3810-193 Aveiro, Portugal
[2] SciLifeLab, Department of Protein Science, KTH Royal Institute of Technology, 114 28 Stockholm, Sweden
[3] Department of Biosciences and Nutrition, Karolinska Institute, 141 83 Stockholm, Sweden
* Correspondence: luisa.helguero@ua.pt
† These authors contributed equally to this study and shared the senior authorship.

Simple Summary: Breast cancer is the most common cancer among women, and it can be classified into subtypes with distinct biology and prognosis. The aim of our bioinformatic study was to assess the potential role of the protein methyltransferase SETD7 in breast cancer by using freely available resources. We saw that SETD7 is differentially expressed across subtypes, which may determine how SETD7 modulates cancer cell biological processes in each subtype. This translates into different prognosis and therapeutic response in patients stratified according to SETD7 levels. SETD7 might provide valuable additional information for discriminating patients based on subtypes and improve therapeutic decisions.

Abstract: SETD7 is a lysine N-methyltransferase that targets many proteins important in breast cancer (BC). However, its role and clinical significance remain unclear. Here, we used online tools and multiple public datasets to explore the predictive potential of *SETD7* expression (high or low quartile) considering BC subtype, grade, stage, and therapy. We also investigated overrepresented biological processes associated with its expression using TCGA-BRCA data. *SETD7* expression was highest in the Her2 (*ERBB2*)-enriched molecular subtype and lowest in the basal-like subtype. For the basal-like subtype specifically, higher *SETD7* was consistently correlated with worse recurrence-free survival ($p < 0.009$). High SETD7-expressing tumours further exhibited a higher rate of *ERBB2* mutation (20% vs. 5%) along with a poorer response to anti-Her2 therapy. Overall, high SETD7-expressing tumours showed higher stromal and lower immune scores. This was specifically related to higher counts of cancer-associated fibroblasts and endothelial cells, but lower B and T cell signatures, especially in the luminal A subtype. Genes significantly associated with SETD7 expression were accordingly overrepresented in immune response processes, with distinct subtype characteristics. We conclude that the prognostic value of SETD7 depends on the BC subtype and that SETD7 may be further explored as a potential treatment-predictive marker for immune checkpoint inhibitors.

Keywords: SETD7; breast cancer; molecular subtypes; survival; gene expression; biological processes

1. Introduction

SETD7 is a lysine N-methyltransferase that monomethylates the histone H3 lysine 4 (K4) and several other nonhistone proteins, including numerous transcription factors and epigenetic regulators (reviewed in [1]). Methylation by SETD7 can modulate a protein's stability, subcellular localization, and/or interactions with other proteins. For example, methylation by SETD7 improves the stability of ERα (*ESR1*) in breast cancer (BC), which may be of relevance to endocrine resistance [2]. SETD7 may also be important to prevent oxidative stress in BC cells by reducing KEAP1 and enhancing the expression of *GSTT2* and

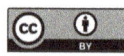

NFE2L2 (Nrf2), and promote metastasis by enhancing *VEGFA* or *RUNX2* expression [3]. On the other hand, SETD7 can methylate oncogenic proteins (DNMT1, E2F1, and HIF1A), leading to their degradation (reviewed in [4]). Data obtained mainly from preclinical models point toward a context-dependent effect mediated by SETD7, and its role in BC remains controversial [4].

Several studies have compared SETD7 mRNA or protein expression between BC and nontumorous tissue using public datasets or in-house cohorts, but with inconclusive results. Some studies showed that *SETD7* mRNA levels are lower in BC [5,6], others that BC has higher SETD7 protein levels [7,8] or that no differences in *SETD7* expression between BC and normal tissue were observed [9]. The discrepancy between the studies also translates to the correlation analysis of SETD7 expression with prognosis. While several studies found that high *SETD7* mRNA levels correlated with better overall survival (OS) [10] or disease-free survival (DFS) [11], others reported that higher SETD7 levels were correlated with shorter OS and DFS [3,7,8]. Breast tumours are classified into distinct molecular subtypes based on gene expression (PAM50) profiles. The subtypes encompass luminal A, luminal B, Her2 (*ERBB2*)-enriched, normal-like, and basal-like subtypes, and exhibit fundamental differences in response to therapy and survival. Notably, in all studies that have analysed public datasets, no clarification as to whether the analysis was done by pooling all BC subtypes was available. Upon considering the number of cases in the studies analysing TCGA data, it appears that all subtypes were pooled, but this remains to be clarified in the other studies.

In a recent systematic review, we were able to associate high SETD7 activity with inhibition of epithelial–mesenchymal transition in all the cancer types where this process had been studied, including BC [4]. Moreover, inhibition of SETD7 function was associated with improved response to DNA-damaging agents in most of the analysed studies [4]. Thus, while effects mediated by SETD7 are cell type- and signalling context-specific, the lack of clarity regarding the role and clinical significance of SETD7 in BC may lead to stagnation in this field of research before clear conclusions can be drawn. Herein, an unbiased systematic analysis of public datasets was carried out. The main goal was to establish the predictive potential of *SETD7* expression in BC considering the impact of clinical factors such as subtype, grade, stage, and therapy on the association between *SETD7* expression and survival outcomes. The mutation frequency of *SETD7* and its target proteins was also investigated. Additionally, we identified the significantly overrepresented biological processes and pathways among the differentially expressed genes that emerge when *SETD7* expression is used to stratify the samples in each breast cancer subtype.

2. Materials and Methods

2.1. Description of Datasets

This study used previously published and publicly available data. No new sequencing or protein expression data were generated. A description of all the datasets that report *SETD7* expression, available for analysis within the different online tools used, is provided in Supplementary Table S1. Since cBioPortal (https://www.cbioportal.org/, v5.1.10, accessed on 5 August 2022) includes TCGA breast cancer data with different release dates, we used the PanCancer Atlas study for all analyses in cBioPortal (v5.1.10).

2.2. Analysis of SETD7 Mutation and Copy Number

SETD7 mutation and copy number were analysed using cBioPortal [12,13]. All datasets including mutation and copy number profiles (Supplementary Table S1) were pooled and analysis was carried out pooling samples from all BC subtypes [14–26], including data from The Metastatic Breast Cancer Project (https://www.mbcproject.org/, accessed on 5 August 2022) Count Me In (https://joincountmein.org/, accessed on 5 August 2022) (MBCproject cBioPortal data version February 2020).

2.3. Analysis of SETD7 Expression Using Online Tools

The analysis of *SETD7* expression in tumour and adjacent normal tissue was performed using RNA-seq data available in the TNMplot [27] online tool (https://www.tnmplot.com, accessed on 26 April 2022). The relationship between *SETD7* mRNA expression and clinicopathological characteristics, genomic alterations, DNA methylation, phosphoproteome, acetylproteome, and total proteome was explored using cBioPortal [12,13] online tool accessed between 20 January and 27 February 2022. RNA-seq and gene-chip data in cBioPortal are based on z-scores relative to all samples precomputed from the expression values in each dataset (fragments per kilobase of exon per million mapped fragments (FPKM), transcripts per million (TPM), or RNA-seq by expectation maximization (RSEM) for RNA-seq and log(microarray) for gene-chip). *SETD7* differential expression was set by comparing upper vs. lower quartiles (high and low expression, respectively). This analysis was done both by pooling all BC subtypes and for each subtype individually.

2.4. Correlation of SETD7 with Breast Cancer Outcomes

KM plotter, cBioPortal, and the Human Protein Atlas (HPA, [28]) were used to study the prognosis value of *SETD7* mRNA or corresponding protein. ROC plotter (https://www.rocplot.org/, accessed on 23 March 2022) [29] was used to study the potential predictive value of SETD7, using the recommended JetSet method [30] and without the 'no outliers' filter. ROC plotter uses 36 publicly available BC datasets that include chemotherapy (n = 2108), endocrine therapy (n = 971), and anti-Her2 (n = 267) treatment data. The patients are grouped into responders or non-responders by taking into consideration either the pathological complete response (n = 1775, incl. 639 responders and 1136 non-responders) or the relapse-free survival (n = 1329, incl. 978 responders and 351 non-responders) data provided by the studies. Differential expression of *SETD7* was set by comparing upper (high expression) vs. lower (low expression) quartiles, with exception of protein data in KM plotter and mRNA data in HPA where the differential expression was automatically set (median). Outcomes (OS, RFS—recurrence/relapse-free survival, PCR—pathological complete response, PFS—progression-free survival, DFS, DSFS—disease-specific free survival, DMFS—distant metastasis-free survival, PPS—palliative performance scale) could be evaluated in specific datasets depending on the patient data available for each dataset. Samples grouped by clinical factors or pooled BC subtypes were analysed.

2.5. Genes Associated with Differential SETD7 mRNA Expression in BC Subtypes

The TCGA-BRCA raw counts and FPKM data were downloaded on 20 March 2022 from NCI Genomic Data Commons (GDC) using the TCGAbiolinks package (version 2.22.4) [31–33] in R (version 4.1.2). SETD7 was defined as highly or lowly expressed based on upper and lower quartiles, respectively. The samples corresponding to the middle quartiles were considered unchanged and therefore removed. Genes with less than 1 FPKM in both high- and low-SETD7 patients were considered not expressed and removed. Genes that were not present in at least a quarter of the samples were also filtered out. This was done based on counts per million using edgeR package (version 3.36.0) [34–36]. The raw counts for the remaining samples and genes were then processed using the default processing pipeline of DESeq2 (package version 1.34.0) [37]. Genes were considered significantly expressed if the Benjamini–Hochberg adjusted *p*-value (or *q*-value) for false-discovery rate (FDR) <0.05 and the absolute value of the log2 fold change >0.4. Principal component analysis (PCA) on gene expression (after variance stabilizing transformation to the count data) was used for data visualization. The infiltrating immune and stromal scores for samples expressing high- and low-SETD7 groups were calculated using immunodeconv (version 2.0.4) package [38]. Significantly differentially expressed genes between the high and low SETD7 groups from each BC subtype were extracted using Venny 2.1 [39]. Gene ontology enrichment analysis was performed using DAVID [40,41]. Genes associated with high- or low-SETD7 groups were analysed regardless of direction (up or down) and also separately in an attempt to distinguish which functional results are a subject of *SETD7* expression. The default parameters with medium stringency were used. Biological processes containing at least two annotations and with adjusted p-value ≤ 0.05 are reported. The ggplot2 (version 3.3.5) [42] and GOplot (version 1.0.2) [43] packages were used for visualization.

3. Results

3.1. Characterization of SETD7 Mutations, Copy Number, and Expression in BC

3.1.1. SETD7 Mutation and Copy Number Profile

The frequency of *SETD7* mutations in BC was explored in publicly available data consisting of 8177 samples from 14 independent studies (whole exome sequencing, targeted sequencing, gene chip) [14–26]. *SETD7* was mutated in only 0.2% of BC cases (7/4378 profiled samples, Supplementary Figure S1A). These rare events corresponded to missense mutations of unknown significance, found randomly across the *SETD7* gene and across subtypes (Supplementary Figure S1B and File S1). *SETD7* copy number was altered with a slightly higher frequency of 12% (972/8177 patients). Shallow deletion (heterogeneous loss) of *SETD7* was observed in 17% of cases (761/4378 profiled samples, Supplementary Figure S1C), whereas deep deletion (deep loss, possibly a homozygous deletion) was only observed in 0.1% (3/4378), low-level gains (a few additional copies, often broad) in 4% (188/4378) and high-level amplification (more copies, often local) in 0.5% (23/4378) of cases (Supplementary Figure S1C). The shallow deletion was more often associated with the basal-like subtype (around 47% for basal-like vs. 35% for Her2-enriched, 21% for luminal A, 33% for luminal B, and 4% for normal-like subtypes). The low-level gain was more often associated with the Her2-enriched subtype (around 13% vs. 5% for basal, 6% for luminal A, 9% for luminal B, and 3% for normal-like subtypes). Overall, the genetic alteration of *SETD7* was not a common occurrence in BC, but a heterogeneous copy number loss was frequent (47%) in basal-like tumours specifically.

3.1.2. Association of SETD7 Expression with Clinical Attributes

To compare the expression of *SETD7* in breast tumours and adjacent normal tissue, we used the publicly available online tool TNMplot comprising RNA-seq data of paired tissue samples from 112 patients. This analysis clearly showed that *SETD7* mRNA is significantly lower in breast tumours compared with the adjacent normal tissue (Figure 1A). Analysis by subtype was not supported by this tool. Next, the expression of *SETD7* was explored in the different BC datasets available from cBioPortal (RNA-seq, gene chip, and mass spectrometry). A significant correlation could be observed between *SETD7* expression and PAM50 subtype (in all datasets except METABRIC [$q = 0.07$], Table 1). *SETD7* mRNA and protein expression were both consistently higher in the Her2-enriched and luminal A subtypes, and lower in the basal subtype (Figures 1B,C and S2, Table 1). The mean differences of each group (Cohen's d) and the confidence interval for TCGA-BRCA data grouped by subtype were further analysed (Supplementary Figure S3). Luminal A vs. Her2-enriched (d = −0.25 [−0.54, 0.04]), luminal B vs. Her2-enriched (d = −0.07 [−0.39, 0.25]), and luminal B vs. luminal A (d = 0.18 [−0.02, 0.38]) differences had a small effect size indicating little or no clinical relevance. However, the differences between normal-like and luminal B (d = −0.49 [−0.92, −0.06]), Her2-enriched (d = −0.56 [−1.03, −0.08]) or basal subtype (d = 0.36 [−0.07, 0.79]) had a medium effect size, and most importantly, luminal A vs. basal (d = 0.67 [0.46, 0.88]) or luminal B vs. basal (d = 0.85 [0.60, 1.10]), and Her2-enriched vs. basal (d = 0.92 [0.60, 1.25]) had strong effect sizes, supportive of relevant clinical differences (Supplementary Figure S3). Luminal B tumours exhibited varying mRNA levels dependent on the dataset (Supplementary Figure S2, Table 1) and low protein levels (Figure 1C). No correlation between *SETD7* differential expression and therapy, tumour grade, or stage was observed in pooled BC samples or when divided by subtype (Supplementary Table S2). In conclusion, our analysis across different large-scale datasets clearly shows that *SETD7* expression is significantly reduced in basal-like BC, which may be related to the copy number loss noted above for basal-like tumours.

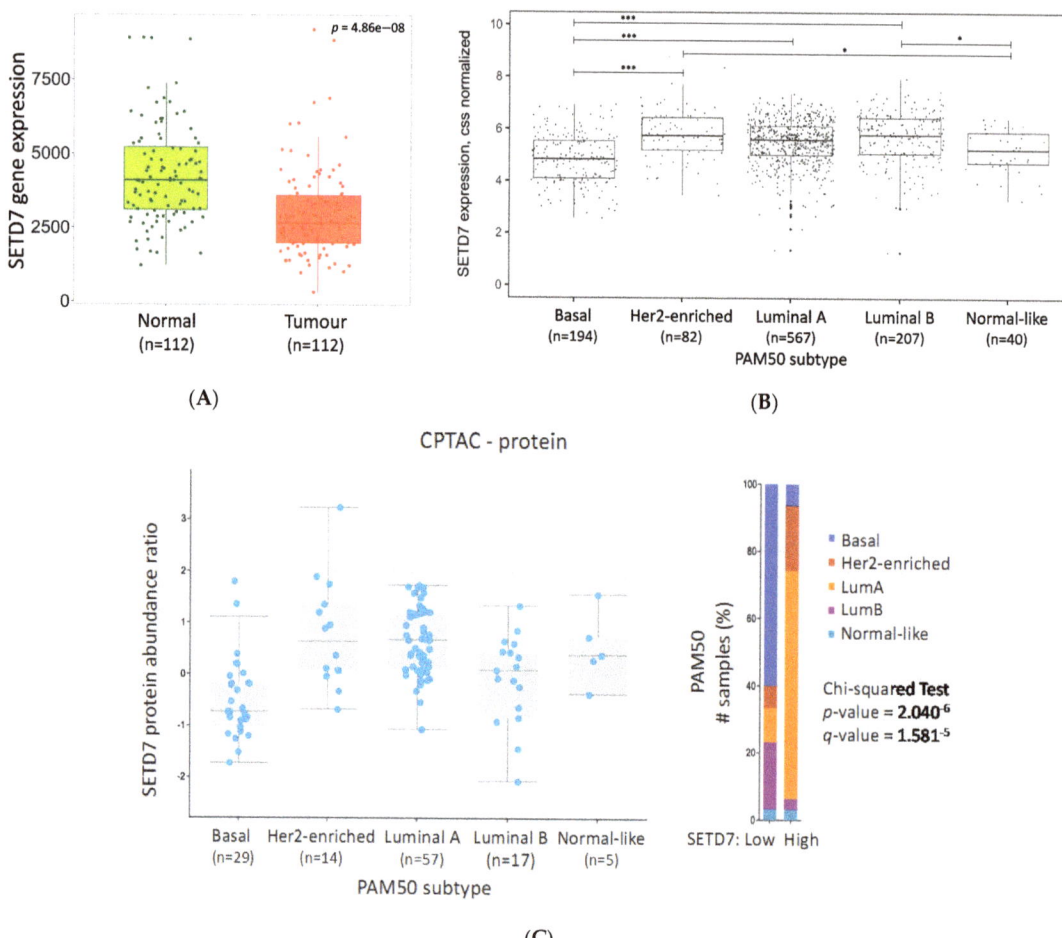

Figure 1. SETD7 expression in breast cancer. (**A**) *SETD7* mRNA expression in tumour and adjacent normal tissue using RNA-seq data available from TNMplot; (**B**) *SETD7* mRNA expression across PAM50 subtypes using TCGA-BRCA data in R. ANOVA followed by Tukey's test: * < 0.05; *** < 0.0001 (**C**) SETD7 protein expression across PAM50 subtypes using CPTAC data from cBioPortal.

3.1.3. Association of SETD7 Expression with Clinically Relevant Signatures

To investigate whether *SETD7* differential expression was correlated with clinically relevant mRNA and protein signatures, we first analysed datasets in cBioPortal where this information was available (hypoxia scores were available for the TCGA PanCancer cohort, and stromal, immune, and stemness scores for CPTAC cohort), and as a second approach, we used a deconvolution method in R to further explore the tumour microenvironment infiltration mRNA signatures in the TCGA-BRCA cohort. High *SETD7* mRNA correlated with lower hypoxia scores [44,45] in pooled samples from all subtypes in the TCGA PanCancer Atlas dataset (Figure 2A, left panel). High SETD7 protein correlated with higher stromal scores [46,47] in CPTAC dataset and high *SETD7* mRNA with cancer-associated fibroblasts (CAFs), endothelial cells, and neutrophil signatures in the TCGA-BRCA dataset (Figure 2B). On the other hand, low *SETD7* mRNA and protein levels were correlated with high xCell immune score and stemness score (CPTAC, pooled samples from all subtypes; Table 2 and Figure 2A, middle and right panels). Further analysis of the xCell immune score showed enrichment of B and T cells (CD8+ T cells) in the low-SETD7 group, while, as mentioned above, enrichment of neutrophils was noted in the high-SETD7 group (TCGA-BRCA; Figure 2B).

Table 1. *SETD7* expression per subtype. Significant values are highlighted in bold. Chi-squared test *p*-value and Benjamini–Hochberg FDR correction *q*-value. NA—not available; nSETD7 DE—number of samples with differentially expressed SETD7; nTotal—total number of samples.

cBioPortal (nSETD7 DE/n Total Samples)	PAM50	Luminal A	Luminal B	Her2-Enriched	Basal	Normal-Like
CPTAC-RNA (61/122)	$p = 1.59^{-5}$ $q = 9.85^{-5}$	High	Low	High	Low	High
CPTAC-protein (61/122)	$p = 2.04^{-6}$ $q = 1.58^{-5}$	High	Low	High	Low	Unchanged
METABRIC (952/2976)	$p = 4.23^{-3}$ $q = 0.07$	High	Unchanged	High	Unchanged	Unchanged
SMC (84/187)	$p = 1.45^{-7}$ $q = 2.33^{-6}$	High	High	High	Low	Unchanged
TCGA PanCancer Atlas (541/1084)	$p < 10^{-10}$ $q < 10^{-10}$	High	High	High	Low	Unchanged

Table 2. SETD7 association with stromal, immune, stemness and hypoxia scores. Significant values are highlighted in bold: Wilcoxon test *p*-value and Benjamini–Hochberg FDR correction *q*-value. NA—not available.

Scores	CPTAC			TCGA PanCancer Atlas			High SETD7 Correlates with
	RNA	Protein		Overall	Luminal A	Luminal B	
	Overall		Luminal A				
xCell Stromal	$p = 4.06^{-4}$ $q = 2.17^{-3}$	$p = 1.26^{-4}$ $q = 8.05^{-4}$	$p = 2.09^{-3}$ $q = 0.01$	NA	NA	NA	High
ESTIMATE Stromal	$p = 1.83^{-3}$ $q = 7.33^{-3}$	$p = 5.96^{-4}$ $q = 2.38^{-3}$	$p = 2.25^{-3}$ $q = 0.01$	NA	NA	NA	High
xCell Immune	$p = 0.01$ $q = 0.03$	$p = 8.83^{-3}$ $q = 0.03$	$p = 0.68$ $q = 0.81$	NA	NA	NA	Low
Stemness	$p = 0.01$ $q = 0.03$	$p = 2.33^{-4}$ $q = 5.96^{-4}$	$p = 0.06$ $q = 0.20$	NA	NA	NA	Low
Buffa Hypoxia	NA	NA	NA	$p < 1.00^{-10}$ $q < 1.00^{-10}$	$p < 1.00^{-10}$ $q < 1.00^{-10}$	$p = 5.82^{-4}$ $q = 0.01$	Low
Winter Hypoxia	NA	NA	NA	$p < 1.00^{-10}$ $q < 1.00^{-10}$	$p = 1.11^{-8}$ $q = 2.51^{-7}$	$p = 6.36^{-4}$ $q = 0.01$	Low

Analysis by molecular subtype revealed that the lower hypoxia scores in high *SETD7* mRNA group was specific for luminal A and B subtypes (Table 2). Likewise, when each subtype was investigated separately, high stromal scores were significantly correlated with high *SETD7* expression in the luminal A subtype (Table 2) whereas enrichment of CAF, endothelial cell, and neutrophil signatures was noted in high-SETD7 samples of all subtypes (Supplementary Figures S4 and S5).

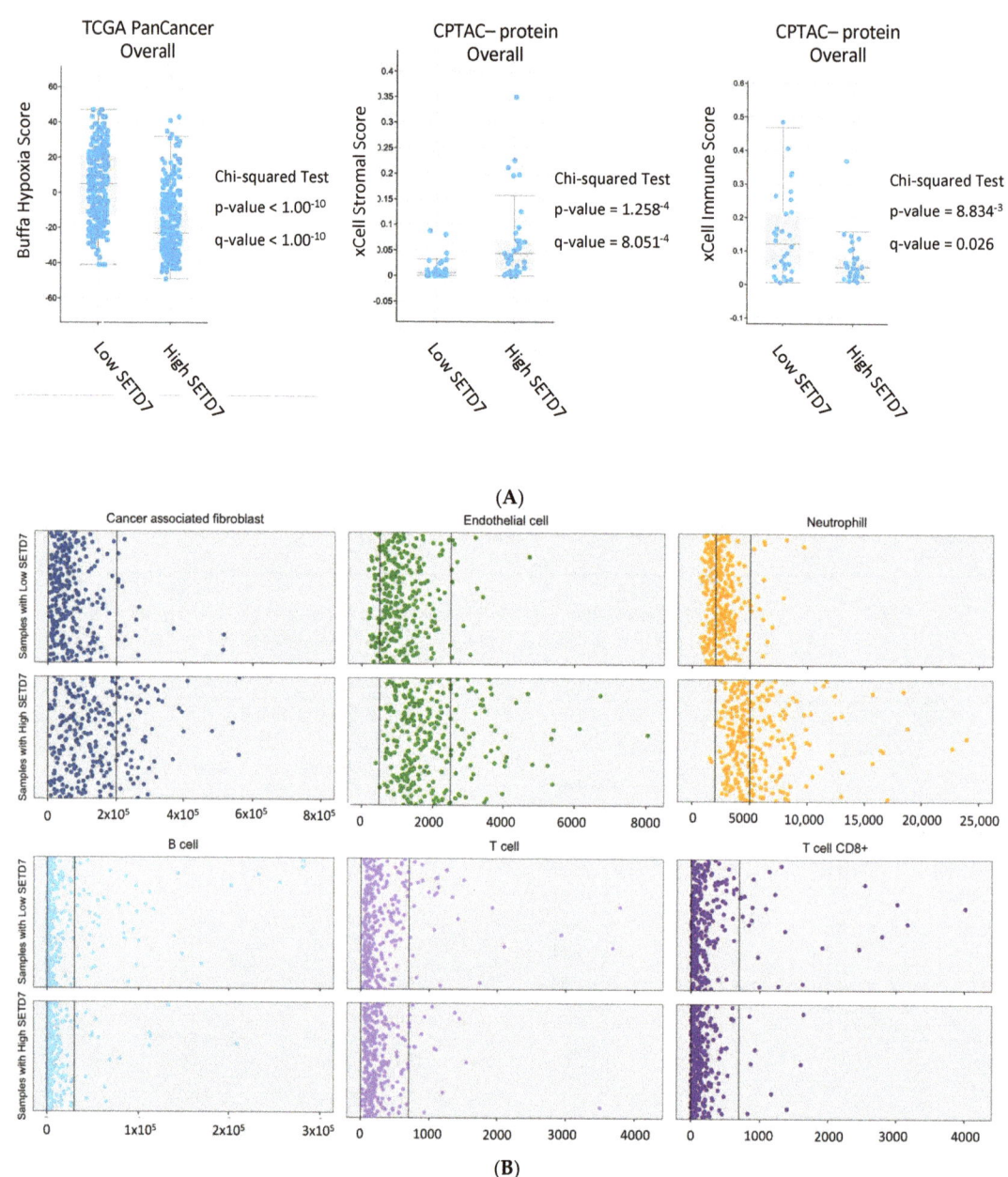

Figure 2. Correlation of *SETD7* differential expression with clinical factors. (**A**) Association of *SETD7* differential expression (high vs. low) with Buffa Hypoxia Score (mRNA), xCell Stromal Score and xCell Immune Score (protein) when pooling all breast cancer types together. Wilcoxon test *p*-value and Benjamini–Hochberg FDR correction *q*-value; (**B**) Association of *SETD7* differential expression (high vs. low) with tissue-infiltrating immune and stromal cell populations using mcp_count method [48] from immunodeconv package and TCGA-BRCA data overall.

In conclusion, we saw that reduced levels of SETD7 are associated with high stemness and immune scores in general, while high expression is associated with increased stromal score, including for CAFs, endothelial cells, and neutrophils, and reduced hypoxia scores in the luminal A subtype specifically.

3.2. Association of SETD7 Expression with Genomic Alterations and DNA Methylation

SETD7 histone methyltransferase can influence chromatin remodelling. The association of differential *SETD7* expression with genomic alterations and DNA methylation was explored in cBioPortal, using the TCGA PanCancer Atlas cohort to investigate associations with genomic alterations and METABRIC to analyse the impact on DNA methylation. No gene was significantly deleted or mutated in either high- or low-SETD7 mRNA groups, even when specific mutation types were queried individually (missense, in-frame, truncating, structural variants, or CNA deletion), although there was a tendency for *TP53* (p53) gene alterations. Significant correlations between *SETD7* differential expression and other genomic alterations (such as amplifications) were observed (Supplementary File S2 and Figure S6). The high-SETD7 group showed higher genomic alterations in *ERBB2* (Her2; 21% event frequency in the high-SETD7 group vs. 6% in the low SETD7 group; Supplementary Figure S6), especially higher copy number amplification (16.42% or 44/268 profiled samples in high SETD7 compared with 4.85% or 13/268 profiled samples in low SETD7 group). On the other hand, the low-SETD7 group showed higher event frequency in the *TP53* gene (c.a. 28% in high SETD7 vs. 48% in low SETD7, respectively; Supplementary Figure S6).

Analysis by molecular subtype did not disclose any significant correlation between *SETD7* differential expression and genomic alterations, although a clear tendency for a higher number of genomic alterations in the *ERBB2* gene in the high-SETD7 group was observed for the Her2-enriched subtype (90% event frequency in high SETD7 vs. 58% in low SETD7. Most of these alterations were copy number amplification (27/29 profiled samples).

SETD7 impacts cancer-related processes, including in BC [4,49], but it was not mutated in BC (as shown above). Therefore, mutations in SETD7 target genes were queried. Forty-two specific genes with known SETD7 target methylation sites were analysed (reviewed in [1,4] and detailed in Supplementary Table S3). Only one mutation in a SETD7 lysine methylation site was found, consisting of a K873E missense mutation in the tumour suppressor *RB1*, in only one sample. No mutations on sites previously reported to compete with SETD7 methylation [4] were identified.

The correlation with general DNA methylation of SETD7 target genes was investigated in the METABRIC dataset, which is the only set with information about DNA methylation. No correlation between *SETD7* differential expression and DNA methylation throughout the genome was observed, either when pooling all BC samples or when stratifying by molecular subtype.

Thus, high *SETD7* expression was related to increased *ERBB2* copy number in the Her2-enriched subtype, but not related with other genetic alterations.

3.3. Gene Expression and Biological Processes Associated with Differential SETD7 mRNA Expression

To avoid heterogeneity, this analysis was carried out on the TCGA data, which is the most powerful gene expression dataset available to date. We retrieved the TCGA-BRCA RNA-seq data, and analysis of differential gene expression between the high-SETD7 and low-SETD7 groups was carried out for each molecular subtype (Supplementary Figure S7A). The normal-like subtype was not included in the analysis due to the low number of samples available. First, the overall gene expression data were validated by the PCA plot clearly separating the basal-like and the Her2-enriched, luminal A and B subtypes, and further showing that the luminal A and B were more similar than the other subtypes, as expected (Supplementary Figure S7B).

Next, the comparison between high- and low-SETD7 groups for each molecular subtype (Venn diagram in Supplementary Figure S8A) disclosed 2834 genes that were commonly associated with *SETD7* expression in all subtypes (Supplementary File S3). Of these, 1699 were highly expressed in the high-SETD7 group and 1133 in the low-SETD7 group.

Only two genes (GPER1 and CYP4F22) were oppositely correlated with *SETD7* expression in different subtypes, being enriched in in low-SETD7 tumours for all subtypes except luminal B where they were upregulated in the high-SETD7 group. The commonly upregulated genes in high-SETD7 groups of all subtypes were overrepresented for biological functions related to protein phosphorylation and ubiquitination. Processes previously associated with SETD7 (reviewed in [4]) also appeared overrepresented in the high-SETD7 groups. These include cellular response to DNA damage stimulus, DNA repair, cell division, cell cycle, and cell migration (Supplementary File S4). The genes upregulated in low-SETD7 tumours, on the other hand, were related to translation and mitochondrial respiration (Supplementary Figure S8B).

Further, the unique genes being differentially expressed between high- or low-SETD7 groups within each subtype were analysed for enrichment of biological pathways (Figures 3 and S9). In luminal A subtype, the pathways related with immune response were overrepresented in low-SETD7 group. The highly expressed genes that related more strongly ($|\log 2 FC| > 1$) with low-SETD7 were mainly immunoglobulins, such as *IGKV2-29* (q-value = 7.39^{-05}, log2FC = -1.57) and other genes which trigger the immune response such as *AZU1* (q-value = 2.24^{-16}, log2FC = -1.81) and *S100A9* (q-value = 2.72^{-11}, log2FC = -1.63) (Supplementary File S3). On the other hand, pathways overrepresented in high-SETD7 tumours were linked to cell adhesion-related pathways (Supplementary Figure S9). These included the genes *FGB* (q-value = 5.99^{-03}, log2FC = 1.37) and *ROBO2* (q-value = 2.54^{-06}, log2FC = 1.32). In the luminal B subtype, DNA repair and response to DNA damage-related pathways were the main biological processes overrepresented in low-SETD7, while the lipid catabolic process was strongly overrepresented in high-SETD7 tumours. Interestingly, magnesium ion transmembrane transport and regulation of insulin secretion involved in cellular response to glucose stimulus were solely overrepresented in the luminal B subtype, where the genes *PNPLA3* (q-value = 5.46^{-03}, log2FC = 1.27) and *ADCY5* (q-value = 4.23^{-03}, log2FC = 1.18) stand out as strongly correlated with SETD7 mRNA expression. In the Her2-enriched subtype, fibroblast migration and extracellular matrix disassembly were overrepresented in low-SETD7 tumours, from which the genes *MMP7* (q-value = 3.25^{-02}, log2FC = -1.32), *KLK5* (q-value = 6.67^{-03}, log2FC = -1.85), and *KLK7* (q-value = 8.63^{-03}, log2FC = -2.31) were strongly regulated ($|\log 2 FC| > 1$). On the other hand, early endosome to late endosome transport was overrepresented in the high-SETD7 group. Finally, in the basal-like subtype, cell differentiation-related pathways were strongly overrepresented in low-SETD7 (Supplementary Figure S9) where keratins stand out (e.g., *KRT13*, q-value = 5.42^{-13}, log2FC = -4.36; *KRT6A*, q-value = 3.21^{-10}, log2FC = -3.56; and *KRT1*, q-value = 8.19^{-08}, log2FC = -2.93), along with other genes, such as *SNAI2* (q-value = 4.82^{-04}, log2FC = -1.13) and *IGF2* (q-value = 1.25^{-02}, log2FC = -1.01). In the high-SETD7 basal-like tumours, the cellular response to DNA damage stimulus and DNA repair-related pathways were overrepresented. Also, *PPARGC1A* (q-value = 1.49^{-03}, log2FC = 1.48), a protein involved in cancer metabolic adaptation to stress, was upregulated.

Some biological processes were shared between subtypes, even though the genes for each subtype were unique (Figure 4A). These included many processes related to immune responses, such as chemotaxis, neutrophil chemotaxis and chemokine-mediated signalling, B cell receptor signalling pathway, and inflammatory response. The genes associated with immune response processes were often associated with low-SETD7 in luminal A and Her2-enriched subtypes and with high-SETD7 in the basal-like subtype (Figure 4B and Supplementary File S4). This aligns with the xCell immune score, B and T cell signatures shown above (Figure 2A,B).

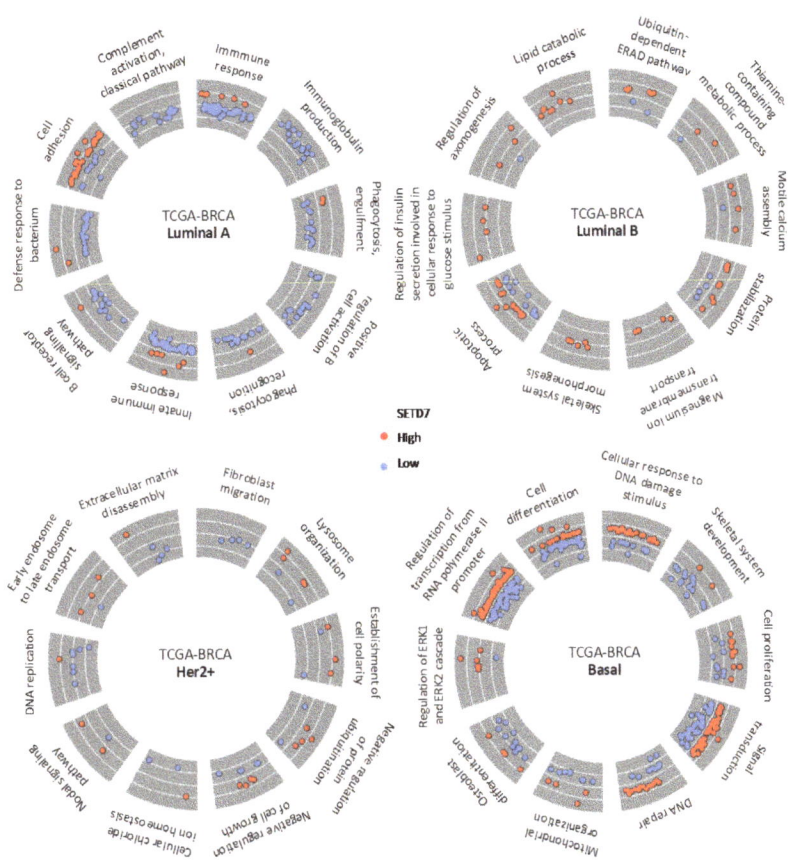

Figure 3. Top 10 biological processes overrepresented among the genes associated with *SETD7* differential expression (high and low) and unique for each subtype.

Next, the expression of genes with reported functional connection to SETD7 was investigated. A list of 83 genes, including the 42 known SETD7 targets plus other genes reported to be associated with SETD7 function, was used to query the genes differentially expressed in high- versus low-SETD7 tumours for each subtype (Figure 5). Interestingly, some of these genes were consistently associated with high-SETD7 (*AR*, *CTNNB1*, *CTNND1*, *EGFR*, *FOXO3*, *HIF1A*, *HK2*, *KAT2B*, *MED1*, *NFE2L2*, *PDPK1*, *PPP1R12A*, *RB1*, *RORA*, *SIRT1*, *SPEN*, *STAT3*, *YAP1*, and *ZEB1*) or low-SETD7 (*E2F1*, *IRF1*, *MMP7*, *MMP9*, *RPL29*, *SUV39H1*, *TAF10*, *TWIST1*, and *ZFHHC8*) independently of the subtype. Others were dependent on the subtype: *CCNA1*, *DNMT1*, *PPARGC1A*, and *TTK* were associated with high-SETD7 and *SNAI2* with low-SETD7 for the basal-like subtype; *LDHA* and *TP53* with high-SETD7 and *ESR1* (ERα) and *SOX2* with low-SETD7 for the Her2-enriched subtype. Moreover, in both luminal A and B subtypes, *ESR1* (ERα) and *PGR* (PR) were associated with high-SETD7, highlighting an association of SETD7 with endocrine treatment-predictive biomarkers.

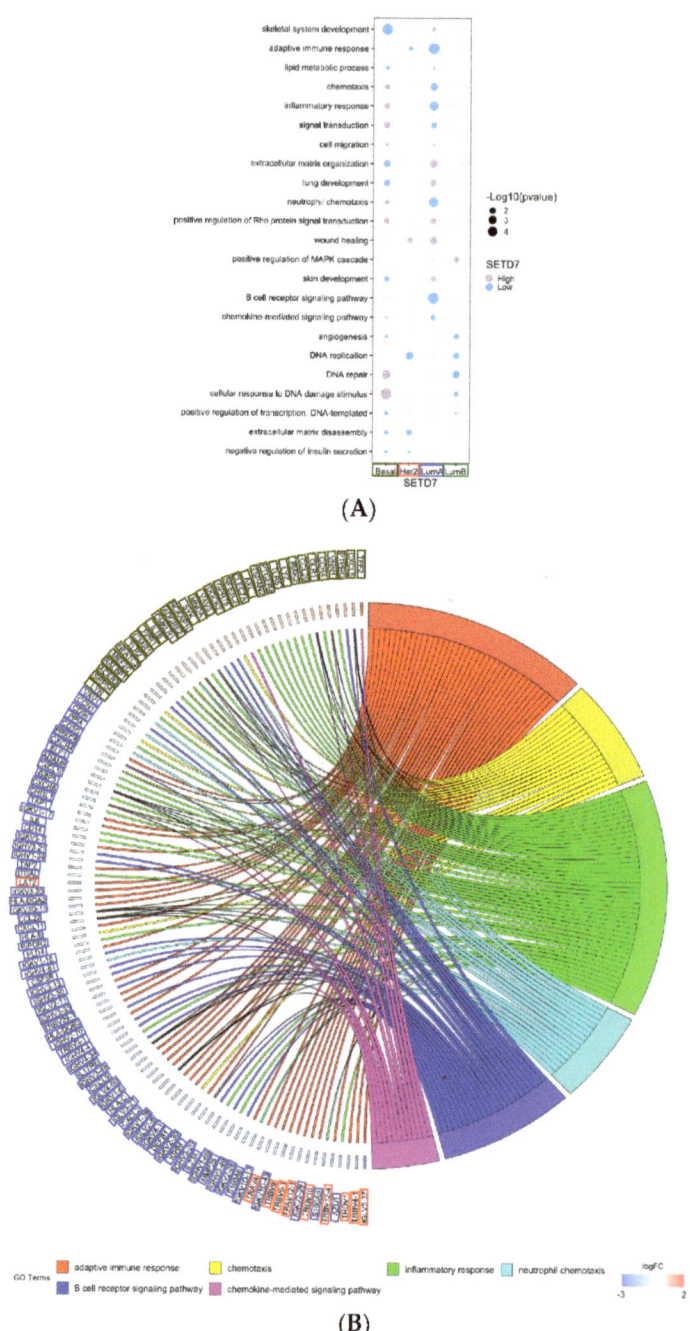

Figure 4. Analysis of the shared biological processes overrepresented among the differentially expressed genes associated with SETD7 (high and low) and unique for each subtype. (**A**) Bubble plot representing all shared biological processes from the unique genes for each subtype; (**B**) GoChord showing all unique genes representing shared immune-related biological processes.

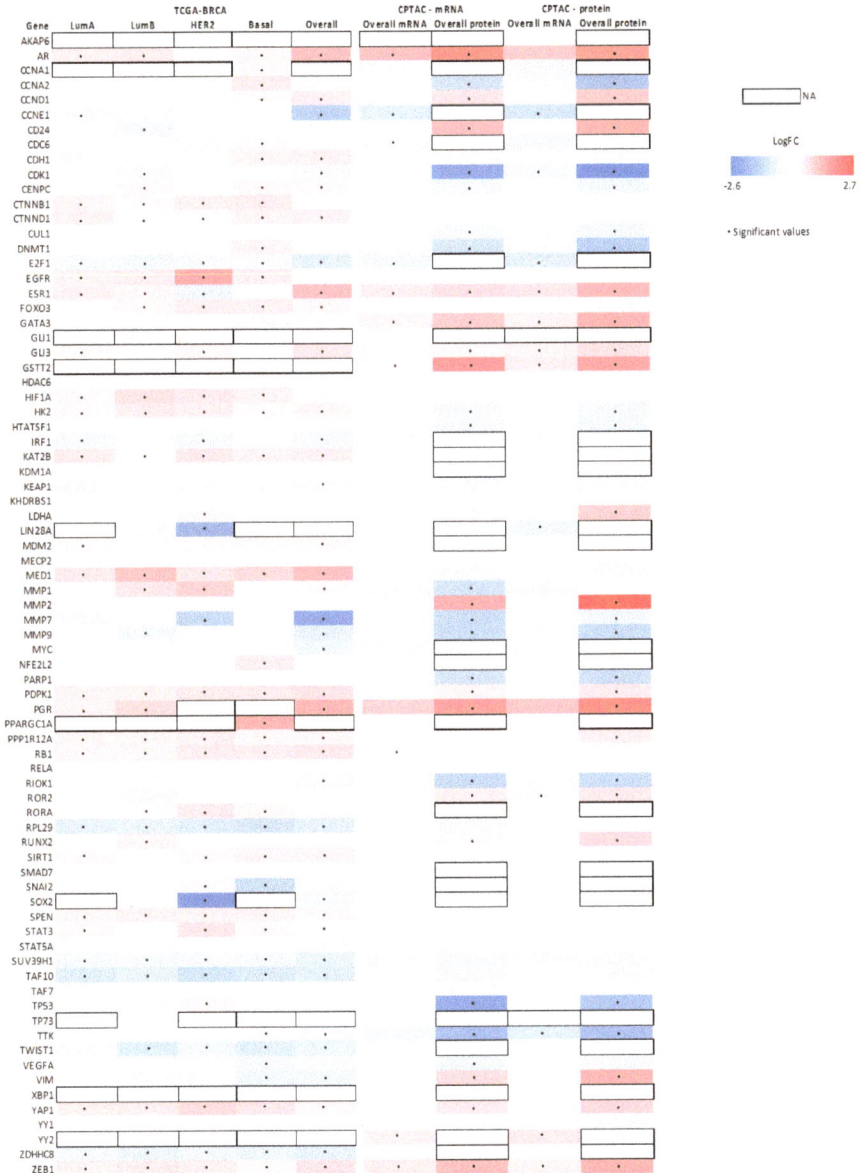

Figure 5. Heatmap showing the association of several genes of interest, including known SETD7 targets, with *SETD7* differential expression using the TCGA-BRCA dataset (analysis performed both by subtype and by pooling all BC samples—overall) and CPTAC dataset (SETD7 stratified by mRNA or protein; analysis performed by pooling all BC—overall). Genes enriched in low-SETD7 group have negative log2 fold change (blue) and the ones enriched in the high-SETD7 group have positive log2 fold change (red). Genes with a significant adjusted *p*-value (Bonferroni post hoc, <0.05) have a star. Genes that were not present for a particular condition are represented as not available (NA, white boxes). Some genes were not detected in any dataset and were excluded from the figure: *ATOH1*, *ESR2* (ERβ), *GATA1*, *NANOG*, *NR1H4* (FXR), and *PDX1*.

In summary, our analysis showed that *SETD7* differential expression is correlated with the expression of different genes depending on the subtype, which may correspond to completely different biological processes (like cell adhesion for luminal A and lysosome organization and early endosome to late endosome transport for Her2-enriched subtype) or shared processes (like immune-related pathways). While no analysis per subtype showed significant results using CPTAC proteome data, it is to be noted that this is a relatively small cohort (total 122 samples), which does not reach a high power when dividing the samples by subtype. Thus, expanding this cohort would be beneficial for further studies.

3.4. Association between SETD7 Expression and Its Target Proteins

SETD7 is a methyltransferase with multiple known target proteins. Thus, the protein levels, phosphorylation, and acetylation patterns of SETD7 targets were investigated in *SETD7*-high and -low groups, respectively. The proteins enriched in high- or low-SETD7 groups (all BC subtypes pooled, mRNA data from TCGA PanCancer Atlas and protein data from CPTAC) were extracted and compared with a list of 42 known SETD7 targets (Supplementary File S5 and Figure S10A). Nineteen targets were not found or were not significantly associated with *SETD7* expression in any dataset (light grey shade in Supplementary Table S3). For low-SETD7 tumours, PARP-1 was present in all datasets from CPTAC; Cullin 1 in the total proteome; centromere protein C, HIV Tat (*HTATSF1*), RIO1, DNMT1, and TTK in total and phosphoproteome; Msx2-interacting protein (*SPEN*), catenin beta-1 (*CTNNB1*), TAF7, PPP1R12A, and SUV39H1 in phosphoproteome; MED1 and YY1 in phosphoproteome and acetylproteome; and Sam68 (*KHDRBS1*) and STAT3 in acetylproteome. For high-SETD7 tumours, PPP1R12A, GLI3, YAP1, and AR were found in total and phosphoproteome from CPTAC; and pRb (*RB1*), RELA, ERα, MECP2, and SPEN in phosphoproteome. AR and ERα were also found in the TCGA PanCancer Atlas data.

When analysing the samples per subtype, only the total proteome showed significant correlations with *SETD7* mRNA or protein levels, mainly in the luminal A subtype (Supplementary Figure S10B), where ERα was associated with high *SETD7* mRNA expression (Supplementary Table S3). No correlations between *SETD7* differential protein levels and phosphoproteome or acetylproteome were observed by subtype.

3.5. Association of SETD7 Expression Levels with Breast Cancer Survival Outcomes

The prognostic value of SETD7 in pooled samples from all BC subtypes was explored using the KMplotter online tool, HPA, and the datasets containing survival data available from cBioPortal. The association of high- or low-SETD7 groups with RFS, DMFS, and OS was variable, varied between datasets, and did not show a clear association with either good or bad prognosis (Supplementary Table S4). This is in line with our recent findings reported in a systematic review [4]. Notably, a cohort analysing only ER (*ESR1*)-negative tumours showed that high-SETD7 was significantly correlated with a poor prognosis. This led us to analyse the influence of clinical factors, including the molecular subtype, on the outcome of patients divided according to high or low *SETD7* expression.

3.5.1. Influence of Histological and Molecular Subtype on Outcomes Associated with SETD7 Expression

Survival outcomes were available in METABRIC and TCGA PanCancer Atlas datasets available at cBioPortal. Luminal A patients from the TCGA PanCancer Atlas cohort (244/499 total samples; RNA-seq data) exhibited a correlation between high *SETD7* mRNA and worse OS (p = 0.044) and PFS (p = 0.032) (Supplementary Table S5). However, when all microarray studies were combined (gene-chip data in KM plotter) high-SETD7 correlated with good DMFS. In the luminal B subtype, high-SETD7 correlated with bad DMFS only in one independent study (Supplementary Table S5). In the basal-like subtype, significant associations between high *SETD7* expression and worse RFS (gene-chip data; all the studies pooled, Figure 6A, left panel; Supplementary Table S5), DMFS and OS (one individual study). Analysis based on high SETD7 protein data [50] in KM plotter also showed that expression was associated with worse OS for ER-negative samples (33/65 total samples, *p* = 0.008; Figure 6A, right panel).

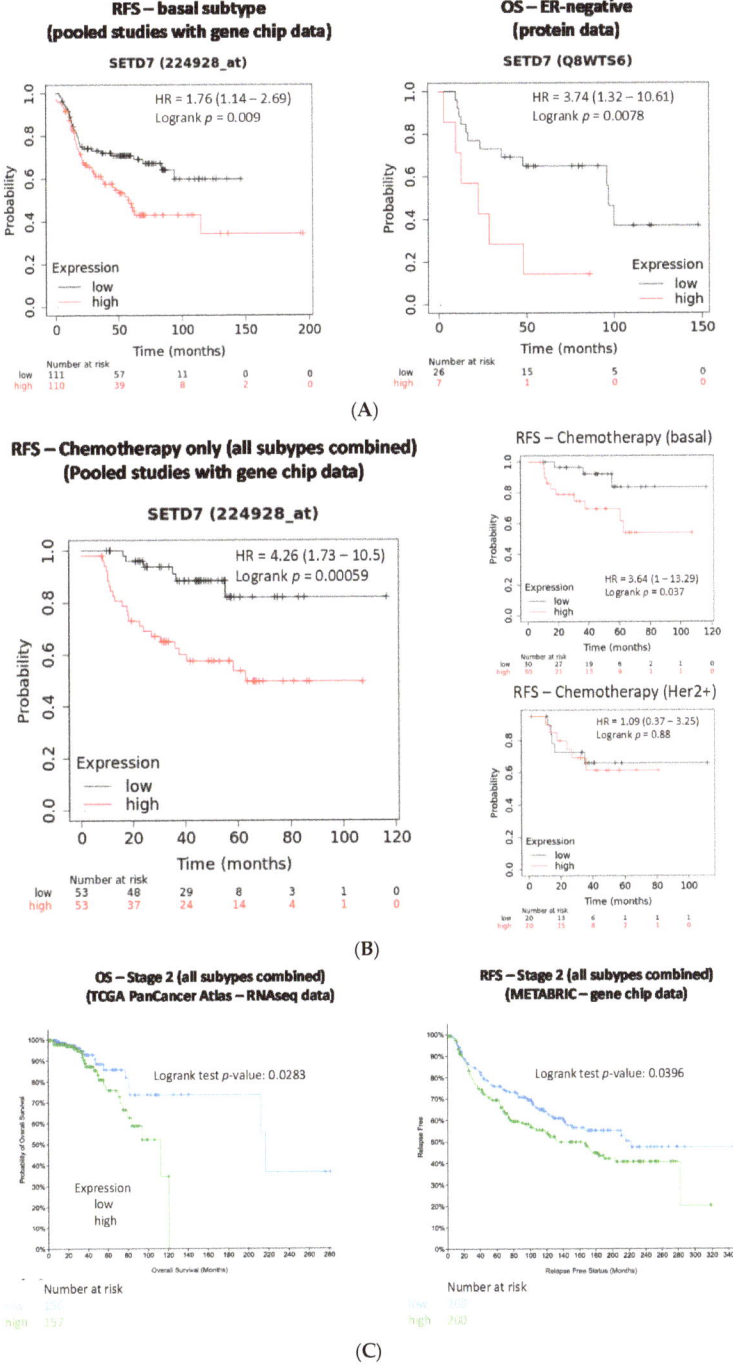

Figure 6. Analysis of the effect of differential SETD7 expression on survival outcomes of BC patients. (**A**) Influence of SETD7 mRNA or protein expression levels on survival outcomes for patients with

the basal-like molecular subtype (left panel) or the ER-negative histological subtype (right panel), respectively; (**B**) Influence of *SETD7* expression levels (mRNA) for RFS outcomes following chemotherapy, combining all subtypes (left panel) or by subtype (right panel); (**C**) Influence of *SETD7* expression levels (mRNA) on survival outcomes for stage 2 tumours, using TCGA PanCancer Atlas (RNA-seq, left panel) or METABRIC cohort (gene chip, right panel). OS—overall survival; RFS—relapse/recurrence-free survival.

In conclusion, strong evidence suggests that expression of *SETD7* is predictive of a poor outcome for patients carrying basal-like tumours, even though this subtype has lower *SETD7* expression in comparison to the luminal A or Her2-enriched subtypes (Figure 1B,C). For all other subtypes, an association between SETD7 expression and survival outcomes remains inconclusive.

3.5.2. Influence of SETD7 Expression on Therapy Outcomes

Pooled gene-chip studies with information about therapy in KM plotter showed that for patients that only received chemotherapy, high *SETD7* mRNA was significantly correlated with bad RFS (106/211 total samples; $p = 0.0006$; Figure 6B, left panel) and DMFS (84/168 total samples; $p = 0.0012$). The same was observed when analysing two of the studies independently (Supplementary Table S6). Most of the patients who received chemotherapy only had basal-like (~60%) or Her2+ (~40%) tumours and, interestingly, high *SETD7* was correlated with worse RFS (Figure 6B, right panels) or DMFS (not shown) only for patients with the basal-like subtype. In patients receiving solely endocrine therapy, high *SETD7* was correlated with worse RFS but in only one study (METABRIC: 495/1025 total samples, $p = 0.0325$; Supplementary Table S6). For patients that had not received any therapy or that had received both endocrine and chemotherapy, the results were inconclusive (Supplementary Table S6). Thus, SETD7 could be a marker of chemoresistance for patients with basal-like tumours.

3.5.3. Influence of Tumour Stage on Outcomes Associated with SETD7 Expression

TCGA data analysed through the HPA showed that high *SETD7* expression (mean expression) was correlated with low survival for stage II patients (609 samples; $p = 0.0003$). The same was observed using cBioPortal, where higher *SETD7* expression was correlated with lower OS (313/628 total samples; $p = 0.0283$; Figure 6C, left panel) and DFS (312/628 total samples; $p = 0.0569$; Supplementary Table S7) for stage 2 in TCGA PanCancer Atlas (confirming the results obtained in the same dataset using HPA; Supplementary Table S7) and lower RFS (400/979 total samples; $p = 0.0396$) for stage 2 in METABRIC (Figure 6C, right panel). High SETD7 protein expression [50] in KM plotter was also correlated with low OS ($p = 0.036$) for stage 2 patients (46/65 total samples; Supplementary Table S7). It is important to note that stage 2 represents ~60% of all BC samples analysed, followed by stage 1 (~30%) and 3 (~10%). Stages 0 and 4 comprise the lowest percentages of tumours in the cohorts studied and analyses on these were limited. Also, most of the stage 2 tumours in these studies were of the luminal subtype (~60%). Even though one might assume these results suggest that SETD7 could serve as a prognostic marker for luminal tumours in stage 2, this was not confirmed when we pooled stage 2 samples of luminal subtypes from TCGA PanCancer or METABRIC cohorts (not shown).

3.5.4. Influence of Tumour Grade, Lymph Node Status, and Metastasis on Survival Outcomes Associated with SETD7 Expression

The influence of BC grade or lymph node status on the correlation of *SETD7* expression with survival outcomes was not clear, since few independent studies allowed this analysis, and the results did not agree (Supplementary Tables S8 and S9). No association between *SETD7* expression (lower vs. upper quartile) and metastasizing tumours was observed using MBC project in cBioPortal (not shown).

3.5.5. Predictive Power of SETD7

Using ROC plotter, no strong association between *SETD7* differential expression and hormone or chemotherapies was observed. However, patients that did not respond to anti-Her2 therapy expressed higher levels of *SETD7* (Figure 7). This may correlate with the higher *ERBB2* mutation rate in patients of the high-SETD7 group.

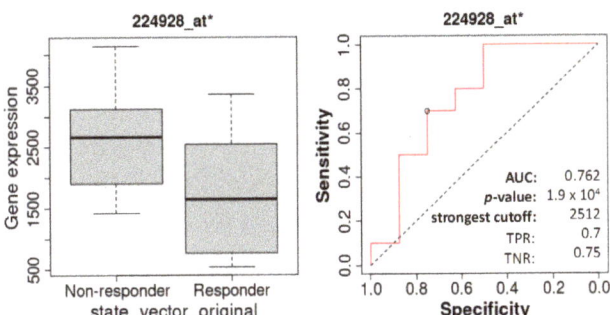

Figure 7. ROCplotter analysis to study the correlation between *SETD7* mRNA expression (microarray data) and 5-year RFS for patients receiving any anti-Her2 therapy (29 responders and 21 non-responders). AUC—area under the curve; TNR—true-negative rate; TPR—true-positive rate.

4. Discussion

Current knowledge on SETD7's impact on BC biology and its prognostic and predictive potential is scarce, with numerous contradictory findings [4,51]. In this work, we systematically analysed public datasets of BC samples to establish if *SETD7* expression is correlated with, or indicative of, diverse clinical conditions. The relevant biological processes associated with expression of *SETD7*, the genes involved, and their clinical significance were also evaluated. Stratification by molecular subtype, which has not previously been performed, showed that *SETD7* expression was dependent on subtype and that distinct processes were related to *SETD7* expression and could be clinically relevant.

Previous studies comparing *SETD7* expression between normal breast tissue and BC have not reported consistent results. We found that *SETD7* is significantly lower in BC than in adjacent normal tissue (TNMplot). This agrees with previous studies analysing mRNA [5,6] but not with studies analysing the protein level [7,8]. We observed a divergent relationship between mRNA and protein levels specifically for the luminal B subtype. This suggests that SETD7 may be regulated post-transcriptionally, possibly by miR-372/373 [52], or post-translationally, possibly through TRIM21 [8]. For the remaining subtypes, *SETD7* mRNA and protein followed the same pattern. We observed a significantly higher expression in the Her2-enriched and luminal A compared with the basal-like subtype, which may be clinically relevant. This differential *SETD7* expression may be related to the higher frequency of *SETD7* gene loss that we noted for the basal-like subtype and, to some extent, the low-level gain of *SETD7* that we observed among the Her2-enriched subtype tumours.

A relationship between SETD7 expression and prognosis was consistent only for patients with basal-like tumours, where high-SETD7 was significantly associated with worse RFS, DMFS, and OS. This aligned with worse OS for ER-negative patients expressing high SETD7 protein and with worse OS and DMFS in basal-like patients treated with chemotherapy. Higher *SETD7* mRNA and protein in Her2-enriched tumours was correlated with increased *ERBB2* amplification and corresponding *ERBB2* mRNA upregulation. This was associated with a significantly lower response to anti-Her-2 therapy in this subgroup. Still, no significant association with disease prognosis was found, but a trend of poorer OS and RFS could be observed in TCGA Pan Cancer Atlas dataset. Regarding luminal tumours, high SETD7 was also correlated with worse RFS, but only in patients receiving endocrine therapy and this association was not sufficiently strong, as the ROC plot did not support a prognostic value.

As the differential expression of *SETD7* between molecular subtypes may be clinically meaningful, we compared the transcriptomes between high- and low-SETD7 groups. This showed how SETD7 differential expression could impact the biology of the different molecular subtypes and reinforced the experimental data showing that SETD7 function is context-dependent [4]. Thus, the hypothesis raised by this study should be validated in clinical specimens and stratified by molecular subtype. Although many genes associated with SETD7 expression were different depending on subtype, in some cases, the same biological processes were overrepresented. This includes many immune-related processes. While immunotherapy has been increasingly used to treat cancer patients, this line of treatment has not been effective in BC, although some success has been noted for the triple-negative breast cancer subtype (mostly comprising the basal-like subtype) [53,54]. Herein, we show that the immune infiltration and response were highly correlated with *SETD7* expression, especially in luminal A and basal-like subtypes. The corresponding genes were primarily upregulated in low-SETD7 luminal A tumours and also correlated with higher xCell Immune score (represented by signatures of B and T cells). Additionally, the upregulation of genes with a functional role in immune evasion (*PD1*, *FOXP3*, *CTLA4*, *IL17B* and the *IL17* receptors *IL17RE* and *IL17RC*) in the low-*SETD7* group of luminal A subtype supports the knowledge that lymphocyte infiltration is associated with worse prognosis in luminal subtypes [55,56]. Immunotherapy is not currently viewed as relevant in luminal A tumours; however, stratification by SETD7 might improve the response rate of immune checkpoint inhibitors. On the contrary, in the basal-like subtype, immune-related genes were upregulated in the high-SETD7 group, and this was correlated with higher T cell infiltration, including of CD8+, as inferred from their gene expression signatures. This usually corresponds to a better prognosis in the basal-like subtype [55,56], and thus suggests that the tumours expressing high SETD7 might benefit from immunotherapy. However, future studies are needed to verify if stratification by SETD7 alone or together with additional markers can improve selection of patients for immunotherapy in subgroups of luminal A and basal-like tumours.

In luminal subtypes, the two gold-standard biomarkers *ESR1* (ERα) and *PGR* (PR) were associated with high SETD7. ERα is the target of endocrine treatments and a primary treatment-predictive marker in breast cancer [57]. However, many ERα-positive tumours develop endocrine resistance, where ERα is active in the absence of ligand. ERα is a known target of SETD7 [2], which stabilizes ERα through methylation in lysine 302. It is not known if this stabilization contributes to endocrine resistance. However, the lower survival of luminal A high-SETD7 patients from the TCGA dataset, along with the upregulation of *RUNX2* and *GPER1* (in luminal B, with reported roles in breast carcinogenesis [58] and endocrine resistance [59]), suggest a role for SETD7 in endocrine resistance. The idea of targeting SETD7 to overcome endocrine resistance thus deserves further testing. This may be specifically relevant for the luminal B subtype, where the most significant biological processes overrepresented in the high-SETD7 (mRNA) group were the ubiquitin-dependent ERAD pathway and the positive regulation of autophagy, which is also linked to the ubiquitin–proteosome system (UPS, also overrepresented). The association with high SETD7 was not strong, but given that these two pathways underly endocrine resistance [60,61], the additive contribution of all these genes to these processes should not be discarded. Autophagy is associated with the suppression of tumour initiation [62] and the survival of dormant BC stem cells and metastatic tumour recurrence [62,63]. Many preclinical studies have shown that autophagy inhibition improves endocrine therapy response [64]. Although the ROC plotter did not find a correlation between high *SETD7* mRNA stratification and 5-year RFS (suggestive of resistance to endocrine therapy), we need to consider that we could not show a correlation between *SETD7* mRNA and protein levels in this subtype. Further, these results deserve further validation, as the majority of patients were treated with tamoxifen.

In the Her2-enriched subtype, lysosome organization and early endosome to late endosome transport were overrepresented in the high-*SETD7* group. Activation of these two biological processes has been linked to anti-Her2 therapy resistance [65,66]. Remarkably, *EGFR* and *ERBB3* were strongly associated with high SETD7 and also connected to anti-Her2 therapy resistance [66]. These results together with the correlation of high SETD7 with higher amplification of *ERBB2* corroborates the ROC plotter results, where high SETD7 was correlated with patients that did not respond well (shorter 5-year RFS) to anti-Her2 therapy. A recent study suggests SORL1 to be a candidate therapeutic target to complement and potentiate anti-Her2 therapy [67]. Indeed, *SORL1* expression was significantly associated with high SETD7 expression, pointing to a potential benefit of targeting SETD7 alone or together with SORL1 in patients with high SETD7 in order to overcome resistance.

A limitation of our study is that multivariable adjustment was unavailable in the tools used to analyse the survival and prognosis value of SETD7. Moreover, information to correct for confounding effects was lacking, which restricts the conclusions that can be drawn about *SETD7* expression as an independent factor of diagnosis or resistance to therapies. Further studies will be needed to validate the clinical impacts.

In previous preclinical studies, SETD7 function has consistently been associated with altered cellular response to DNA damage stimulus, including hypoxia and oxidative stress and independently of *TP53* status [4]. Genes related to the cellular response to DNA damage stimulus and DNA repair were common to all subtypes (Supplementary Files S3 and S4). Two of the major players in the DNA damage response pathway, *ATR* and *ATM* were highly expressed in the high-SETD7 group in all subtypes. This indicates that chemotherapy might be less efficient in tumours expressing high SETD7. This was also supported by the poor prognosis associated with SETD7 expression when analysing all BC subtypes from TCGA. When analysis was carried out by BC subtype, the basal-like subtype also showed unique genes associated with *SETD7* expression and strongly overrepresented in cellular response to DNA damage and DNA repair-related pathways were. This was in line with poor outcome after chemotherapy for patients with basal-like tumours expressing high SETD7. In the future and based on previous findings showing that inhibition of SETD7 in other types of cancer improves response to chemotherapy [10,68–72], it would be interesting to explore if this subgroup of patients could benefit from targeting SETD7 with inhibitors to improve chemotherapy response.

5. Conclusions

SETD7 expression appears strongly associated with tumour stromal and immune signatures and related to therapy resistance. In the basal-like BC subtype, high *SETD7* expression was consistently predictive of bad prognosis, and this group was enriched in immune signatures. The unique genes associated with *SETD7* expression were strongly overrepresented in cellular response to DNA damage and DNA repair-related pathways, and this was aligned with poor outcome after chemotherapy. Future studies should focus on the identification of the differentially expressed genes that could constitute markers to aid decisions on prescribing immune therapy and test if inhibiting SETD7 improves basal-like response to chemotherapy. In the Her2-enriched subtype, high SETD7 may also have a predictive value, since SETD7 expression was associated with *ERBB2* copy number amplification and worse response to anti-Her2 therapy, as well as upregulation of EGFR, HER-3, and overrepresentation of such biological processes as lysosome organization and early endosome to late endosome transport known to be underlying mechanisms of anti-Her-2 therapy resistance. In the luminal subtype, high SETD7 expression was associated with higher *ESR1* (ERα), *PGR* (PR), *RUNX2* and *GPER1*, which together with previous findings on the role of SETD7 maintaining ERα protein stability and activity, highlight the need for further studies on the role of SETD7 in endocrine resistance. Still, no consistent relationship with prognosis was found, except for worse OS in tumours with high SETD7 and treated with endocrine therapy.

In summary, this study emphasizes that there is clinical potential in the study of SETD7, which must be evaluated in the context of the BC molecular subtype.

Supplementary Materials: The following supporting information can be downloaded at https://www.mdpi.com/article/10.3390/cancers14246029/s1. Figure S1: *SETD7* genomic alterations in breast cancer using cBioPortal; Figure S2: *SETD7* mRNA expression in breast cancer PAM50 subtypes using cBioPortal datasets; Figure S3: Mean differences of each comparison done in Figure 1B and the confidence intervals associated with it; Figure S4: Predicted infiltration of cancer-associated fibroblasts (CAFs), endothelial cells and cytotoxicity score in samples with differential SETD7 mRNA expression (high vs. low) from different breast cancer PAM50 subtypes; Figure S5: Predicted infiltration of immune cells in samples with differential *SETD7* mRNA expression (high vs. low) from different breast cancer PAM50 subtypes; Figure S6: Genomic alterations associated with *SETD7* mRNA differential expression from TCGA PanCancer atlas in cBioPortal; Figure S7: TCGA-BRCA data processing; Figure S8: Analysis of genes associated with *SETD7* mRNA differential expression per subtype from TCGA-BRCA; Figure S9: Top 10 biological processes overrepresented by the genes associated with *SETD7* differential expression (high and low distinctly) and unique for each subtype; Figure S10: Analysis of proteins associated with SETD7 protein differential expression using CPTAC; Table S1: Breast cancer datasets with *SETD7* expression (mRNA or protein), mutation or copy number information.; Table S2: Association of *SETD7* expression with therapy, grade and stage using datasets in cBioPortal; Table S3: Association of *SETD7* differential expression and known SETD7 targets and their methylation sites and other sites known to compete with SETD7 methylation; Table S4: *SETD7* association with survival outcomes; Table S5: Prognosis associated with high SETD7 in BC subtypes; Table S6: Prognosis associated with high *SETD7* in BC considering therapy; Table S7: Prognosis associated with high SETD7 in BC considering stage; Table S8: Prognosis associated with high *SETD7* in BC considering grade; Table S9: Prognosis associated with high SETD7 in BC considering lymph node status; Supplementary File S1: Mutations in SETD7 gene; Supplementary File S2: Genomic alterations correlating with *SETD7* differential expression; Supplementary File S3: List of significant genes per subtype and common to all subtypes; Supplementary File S4: Biological processes list; Supplementary File S5: Proteome enriched in high or low SETD7 protein from CPTAC [2,68,73–110].

Author Contributions: Conceptualization, L.A.H., C.W. and F.L.M.; methodology, F.L.M. and L.S.; formal analysis, F.L.M.; investigation, F.L.M.; data curation, F.L.M.; writing—original draft preparation, F.L.M.; writing—review and editing, F.L.M., L.A.H., C.W. and L.S.; supervision, L.A.H. and C.W. All authors have read and agreed to the published version of the manuscript.

Funding: This research was funded by iBiMED research unit UIDB/04501/2020 and UIDP/04501/2020, MEDISIS (CENTRO-01-0246-FEDER-000018) supported by Comissão de Coordenação e Desenvolvimento Regional do Centro. FLM thanks the Portuguese Science and Technology Foundation—FCT for her PhD scholarship SFRH/BD/117818/2016; C.W acknowledges the Swedish Cancer Society (21 1632 Pj), Karolinska Institute PhD for support for L.S. (KID 2021-00501) and Region Stockholm (HMT RS2021-0316).

Institutional Review Board Statement: Not applicable.

Informed Consent Statement: Not applicable.

Data Availability Statement: Not applicable.

Acknowledgments: The results shown here are in part based upon data generated by the TCGA Research Network: https://www.cancer.gov/tcga, accessed on 5 August 2022. We would like to thank Madeleine Birgersson for the helpful discussions that contributed to the development of this project.

Conflicts of Interest: The authors declare no conflict of interest.

References

1. Batista, I.D.A.A.; Helguero, L.A. Biological Processes and Signal Transduction Pathways Regulated by the Protein Methyltransferase SETD7 and Their Significance in Cancer. *Signal Transduct. Target. Ther.* **2018**, *3*, 19. [CrossRef] [PubMed]
2. Subramanian, K.; Jia, D.; Kapoor-Vazirani, P.; Powell, D.R.; Collins, R.E.; Sharma, D.; Peng, J.; Cheng, X.; Vertino, P.M. Regulation of Estrogen Receptor Alpha by the SET7 Lysine Methyltransferase. *Mol. Cell* **2008**, *30*, 336–347. [CrossRef] [PubMed]

3. Huang, R.; Li, X.; Yu, Y.; Ma, L.; Liu, S.; Zong, X.; Zheng, Q. SETD7 Is a Prognosis Predicting Factor of Breast Cancer and Regulates Redox Homeostasis. *Oncotarget* **2017**, *8*, 94080–94090. [CrossRef]
4. Monteiro, F.L.; Williams, C.; Helguero, L.A. A Systematic Review to Define the Multi-Faceted Role of Lysine Methyltransferase SETD7 in Cancer. *Cancers* **2022**, *14*, 1414. [CrossRef] [PubMed]
5. Gu, Y.; Wang, X.; Liu, H.; Li, Q.; Yu, W.; Ma, Q. SET7/9 Promotes Hepatocellular Carcinoma Progression through Regulation of E2F1. *Oncol. Rep.* **2018**, *40*, 1863–1874. [CrossRef] [PubMed]
6. Song, Y.; Zhang, J.; Tian, T.; Fu, X.; Wang, W.; Li, S.; Shi, T.; Suo, A.; Ruan, Z.; Guo, H.; et al. SET7/9 Inhibits Oncogenic Activities through Regulation of Gli-1 Expression in Breast Cancer. *Tumor Biol.* **2016**, *37*, 9311–9322. [CrossRef]
7. Zhang, Y.; Liu, J.; Lin, J.; Zhou, L.; Song, Y.; Wei, B.; Luo, X.; Chen, Z.; Chen, Y.; Xiong, J.; et al. The Transcription Factor GATA1 and the Histone Methyltransferase SET7 Interact to Promote VEGF-Mediated Angiogenesis and Tumor Growth and Predict Clinical Outcome of Breast Cancer. *Oncotarget* **2016**, *7*, 9859–9875. [CrossRef] [PubMed]
8. Si, W.; Zhou, J.; Zhao, Y.; Zheng, J.; Cui, L. SET7/9 Promotes Multiple Malignant Processes in Breast Cancer Development via RUNX2 Activation and Is Negatively Regulated by TRIM21. *Cell Death Dis.* **2020**, *11*, 151. [CrossRef]
9. Duan, B.; Bai, J.; Qiu, J.; Wang, J.; Tong, C.; Wang, X.; Miao, J.; Li, Z.; Li, W.; Yang, J.; et al. Histone-Lysine N-Methyltransferase SETD7 Is a Potential Serum Biomarker for Colorectal Cancer Patients. *EBioMedicine* **2018**, *37*, 134–143. [CrossRef]
10. Lezina, L.; Aksenova, V.; Fedorova, O.; Malikova, D.; Shuvalov, O.; Antonov, A.V.; Tentler, D.; Garabadgiu, A.V.; Melino, G.; Barlev, N.A. KMT Set7/9 Affects Genotoxic Stress Response via the Mdm2 Axis. *Oncotarget* **2015**, *6*, 25843–25855. [CrossRef]
11. Montenegro, M.F.; Sánchez-Del-Campo, L.; González-Guerrero, R.; Martínez-Barba, E.; Piñero-Madrona, A.; Cabezas-Herrera, J.; Rodríguez-López, J.N. Tumor Suppressor SET9 Guides the Epigenetic Plasticity of Breast Cancer Cells and Serves as an Early-Stage Biomarker for Predicting Metastasis. *Oncogene* **2016**, *35*, 6143–6152. [CrossRef] [PubMed]
12. Gao, J.; Aksoy, B.A.; Dogrusoz, U.; Dresdner, G.; Gross, B.; Sumer, S.O.; Sun, Y.; Jacobsen, A.; Sinha, R.; Larsson, E.; et al. Integrative Analysis of Complex Cancer Genomics and Clinical Profiles Using the CBioPortal. *Sci. Signal.* **2013**, *6*, pl1. [CrossRef] [PubMed]
13. Cerami, E.; Gao, J.; Dogrusoz, U.; Gross, B.E.; Sumer, S.O.; Aksoy, B.A.; Jacobsen, A.; Byrne, C.J.; Heuer, M.L.; Larsson, E.; et al. The CBio Cancer Genomics Portal: An Open Platform for Exploring Multidimensional Cancer Genomics Data. *Cancer Discov.* **2012**, *2*, 401–404. [CrossRef] [PubMed]
14. Krug, K.; Jaehnig, E.J.; Satpathy, S.; Blumenberg, L.; Karpova, A.; Anurag, M.; Miles, G.; Mertins, P.; Geffen, Y.; Tang, L.C.; et al. Proteogenomic Landscape of Breast Cancer Tumorigenesis and Targeted Therapy. *Cell* **2020**, *183*, 1436–1456.e31. [CrossRef] [PubMed]
15. Curtis, C.; Shah, S.P.; Chin, S.F.; Turashvili, G.; Rueda, O.M.; Dunning, M.J.; Speed, D.; Lynch, A.G.; Samarajiwa, S.; Yuan, Y.; et al. The Genomic and Transcriptomic Architecture of 2,000 Breast Tumours Reveals Novel Subgroups. *Nature* **2012**, *486*, 346–352. [CrossRef] [PubMed]
16. Liu, J.; Lichtenberg, T.; Hoadley, K.A.; Poisson, L.M.; Lazar, A.J.; Cherniack, A.D.; Kovatich, A.J.; Benz, C.C.; Levine, D.A.; Lee, A.V.; et al. An Integrated TCGA Pan-Cancer Clinical Data Resource to Drive High-Quality Survival Outcome Analytics. *Cell* **2018**, *173*, 400–416.e11. [CrossRef]
17. Lefebvre, C.; Bachelot, T.; Filleron, T.; Pedrero, M.; Campone, M.; Soria, J.C.; Massard, C.; Lévy, C.; Arnedos, M.; Lacroix-Triki, M.; et al. Mutational Profile of Metastatic Breast Cancers: A Retrospective Analysis. *PLoS Med.* **2016**, *13*, e1002201. [CrossRef]
18. Razavi, P.; Chang, M.T.; Xu, G.; Bandlamudi, C.; Ross, D.S.; Vasan, N.; Cai, Y.; Bielski, C.M.; Donoghue, M.T.A.; Jonsson, P.; et al. The Genomic Landscape of Endocrine-Resistant Advanced Breast Cancers. *Cancer Cell* **2018**, *34*, 427–438.e6. [CrossRef]
19. Razavi, P.; Dickler, M.N.; Shah, P.D.; Toy, W.; Brown, D.N.; Won, H.H.; Li, B.T.; Shen, R.; Vasan, N.; Modi, S.; et al. Alterations in PTEN and ESR1 Promote Clinical Resistance to Alpelisib plus Aromatase Inhibitors. *Nat. Cancer* **2020**, *1*, 382. [CrossRef]
20. Nixon, M.J.; Formisano, L.; Mayer, I.A.; Estrada, M.V.; González-Ericsson, P.I.; Isakoff, S.J.; Forero-Torres, A.; Won, H.; Sanders, M.E.; Solit, D.B.; et al. PIK3CA and MAP3K1 Alterations Imply Luminal A Status and Are Associated with Clinical Benefit from Pan-PI3K Inhibitor Buparlisib and Letrozole in ER+ Metastatic Breast Cancer. *NPJ Breast Cancer* **2019**, *5*, 31. [CrossRef]
21. Pareja, F.; Brown, D.N.; Lee, J.Y.; Paula, A.D.C.; Selenica, P.; Bi, R.; Geyer, F.C.; Gazzo, A.; da Silva, E.M.; Vahdatinia, M.; et al. Whole-Exome Sequencing Analysis of the Progression from Non–Low-Grade Ductal Carcinoma in Situ to Invasive Ductal Carcinoma. *Clin. Cancer Res.* **2020**, *26*, 3682–3693. [CrossRef] [PubMed]
22. Kan, Z.; Ding, Y.; Kim, J.; Jung, H.H.; Chung, W.; Lal, S.; Cho, S.; Fernandez-Banet, J.; Lee, S.K.; Kim, S.W.; et al. Multi-Omics Profiling of Younger Asian Breast Cancers Reveals Distinctive Molecular Signatures. *Nat. Commun.* **2018**, *9*, 1725. [CrossRef]
23. Shah, S.P.; Roth, A.; Goya, R.; Oloumi, A.; Ha, G.; Zhao, Y.; Turashvili, G.; Ding, J.; Tse, K.; Haffari, G.; et al. The Clonal and Mutational Evolution Spectrum of Primary Triple Negative Breast Cancers. *Nature* **2012**, *486*, 395–399. [CrossRef] [PubMed]
24. Banerji, S.; Cibulskis, K.; Rangel-Escareno, C.; Brown, K.K.; Carter, S.L.; Frederick, A.M.; Lawrence, M.S.; Sivachenko, A.Y.; Sougnez, C.; Zou, L.; et al. Sequence Analysis of Mutations and Translocations across Breast Cancer Subtypes. *Nature* **2012**, *486*, 405–409. [CrossRef] [PubMed]
25. Stephens, P.J.; Tarpey, P.S.; Davies, H.; Van Loo, P.; Greenman, C.; Wedge, D.C.; Nik-Zainal, S.; Martin, S.; Varela, I.; Bignell, G.R.; et al. The Landscape of Cancer Genes and Mutational Processes in Breast Cancer. *Nature* **2012**, *486*, 400. [CrossRef] [PubMed]
26. Li, Q.; Jiang, B.; Guo, J.; Shao, H.; Del Priore, I.S.; Chang, Q.; Kudo, R.; Li, Z.; Razavi, P.; Liu, B.; et al. INK4 Tumor Suppressor Proteins Mediate Resistance to CDK4/6 Kinase Inhibitors. *Cancer Discov.* **2022**, *12*, 356–371. [CrossRef]

27. Bartha, Á.; Győrffy, B. TNMplot.Com: A Web Tool for the Comparison of Gene Expression in Normal, Tumor and Metastatic Tissues. *Int. J. Mol. Sci.* **2021**, *22*, 2622. [CrossRef]
28. Thul, P.J.; Lindskog, C. The Human Protein Atlas: A Spatial Map of the Human Proteome. *Protein Sci.* **2018**, *27*, 233–244. [CrossRef]
29. Fekete, J.T.; Győrffy, B. ROCplot.Org: Validating Predictive Biomarkers of Chemotherapy/Hormonal Therapy/Anti-HER2 Therapy Using Transcriptomic Data of 3,104 Breast Cancer Patients. *Int. J. Cancer* **2019**, *145*, 3140–3151. [CrossRef]
30. Li, Q.; Birkbak, N.J.; Gyorffy, B.; Szallasi, Z.; Eklund, A.C. Jetset: Selecting the Optimal Microarray Probe Set to Represent a Gene. *BMC Bioinform.* **2011**, *12*, 474. [CrossRef]
31. Mounir, M.; Lucchetta, M.; Silva, T.C.; Olsen, C.; Bontempi, G.; Chen, X.; Noushmehr, H.; Colaprico, A.; Papaleo, E. New Functionalities in the TCGAbiolinks Package for the Study and Integration of Cancer Data from GDC and GTEx. *PLoS Comput. Biol.* **2019**, *15*, e1006701. [CrossRef] [PubMed]
32. Colaprico, A.; Silva, T.C.; Olsen, C.; Garofano, L.; Cava, C.; Garolini, D.; Sabedot, T.S.; Malta, T.M.; Pagnotta, S.M.; Castiglioni, I.; et al. TCGAbiolinks: An R/Bioconductor Package for Integrative Analysis of TCGA Data. *Nucleic Acids Res.* **2016**, *44*, e71. [CrossRef] [PubMed]
33. Silva, T.C.; Colaprico, A.; Olsen, C.; D'Angelo, F.; Bontempi, G.; Ceccarelli, M.; Noushmehr, H. TCGA Workflow: Analyze Cancer Genomics and Epigenomics Data Using Bioconductor Packages. *F1000Research* **2016**, *5*, 1542. [CrossRef] [PubMed]
34. Robinson, M.D.; McCarthy, D.J.; Smyth, G.K. EdgeR: A Bioconductor Package for Differential Expression Analysis of Digital Gene Expression Data. *Bioinformatics* **2010**, *26*, 139–140. [CrossRef] [PubMed]
35. McCarthy, D.J.; Chen, Y.; Smyth, G.K. Differential Expression Analysis of Multifactor RNA-Seq Experiments with Respect to Biological Variation. *Nucleic Acids Res.* **2012**, *40*, 4288–4297. [CrossRef]
36. Chen, Y.; Lun, A.T.L.; Smyth, G.K.; Burden, C.J.; Ryan, D.P.; Khang, T.F.; Lianoglou, S. From Reads to Genes to Pathways: Differential Expression Analysis of RNA-Seq Experiments Using Rsubread and the EdgeR Quasi-Likelihood Pipeline. *F1000Research* **2016**, *5*, 1438.
37. Love, M.I.; Huber, W.; Anders, S. Moderated Estimation of Fold Change and Dispersion for RNA-Seq Data with DESeq2. *Genome Biol.* **2014**, *15*, 550. [CrossRef] [PubMed]
38. Sturm, G.; Finotello, F.; Petitprez, F.; Zhang, J.D.; Baumbach, J.; Fridman, W.H.; List, M.; Aneichyk, T. Comprehensive Evaluation of Transcriptome-Based Cell-Type Quantification Methods for Immuno-Oncology. *Bioinformatics* **2019**, *35*, i436–i445. [CrossRef]
39. Oliveros, J.C. VENNY. An Interactive Tool for Comparing Lists with Venn's Diagrams. Available online: https://bioinfogp.cnb.csic.es/tools/venny/ (accessed on 24 March 2022).
40. Huang, D.W.; Sherman, B.T.; Lempicki, R.A. Systematic and Integrative Analysis of Large Gene Lists Using DAVID Bioinformatics Resources. *Nat. Protoc.* **2008**, *4*, 44–57. [CrossRef]
41. Huang, D.W.; Sherman, B.T.; Lempicki, R.A. Bioinformatics Enrichment Tools: Paths toward the Comprehensive Functional Analysis of Large Gene Lists. *Nucleic Acids Res.* **2009**, *37*, 1–13. [CrossRef]
42. Wickham, H. *Ggplot2: Elegant Graphics for Data Analysis*; Springer: New York, NY, USA, 2016.
43. Walter, W.; Sánchez-Cabo, F.; Ricote, M. GOplot: An R Package for Visually Combining Expression Data with Functional Analysis. *Bioinformatics* **2015**, *31*, 2912–2914. [CrossRef]
44. Winter, S.C.; Buffa, F.M.; Silva, P.; Miller, C.; Valentine, H.R.; Turley, H.; Shah, K.A.; Cox, G.J.; Corbridge, R.J.; Homer, J.J.; et al. Relation of a Hypoxia Metagene Derived from Head and Neck Cancer to Prognosis of Multiple Cancers. *Cancer Res.* **2007**, *67*, 3441–3449. [CrossRef]
45. Buffa, F.M.; Harris, A.L.; West, C.M.; Miller, C.J. Large Meta-Analysis of Multiple Cancers Reveals a Common, Compact and Highly Prognostic Hypoxia Metagene. *Br. J. Cancer* **2010**, *102*, 428. [CrossRef]
46. Yoshihara, K.; Shahmoradgoli, M.; Martínez, E.; Vegesna, R.; Kim, H.; Torres-Garcia, W.; Treviño, V.; Shen, H.; Laird, P.W.; Levine, D.A.; et al. Inferring Tumour Purity and Stromal and Immune Cell Admixture from Expression Data. *Nat. Commun.* **2013**, *4*, 2612. [CrossRef] [PubMed]
47. Aran, D.; Hu, Z.; Butte, A.J. XCell: Digitally Portraying the Tissue Cellular Heterogeneity Landscape. *Genome Biol.* **2017**, *18*, 220. [CrossRef] [PubMed]
48. Becht, E.; Giraldo, N.A.; Lacroix, L.; Buttard, B.; Elarouci, N.; Petitprez, F.; Selves, J.; Laurent-Puig, P.; Sautès-Fridman, C.; Fridman, W.H.; et al. Estimating the Population Abundance of Tissue-Infiltrating Immune and Stromal Cell Populations Using Gene Expression. *Genome Biol.* **2016**, *17*, 218. [CrossRef]
49. Daks, A.; Vasileva, E.; Fedorova, O.; Shuvalov, O.; Barlev, N.A. The Role of Lysine Methyltransferase SET7/9 in Proliferation and Cell Stress Response. *Life* **2022**, *12*, 362. [CrossRef]
50. Tang, W.; Zhou, M.; Dorsey, T.H.; Prieto, D.A.; Wang, X.W.; Ruppin, E.; Veenstra, T.D.; Ambs, S. Integrated Proteotranscriptomics of Breast Cancer Reveals Globally Increased Protein-MRNA Concordance Associated with Subtypes and Survival. *Genome Med.* **2018**, *10*, 94. [CrossRef] [PubMed]
51. Gu, Y.; Zhang, X.; Yu, W.; Dong, W. Oncogene or Tumor Suppressor: The Coordinative Role of Lysine Methyltransferase SET7/9 in Cancer Development and the Related Mechanisms. *J. Cancer* **2022**, *13*, 623–640. [CrossRef] [PubMed]
52. Wang, L.Q.; Yu, P.; Li, B.; Guo, Y.H.; Liang, Z.R.; Zheng, L.L.; Yang, J.H.; Xu, H.; Liu, S.; Zheng, L.S.; et al. MiR-372 and MiR-373 Enhance the Stemness of Colorectal Cancer Cells by Repressing Differentiation Signaling Pathways. *Mol. Oncol.* **2018**, *12*, 1949–1964. [CrossRef] [PubMed]

53. Schmid, P.; Adams, S.; Rugo, H.S.; Schneeweiss, A.; Barrios, C.H.; Iwata, H.; Diéras, V.; Hegg, R.; Im, S.-A.; Shaw Wright, G.; et al. Atezolizumab and Nab-Paclitaxel in Advanced Triple-Negative Breast Cancer. *N. Engl. J. Med.* **2018**, *379*, 2108–2121. [CrossRef] [PubMed]
54. Schmid, P.; Cortes, J.; Pusztai, L.; McArthur, H.; Kümmel, S.; Bergh, J.; Denkert, C.; Park, Y.H.; Hui, R.; Harbeck, N.; et al. Pembrolizumab for Early Triple-Negative Breast Cancer. *N. Engl. J. Med.* **2020**, *382*, 810–821. [CrossRef] [PubMed]
55. Pellegrino, B.; Hlavata, Z.; Migali, C.; De Silva, P.; Aiello, M.; Willard-Gallo, K.; Musolino, A.; Solinas, C. Luminal Breast Cancer: Risk of Recurrence and Tumor-Associated Immune Suppression. *Mol. Diagnosis Ther.* **2021**, *25*, 409–424. [CrossRef] [PubMed]
56. Goldberg, J.; Pastorello, R.G.; Vallius, T.; Davis, J.; Cui, Y.X.; Agudo, J.; Waks, A.G.; Keenan, T.; McAllister, S.S.; Tolaney, S.M.; et al. The Immunology of Hormone Receptor Positive Breast Cancer. *Front. Immunol.* **2021**, *12*, 1515. [CrossRef] [PubMed]
57. Frigo, D.E.; Bondesson, M.; Williams, C. Nuclear Receptors: From Molecular Mechanisms to Therapeutics. *Essays Biochem.* **2021**, *65*, 847. [CrossRef] [PubMed]
58. Wysokinski, D.; Blasiak, J.; Pawlowska, E. Role of RUNX2 in Breast Carcinogenesis. *Int. J. Mol. Sci.* **2015**, *16*, 20969–20993. [CrossRef] [PubMed]
59. Pepermans, R.A.; Prossnitz, E.R. ERα-Targeted Endocrine Therapy, Resistance and the Role of GPER. *Steroids* **2019**, *152*, 108493. [CrossRef]
60. Direito, I.; Fardilha, M.; Helguero, L.A. Contribution of the Unfolded Protein Response to Breast and Prostate Tissue Homeostasis and Its Significance to Cancer Endocrine Response. *Carcinogenesis* **2018**, *40*, 203–215. [CrossRef]
61. Direito, I.; Monteiro, L.; Melo, T.; Figueira, D.; Lobo, J.; Enes, V.; Moura, G.; Henrique, R.; Santos, M.A.S.; Jerónimo, C.; et al. Protein Aggregation Patterns Inform about Breast Cancer Response to Antiestrogens and Reveal the RNA Ligase RTCB as Mediator of Acquired Tamoxifen Resistance. *Cancers* **2021**, *13*, 3195. [CrossRef]
62. La Belle Flynn, A.; Schiemann, W.P. Autophagy in Breast Cancer Metastatic Dormancy: Tumor Suppressing or Tumor Promoting Functions? *J. Cancer Metastasis Treat.* **2019**, *2019*, 43. [CrossRef] [PubMed]
63. Vera-Ramirez, L.; Vodnala, S.K.; Nini, R.; Hunter, K.W.; Green, J.E. Autophagy Promotes the Survival of Dormant Breast Cancer Cells and Metastatic Tumour Recurrence. *Nat. Commun.* **2018**, *9*, 1944. [CrossRef]
64. Cook, K.L.; Shajahan, A.N.; Clarke, R. Autophagy and Endocrine Resistance in Breast Cancer. *Expert Rev. Anticancer Ther.* **2011**, *11*, 1283. [CrossRef] [PubMed]
65. Mishra, A.; Hourigan, D.; Lindsay, A.J. Inhibition of the Endosomal Recycling Pathway Downregulates HER2 Activation and Overcomes Resistance to Tyrosine Kinase Inhibitors in HER2-Positive Breast Cancer. *Cancer Lett.* **2022**, *529*, 153–167. [CrossRef]
66. Hunter, F.W.; Barker, H.R.; Lipert, B.; Rothé, F.; Gebhart, G.; Piccart-Gebhart, M.J.; Sotiriou, C.; Jamieson, S.M.F. Mechanisms of Resistance to Trastuzumab Emtansine (T-DM1) in HER2-Positive Breast Cancer. *Br. J. Cancer* **2019**, *122*, 603–612. [CrossRef]
67. Pietilä, M.; Sahgal, P.; Peuhu, E.; Jäntti, N.Z.; Paatero, I.; Närvä, E.; Al-Akhrass, H.; Lilja, J.; Georgiadou, M.; Andersen, O.M.; et al. SORLA Regulates Endosomal Trafficking and Oncogenic Fitness of HER2. *Nat. Commun.* **2019**, *10*, 2340. [CrossRef] [PubMed]
68. Kontaki, H.; Talianidis, I. Lysine Methylation Regulates E2F1-Induced Cell Death. *Mol. Cell* **2010**, *39*, 152–160. [CrossRef] [PubMed]
69. Lezina, L.; Aksenova, V.; Ivanova, T.; Purmessur, N.; Antonov, A.V.; Tentler, D.; Fedorova, O.; Garabadgiu, A.V.; Talianidis, I.; Melino, G.; et al. KMTase Set7/9 Is a Critical Regulator of E2F1 Activity upon Genotoxic Stress. *Cell Death Differ.* **2014**, *21*, 1889–1899. [CrossRef]
70. Daks, A.; Mamontova, V.; Fedorova, O.; Petukhov, A.; Shuvalov, O.; Parfenyev, S.; Netsvetay, S.; Venina, A.; Kizenko, A.; Imyanitov, E.; et al. Set7/9 Controls Proliferation and Genotoxic Drug Resistance of NSCLC Cells. *Biochem. Biophys. Res. Commun.* **2021**, *572*, 41–48. [CrossRef] [PubMed]
71. Chuikov, S.; Kurash, J.K.; Wilson, J.R.; Xiao, B.; Justin, N.; Ivanov, G.S.; McKinney, K.; Tempst, P.; Prives, C.; Gamblin, S.J.; et al. Regulation of P53 Activity through Lysine Methylation. *Nature* **2004**, *432*, 353–360. [CrossRef]
72. Wang, C.; Shu, L.; Zhang, C.; Li, W.; Wu, R.; Guo, Y.; Yang, Y.; Kong, A.N. Histone Methyltransferase Setd7 Regulates Nrf2 Signaling Pathway by Phenethyl Isothiocyanate and Ursolic Acid in Human Prostate Cancer Cells. *Mol. Nutr. Food Res.* **2018**, *62*, e1700840. [CrossRef]
73. Dhayalan, A.; Kudithipudi, S.; Rathert, P.; Jeltsch, A. Specificity Analysis-Based Identification of New Methylation Targets of the SET7/9 Protein Lysine Methyltransferase. *Chem. Biol.* **2011**, *18*, 111–120. [CrossRef]
74. Ko, S.; Ahn, J.; Song, C.S.; Kim, S.; Knapczyk-Stwora, K.; Chatterjee, B. Lysine Methylation and Functional Modulation of Androgen Receptor by Set9 Methyltransferase. *Mol. Endocrinol.* **2011**, *25*, 433–444. [CrossRef] [PubMed]
75. Gaughan, L.; Stockley, J.; Wang, N.; McCracken, S.R.; Treumann, A.; Armstrong, K.; Shaheen, F.; Watt, K.; McEwan, I.J.; Wang, C.; et al. Regulation of the androgen receptor by SET9-mediated methylation. *Nucleic Acids Res.* **2010**, *39*, 1266–1279. [CrossRef] [PubMed]
76. Shen, C.; Wang, D.; Liu, X.; Gu, B.; Du, Y.; Wei, F.; Cao, L.; Song, B.; Lu, X.; Yang, Q.; et al. SET7/9 regulates cancer cell proliferation by influencing β-catenin stability. *FASEB J.* **2015**, *29*, 4313–4323. [CrossRef] [PubMed]
77. Estève, P.-O.; Chin, H.G.; Benner, J.; Feehery, G.R.; Samaranayake, M.; Horwitz, G.A.; Jacobsen, S.E.; Pradhan, S. Regulation of DNMT1 stability through SET7-mediated lysine methylation in mammalian cells. *Proc. Natl. Acad. Sci. USA* **2009**, *106*, 5076–5081. [CrossRef] [PubMed]

78. Xie, Q.; Bai, Y.; Wu, J.; Sun, Y.; Wang, Y.; Zhang, Y.; Mei, P.; Yuan, Z. Methylation-mediated regulation of E2F1 in DNA damage-induced cell death. *J. Recept. Signal Transduct.* **2011**, *31*, 139–146. [CrossRef]
79. Calnan, D.R.; Webb, A.E.; White, J.L.; Stowe, T.R.; Goswami, T.; Shi, X.; Espejo, A.; Bedford, M.T.; Gozani, O.; Gygi, S.P.; et al. Methylation by Set9 modulates FoxO3 stability and transcriptional activity. *Aging* **2012**, *4*, 462–479. [CrossRef]
80. Xie, Q.; Hao, Y.; Tao, L.; Peng, S.; Rao, C.; Chen, H.; You, H.; Dong, M.; Yuan, Z. Lysine methylation of FOXO3 regulates oxidative stress-induced neuronal cell death. *EMBO Rep.* **2012**, *13*, 371–377. [CrossRef] [PubMed]
81. Fu, L.; Wu, H.; Cheng, S.Y.; Gao, D.; Zhang, L.; Zhao, Y. Set7 mediated Gli3 methylation plays a positive role in the activation of Sonic Hedgehog pathway in mammals. *eLife* **2016**, *5*, e15690. [CrossRef]
82. Kim, Y.; Nam, H.J.; Lee, J.; Park, D.Y.; Kim, C.; Yu, Y.S.; Kim, D.; Park, S.W.; Bhin, J.; Hwang, D.; et al. Methylation-dependent regulation of HIF-1α stability restricts retinal and tumour angiogenesis. *Nat. Commun.* **2016**, *7*, 10347. [CrossRef]
83. Pagans, S.; Kauder, S.E.; Kaehlcke, K.; Sakane, N.; Schroeder, S.; Dormeyer, W.; Trievel, R.C.; Verdin, E.; Schnolzer, M.; Ott, M. The Cellular Lysine Methyltransferase Set7/9-KMT7 Binds HIV-1 TAR RNA, Monomethylates the Viral Transactivator Tat, and Enhances HIV Transcription. *Cell Host Microbe* **2010**, *7*, 234–244. [CrossRef] [PubMed]
84. Ali, I.; Ramage, H.; Boehm, D.; Dirk, L.M.; Sakane, N.; Hanada, K.; Pagans, S.; Kaehlcke, K.; Aull, K.; Weinberger, L.; et al. The HIV-1 Tat Protein Is Monomethylated at Lysine 71 by the Lysine Methyltransferase KMT7. *J. Biol. Chem.* **2016**, *291*, 16240–16248. [CrossRef] [PubMed]
85. Masatsugu, T.; Yamamoto, K. Multiple lysine methylation of PCAF by Set9 methyltransferase. *Biochem. Biophys. Res. Commun.* **2009**, *381*, 22–26. [CrossRef] [PubMed]
86. Vasileva, E.; Shuvalov, O.; Petukhov, A.; Fedorova, O.; Daks, A.; Nader, R.; Barlev, N. KMT Set7/9 is a new regulator of Sam68 STAR-protein. *Biochem. Biophys. Res. Commun.* **2020**, *525*, 1018–1024. [CrossRef] [PubMed]
87. Kim, S.-K.; Lee, H.; Han, K.; Kim, S.C.; Choi, Y.; Park, S.-W.; Bak, G.; Lee, Y.; Choi, J.K.; Kim, T.-K.; et al. SET7/9 Methylation of the Pluripotency Factor LIN28A Is a Nucleolar Localization Mechanism that Blocks let-7 Biogenesis in Human ESCs. *Cell Stem Cell* **2014**, *15*, 735–749. [CrossRef] [PubMed]
88. Balasubramaniyan, N.; Ananthanarayanan, M.; Suchy, F.J. Direct methylation of FXR by Set7/9, a lysine methyltransferase, regulates the expression of FXR target genes. *Am. J. Physiol. Liver Physiol.* **2012**, *302*, G937–G947. [CrossRef] [PubMed]
89. Kassner, I.; Andersson, A.; Fey, M.; Tomas, M.; Ferrando-May, E.; Hottiger, M.O. SET7/9-dependent methylation of ARTD1 at K508 stimulates poly-ADP-ribose formation after oxidative stress. *Open Biol.* **2013**, *3*, 120173. [CrossRef]
90. Maganti, A.V.; Maier, B.; Tersey, S.A.; Sampley, M.L.; Mosley, A.L.; Özcan, S.; Pachaiyappan, B.; Woster, P.M.; Hunter, C.S.; Stein, R.; et al. Transcriptional Activity of the Islet β Cell Factor Pdx1 Is Augmented by Lysine Methylation Catalyzed by the Methyltransferase Set7/9. *J. Biol. Chem.* **2015**, *290*, 9812–9822. [CrossRef]
91. Aguilo, F.; Li, S.; Balasubramaniyan, N.; Sancho, A.; Benko, S.; Zhang, F.; Vashisht, A.; Rengasamy, M.; Andino, B.; Chen, C.-H.; et al. Deposition of 5-Methylcytosine on Enhancer RNAs Enables the Coactivator Function of PGC-1α. *Cell Rep.* **2016**, *14*, 479–492. [CrossRef] [PubMed]
92. Cho, H.-S.; Suzuki, T.; Dohmae, N.; Hayami, S.; Unoki, M.; Yoshimatsu, M.; Toyokawa, G.; Takawa, M.; Chen, T.; Kurash, J.K.; et al. Demethylation of RB Regulator MYPT1 by Histone Demethylase LSD1 Promotes Cell Cycle Progression in Cancer Cells. *Cancer Res* **2011**, *71*, 655–660. [CrossRef]
93. Carr, S.M.; Munro, S.; Kessler, B.; Oppermann, U.; La Thangue, N.B. Interplay between lysine methylation and Cdk phosphorylation in growth control by the retinoblastoma protein. *EMBO J.* **2010**, *30*, 317–327. [CrossRef] [PubMed]
94. Munro, S.; Khaire, N.; Inche, A.; Carr, S.; La Thangue, N.B. Lysine methylation regulates the pRb tumour suppressor protein. *Oncogene* **2010**, *29*, 2357–2367. [CrossRef] [PubMed]
95. Ea, C.-K.; Baltimore, D. Regulation of NF-κB activity through lysine monomethylation of p65. *Proc. Natl. Acad. Sci. USA* **2009**, *106*, 18972–18977. [CrossRef] [PubMed]
96. Yang, X.-D.; Huang, B.; Li, M.; Lamb, A.; Kelleher, N.L.; Chen, L.-F. Negative regulation of NF-κB action by Set9-mediated lysine methylation of the RelA subunit. *EMBO J.* **2009**, *28*, 1055–1066. [CrossRef] [PubMed]
97. Hong, X.; Huang, H.; Qiu, X.; Ding, Z.; Feng, X.; Zhu, Y.; Zhuo, H.; Hou, J.; Zhao, J.; Cai, W.; et al. Targeting posttranslational modifications of RIOK1 inhibits the progression of colorectal and gastric cancers. *eLife* **2018**, *7*, e29511. [CrossRef]
98. Song, H.; Chu, J.W.; Park, S.C.; Im, H.; Park, I.-G.; Kim, H.; Lee, J.M. Isoform-Specific Lysine Methylation of RORα2 by SETD7 Is Required for Association of the TIP60 Coactivator Complex in Prostate Cancer Progression. *Int. J. Mol. Sci.* **2020**, *21*, 1622. [CrossRef] [PubMed]
99. Hamidi, T.; Singh, A.K.; Veland, N.; Vemulapalli, V.; Chen, J.; Hardikar, S.; Bao, J.; Fry, C.J.; Yang, V.; Lee, K.A.; et al. Identification of Rpl29 as a major substrate of the lysine methyltransferase Set7/9. *J. Biol. Chem.* **2018**, *293*, 12770–12780. [CrossRef]
100. Liu, X.; Wang, D.; Zhao, Y.; Tu, B.; Zheng, Z.; Wang, L.; Wang, H.; Gu, W.; Roeder, R.G.; Zhu, W.-G. Methyltransferase Set7/9 regulates p53 activity by interacting with Sirtuin 1 (SIRT1). *Proc. Natl. Acad. Sci. USA* **2011**, *108*, 1925–1930. [CrossRef] [PubMed]
101. Elkouris, M.; Kontaki, H.; Stavropoulos, A.; Antonoglou, A.; Nikolaou, K.C.; Samiotaki, M.; Szantai, E.; Saviolaki, D.; Brown, P.J.; Sideras, P.; et al. SET9-Mediated Regulation of TGF-β Signaling Links Protein Methylation to Pulmonary Fibrosis. *Cell Rep.* **2016**, *15*, 2733–2744. [CrossRef]
102. Fang, L.; Zhang, L.; Wei, W.; Jin, X.; Wang, P.; Tong, Y.; Li, J.; Du, J.X.; Wong, J. A Methylation-Phosphorylation Switch Determines Sox2 Stability and Function in ESC Maintenance or Differentiation. *Mol. Cell* **2014**, *55*, 537–551. [CrossRef]

103. Stark, G.R.; Wang, Y.; Lu, T. Lysine methylation of promoter-bound transcription factors and relevance to cancer. *Cell Res.* **2010**, *21*, 375–380. [CrossRef] [PubMed]
104. Wang, D.; Zhou, J.; Liu, X.; Lu, D.; Shen, C.; Du, Y.; Wei, F.-Z.; Song, B.; Lu, X.; Yu, Y.; et al. Methylation of SUV39H1 by SET7/9 results in heterochromatin relaxation and genome instability. *Proc. Natl. Acad. Sci. USA* **2013**, *110*, 5516–5521. [CrossRef] [PubMed]
105. Couture, J.-F.; Collazo, E.; Hauk, G.; Trievel, R.C. Structural basis for the methylation site specificity of SET7/9. *Nat. Struct. Mol. Biol.* **2006**, *13*, 140–146. [CrossRef]
106. Kouskouti, A.; Scheer, E.; Staub, A.; Tora, L.; Talianidis, I. Gene-Specific Modulation of TAF10 Function by SET9-Mediated Methylation. *Mol. Cell* **2004**, *14*, 175–182. [CrossRef] [PubMed]
107. Ivanov, G.S.; Ivanova, T.; Kurash, J.; Ivanov, A.; Chuikov, S.; Gizatullin, F.; Herrera-Medina, E.M.; Rauscher, F.; Reinberg, D.; Barlev, N.A. Methylation-Acetylation Interplay Activates p53 in Response to DNA Damage. *Mol. Cell. Biol.* **2007**, *27*, 6756–6769. [CrossRef] [PubMed]
108. Oudhoff, M.; Freeman, S.A.; Couzens, A.L.; Antignano, F.; Kuznetsova, E.; Min, P.H.; Northrop, J.P.; Lehnertz, B.; Barsyte-Lovejoy, D.; Vedadi, M.; et al. Control of the Hippo Pathway by Set7-Dependent Methylation of Yap. *Dev. Cell* **2013**, *26*, 188–194. [CrossRef]
109. Zhang, W.J.; Wu, X.N.; Shi, T.T.; Xu, H.T.; Yi, J.; Shen, H.F.; Huang, M.F.; Shu, X.Y.; Wang, F.F.; Peng, B.L.; et al. Regulation of Transcription Factor Yin Yang 1 by SET7/9-Mediated Lysine Methylation. *Sci. Rep.* **2016**, *6*, 21718. [CrossRef]
110. Wu, X.-N.; Shi, T.-T.; He, Y.; Wang, F.-F.; Sang, R.; Ding, J.-C.; Zhang, W.; Shu, X.-Y.; Shen, H.-F.; Yi, J.; et al. Methylation of transcription factor YY2 regulates its transcriptional activity and cell proliferation. *Cell Discov.* **2017**, *3*, 17035. [CrossRef] [PubMed]

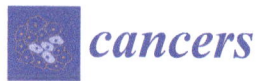

Article

Survival in Breast Cancer Patients with Bone Metastasis: A Multicenter Real-World Study on the Prognostic Impact of Intensive Postoperative Bone Scan after Initial Diagnosis of Breast Cancer (CSBrS-023)

Liu Yang [1], Wei Du [1], Taobo Hu [1], Miao Liu [1], Li Cai [2], Qiang Liu [3], Zhigang Yu [4], Guangyu Liu [5,*] and Shu Wang [1,*]

1. Department of Breast Disease Center, Peking University People's Hospital, Beijing 100044, China
2. Department of Breast Oncology, Harbin Medical University Cancer Hospital, Harbin 150000, China
3. Department of Breast Surgery, Sun Yai-Sen Memorial Hospital, Guangzhou 510120, China
4. Department of Breast Surgery, The Second Hospital of Shandong University, Jinan 250021, China
5. Department of Breast Surgery, Fudan University Shanghai Cancer Center, Shanghai 200032, China
* Correspondence: liugy688@163.com (G.L.); shuwang@pkuph.edu.cn (S.W.); Tel.: +86-216-417-2585 (ext. 200032) (G.L.); +86-108-832-4010 (ext. 100044) (S.W.)

Simple Summary: The bone scan (BS) is widely used in follow-up to detect bone metastasis (BM) in breast cancer (BC) patients presenting bone-related symptoms after surgery. However, it remains controversial whether asymptomatic BS (intensive postoperative BS) screening could be translated into a survival benefit. Therefore, we conducted this multicenter real-world study to understand the prognostic impact of intensive postoperative BS screening among 1059 Chinese patients with BM during the years 2005–2013. This study showed that intensive postoperative BS screening was an independent prognostic factor and prolonged the survival in patients with BC with BM. The prognostic value of intensive BS screening was consistently favorable for survival in patients at clinical high-risk. These findings suggested that intensive BS screening was important for improving survival, and should be recommended for postoperative surveillance, especially for patients with a high risk of recurrence and metastasis.

Abstract: The prognostic value of intensive postoperative bone scan (BS) screening, which is performed in asymptomatic patients with breast cancer (BC) after surgery, remained unclear. Patients diagnosed with BC with bone metastasis (BM) from five medical centers in China during the years 2005–2013 were retrospectively collected. Propensity score matching (PSM) was performed to balance the baseline characteristics. The survival outcomes were overall survival (OS) and overall survival after BM (OSABM). Among 1059 eligible patients, 304 underwent intensive postoperative BS while 755 did not. During a median follow-up of 6.67 years (95%CI 6.45, 7.21), intensive postoperative BS prolonged the median OS by 1.63 years (Log-Rank $p = 0.006$) and OSABM by 0.66 years (Log-Rank $p = 0.002$). Intensive postoperative BS was an independent prognostic factor for both OS (adjusted HR 0.77, 95%CI 0.64, 0.93, adjusted $p = 0.006$) and OSABM (adjusted HR 0.71, 95%CI 0.60, 0.86, adjusted $p < 0.001$). The prognostic value of intensive postoperative BS was consistently favorable for OS among clinical high-risk patients, including those with ages younger than 50, stage II, histology grade G3 and ER-Her2- subtype. This multicenter real-world study showed that intensive postoperative BS screening improved survival for BC patients with BM and should probably be recommended for postoperative surveillance, especially for patients at clinical high-risk.

Keywords: breast cancer; bone metastases; bone scan; follow-up; prognosis; survival

Citation: Yang, L.; Du, W.; Hu, T.; Liu, M.; Cai, L.; Liu, Q.; Yu, Z.; Liu, G.; Wang, S. Survival in Breast Cancer Patients with Bone Metastasis: A Multicenter Real-World Study on the Prognostic Impact of Intensive Postoperative Bone Scan after Initial Diagnosis of Breast Cancer (CSBrS-023). Cancers 2022, 14, 5835. https://doi.org/10.3390/cancers14235835

Academic Editor: Samuel C. Mok

Received: 12 July 2022
Accepted: 23 November 2022
Published: 26 November 2022

Publisher's Note: MDPI stays neutral with regard to jurisdictional claims in published maps and institutional affiliations.

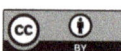

Copyright: © 2022 by the authors. Licensee MDPI, Basel, Switzerland. This article is an open access article distributed under the terms and conditions of the Creative Commons Attribution (CC BY) license (https://creativecommons.org/licenses/by/4.0/).

1. Introduction

Breast cancer (BC) is the most commonly diagnosed malignant cancer in women [1], and bone is the most common distant metastatic site [2–4]. The bone scan (BS), a conventional and cost-effective modality for detecting the entire skeleton in one examination [5,6], is widely used in postoperative follow-up for surveillance of bone metastasis (BM) in BC patients presenting related symptoms after surgery. However, current guidelines do not recommend intensive BS screening, which is referred to BS screening in asymptomatic patients, without specific findings on clinical examination before a diagnosis of BM.

The prognostic value of intensive postoperative BS remains unclear. Two well-designed randomized controlled trials, GIVIO (Interdisciplinary Group for Cancer Care Evaluation) trials [7], as well as Rosselli del Turco trials [8], and the Cochrane meta-analysis [9] demonstrated that intensive follow-up (imaging examinations including BS and laboratory tests) does not improve overall survival compared to clinical follow-up (physical examinations and annual mammography). Hence the American Society of Clinical Oncology (ASCO) [10], National Comprehensive Cancer Network (NCCN) [11] and European Society for Medical Oncology (ESMO) [12] do not recommend an intensive follow-up including BS.

It is important to note that the two trials were conducted almost three decades ago when advanced postoperative screening methods and palliative therapeutic options were scarce. Moreover, oncologists at that time lacked an adequate understanding of the intrinsic biological characteristics of BC. Recently, new regimens of systemic chemotherapy [13,14] and endocrine therapy [15] have made considerable progress in increasing patients' survival with far-advanced cancer. Anti-Her2 (human epidermal growth factor receptor 2) therapy increased the prognosis of patients with Her2-positive metastatic BC [16,17]. Bone-modifying agents, such as bisphosphonates [18] and denosumab [19], slowed down the progression of skeletal-related events, thus promoting the quality of life.

It is possible that recent improvements in diagnostics and treatments could promote earlier detection and effective treatment of BM, important for improving survival. Therefore, we conducted this multicenter real-world study to understand the prognostic factors of BC patients with BM, especially the prognostic impact of an intensive postoperative BS after initial diagnosis of BC.

2. Materials and Methods

2.1. Design and Patients

According to Chinese Society of Breast Surgery (CSBrS), this multicenter real-world study was conducted by five medical centers in China. This study has been registered in Clinicaltrials.gov as NCT03924609 on 23 April 2019 and approved by the Ethics Committee of the People's Hospital of Peking University (No. 2021PHB071-001). As this study was a retrospective study and all data were performed anonymously, the need for informed consent from patients was waived. All data generated or analyzed during the study are included in the published paper.

Patients eligible were required to have a histology-confirmed diagnosis of invasive BC and undergo curative-intent primary therapy. The diagnosis of BM must be supported by pathological or imaging evidence. The following cases were not eligible: (1) with other malignant primary cancer; (2) de novo stage IV BC; (3) incomplete and ambiguous clinical and pathological records.

2.2. Clinicopathological Factors

Clinicopathological factors of eligible patients were extracted from the standardized case report forms. Intensive postoperative BS was defined as at least one asymptomatic postoperative BS screening after initial diagnosis of BC before a diagnosis of BM. Clinical postoperative BS was referred to postoperative BS screening only performed in patients presenting bone-related symptoms. Primary tumor staging was defined according to the criteria of the TNM (tumor-nodal-metastasis) staging system by AJCC (American Joint

Committee on Cancer) [20]. The histology type of BC was defined according to criteria from the WHO (World Health Organization) [21]. The molecular subtypes of BC were classified based on the expression of the estrogen receptor (ER) and Her2 according to ASCO/CAP (American Society of Clinical Oncology/College of American Pathologists) [22,23]. Based on the timing of BM and visceral metastasis (VM), the pattern of distant metastasis was mainly divided into the following types: (1) BM only: only diagnosed with BM; (2) BM with VM: diagnosed with BM and VM simultaneously; (3) BM to VM: first diagnosed with BM, followed by VM; (4) VM to BM: first diagnosed with VM, followed by BM.

2.3. Follow-Up and Outcomes Definition

Follow-up was conducted by telephone or clinical visit from the date of diagnosis of BM until death. The follow-up information was obtained from the databases of the participating medical centers. The survival endpoints were overall survival (OS), which was calculated from the date BC was diagnosed to the date of death, and overall survival after diagnosis of bone metastasis (OSABM), which was calculated from the date BM was diagnosed to the date of death. The length of bone-metastasis free interval (BMFI) was also retrospectively observed, which was calculated as the time from diagnosis of BC to initial BM.

2.4. Propensity Score Matching (PSM)

When comparing survival between patients who underwent an intensive postoperative BS and those who underwent a clinical postoperative BS, propensity score matching was used to balance the baseline characteristics. We performed a 1:2 nearest-neighbor matching procedure within a caliper of 0.02 and all clinic and pathological factors were included in the matching model. Balance between the two groups before and after matching was assessed using standardized mean differences (SMD) and p-value by chi-square test or t test. SMD > 0.20 or p-value < 0.05 were considered imbalanced.

2.5. Statistical Analysis

Continuous variables were reported as mean and standard deviation, whereas categorical variables were reported as percentage. Statistical differences in the distribution of continuous and categorical variables were conducted by t-test and chi-square test, respectively. The statistical differences in the distribution of BMFI in various subgroups according to TNM stage and molecular subtype of BC were tested using the Kruskal–Wallis method.

Survival analysis was performed using the Kaplan–Meier method before and after PSM, thus median survival time was estimated and the Log-rank test was used for comparisons between groups. After PSM, univariate and multivariate Cox proportional hazards regression analyses and associated 95% confidence intervals (95%CI) were used to assess whether the hazard risks of survival endpoints in patients varied by certain clinical or pathological factors. Factors that showed a univariate connection with survival (p-value < 0.20) or considered clinically relevant were entered into the multivariate Cox proportional hazard regression model. Interaction terms were tested using the qualitative method and the univariate stratified Cox proportional hazard regression model, which were used to investigate whether the association between postoperative follow-up strategies and survival outcomes differed according to all clinical and pathological factors. Two-tailed p-values < 0.05 were considered statistically significant. All analyses were conducted using R*64 4.0.0 (Beijing, China, http://Rproject.org, accessed on 10 January 2022) and IBM SPSS Statistics 25.

3. Results

3.1. Patient Characteristics

From February 2005 to December 2013, we retrospectively identified 1425 patients with BC with BM from five medical centers in China. Excluding 239 patients with de novo stage IV BC and 127 with incomplete clinicopathological records, 1059 eligible patients were included in the analyses. The flow chart of the process of patients' enrollment and analyses is presented in Figure 1.

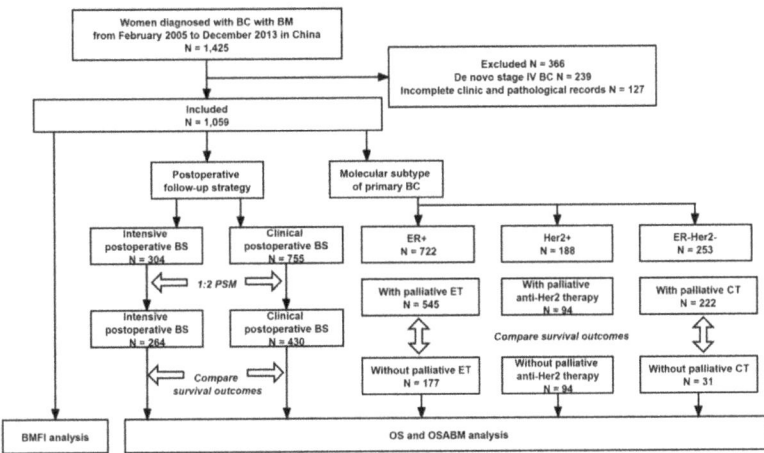

Figure 1. Flowchart of the process of patient's enrollment and analyses. Abbreviations: BC = breast cancer; BM = bone metastasis; BMFI = bone metastasis-free interval; BS = bone scan; CT = chemotherapy; ER = estrogen receptor; Her2 = Human epidermal growth factor receptor 2; ET = endocrine therapy; OS = overall survival; OSABM = overall survival after diagnosis of bone metastasis; PSM = propensity scores matching.

Among 1059 eligible patients, 304 underwent an intensive postoperative BS while 755 underwent a clinical postoperative BS. The median time when a patient received the first intensive postoperative BS was 2.5 years after initial diagnosis of BC. Baseline characteristics in the two groups stratified by postoperative follow-up strategy were balanced after PSM (shown in Table 1).

Table 1. Clinicopathological characteristics of eligible patients (N = 1059) stratified by postoperative follow-up strategy (Clinical postoperative BS vs. Intensive postoperative BS) before and after PSM.

Clinicopathological Characteristics		Before PSM				After PSM			
		Clinical $n = 755$	Intensive $n = 304$	P	SMD	Clinical $n = 430$	Intensive $n = 264$	P	SMD
Age * (mean (SD))		51.66 (10.42)	51.76 (11.04)	0.891	0.009	51.08 (10.32)	51.48 (11.06)	0.633	0.037
Year of diagnosis of BM (%)	2010~2013	474 (62.8)	218 (71.7)	0.007	0.191	296 (68.8)	183 (69.3)	0.961	0.010
	2005~2009	281 (37.2)	86 (28.3)			134 (31.2)	81 (30.7)		
Histology type (%)	Ductal	661 (87.5)	258 (84.9)	0.260	0.128	376 (87.4)	235 (89.0)	0.796	0.080
	Lobular	21 (2.8)	16 (5.3)			15 (3.5)	8 (3.0)		
	Mixed	31 (4.1)	13 (4.3)			21 (4.9)	9 (3.4)		
	Other **	42 (5.6)	17 (5.6)			18 (4.2)	12 (4.5)		
Histology grade (%)	G1	129 (17.1)	28 (9.2)	<0.001	0.406	47 (10.9)	27 (10.2)	0.417	0.103
	G2	374 (49.5)	117 (38.5)			203 (47.2)	113 (42.8)		
	G3	252 (33.4)	159 (52.3)			180 (41.9)	124 (47.0)		
TNM (%)	Stage I	89 (11.8)	38 (12.5)	0.886	0.033	49 (11.4)	32 (12.1)	0.744	0.060
	Stage II	314 (41.6)	129 (42.4)			171 (39.8)	111 (42.0)		
	Stage III	352 (46.6)	137 (45.1)			210 (48.8)	121 (45.8)		
Molecular subtype (%)	ER+Her2-	443 (58.7)	175 (57.6)	0.139	0.153	253 (58.8)	155 (58.7)	0.922	0.054
	ER+Her2+	74 (9.8)	30 (9.9)			50 (11.6)	29 (11.0)		
	ER-Her2+	51 (6.8)	33 (10.9)			30 (7.0)	22 (8.3)		
	ER-Her2-	187 (24.8)	66 (21.7)			97 (22.6)	58 (22.0)		
Distant metastatic pattern (%)	BM only	217 (28.7)	64 (21.1)	0.003	0.251	102 (23.7)	59 (22.3)	0.780	0.081
	BM to VM	183 (24.2)	67 (22.0)			102 (23.7)	65 (24.6)		
	BM with VM	277 (36.7)	121 (39.8)			173 (40.2)	101 (38.3)		
	VM to BM	78 (10.3)	52 (17.1)			53 (12.3)	39 (14.8)		
BMFI (%)	≤1 year	82 (10.9)	21 (6.9)	0.064	0.139	39 (9.1)	21 (8.0)	0.713	0.040
	>1 year	673 (89.1)	283 (93.1)			391 (90.9)	243 (92.0)		

Table 1. Cont.

Clinicopathological Characteristics		Before PSM				After PSM			
		Clinical $n = 755$	Intensive $n = 304$	P	SMD	Clinical $n = 430$	Intensive $n = 264$	P	SMD
Site of osseous lesion (%)	Appendicular	122 (16.2)	55 (18.1)	0.204	0.123	72 (16.7)	44 (16.7)	0.653	0.072
	Axial	235 (31.1)	78 (25.7)			129 (30.0)	71 (26.9)		
	Mixed	398 (52.7)	171 (56.2)			229 (53.3)	149 (56.4)		
Number of osseous lesion (%)	Multiple	595 (78.8)	237 (78.0)	0.825	0.021	339 (78.8)	207 (78.4)	0.970	0.010
	Solitary	160 (21.2)	67 (22.0)			91 (21.2)	57 (21.6)		
Palliative treatment on BM									
Surgery to bone (%)	No	731 (96.8)	297 (97.7)	0.573	0.054	416 (96.7)	257 (97.3)	0.824	0.036
	Yes	24 (3.2)	7 (2.3)			14 (3.3)	7 (2.7)		
Radiotherapy (%)	No	357 (47.3)	168 (55.3)	0.023	0.160	211 (49.1)	139 (52.7)	0.402	0.072
	Yes	398 (52.7)	136 (44.7)			219 (50.9)	125 (47.3)		
Endocrine therapy (%)	No	333 (44.1)	128 (42.1)	0.599	0.040	186 (43.3)	109 (41.3)	0.667	0.040
	Yes	422 (55.9)	176 (57.9)			244 (56.7)	155 (58.7)		
Chemotherapy (%)	No	119 (15.8)	36 (11.8)	0.124	0.114	56 (13.0)	34 (12.9)	1.000	0.004
	Yes	636 (84.2)	268 (88.2)			374 (87.0)	230 (87.1)		
Anti-Her2 therapy (%)	No	698 (92.5)	267 (87.8)	0.023	0.155	389 (90.5)	237 (89.8)	0.868	0.023
	Yes	57 (7.5)	37 (12.2)			41 (9.5)	27 (10.2)		
Bone-Modifying therapy (%)	No	263 (34.8)	96 (31.6)	0.347	0.069	135 (31.4)	84 (31.8)	0.974	0.009
	Yes	492 (65.2)	208 (68.4)			295 (68.6)	180 (68.2)		

* Age at diagnosis of breast cancer with bone metastasis. ** Other histological types of invasive breast cancer in addition to infiltrating ductal or lobular carcinoma according to WHO criteria. Abbreviations: BM = bone metastasis; BMFI = bone metastasis-free interval; BS = bone scan; ER = estrogen receptor; Her2 = Human epidermal growth factor receptor 2; PSM = propensity scores matching; SD = standard deviation; SMD = standardized mean differences; VM = visceral metastasis.

3.2. The Impact of an Intensive Postoperative BS on Survival

Follow-up was regularly performed until December 2018. During a median follow-up of 6.67 years (95%CI 6.45, 7.21), 759 out of 1059 eligible patients were dead: 197 in the intensive postoperative BS group and 562 in the clinical postoperative BS group. Before PSM, both median OS and OSABM of patients with an intensive postoperative BS were longer than those with a clinical postoperative BS (median OS, 7.99 vs. 6.61 years, Log-Rank $p = 0.003$, Figure 2A; median OSABM, 3.16 vs. 2.57 years, Log-Rank $p = 0.003$, Figure 2C). After PSM, both OS and OSABM benefits were still statistically significant in patients with an intensive postoperative BS (median OS, 7.88 vs. 6.25 years, Log-Rank $p = 0.006$, Figure 2B; median OSABM, 3.16 vs. 2.50 years, Log-Rank $p = 0.002$, Figure 2D).

3.3. Univariate and Multivariate Analysis of Factors Influencing Survival

When adjusting clinicopathological covariates after PSM, intensive postoperative BS was a favorable prognostic factor for both OS and OSABM of patients with BC with BM and reduced the risk of mortality by 23% (OS, adjusted HR 0.77, 95%CI 0.64, 0.93, adjusted $p = 0.006$; OSABM, adjusted HR 0.71, 95%CI 0.60, 0.86, adjusted $p < 0.001$). Histology type, TNM stage, distant metastatic pattern and palliative endocrine therapy were also independent prognostic factors for both OS and OSABM. Additionally, BMFI and age at diagnosis of BM were independent prognostic factors of OS and OSABM, respectively. The results of univariate and multivariate analysis of clinicopathological factors affecting OS and OSABM among eligible patients after PSM are listed in Table 2.

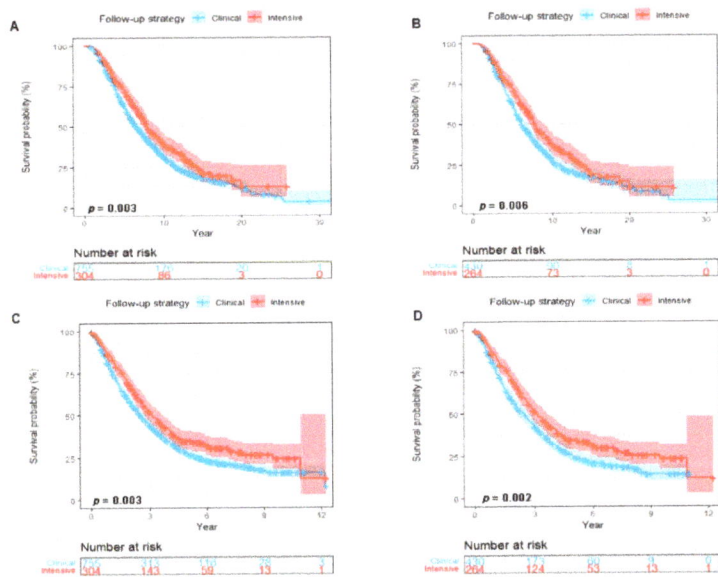

Figure 2. Kaplan–Meier curves showing a comparison of survival among patients with breast cancer with BM according to postoperative follow-up strategy (Intensive postoperative BS vs. Clinical postoperative BS). OS curves before (**A**) and after (**B**) PSM. OSABM curves before (**C**) and after (**D**) PSM. Abbreviations: BS = bone scan; BM = bone metastasis; OS = overall survival; OSABM = overall survival after diagnosis of bone metastasis; PSM = propensity scores matching.

Table 2. Univariate and multivariate analysis of clinicopathological factors affecting OS and OSABM among eligible patients (N = 694) after PSM.

Clinicopathological Factor	No.	Events	OS						OSABM					
			Univariate			Multivariate			Univariate			Multivariate		
			Crude HR	95%CI	Crude p Value	Adjusted HR	95%CI	Adjusted p Value	Crude HR	95%CI	Crude p Value	Adjusted HR	95%CI	Adjusted p Value
Follow-up strategy														
Clinical postoperative BS	430	326	0.77	0.64,0.93	0.006	0.77	0.64,0.93	0.006	0.75	0.63,0.90	0.002	0.71	0.60,0.86	<0.001
Intensive postoperative BS	264	175												
Age * (year)														
<=50	312	210	0.98	0.82,1.18	0.846	Not selected			1.26	1.06,1.51	0.011	1.23	1.03,1.47	0.026
>50	382	291												
Year of diagnosis of BM														
2005–2009	215	172	0.85	0.71,1.02	0.084	0.85	0.74,1.03	0.098	0.96	0.79,1.15	0.635	Not selected		
2010–2013	479	329												
Histology type					0.001			<0.001			0.025			0.002
Ductal	611	449	Ref.			Ref.			Ref.			Ref.		
Lobular	23	18	1.21	0.76,1.94	0.424	1.01	0.62,1.65	0.969	0.92	0.58,1.48	0.738	0.87	0.53,1.41	0.564
Mixed	30	20	0.85	0.54,1.34	0.487	0.76	0.48,1.21	0.254	0.94	0.60,1.47	0.787	0.79	0.50,1.26	0.325
Other **	30	14	0.32	0.18,0.55	<0.001	0.30	0.17,0.52	<0.001	0.44	0.26,0.74	0.002	0.36	0.21,0.62	<0.001
Histology grade					0.411						0.659			
G1	74	61	Ref.						Ref.					
G2	316	225	1.04	0.78,1.38	0.809	Not selected			0.92	0.70,1.23	0.583	Not selected		
G3	304	215	1.16	0.87,1.54	0.317				1.00	0.76,1.33	0.981			
TNM stage					<0.001			0.002			0.003			0.002
Stage I	81	58	Ref.			Ref.			Ref.			Ref.		
Stage II	282	192	1.09	0.81,1.46	0.584	1.09	0.81,1.46	0.593	1.09	0.81,1.46	0.582	1.19	0.89,1.60	0.247
Stage III	331	251	1.56	1.17,2.08	0.003	1.48	1.11,1.99	0.009	1.44	1.08,1.92	0.012	1.56	1.16,2.09	0.003
Molecular subtype					<0.001			0.178			<0.001			0.310
ER+Her2-	408	275	Ref.			Ref.			Ref.			Ref.		
ER+Her2+	79	60	1.47	1.11,1.95	0.007	1.23	0.92,1.64	0.156	1.23	0.93,1.63	0.145	0.95	0.72,1.27	0.739
ER-Her2+	52	42	2.53	1.82,3.51	<0.001	1.42	0.98,2.05	0.065	1.95	1.41,2.71	<0.001	1.27	0.89,1.83	0.194
ER-Her2-	155	124	1.50	1.21,1.86	<0.001	1.17	0.91,1.49	0.218	1.63	1.31,2.01	<0.001	1.21	0.95,1.55	0.126
Distant metastatic pattern					<0.001			<0.001			<0.001			<0.001
BM only	161	84	Ref.			Ref.			Ref.			Ref.		
BM with VM	274	227	2.04	1.59,2.63	<0.001	2.01	1.55,2.62	<0.001	2.36	1.83,3.04	<0.001	2.32	1.79,3.01	<0.001
BM to VM	167	110	1.34	1.01,1.79	0.042	1.34	1.00,1.81	0.052	1.22	0.91,1.62	0.181	1.27	0.95,1.71	0.108
VM to BM	92	80	1.64	1.20,2.23	0.002	1.89	1.37,2.61	<0.001	3.03	2.23,4.13	<0.001	3.43	2.49,4.73	<0.001

Table 2. Cont.

Clinicopathological Factor	No.	Events	OS						OSABM					
			Univariate			Multivariate			Univariate			Multivariate		
			Crude HR	95%CI	Crude p Value	Adjusted HR	95%CI	Adjusted p Value	Crude HR	95%CI	Crude p Value	Adjusted HR	95%CI	Adjusted p Value
BMFI (year) ≤1 >1	60 634	45 456	0.29	0.21,0.39	<0.001	0.29	0.21,0.41	<0.001	0.75	0.55,1.02	0.062	0.80	0.58,1.10	0.799
Site of osseous lesion Appendicular Axial Mixed	116 200 378	75 135 291	Ref. 1.26 1.45	Ref. 0.95,1.68 1.12,1.87	0.014 0.107 0.004	Ref. 1.14 1.38	Ref. 0.85,1.52 1.02,1.85	0.090 0.377 0.035	Ref. 1.14 1.52	Ref. 0.86,1.51 1.18,1.96	0.001 0.370 0.001	Ref. 1.09 1.36	Ref. 0.82,1.45 1.01,1.81	0.078 0.561 0.040
Number of osseous lesion Solitary Multiple	148 546	101 400	1.29	1.04,1.61	0.022	0.98	0.74,1.30	0.908	1.37	1.10,1.71	0.005	1.12	0.85,1.48	0.437
Surgery to bone No Yes	673 21	487 14	0.60	0.35,1.02	0.059	0.64	0.37,1.10	0.107	0.71	0.42,1.21	0.213	Not selected		
Palliative radiotherapy No Yes	350 344	242 259	1.10	0.92,1.31	0.289	Not selected			1.08	0.91,1.29	0.388	Not selected		
Palliative endocrine therapy No Yes	295 399	218 283	0.61	0.51,0.73	<0.001	0.62	0.50,0.78	<0.001	0.62	0.52,0.75	<0.001	0.68	0.55,0.85	0.001
Palliative chemotherapy No Yes	90 604	62 439	0.64	0.72,1.22	0.635	Not selected			0.94	0.72,1.23	0.668	Not selected		
Palliative anti-Her2 therapy No Yes	626 68	452 49	1.14	0.85,1.54	0.375	Not selected			0.85	0.63,1.14	0.273	Not selected		
Bone-Modifying therapy No Yes	219 475	141 360	1.04	0.86,1.26	0.697	Not selected			0.99	0.81,1.20	0.901	Not selected		

* Age at diagnosis of breast cancer with bone metastasis. ** Other histological types of invasive breast cancer in addition to infiltrating ductal or lobular carcinoma according to WHO criteria. Abbreviations: BM = bone metastasis; BMFI = bone metastasis-free interval; BS = bone scan; 95%CI = 95% confidence interval; ER = estrogen receptor; Her2 = Human epidermal growth factor receptor 2; HR = hazard ratio; OS = overall survival; OSABM = overall survival after bone metastasis; PSM = propensity scores matching; Ref. = reference; VM = visceral metastasis.

3.4. Interaction and Univariate Stratified Analysis of the Impact of an Intensive Postoperative BS on Survival

As shown in Figure 3, eligible patients were stratified by all clinicopathological factors and palliative treatment methods on BM to explore the relationship between postoperative follow-up strategy and survival after PSM. The prognostic value of an intensive postoperative BS was consistently favorable for OS among BC patients at clinical high-risk, including an age at diagnosis of BM younger than 50, TNM stage II, histology grade G3 and ER-Her2-subtype (Figure 3A). Similarly, as for OSABM, the favorable prognostic value of an intensive postoperative BS was also significant in patients at clinical high-risk, including TNM stage II, histology grade G3 and ER-Her2-subtype (Figure 3B).

3.5. The Impact of Palliative Treatments on Survival Stratified by Molecular Subtype

From the point of molecular subtypes of BC, we observed the association between palliative treatments and survival of patients with BM. For patients with a Her2+ BC, 50% (94/188) received palliative anti-Her2 therapy. Palliative anti-Her2 therapy prolonged median OS by 2.4 years (Log-Rank p = 0.002; HR 0.60, 95%CI 0.43, 0.83; Figure 4A) and OSABM by 1.6 years (Log-Rank p < 0.001; HR 0.49, 95%CI 0.35, 0.68; Figure 4B) among Her2+ patients. For patients with an ER + BC, 75.5% (545/722) underwent palliative endocrine therapy. Palliative endocrine therapy improved both OS (Log-Rank p < 0.001; HR 0.70, 95%CI 0.57, 0.86; Figure 4C) and OSABM (Log-Rank p = 0.007; HR 0.75, 95%CI 0.61, 0.92; Figure 4D) for this subgroup of patients. In addition, 87.7% (222/253) of patients with an ER-HER2-BC received palliative chemotherapy. However, palliative chemotherapy converted into neither OS (Log-Rank p = 0.300; HR 0.81, 95%CI 0.53, 1.24; Figure 4E) nor OSABM (Log-Rank p = 0.070; HR 0.68, 95%CI 0.45, 1.04; Figure 4F) benefits for ER-Her2-patients.

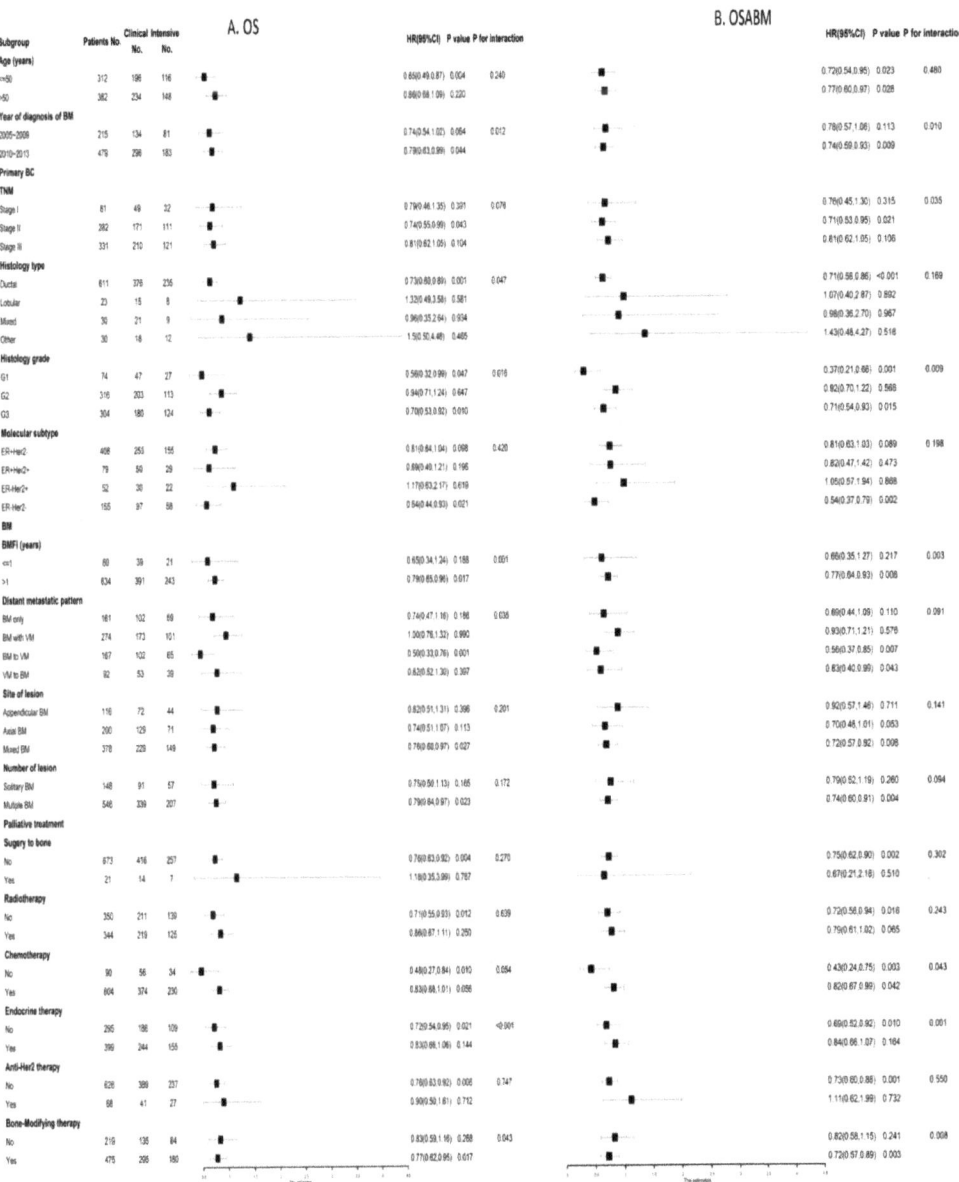

Figure 3. Forest plots of interaction and univariate subgroup analyses on the association between postoperative follow-up strategies (Intensive postoperative BS vs. Clinical postoperative BS) and (**A**) OS and (**B**) OSABM of patients with breast cancer with BM after PSM. Abbreviations: BS = bone scan; BM = bone metastasis; BMFI = bone metastasis-free interval; 95%CI = 95% confidence interval; ER = estrogen receptor; Her2 = Human epidermal growth factor receptor 2; HR = hazard risk; No. = Numbers of patients; OS = overall survival; OSABM = overall survival after bone metastasis; PSM = propensity scores matching.

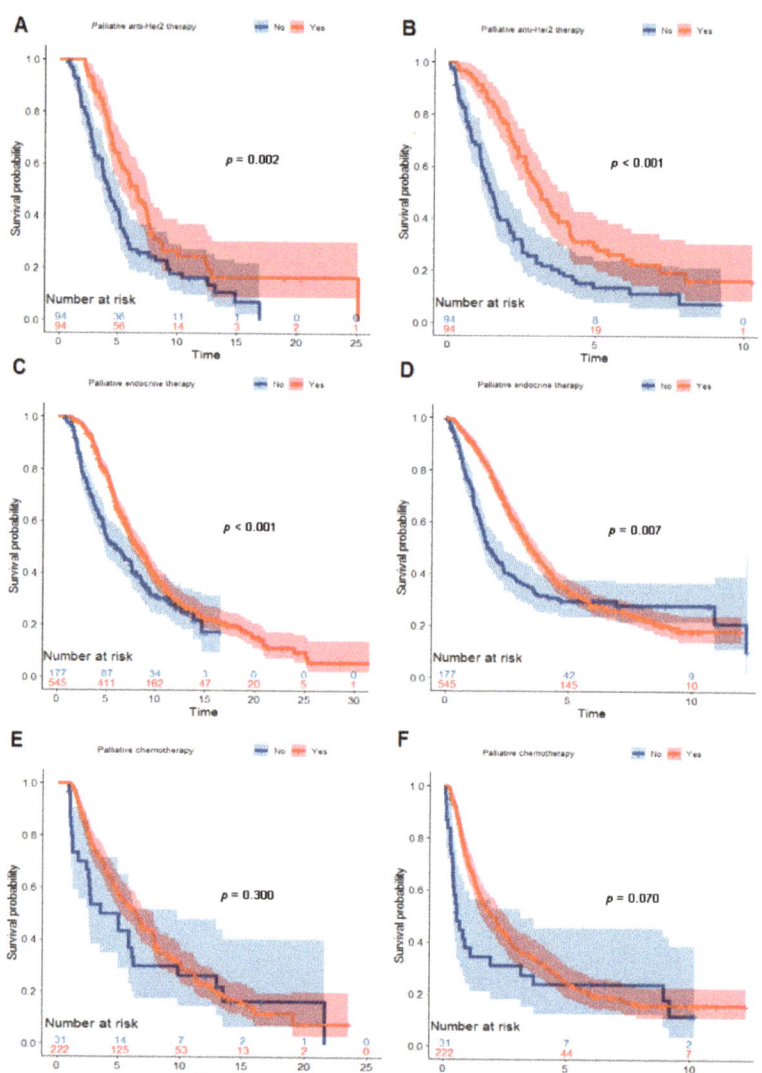

Figure 4. Kaplan–Meier curves showing a comparison of survival time among patients with breast cancer with BM according to molecular subtype and palliative treatment. Curves for OS (**A**) and OSABM (**B**) of patients with a Her2+ breast cancer stratified by palliative anti-Her2 therapy. Curves for OS (**C**) and OSABM (**D**) of patients with an ER+ breast cancer stratified by palliative endocrine therapy. Curves for OS € (**E**) and OSABM (**F**) of patients with an ER-Her2-breast cancer stratified by palliative chemotherapy. Abbreviations: BM = bone metastasis; ER = estrogen receptor; Her2 = Human epidermal growth factor receptor 2; OS = overall survival; OSABM = overall survival after diagnosis of bone metastasis.

3.6. The Association of BMFI with BC Stage and Molecular Subtype

The median BMFI was 3.08 years for 1059 eligible patients. However, as shown in Figure 5, BC patients with a different TNM stage and molecular subtype presented specific distributions of the length of BMFI. The median BMFI was 3.29 years for patients at stage I-II and 2.13 years for patients at stage III ($p < 0.001$, Figure 5C). The annual incidence of BM reached a peak at the second year after initial diagnosis of BC among patients at stage III

(24.5%, 120/489), the third year among patients at stage II (19.0%, 84/443), while the fourth year among patients at stage I (18.1%, 23/127, Figure 5A). The median BMFI was 3.38, 2.88 and 2.30 years for patients with an ER+, ER-Her2- and Her2+ BC, respectively ($p < 0.001$, Figure 5D). Compared with ER+ and ER-Her2-, patients with a Her2+ BC progressed to BM more rapidly. The cumulative incidence of BM (two years after initial diagnosis of BC) was 26.6% (192/722) for ER+ patients and 34.4% (87/253) for ER-Her2-patients; however, it was 42.0% (79/188) for Her2+ patients (Figure 5B).

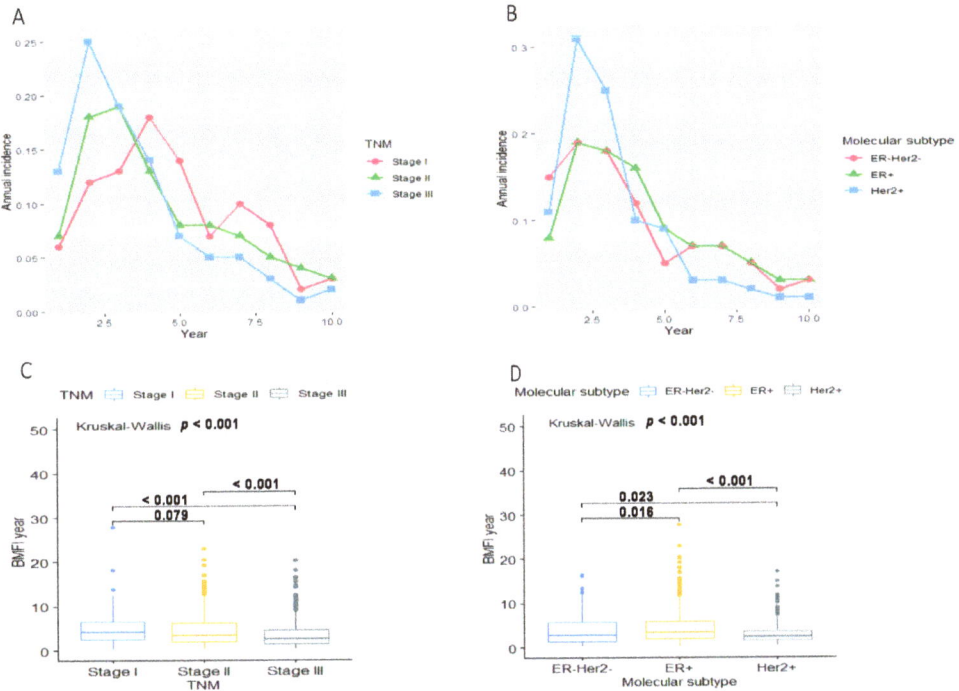

Figure 5. Annual incidence of BM for overall eligible patients (N = 1059) in groups stratified by (**A**) TNM stage and (**B**) molecular subtype. The distribution of BMFI for overall eligible patients (N = 1059) in groups stratified by (**C**) TNM stage and (**D**) molecular subtype. Abbreviations: BM = bone metastasis; BMFI = bone metastasis-free survival; ER = estrogen receptor; Her2 = Human epidermal growth factor receptor 2.

4. Discussion

This multicenter real-world study showed an intensive postoperative BS improved survival for BC patients with BM. In the point of molecular subtypes of BC, palliative anti-Her2 therapy and endocrine therapy improved both OS and OSABM among patients with a Her2+ and ER+ BC, respectively. These results indicated that the intensive postoperative BS and phenotype-specific palliative systemic treatments were important for improving survival of patients with BM.

Currently, ASCO, NCCN and ESMO guidelines do not recommend an intensive postoperative BS for BC patients [10–12]. However, in clinical practice, there are substantial variations in adherence to guideline recommendations. Intensive follow-up is a widespread reality that costs 2.2–3.6 times more than follow-up suggested by guidelines [24]. In a large population-based retrospective longitudinal study ($n = 11,219$) of women in Canada, 8.7–14.6% of women underwent BS screening in each follow-up year, and about half of them had greater than ASCO guideline-recommended surveillance imaging for metastatic diseases [25]. In line with these results, Surveillance, Epidemiology, and End Results

(SEER)-Medicare database showed that 13.3% of 37,967 patients underwent at least one BS screening in the first year of follow-up [26]. Similarly, in our study, 28.7% (304/1059) of patients received an intensive postoperative BS. There are several possible reasons for the overuse of intensive BS imaging. First, the patient-driven anxiety and the feeling of reassurance induced by intensive postoperative surveillance, including the BS. Stemmler et al. have examined 801 questionnaires of German women with a history of BC and reported that more than 47.8% of them needed an intensive schedule, which increased their feeling of security [27]. Second, patients with early or limited metastatic recurrence may be curable; thus, the monitoring of asymptomatic patients could result in better efficacy of BC treatment, at least in theory, when tumor burden is low [26]. Third, all the high-level evidence was conducted almost 30 years ago in an era of outdated technology and limited therapeutic options. Current evidence demonstrated that improvements in diagnostics and treatments could improve the survival of patients with metastatic BC, especially with more detailed subtype classification and corresponding efficient target therapies [13–15,17]. However, there are no current well-designed trials to verify this issue. To the best of our knowledge, this is the first study that observed the prognostic value of an intensive postoperative BS in patients with BC with BM.

In our study, an intensive postoperative BS resulted in an independent prognostic factor of OS and OSABM among patients with BC with BM. It was worth noticing that 85.4% (904/1059) of patients received palliative chemotherapy, and 66.1% (700/1059) received bone-modifying therapy. In addition, 75.5% (545/722) of ER+ patients received palliative endocrine therapy and 50% (94/188) of Her2+ patients received palliative anti-Her2 therapy. The strength of these treatments was much stronger than it was decades ago. Palliative endocrine therapy had been identified as an independent prognostic factor for OS as well as OSABM, and palliative anti-Her2 therapy also improved OS and OSABM of patients with Her2+ BC. For ER-Her2-patients, palliative systemic chemotherapy increased 5-year OS by 14.3% (57.7% vs. 43.4%) and 2-year OSABM by 18.7% (49.7% vs. 31.0%) compared with the patients who did not receive palliative chemotherapy. This evidence suggested that intensive detection and effective phenotype-specific systemic intervention for BM could be translated into a survival benefit.

In order to make intensive postoperative BSs more cost-effective, we selected high-risk patients based on stratified analysis. A higher tumor burden led to a higher risk of distant metastasis [28–31]. Our study showed that the patients at stage II-III progressed to BM more rapidly compared with those at stage I. It was worth nothing that an intensive postoperative BS particularly improved survival of patients at stage II. Consequently, it was rational to suggest patients with a heavy local tumor burden receive intensive postoperative BS screening. From an intrinsic biological point of view, early BC presents special metastatic behaviors [32,33], so postoperative monitoring strategies should vary accordingly. The ER-Her2-subtype, with a dramatically increased risk of distant relapse [34], accounted for 23.9% (253/1059) of patients in our study. An intensive postoperative BS improved OS as well as OSABM among ER-Her2-patients. Thus, we assumed that an intensive postoperative BS for ER-Her2-patients might be of significance. However, an intensive postoperative BS did not convert into a survival benefit in Her2+ patients. It is possible that this was due to limited Her2 status detection techniques and therapeutic options, even though early postoperative detection of BM was performed. In our study, 367 out of 1059 patients were diagnosed with BM before 2009, when Her2 status detection techniques were not commonly used in China, and trastuzumab was not widely implemented for relapse patients.

It is also worth noting that for all eligible patients, 26.5% (281/1059) were diagnosed with BM only, 37.6% (398/1059) were BM with VM, 23.6% (250/1059) were BM followed by VM, and 12.3% (130/1059) were VM followed by BM. There is probably a certain percent of patients classified as BM with VM who developed BM first and then progressed to VM but were not detected when simple BM originated. Previous studies showed that 26% to 50% of patients with early BC developed bone metastasis as the first site of distant relapse [4]. Consequently, early detection and treatment of BM may prolong the interval to visceral metastasis. As predicted, according to interaction and univariate stratified subgroup analysis, an intensive postoperative BS could improve OS for patients with "BM to VM", thus supporting the idea that early detection and early treatment are effective.

This multicenter real-world study showed that an intensive postoperative BS should probably be recommended as a follow-up strategy for patients with BC with BM. The main limitation of the present study is the retrospective study design. When evaluating the prognostic value of an intensive postoperative BS, cost-effectiveness and quality of life were not included in the analyses. Future studies with a randomized design are warranted to get an explicit estimation.

5. Conclusions

This multicenter real-world study showed that intensive postoperative BS screening improved survival for BC patients with BM, and should be recommended for postoperative surveillance, especially for patients at clinical high-risk.

Author Contributions: Conceptualization, G.L. and S.W.; methodology, L.Y., W.D., T.H., G.L. and S.W.; software, L.Y., W.D. and T.H.; validation, G.L. and S.W.; formal analysis, L.Y., W.D. and T.H.; investigation, G.L. and S.W.; resources, L.Y., W.D., M.L., L.C., Z.Y., Q.L., G.L. and S.W.; data curation, L.Y., G.L. and S.W.; writing—original draft preparation, L.Y.; writing—review and editing, L.Y., G.L. and S.W.; visualization, L.Y. and T.H.; supervision, G.L. and S.W.; project administration, G.L. and S.W.; funding acquisition, S.W. All authors have read and agreed to the published version of the manuscript.

Funding: This study was funded by the Ministry of Science and Technology of People's Republic of China (Grant No. 2016YFC0901302), the National Natural Science Foundation of China (Grant No. 92059105, 82002979), and the Beijing Municipal Natural Science Foundation (Grant No. 7202212).

Institutional Review Board Statement: The study was conducted in accordance with the Declaration of Helsinki, and approved by the Ethics Committee of the People's Hospital of Peking University (No. 2021PHB071-001).

Informed Consent Statement: As this study was a retrospective study and all data analyses were performed anonymously, the need for patient consent was waived.

Data Availability Statement: All data generated or analyzed during the study are included in the published paper.

Acknowledgments: The authors would like to acknowledgement the member units of CSBrS for data collection: Department of Breast Oncology, Harbin Medical University Cancer Hospital; Department of Breast Surgery, Sun Yai-Sen Memorial Hospital; Department of Breast Surgery, Fudan University Shanghai Cancer Center; Department of Breast Surgery, The Second Hospital of Shandong University.

Conflicts of Interest: The authors declare no conflict of interest.

References

1. Bray, F.; Ferlay, J.; Soerjomataram, I.; Siegel, R.L.; Torre, L.A.; Jemal, A. Global cancer statistics 2018: GLOBOCAN estimates of incidence and mortality worldwide for 36 cancers in 185 countries. *CA Cancer J. Clin.* **2018**, *68*, 394–424. [CrossRef] [PubMed]
2. Coleman, R.E. Metastatic bone disease: Clinical features, pathophysiology and treatment strategies. *Cancer Treat. Rev.* **2001**, *27*, 165–176. [CrossRef] [PubMed]
3. Cetin, K.; Christiansen, C.F.; Svaerke, C.; Jacobsen, J.B.; Sørensen, H.T. Survival in patients with breast cancer with bone metastasis: A Danish population-based cohort study on the prognostic impact of initial stage of disease at breast cancer diagnosis and length of the bone metastasis-free interval. *BMJ Open* **2015**, *5*, e007702. [CrossRef]
4. Hamaoka, T.; Madewell, J.E.; Podoloff, D.A.; Hortobagyi, G.N.; Ueno, N.T. Bone imaging in metastatic breast cancer. *J. Clin. Oncol.* **2004**, *22*, 2942–2953. [CrossRef]
5. Hildebrandt, M.G.; Gerke, O.; Baun, C.; Falch, K.; Hansen, J.A.; Farahani, Z.A.; Petersen, H.; Larsen, L.B.; Duvnjak, S.; Buskevica, I.; et al. [18F]Fluorodeoxyglucose (FDG)-Positron Emission Tomography (PET)/Computed Tomography (CT) in Suspected Recurrent Breast Cancer: A Prospective Comparative Study of Dual-Time-Point FDG-PET/CT, Contrast-Enhanced CT, and Bone Scintigraphy. *J. Clin. Oncol.* **2016**, *34*, 1889–1897. [CrossRef] [PubMed]

6. Cook, G.J.; Azad, G.K.; Goh, V. Imaging Bone Metastases in Breast Cancer: Staging and Response Assessment. *J. Nucl. Med.* **2016**, *57* (Suppl. 1), 27S–33S. [CrossRef]
7. Ghezzi, P.; Magnanini, S.; Rinaldini, M.; Berardi, F.; Di Biagio, G.; Testare, F.; Tavoni, N.; Schittulli, F.; D'Amico, C.; Pedicini, T.; et al. Impact of follow-up testing on survival and health-related quality of life in breast cancer patients. A multicenter randomized controlled trial. The GIVIO Investigators. *JAMA* **1974**, *271*, 1587–1592. [CrossRef] [PubMed]
8. Palli, D.; Russo, A.; Saieva, C.; Ciatto, S.; Del Turco, M.R.; Distante, V.; Pacini, P. Intensive vs clinical follow-up after treatment of primary breast cancer: 10-year update of a randomized trial. National Research Council Project on Breast Cancer Follow-up. *JAMA* **1999**, *281*, 1586. [CrossRef]
9. Moschetti, I.; Cinquini, M.; Lambertini, M.; Levaggi, A.; Liberati, A. Follow-up strategies for women treated for early breast cancer. *Cochrane Database Syst. Rev.* **2016**, *5*, CD001768. [CrossRef]
10. Khatcheressian, J.L.; Hurley, P.; Bantug, E.; Esserman, L.J.; Grunfeld, E.; Halberg, F.; Hantel, A.; Henry, N.L.; Muss, H.B.; Smith, T.J.; et al. Breast cancer follow-up and management after primary treatment: American Society of Clinical Oncology clinical practice guideline update. *J. Clin. Oncol.* **2013**, *31*, 961–965. [CrossRef]
11. Gradishar, W.J.; Anderson, B.O.; Abraham, J.; Aft, R.; Agnese, D.; Allison, K.H.; Blair, S.L.; Burstein, H.J.; Dang, C.; Elias, A.D.; et al. Breast Cancer, Version 3.2020, NCCN Clinical Practice Guidelines in Oncology. *J. Natl. Compr. Canc. Netw.* **2020**, *18*, 452–478. [CrossRef] [PubMed]
12. Cardoso, F.; Kyriakides, S.; Ohno, S.; Penault-Llorca, F.; Poortmans, P.; Rubio, I.T.; Zackrisson, S.; Senkus, E.; ESMO Guidelines Committee. Primary breast cancer: ESMO Clinical Practice Guidelines for diagnosis, treatment and follow-up. *Ann. Oncol.* **2019**, *30*, 1194–1220. [CrossRef] [PubMed]
13. Kalinsky, K.; Diamond, J.; Vahdat, L.; Tolaney, S.; Juric, D.; O'Shaughnessy, J.; Moroose, R.; Mayer, I.; Abramson, V.; Goldenberg, D.; et al. Sacituzumab govitecan in previously treated hormone receptor- positive/HER2-negative metastatic breast cancer: Final results from a phase I/II, single-arm, basket trial. *Ann. Oncol.* **2020**, *31*, 1709–1718. [CrossRef]
14. Robson, M.E.; Tung, N.; Conte, P.; Im, S.-A.; Senkus, E.; Xu, B.; Masuda, N.; Delaloge, S.; Li, W.; Armstrong, A.; et al. OlympiAD final overall survival and tolerability results: Olaparib versus chemotherapy treatment of physician's choice in patients with a germline BRCA mutation and HER2-negative metastatic breast cancer. *Ann. Oncol.* **2019**, *30*, 558–566. [CrossRef] [PubMed]
15. Turner, N.C.; Slamon, D.J.; Ro, J.; Bondarenko, I.; Im, S.-A.; Masuda, N.; Colleoni, M.; DeMichele, A.; Loi, S.; Verma, S.; et al. Overall Survival with Palbociclib and Fulvestrant in Advanced Breast Cancer. *N. Engl. J. Med.* **2018**, *379*, 1926–1936. [CrossRef] [PubMed]
16. Swain, S.M.; Kim, S.-B.; Cortés, J.; Ro, J.; Semiglazov, V.; Campone, M.; Ciruelos, E.; Ferrero, J.-M.; Schneeweiss, A.; Knott, A.; et al. Pertuzumab, trastuzumab, and docetaxel for HER2-positive metastatic breast cancer (CLEOPATRA study): Overall survival results from a randomised, double-blind, placebo-controlled, phase 3 study. *Lancet Oncol.* **2013**, *14*, 461–471. [CrossRef]
17. Perez, E.A.; Barrios, C.; Eiermann, W.; Toi, M.; Im, Y.-H.; Conte, P.; Martin, M.; Pienkowski, T.; Pivot, X.; Burris, H.A.; et al. Trastuzumab Emtansine with or Without Pertuzumab Versus Trastuzumab Plus Taxane for Human Epidermal Growth Factor Receptor 2-Positive, Advanced Breast Cancer: Primary Results from the Phase III MARIANNE Study. *J. Clin. Oncol.* **2017**, *35*, 141–148. [CrossRef]
18. O'Carrigan, B.; Wong, M.H.; Willson, M.L.; Stockler, M.R.; Pavlakis, N.; Goodwin, A. Bisphosphonates and other bone agents for breast cancer. *Cochrane Database Syst. Rev.* **2017**, *10*, Cd003474. [CrossRef]
19. Fizazi, K.; Carducci, M.; Smith, M.; Damião, R.; Brown, J.; Karsh, L.; Milecki, P.; Shore, N.; Rader, M.; Wang, H.; et al. Denosumab versus zoledronic acid for treatment of bone metastases in men with castration-resistant prostate cancer: A randomised, double-blind study. *Lancet* **2011**, *377*, 813–822. [CrossRef]
20. Giuliano, A.E.; Edge, S.B.; Hortobagyi, G.N. Eighth Edition of the AJCC Cancer Staging Manual: Breast Cancer. *Ann. Surg. Oncol.* **2018**, *25*, 1783–1785. [CrossRef]
21. Frank, G.A.; Danilova, N.V.; Andreeva, I.I.; Nefedova, N.A. WHO classification of tumors of the breast, 2012. *Arkh. Patol.* **2013**, *75*, 53–63.
22. Wolff, A.C.; Hammond, M.E.H.; Hicks, D.G.; Dowsett, M.; McShane, L.M.; Allison, K.H.; Allred, D.C.; Bartlett, J.M.S.; Bilous, M.; Fitzgibbons, P.; et al. Recommendations for human epidermal growth factor receptor 2 testing in breast cancer: American Society of Clinical Oncology/College of American Pathologists clinical practice guideline update. *J. Clin. Oncol.* **2013**, *31*, 3997–4013. [CrossRef] [PubMed]
23. Dowsett, M.; Nielsen, T.O.; A'Hern, R.; Bartlett, J.; Coombes, R.C.; Cuzick, J.; Ellis, M.; Henry, N.L.; Hugh, J.C.; Lively, T.; et al. Estrogen and Progesterone Receptor Testing in Breast Cancer: American Society of Clinical Oncology/College of American Pathologists Guideline Update. *Arch. Pathol. Lab. Med.* **2020**, *144*, 545–563. [CrossRef]
24. Mille, D.; Roy, T.; Carrère, M.-O.; Ray, I.; Ferdjaoui, N.; Späth, H.-M.; Chauvin, F.; Philip, T. Economic impact of harmonizing medical practices: Compliance with clinical practice guidelines in the follow-up of breast cancer in a French Comprehensive Cancer Center. *J. Clin. Oncol.* **2000**, *18*, 1718–1724. [CrossRef]
25. Grunfeld, E.; Hodgson, D.C.; Del Giudice, M.E.; Moineddin, R. Population-based longitudinal study of follow-up care for breast cancer survivors. *J. Oncol. Pract.* **2010**, *6*, 174–181. [CrossRef] [PubMed]
26. Keating, N.L.; Landrum, M.B.; Guadagnoli, E.; Winer, E.P.; Ayanian, J.Z. Surveillance testing among survivors of early-stage breast cancer. *J. Clin. Oncol.* **2007**, *25*, 1074–1081. [CrossRef]

27. Hans-Joachim, S.; Dorit, L.; Petra, S.; Ingo, B.; Steffen, K.; Alexander, F.P.; Wilhelm, B.M.; Margrit, G.; Ursula, G.-P.; Verena, H.; et al. The reality in the surveillance of breast cancer survivors-results of a patient survey. *Breast Cancer* **2008**, *1*, 17–23. [CrossRef]
28. Lee, J.E.; Park, S.-S.; Han, W.; Kim, S.W.; Shin, H.J.; Choe, K.J.; Oh, S.K.; Youn, Y.-K.; Noh, N.-Y.; Kim, S.-W. The clinical use of staging bone scan in patients with breast carcinoma: Reevaluation by the 2003 American Joint Committee on Cancer staging system. *Cancer* **2005**, *104*, 499–503. [CrossRef]
29. Lee, Y.T. Bone scanning in patients with early breast carcinoma: Should it be a routine staging procedure? *Cancer* **1981**, *47*, 486–495. [CrossRef]
30. Brar, H.S.; Sisley, J.F.; Johnson, R.H. Value of preoperative bone and liver scans and alkaline phosphatase in the evaluation of breast cancer patients. *Am. J. Surg.* **1993**, *165*, 221–223. [CrossRef]
31. Lewin, A.A.; Moy, L.; Baron, P.; Didwania, A.D.; Diflorio-Alexander, R.M.; Hayward, J.H.; Le-Petross, H.T.; Newell, M.S.; Rewari, A.; Scheel, J.R.; et al. ACR Appropriateness Criteria(®) Stage I Breast Cancer: Initial Workup and Surveillance for Local Recurrence and Distant Metastases in Asymptomatic Women. *J. Am. Coll. Radiol.* **2017**, *14*, S282–S292. [CrossRef] [PubMed]
32. Buonomo, O.C.; Caredda, E.; Portarena, I.; Vanni, G.; Orlandi, A.; Bagni, C.; Petrella, G.; Palombi, L.; Orsaria, P. New insights into the metastatic behavior after breast cancer surgery, according to well-established clinicopathological variables and molecular subtypes. *PLoS ONE* **2017**, *12*, e0184680. [CrossRef] [PubMed]
33. Kennecke, H.; Yerushalmi, R.; Woods, R.; Cheang, M.C.U.; Voduc, D.; Speers, C.H.; Nielsen, T.O.; Gelmon, K. Metastatic behavior of breast cancer subtypes. *J. Clin. Oncol.* **2010**, *28*, 3271–3277. [CrossRef] [PubMed]
34. Lin, N.U.; Vanderplas, A.; Hughes, M.E.; Theriault, R.L.; Edge, S.B.; Wong, Y.-N.; Blayney, D.W.; Niland, J.C.; Winer, E.P.; Weeks, J.C. Clinicopathologic features, patterns of recurrence, and survival among women with triple-negative breast cancer in the National Comprehensive Cancer Network. *Cancer* **2012**, *118*, 5463–5472. [CrossRef]

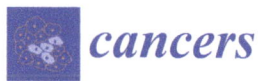

Article

Immune-Related Gene Signatures to Predict the Effectiveness of Chemoimmunotherapy in Triple-Negative Breast Cancer Using Exploratory Subgroup Discovery

Olha Kholod [1], William I. Basket [1], Jonathan B. Mitchem [1,2,3,4], Jussuf T. Kaifi [1,2,3,4], Richard D. Hammer [1,4,5,6], Christos N. Papageorgiou [4,6] and Chi-Ren Shyu [1,7,*]

1. MU Institute for Data Science and Informatics, University of Missouri, Columbia, MO 65212, USA
2. Department of Surgery, School of Medicine, University of Missouri, Columbia, MO 65212, USA
3. Harry S. Truman Memorial Veterans' Hospital, Columbia, MO 65201, USA
4. Ellis Fischel Cancer Center, University of Missouri, Columbia, MO 65211, USA
5. Department of Pathology & Anatomical Sciences, School of Medicine, University of Missouri, Columbia, MO 65212, USA
6. Department of Medicine, School of Medicine, University of Missouri, Columbia, MO 65212, USA
7. Department of Electrical Engineering & Computer Science, University of Missouri, Columbia, MO 65212, USA
* Correspondence: shyuc@missouri.edu

Citation: Kholod, O.; Basket, W.I.; Mitchem, J.B.; Kaifi, J.T.; Hammer, R.D.; Papageorgiou, C.N.; Shyu, C.-R. Immune-Related Gene Signatures to Predict the Effectiveness of Chemoimmunotherapy in Triple-Negative Breast Cancer Using Exploratory Subgroup Discovery. *Cancers* 2022, *14*, 5806. https://doi.org/10.3390/cancers14235806

Academic Editor: Enrico Cassano

Received: 6 November 2022
Accepted: 23 November 2022
Published: 25 November 2022

Publisher's Note: MDPI stays neutral with regard to jurisdictional claims in published maps and institutional affiliations.

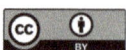

Copyright: © 2022 by the authors. Licensee MDPI, Basel, Switzerland. This article is an open access article distributed under the terms and conditions of the Creative Commons Attribution (CC BY) license (https://creativecommons.org/licenses/by/4.0/).

Simple Summary: Chemoimmunotherapy combinations have transformed the treatment landscape for patients with triple-negative breast cancer (TNBC). However, the discovery of immune-related biomarkers is needed to optimally identify patients requiring the addition of immune-checkpoint inhibitors (ICIs) to chemotherapy. In this study, we identified immune-related gene signatures via exploratory subgroup discovery algorithm that substantially increase the odds of partial remission for TNBC patients on anti-PD-L1+chemotherapy regimen. We have also uncovered distinct cell populations for TNBC patients with various treatment outcomes. Our framework may result in better risk stratification for TNBC patients that undergo chemoimmunotherapy and lead to overall improvement of their health outcomes in the future.

Abstract: Triple-negative breast cancer (TNBC) is an aggressive subtype of breast cancer with limited therapeutic options. Although immunotherapy has shown potential in TNBC patients, clinical studies have only demonstrated a modest response. Therefore, the exploration of immunotherapy in combination with chemotherapy is warranted. In this project we identified immune-related gene signatures for TNBC patients that may explain differences in patients' outcomes after anti-PD-L1+chemotherapy treatment. First, we ran the exploratory subgroup discovery algorithm on the TNBC dataset comprised of 422 patients across 24 studies. Secondly, we narrowed down the search to twelve homogenous subgroups based on tumor mutational burden (TMB, low or high), relapse status (disease-free or recurred), tumor cellularity (high, low and moderate), menopausal status (pre- or post) and tumor stage (I, II and III). For each subgroup we identified a union of the top 10% of genotypic patterns. Furthermore, we employed a multinomial regression model to predict significant genotypic patterns that would be linked to partial remission after anti-PD-L1+chemotherapy treatment. Finally, we uncovered distinct immune cell populations (T-cells, B-cells, Myeloid, NK-cells) for TNBC patients with various treatment outcomes. CD4-Tn-LEF1 and CD4-CXCL13 T-cells were linked to partial remission on anti-PD-L1+chemotherapy treatment. Our informatics pipeline may help to select better responders to chemoimmunotherapy, as well as pinpoint the underlying mechanisms of drug resistance in TNBC patients at single-cell resolution.

Keywords: triple-negative breast cancer; exploratory subgroup discovery; chemoimmunotherapy

1. Introduction

Triple-negative breast cancer (TNBC) occurs in about 10 to 20% of diagnosed breast cancers and defined by the absence or minimal expression of estrogen receptor (ER), progesterone receptor (PR) and epidermal growth factor receptor 2 (HER2) [1,2]. Due to its aggressive clinical phenotype and limited response to hormonal therapy, one in three TNBC patients will likely to relapse within the first three years of primary diagnosis [3]. Although numerous therapeutic agents have been evaluated for the treatment of early TNBC [4], only Olaparib has been approved for the treatment of the small group of patients with high-risk TNBC harboring germline BRCA1 or BRCA2 pathogenic variants in the adjuvant setting [5]. The emergence of cancer immunotherapy, however, is altering the paradigm in TNBC treatment.

TNBC, unlike other breast cancer subtypes, has high tumor mutational burden (TMB), which has been correlated with responsiveness to immune checkpoint inhibitors (ICIs) [6]. Indeed, checkpoint inhibition with the anti-PD1 antibody Pembrolizumab has been approved for advanced-stage, PD-L1 positive TNBC due to improved outcomes when combined with frontline chemotherapy [7]. Interestingly, ICIs are more effective in treating TNBC when given early in the course of the disease, which may be a result of immune escape mechanisms emerging as the condition progresses [8]. More recently, results from the KEYNOTE-522 trial indicated that adding checkpoint inhibition in the early stage setting does in fact improve long-term outcomes [9]. However, subgroup analyses did not pinpoint any strongly predictive biomarkers. For example, PD-L1 expression did not distinguish responders from non-responders in the early setting, with both PD-L1-negative and PD-L1-positive patients obtaining a benefit from Pembrolizumab. Moreover, the addition of immunotherapy increased adverse effects (AEs) [10]. In another study—IMPASSION131– the combination of Paclitaxel with the PD-L1 inhibitor Atezolizumab failed to improve progression-free survival (PFS) or overall survival (OS) in TNBC patients [11]. These findings could be due to imbalances in prognostic features or accidental discoveries in a relatively small trial. Therefore, the exploration of immune-related biomarkers is needed to optimally identify patients requiring the addition of ICIs to chemotherapy [12,13].

In this work we determined homogenous TNBC subgroups based on both phenotypic and genotypic parameters using exploratory subgroup mining. We have also identified significant predictors that increase chances of partial remission in TNBC patients on chemoimmunotherapy treatment using multinomial regression model on TNBC scRNA-seq dataset. Lastly, we uncovered distinct immune cell populations (T-cells, B-cells, Myeloid, NK-cells) for TNBC patients with various treatment outcomes. We interpreted our results using biomedical knowledge, including findings from existing clinical trials, immunohistochemistry experiments and functional characterization of specific genes. The proposed informatics pipeline may assist health care professionals in the selection of chemoimmunotherapy responders, as well as determine the underlying causes of drug resistance in TNBC patients at a single-cell level and resolution.

2. Materials and Methods

2.1. Data Mapping

In this study we employed two datasets. Each dataset consisted of multiple phenotypic (either categorical or continuous) and genotypic (continuous only) variables. Each categorical variable was labeled based on the National Comprehensive Cancer Network (NCCN) Guidelines in Oncology [14]. For example, relapse-free status was categorized as (1) disease-free or (2) recurred. Continuous variables were converted into categoric variables by grouping values into several categories. For example, normalized gene expression values were categorized as (1) downregulated, (2) upregulated, or (3) non-differentially expressed.

The first TNBC dataset comprised of 422 patients. These patients were selected from 24 breast cancer studies available at the cBioPortal platform [15]. The final dataset included breast cancer patients based on the following immunohistochemical profile: ER-negative, PR-negative and HER2-negative. This dataset consisted of 12 phenotypic variables, including clinical-pathologic data (age at diagnosis, menopausal status, tumor type, tumor stage, tumor cellularity, histologic grade, TMB), treatment regimen (chemotherapy, radiotherapy, hormone therapy) and survival status (overall survival status, relapse-free status). There were 1067 genotypic variables in the form of normalized gene expression values derived from human immunome (immune-related genes) and human kinome (protein kinase genes).

The second TNBC dataset consisted of scRNA-seq profiles for 22 TNBC patients that underwent chemotherapy (*Pactilaxel*) or chemoimmunotherapy treatment (*Paclitaxel* with *Atezolizumab*) [16]. For this study we selected six phenotypic variables, including information about treatment timeline (pre-, post-treatment, progression), tissue type (tumor or blood), tumor site (brain, breast, chest wall, liver, lymph nodes), treatment type (anti-PD-L1+chemotherapy or chemotherapy only), treatment response (partial response (PR), stable disease (SD), progressive disease (PD) and cell cluster (T-cells, B-cells, Myeloid, NK-cells)). We used the same genotypic variables as in the TNBC subgroup discovery dataset.

2.2. The Informatics Pipeline

Our informatics pipeline has three modules: (1) exploratory subgroup discovery, (2) inference module based on multinomial regression model and (3) immune cell populations discovery. Our goal was two-fold: (1) to identify significant genes from exploratory subgroup discovery that increase odds of having partial remission after anti-PD-L1+chemotherapy treatment and (2) to uncover unique immune cell populations for TNBC subgroups with various treatment outcomes.

The main goal of exploratory subgroup discovery module was to determine homogenous patient subgroups based on expanatory phenotypic characteristics (Module A on Figure 1), where prevailing number of patients in that subgroup exemplify distinctive genotypic patterns (Module B on Figure 1). Each genotypic pattern had been represented as a combination of differentially expressed genes. For example, the genotypic pattern may consist of three genes: upregulated EGFR, downregulated MTOR and upregulated MAPK1 genes. On the first step, the algorithm determines the base subgroup (e.g., Chemotherapy = Yes) contingent on the most significant contrast against the rest of the population. On the next inclusion step it adds a new phenotypic variable, e.g., TMB = High, to the previous subgroup to generate a more focused subgroup (Chemotherapy = Yes and TMB = High). Subsequently, the exclusion step is employed to remove a less relevant inclusion move after each inclusion step. The exploratory search selects multiple paths that form multiple subgroups and have equally relevant genotypic patterns within each subgroup. When the algorithm reaches the most focused subgroup with the highest contrast score that cannot be further increased, the search would be terminated. Support [17] and growth rate [18] were used to measure the frequency for a specific genotypic pattern in the homogenous subgroup. We then applied a J-value [19] to prioritize each subgroup based on the relevance (contrasts) for all patterns in each subgroup [20].

To find significant predictors of partial remission on anti-PD-L1+chemotherapy regimen, we employed multinomial regression model (Module C on Figure 1) on the scRNA-seq TNBC dataset. The outcome variable was categorical and represented as a combination of treatment response, treatment timeline, and treatment type. For example, the level of outcome variable can be encoded as *SD-Post_treatment-Chemo* meaning that a fraction of TNBC patients achieved stable disease after treatment with chemotherapy only. Overall, there were ten levels of outcome variable. We set *PD-Post_treatment-Chemo*—progressive disease after chemotherapy—as a baseline for the model. The continuous covariates were encoded as genes with normalized gene expression values identified as a top 10% of genotypic patterns in the exploratory subgroup discovery stage. We used the multinom function from the nnet package [21] to estimate a multinomial logistic regression model. We computed p-values via two-tailed z-test to identify significant predictors of response to anti-PD-L1+chemotherapy treatment.

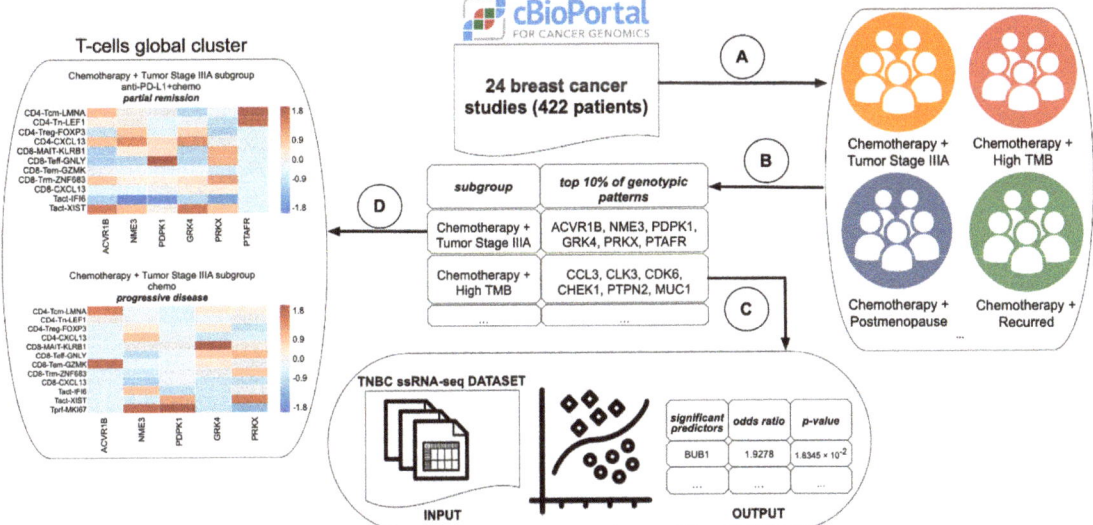

Figure 1. The informatics pipeline. Modules (**A**) and (**B**)—the exploratory subgroup discovery process, Module (**C**)—the inference module based on multinomial regression model, Module (**D**)—immune cell populations discovery.

The immune cell populations discovery module (Module D on Figure 1) determined distinct immune cell populations (T-cells, B-cells, Myeloid, NK-cells) for TNBC patients with various treatment outcomes. Each TNBC subgroup had two conditions: (1) anti-PD-L1+chemotherapy, post treatment, partial remission and (2) chemotherapy, post treatment, PD. Using the top 10% of genotypic patterns from exploratory mining stage as an input, we generated heatmap plots for each condition in every TNBC subgroup of interest. For example, NME3 gene was represented as a geometric mean of NME3 expression values in CD4-Tcm-LMNA cells [22]. Finally, we compared immune cell populations in these two conditions to identify mutually exclusive cell populations that were associated with either partial remission after anti-PD-L1+chemotherapy treatment or progressive disease after chemotherapy treatment.

3. Results

3.1. The Identification of Homogenous TNBC Subgroups

First, we ran the exploratory subgroup discovery algorithm on the TNBC dataset described in Section 2.1. The algorithm revealed 11,944 subgroups. We focused our analysis of the 460 subgroups where TNBC patients had undergone chemotherapy. On the next step, we narrowed down the search to twelve homogenous subgroups based on TMB (low or high), relapse status (disease-free or recurred), tumor cellularity (high, low and moderate), menopausal status (pre- or post) and tumor stage (I, II and III). Since the lengths of genotypic patterns vary (up to 5 genes), we decided to make a union of top 10% of genotypic patterns for each subgroup of interest. Let us assume that each genotypic pattern is a set of elements, where each element is a unique differentially expressed gene (e.g., upregulated *MTOR* gene). The union would represent a set of a collection of genotypic patterns, where each element would not be repetitive. These genotypic patterns were used as covariates for the multinomial regression model in the next section.

3.2. Significant Predictors of Partial Remission after Anti-PD-L1+Chemotherapy

The multinomial regression model on scRNA-seq TNBC dataset was able to identify significant predictors from exploratory subgroup discovery results that increase odds of having partial remission after anti-PD-L1+chemotherapy treatment versus progressive disease after chemotherapy (Table 1).

Table 1. Significant predictors that increase odds of partial remission after anti-PD-L1+chemotherapy identified by our informatics pipeline.

Subgroups	Predictors	Coefficients	p-Values	Odds Ratio
Chemotherapy (Yes) TMB (High)	ACVR1B	0.4506	0.0136	1.5692
	PDPK1	0.1271	0.0169	1.1355
Chemotherapy (Yes) TMB (Low)	CLK3	0.1402	0.0017	1.1505
	TAOK2	0.6603	<0.0001	1.9354
Chemotherapy (Yes) Relapse Status (Disease Free)	CDK9	0.4152	<0.0001	1.5146
	CFP	0.2368	0.0438	1.2673
	VRK3	0.1591	0.0011	1.1725
Chemotherapy (Yes) Relapse Status (Recurred)	BUB1	0.6563	0.0183	1.9278
	BAZ1B	0.3529	<0.0001	1.4232
Chemotherapy (Yes) Tumor Cellularity (High)	PDIK1L	0.6405	1.3243×10^{-5}	1.8974
	KIR2DL4	1.8931	0.0094	6.6403
	MAPK3	0.8886	<0.0001	2.4319
	STK24	0.2842	<0.0001	1.3287
Chemotherapy (Yes) Tumor Cellularity (Low)	IFI16	0.0665	0.0205	1.0688
	CSK	0.2397	<0.0001	1.2709
	TAP2	0.2165	0.0185	1.2417
	TIGIT	0.5160	<0.0001	1.6754
Chemotherapy (Yes) Menopausal Status (Pre)	CCR6	0.1307	0.0023	1.1396
	BCL10	0.1222	0.0064	1.1300
	PRKCA	0.9982	<0.0001	2.7135
	EPHB6	0.8559	<0.0001	2.3536
	IFNAR2	0.4546	6.4298×10^{-6}	1.5756
Chemotherapy (Yes) Menopausal Status (Post)	PDIK1L	0.4952	0.0003	1.6409
	RPS6KA5	0.2836	<0.0001	1.3279
	IKZF2	0.4714	<0.0001	1.6023
Chemotherapy (Yes) Tumor Stage (I)	RIOK3	0.1683	2.4615×10^{-5}	1.1833
Chemotherapy (Yes) Tumor Stage (II)	PRKCA	1.0213	<0.0001	2.7770
Chemotherapy (Yes) Tumor Stage (III)	IFIH1	0.3366	1.2977×10^{-5}	0.1773
	CDKL5	0.7786	0.0066	2.1785

Next, we highlight the importance of identified phenotypic features from Table 1 for TNBC patient outcomes. Using literature, high-TMB TNBC status may benefit specifically from ICIs in combination with chemotherapy [23] or ICIs alone [24]. TNBC patients have high TMB due to accumulation of genomic instability, which leads to the production neoantigens, thereby resulting in strong effector cell responses [25]. TNBC tumors have a "hot tumor phenotype", which characterized by a high degree of immune infiltration and associated with improved survival outcomes regardless of tumor stage, molecular subtype, PD-L1 status, age and treatment schedule [26]. The IMpassion130 trial tested immunotherapy agent Durvalumab in combination with chemotherapy or chemotherapy alone on 149 early stage TNBC patients. Median TMB was significantly higher in patients with pathologic complete response (pCR) (median 1.87 versus 1.39, $p = 0.005$), and odds ratios for pCR per mut/MB were 2.06 (95% CI 1.33–3.20) among all patients, 1.77 (95% CI 1.00–3.13) in the Durvalumab arm, and 2.82 (95% CI 1.21–6.54) in the chemotherapy arm. Interestingly, the association between pCR and TMB was more pronounced in patients treated with chemotherapy alone. The KEYNOTE-119 trial evaluated metastatic TNBC patients treated with Pembrolizumab monotherapy versus chemotherapy. The positive association was observed between TMB and clinical response to Pembrolizumab (ORR

$p = 0.154$, PSF $p = 0.014$, OS $p = 0.018$) but not to chemotherapy (ORR $p = 0.114$, PFS $p = 0.478$, OS $p = 0.906$). ORR and hazard ratio (HR) for OS also suggested a trend towards increased benefit with Pembrolizumab versus chemotherapy in TNBC patients with high TMB. This clinical trial was constrained by the small sample size and low number of TMB-high cases.

In terms of relapse status, one study suggested that rapid versus late relapse in TNBC might be characterized by unique clinical and genomic features [27]. Both 'rapid relapse' (rrTNBC) and 'late relapse' (lrTNBC) groups had significantly lower expression of immune-related genes. Intriguingly, lrTNBCs were enriched for luminal signatures. There was no difference in TMB or percent genome altered across investigated subgroups of TNBC patients.

In connection to menopausal status, TNBC was observed primarily in postmenopausal patients [28]. The overexpression of the p53 protein, a significantly higher Ki-67 proliferation index value, and a higher nuclear grade was detected in TNBC premenopausal patients. A multivariate analysis estimated that menopausal status, nodal status, and tumor size were significant contributors for disease-free survival (DFS) in TNBC cases.

We had also discovered novel phenotypic features in TNBC subgroups, such as tumor cellularity and tumor stage. The evaluation of tumor cellularity, defined as the percentage of invasive tumor comprised of tumor cells, may represent an informative histologic measure of the differential response of TNBC to chemoimmunotherapy. To classify the severity of a malignant disease in a particular patient, the tumor staging system is employed during the course of disease. This system is essential in optimizing cancer patients treatment options and their risk stratification. Therefore, these features can be important in the design and analysis of intervention studies, including randomized clinical trials, to better assess their prognostic utility for TNBC patients.

3.3. Differences in Immune Cell Populations for Discovered TNBC Subgroups

This section described immune cell populations that were discovered in scRNA-seq TNBC data based on genotypic patterns from exploratory mining stage. We interpreted our results using biomedical knowledge, including findings from existing clinical trials, immunohistochemistry experiments and functional characterization of specific genes. The summary of our findings is presented in Table 2.

Table 2. Immune cell populations that are linked to the specific TNBC outcome determined by our informatics pipeline.

Condition	T-Cells	B-Cells	Myeloid Cells	NK-Cells
anti-PD-L1 post treatment partial remission	CD4-Tn-LEF1 CD4-CXCL13	-	-	ILC3-AREG ILC3-IL7R
chemo post treatment progressive disease	Tact-IFI6	pB-IGHG1	cDC1-CLEC9A macro-CFD macro-FOLR2 macro-MKI67 macro-SPP1 macro-TUBA1B mono-FCN1 mono-S100A89 mono-SMIM25	ILC1-VCAM1

3.3.1. T-Cells Global Cluster

The proliferative MKI67$^+$ T-cells (Tprf-MKI67) were exclusively present in TNBC patients achieving progressive disease after chemotherapy. Based on literature findings, the expression of MKI67 gene was significantly correlated with lymph node metastases, tumor invasion and adverse survival outcome in TNBC [29]. In addition, more unfavourable survival outcomes in breast cancer patients with recurrent lesions were significantly correlated with high Ki-67 immunohistochemical expression levels (hazard ratio 2.307; 95% confidence interval 1.207–4.407, p-value = 0.011) [30]. Therefore, MKI67 may be an important biomarker of predictive and prognostic value in TNBC.

CD4-Tn-LEF1 and CD4-CXCL13 T-cells were linked to partial remission after anti-PD-L1+chemotherapy treatment. Importantly, these CD4$^+$ T-cells express very high amounts of PD-1 and other co-stimulatory and inhibitory receptors. Therefore, they instrumental to B-cells for efficient antibody responses and their presence in tumor samples is often correlated with a better outcome in patients with solid tumors [31]. Based on biomedical literature, the presence of CD4-CXCL13 T-cells in TNBC tumors responsive to chemoimmunotherapy was detected through immunohistochemistry staining [16,32]. In addition to CXCL13$^+$ T-cells, naïve LEF1$^+$ T-cells (Tn-LEF1) were also linked to a favorable response to both anti-PD-L1+chemotherapy and chemotherapy. In a recent study, the magnitude of lymphocytic infiltration was assessed by a four-gene signature—HLF, CXCL13, SULT1E1 and GBP1, which was indicative of favourable outcome in TNBC after neoadjuvant therapy. This signature may help to identify early stage TNBC patients and being a novel prognostic biomarker of this aggressive disease [33].

The activated IFI6$^+$ T-cells (Tact-IFI6) were linked to progressive disease after chemotherapy. The poor metastasis-free survival in breast cancer patients was linked to upregulation of mitochondrial antiapoptotic protein IFI6 that might be involved in regulation of mitochondrial ROS production [34]. Therefore, to improve clinical outcomes in breast cancer patients, the deactivation of mitochondrial functions of IFI6 is paramount.

3.3.2. B-Cells Global Cluster

The MKI67$^+$ follicular B-cells (Bfoc-MKI67), NEIL1$^+$ follicular B-cells (Bfoc-NEIL1) and MKI67$^+$ memory B-cells (Bmem-MKI67) were exclusively present in TNBC patients with partial remission after anti-PD-L1+chemotherapy treatment. Based on biomedical literature, follicular B-cells was associated with favorable outcomes for TCGA patients with breast cancer [35]. The naïve B-cells, memory B-cells and follicular B-cells were present primarily in patients responsive to chemoimmunotherapy but not in patients responsive to chemotherapy treatment [16]. In regard with Bfoc-NEIL1 cell population, NEIL1 implicated in repair of oxidative damage associated with DNA replication or transcription [36]. Reduction in NEIL1 expression was associated with a poorer outcome in patients with breast invasive carcinoma [37]. Hence, NEIL1 could be a promising biomarker for TNBC patients that consider chemoimmunotherapy treatment.

Plasma IGHG1$^+$ B-cells (pB-IGHG1) were linked to progressive disease after chemotherapy treatment. In TNBC, the expression of IGHG1 indicated the most significant prognostic value compared to trivial clinicopathological parameters [38]. Intriguingly, IGHG1 expression in B-cells and plasma cells could be associated with immune evasion and tumor cell proliferation in breast malignancies [39]. These data may imply that B cells or plasma cells could have pro-tumoral roles under particular conditions; however, the factors influencing the emergence of this pathologic phenotype and the roles played by B cells and plasma cells in these contexts remains unclear.

3.3.3. Myeloid Cells Global Cluster

The MMP9$^+$ macrophages (macro-MMP9) were exclusively present in TNBC patients with partial remission after anti-PD-L1+chemotherapy treatment. The literature search revealed that MMPs have a intricate role in cancer progression and may exert both pro- and antitumorigenic activities [40]. Although MMP expression has been linked to tumor progression in various cancer types including breast cancer [41], clinical trials investigating the effect of broad-spectrum MMP inhibitors have failed, and in some cases, patients treated with these inhibitors even progressed after treatment comparing to control placebo group [42]. Indeed, the overexpression of MMP9 results in increased production of antiangiogenic fragments, decreased angiogenesis, and therapeutic effects of established breast cancer [43]. In another study, gene transfer of MMP-9 to ex vivo breast cancer tumors caused tumor regression via increased neutrophil infiltration and an activation of tumor-associated macrophages (TAMs) [44]. Therefore, MMP9 can serve as a biomarker for predicting tumor regression in TNBC.

The macro-CCL2, macro-CX3CR1, macro-IFI27, macro-IGFBP7, macro-IL1B9, macro-MGP and macro-SLC40A1 cells were exclusively present in TNBC patients achieving progressive disease after chemotherapy. Based on biomedical findings, CCL2 expression in breast carcinomas was highly associated with macrophage infiltration, and its expression was correlated with poor prognosis in breast cancer patients [45]. In another study, chemokine receptor CX3CR1 showed a role in angiogenic macrophage survival in the tumor microenvironment contributing to tumor metastasis [46]. In a similar fashion, IFI27 overexpression was shown to impair the tamoxifen-induced apoptosis in breast cancer cells [47]. Finally, IL1B signalling contributed to breast cancer metastasis by enhancing tumor cell motility and inhibiting cell proliferation [48]. These findings highlight the importance of CCL2, CX3CR1, IFI27 and IL1B expressed in macrophages in progression of TNBC.

The CLEC9A$^+$ dendritic cells (cDC1-CLEC9A), macro-CFD, macro-FOLR2, macro-MKI67, macro-SPP1, macro-TUBA1B, FCN1$^+$ monocytes (mono-FCN1), mono-S100A89 and mono-SMIM25 cells were linked to progressive disease after chemotherapy treatment. Notably, CFD functioned as an enhancer of tumor proliferation and cancer stem cell properties in breast cancers [49]. In another study, SPP1-associated macrophages in the tumor-adipose microenvironment facilitate breast cancer progression [50]. Interestingly, S100A8/A9, which are calcium-binding proteins that are secreted primarily by granulocytes and monocytes, may be associated with the loss of estrogen receptor and may be involved in the poor prognosis of Her2$^+$/basal-like subtypes of breast cancer. Therefore, myeloid cell populations expressing CFD, SPP1 and S100A89 might be crucial biomarkers of poor treatment response in TNBC.

3.3.4. NK-Cells Global Cluster

The CNOT2$^+$ group 2 innate lymphoid cells (ILC2-CNOT2) were exclusively present in TNBC patients achieving partial remission after anti-PD-L1+chemotherapy treatment. Indeed, ILC2s involved in both anti-tumor and pro-tumoral immunity in a variety of human cancers [51]. In terms of pro-tumoral immunity, the promotion of tumor growth and metastasis is achieved by crosstalk between ILC2s and tumor microenviroment (TME) [52]. In addition, the ILC2s trigger the apoptosis of tumor cells by recruiting and activating eosinophils [53], CXCL1L/CXCL2L molecules and macrophages with M1 profile [54].

The ZNF683$^+$ group 1 innate lymphoid cells (ILC1-ZNF683) cells were exclusively present in TNBC patients achieving progressive disease after chemotherapy. The biomedical literature demonstrates that ILC1 cells involved in inhibiting the antitumoral immune response, enabling the differential tumor infiltration of ILC1 cells in patients to improve the levaraging of immunity in cancer therapies [55]. However, the role of ZNF683 gene in particular remains elusive.

ILC3-AREG and ILC3-IL7R cells were linked to partial remission after anti-PD-L1 +chemotherapy treatment. It had been shown that ILC3-IL7R could predict a favorable response to both treatment regimens, indicating its potential role in effective antitumor immunity [16]. In contrary, ILC1-VCAM1 cells were linked to progressive disease after chemotherapy treatment. Recent studies have shown that vascular cell adhesion molecule-1 (VCAM1) is aberrantly expressed in breast cancer cells and mediates prometastatic tumor-stromal interactions [56]. Therefore, AREG$^+$, IL7R$^+$ and VCAM1$^+$ innate lymphoid cells can help determine prognosis for breast cancer patients.

4. Discussion

The analysis of the TNBC scRNA-seq data revealed distinct immune cell populations that are linked to either partial remission after anti-PD-L1+chemotherapy or progressive disease after chemotherapy only. In terms of T-cells, CD4-Tn-LEF1 and CD4-CXCL13 T-cells were linked to partial remission after anti-PD-L1+chemotherapy treatment, while Tact-IFI6 T-cells were linked to progressive disease after chemotherapy. The naïve B-cells, memory B-cells and follicular B-cells were mainly enriched in tumors responsive to chemoimmunotherapy but not in tumors responsive to chemotherapy treatment. The MMP9$^+$ macrophages (macro-MMP9) were exclusively present in TNBC patients with partial remission after anti-PD-L1+chemotherapy treatment, while heterogenous population of macrophages, including macro-CCL2, macro-CX3CR1, macro-IFI27, macro-IGFBP7, macro-IL1B9, macro-MGP and macro-SLC40A1 cells were exclusively present in TNBC patients achieving progressive disease after chemotherapy. Finally, group 3 innate lymphoid cells (ILC3-AREG and ILC3-IL7R) were linked to partial remission after anti-PD-L1+chemotherapy treatment, while ZNF683$^+$ group 1 innate lymphoid cells (ILC1-ZNF683) cells were exclusively present in TNBC patients achieving progressive disease after chemotherapy. Each of these cell populations have distinctive genetic markers that could be useful therapeutic targets for chemoimmunotherapy.

The role of T follicular helper and B-cell crosstalk in tumor immunity has been extensively studied over the last decade. Accumulating evidence suggests that tumor infiltrated lymphocyte (TIL) subpopulations (CD4, CD8, and CD19/20) constitute of both suppressive (pro-tumor) or effector (anti-tumor) phenotypes whose functions are influenced by the surrounding TME [57]. Natural or treatment-induced immune activation or suppression may determine the balance between pro- or anti-tumor immune cell crosstalk within a given tumor. Key anti-tumor effector activities include antibody-dependent cell cytotoxicity, complement activation, antibody-mediated tumor cell phagocytosis, antigen presentation, T cell activation, cytokine secretion, and direct tumor killing by TIL, including CD8, NK, B cells, and/or macrophages [58].

Despite of significant survival advantages that could be achieved after treatment with chemoimmunotherapy, most TNBC patients would not benefit. Therefore, more and more attention has been paid to the identification and development of biomarkers for the response of chemoimmunotherapy in recent years. Our informatics pipeline identified novel phenotypic and genotypic predictors in unsupervised manner that indicative of favorable outcome after chemoimmunotherapy. These predictors could be important biomarkers in the design and analysis of intervention studies and ultimately could help to optimize therapy decisions for TNBC patients. In addition, it may help to select better responders to chemoimmunotherapy, as well as pinpoint the underlying mechanisms of drug resistance in TNBC patients at single-cell resolution.

5. Conclusions

To tackle patient heterogeneity, chemoimmunotherapy combinations represent a feasible alternative for TNBC patients. However, matching patient subgroups to effective treatments that increase their chance of survival remains a challenging endeavor. In this work, we augmented our exploratory subgroup discovery algorithm to identify TNBC subpopulations that may benefit from chemoimmunotherapy. Specifically, we identified immune-related gene signatures that increased the likelihood of partial remission after anti-PD-L1+chemotherapy regimen versus progressive disease after chemotherapy in TNBC patients. Our novel informatics pipeline identified immune cell populations that associated with various treatment outcomes in TNBC. We also showed the importance of TMB and menopausal status among the investigated TNBC subgroups. The potential limitations include the usage of two disjoint datasets and the absence of outcome variable for immunotherapy outcomes in TCGA datasets. Further validation of our computational results in wet-lab studies would be a significant step toward improving survival outcomes for TNBC patients.

Author Contributions: Conceptualization, O.K. and C.-R.S.; methodology, O.K.; software, W.I.B.; validation, O.K. and C.-R.S.; formal analysis, O.K., W.I.B. and C.-R.S.; data curation, O.K.; writing—original draft preparation, O.K. and C.-R.S.; writing—review and editing, C.-R.S., J.B.M., J.T.K., R.D.H. and C.N.P.; visualization, O.K.; supervision, C.-R.S. and J.B.M.; project administration, C.-R.S.; funding acquisition, C.-R.S. All authors have read and agreed to the published version of the manuscript.

Funding: This research study was funded by University of Missouri Institute for Data Science and Informatics to O.K and W.I.B. and Data-Driven and Artificial Intelligence Initiatives to C.-R.S., O.K. and C.-R.S. were funded by Shumaker Endowment for Bioinformatics. J.B.M. received funding from the Department of Veteran's Affairs (K2BX004346-01A1). The content is solely the responsibility of the authors and does not necessarily represent the official views of the Department of Veterans' Affairs. The funding bodies had no role in the study design; in the collection, analysis, interpretation of data; or in the writing of the manuscript.

Institutional Review Board Statement: Not applicable.

Informed Consent Statement: Not applicable.

Data Availability Statement: The TCGA dataset is available online at https://www.cbioportal.org (accessed on 22 August 2022). The scRNA-seq TNBC dataset is available online at http://tnbc_pd-l1.cancer-pku.cn (accessed on 22 August 2022).

Acknowledgments: We appreciate the critical input of members from Interdisciplinary Data Analytics and Search (iDAS) Laboratory at University of Missouri, Columbia.

Conflicts of Interest: The authors declare no conflict of interest.

References

1. Moss, J.L.; Tatalovich, Z.; Zhu, L.; Morgan, C.; Cronin, K.A. Triple-negative breast cancer incidence in the United States: Ecological correlations with area-level sociodemographics, healthcare, and health behaviors. *Breast Cancer* **2020**, *28*, 82–91. [CrossRef]
2. Lehmann, B.D.; Pietenpol, J.A. Identification and use of biomarkers in treatment strategies for triple-negative breast cancer subtypes. *J. Pathol.* **2014**, *232*, 142–150. [CrossRef]
3. Gupta, G.K.; Collier, A.L.; Lee, D.; Hoefer, R.A.; Zheleva, V.; Van Reesema, L.L.S.; Tang-Tan, A.M.; Guye, M.L.; Chang, D.Z.; Winston, J.S.; et al. Perspectives on Triple-Negative Breast Cancer: Current Treatment Strategies, Unmet Needs, and Potential Targets for Future Therapies. *Cancers* **2020**, *12*, 2392. [CrossRef]
4. Tarantino, P.; Corti, C.; Schmid, P.; Cortes, J.; Mittendorf, E.A.; Rugo, H.; Tolaney, S.M.; Bianchini, G.; Andrè, F.; Curigliano, G. Immunotherapy for early triple negative breast cancer: Research agenda for the next decade. *NPJ Breast Cancer* **2022**, *8*, 23. [CrossRef]
5. Tutt, A.N.; Garber, J.E.; Kaufman, B.; Viale, G.; Fumagalli, D.; Rastogi, P.; Gelber, R.D.; de Azambuja, E.; Fielding, A.; Balmaña, J.; et al. Adjuvant Olaparib for Patients with BRCA1- or BRCA2-Mutated Breast Cancer. *N. Engl. J. Med.* **2021**, *384*, 2394–2405. [CrossRef]
6. O'Meara, T.A.; Tolaney, S.M. Tumor mutational burden as a predictor of immunotherapy response in breast cancer. *Oncotarget* **2021**, *12*, 394–400. [CrossRef]
7. Cortes, J.; Cescon, D.W.; Rugo, H.S.; Nowecki, Z.; Im, S.-A.; Yusof, M.M.; Gallardo, C.; Lipatov, O.; Barrios, C.H.; Holgado, E.; et al. Pembrolizumab plus chemotherapy versus placebo plus chemotherapy for previously untreated locally recurrent inoperable or metastatic triple-negative breast cancer (KEYNOTE-355): A randomised, placebo-controlled, double-blind, phase 3 clinical trial. *Lancet* **2020**, *396*, 1817–1828. [CrossRef]
8. Hutchinson, K.E.; Yost, S.E.; Chang, C.-W.; Johnson, R.M.; Carr, A.R.; McAdam, P.R.; Halligan, D.L.; Chang, C.-C.; Schmolze, D.; Liang, J.; et al. Comprehensive Profiling of Poor-Risk Paired Primary and Recurrent Triple-Negative Breast Cancers Reveals Immune Phenotype Shifts. *Clin. Cancer Res.* **2020**, *26*, 657–668. [CrossRef]
9. Schmid, P.; Cortes, J.; Dent, R.; Pusztai, L.; McArthur, H.; Kümmel, S.; Bergh, J.; Denkert, C.; Park, Y.H.; Hui, R.; et al. VP7-2021: KEYNOTE-522: Phase III study of neoadjuvant pembrolizumab + chemotherapy vs. placebo + chemotherapy, followed by adjuvant pembrolizumab vs. placebo for early-stage TNBC. *Ann. Oncol.* **2021**, *32*, 1198–1200. [CrossRef]
10. Criscitiello, C.; Corti, C.; Pravettoni, G.; Curigliano, G. Managing side effects of immune checkpoint inhibitors in breast cancer. *Crit. Rev. Oncol. Hematol.* **2021**, *162*, 103354. [CrossRef]
11. Miles, D.; Gligorov, J.; André, F.; Cameron, D.; Schneeweiss, A.; Barrios, C.; Xu, B.; Wardley, A.; Kaen, D.; Andrade, L.; et al. Primary results from IMpassion131, a double-blind, placebo-controlled, randomised phase III trial of first-line paclitaxel with or without atezolizumab for unresectable locally advanced/metastatic triple-negative breast cancer. *Ann. Oncol. Off. J. Eur. Soc. Med. Oncol.* **2021**, *32*, 994–1004. [CrossRef]
12. Davis, A.A.; Patel, V.G. The role of PD-L1 expression as a predictive biomarker: An analysis of all US Food and Drug Administration (FDA) approvals of immune checkpoint inhibitors. *J. Immunother. Cancer* **2019**, *7*, 278. [CrossRef]

13. Cristescu, R.; Aurora-Garg, D.; Albright, A.; Xu, L.; Liu, X.Q.; Loboda, A.; Lang, L.; Jin, F.; Rubin, E.H.; Snyder, A.; et al. Tumor mutational burden predicts the efficacy of pembrolizumab monotherapy: A pan-tumor retrospective analysis of participants with advanced solid tumors. *J. Immunother. Cancer* **2022**, *10*, e003091. [CrossRef]
14. Gradishar, W.J.; Anderson, B.O.; Abraham, J.; Aft, R.; Agnese, D.; Allison, K.H.; Blair, S.L.; Burstein, H.J.; Dang, C.; Elias, A.D.; et al. Breast Cancer, Version 3.2020, NCCN Clinical Practice Guidelines in Oncology. *J. Natl. Compr. Cancer Netw. JNCCN* **2020**, *18*, 452–478. [CrossRef]
15. Gao, J.; Aksoy, B.A.; Dogrusoz, U.; Dresdner, G.; Gross, B.E.; Sumer, S.O.; Sun, Y.; Jacobsen, A.; Sinha, R.; Larsson, E.; et al. Integrative Analysis of Complex Cancer Genomics and Clinical Profiles Using the cBioPortal. *Sci. Signal.* **2013**, *6*, pl1. [CrossRef]
16. Zhang, Y.; Chen, H.; Mo, H.; Hu, X.; Gao, R.; Zhao, Y.; Liu, B.; Niu, L.; Sun, X.; Yu, X.; et al. Single-cell analyses reveal key immune cell subsets associated with response to PD-L1 blockade in triple-negative breast cancer. *Cancer Cell* **2021**, *39*, 1578–1593.e8. [CrossRef]
17. Agrawal, R.; Srikant, R. Fast Algorithms for Mining Association Rules in Large Databases. In Proceedings of the 20th International Conference on Very Large Data Bases, VLDB '94, Santiago de Chile, Chile, 12–15 September 1994; Morgan Kaufmann Publishers Inc.: Burlington, MA, USA, 1994; pp. 487–499.
18. Dong, G.; Li, J. Efficient mining of emerging patterns: Discovering trends and differences. In Proceedings of the Fifth ACM SIGKDD International Conference on Knowledge Discovery and Data Mining, KDD '99, San Diego, CA, USA, 15–18 August 1999; Association for Computing Machinery: New York, NY, USA, 1999; pp. 43–52. [CrossRef]
19. Egghe, L. Theory and practise of the g-index. *Scientometrics* **2006**, *69*, 131–152. [CrossRef]
20. Liu, D.; Baskett, W.; Beversdorf, D.; Shyu, C.-R. Exploratory Data Mining for Subgroup Cohort Discoveries and Prioritization. *IEEE J. Biomed. Health Inform.* **2020**, *24*, 1456–1468. [CrossRef]
21. Nnet: Feed-Forward Neural Networks and Multinomial Log-Linear Models Version 7.3-17 from CRAN. Available online: https://rdrr.io/cran/nnet/ (accessed on 2 September 2022).
22. Azizi, E.; Carr, A.J.; Plitas, G.; Cornish, A.E.; Konopacki, C.; Prabhakaran, S.; Nainys, J.; Wu, K.; Kiselovas, V.; Setty, M.; et al. Single-Cell Map of Diverse Immune Phenotypes in the Breast Tumor Microenvironment. *Cell* **2018**, *174*, 1293–1308.e36. [CrossRef]
23. Karn, T.; Denkert, C.; Weber, K.; Holtrich, U.; Hanusch, C.; Sinn, B.; Higgs, B.; Jank, P.; Sinn, H.; Huober, J.; et al. Tumor mutational burden and immune infiltration as independent predictors of response to neoadjuvant immune checkpoint inhibition in early TNBC in GeparNuevo. *Ann. Oncol. Off. J. Eur. Soc. Med. Oncol.* **2020**, *31*, 1216–1222. [CrossRef]
24. Winer, E.P.; Lipatov, O.; Im, S.-A.; Goncalves, A.; Muñoz-Couselo, E.; Lee, K.S.; Schmid, P.; Testa, L.; Witzel, I.; Ohtani, S.; et al. Association of tumor mutational burden (TMB) and clinical outcomes with pembrolizumab (pembro) versus chemotherapy (chemo) in patients with metastatic triple-negative breast cancer (mTNBC) from KEYNOTE-119. *J. Clin. Oncol.* **2020**, *38* (Suppl. 15), 1013. [CrossRef]
25. El Bairi, K.; Haynes, H.R.; Blackley, E.; Fineberg, S.; Shear, J.; Turner, S.; de Freitas, J.R.; Sur, D.; Amendola, L.C.; Gharib, M.; et al. The tale of TILs in breast cancer: A report from The International Immuno-Oncology Biomarker Working Group. *NPJ Breast Cancer* **2021**, *7*, 150. [CrossRef]
26. Thomas, A.; Routh, E.; Pullikuth, A.; Jin, G.; Su, J.; Chou, J.W.; Hoadley, K.; Print, C.; Knowlton, N.; Black, M.A.; et al. Tumor mutational burden is a determinant of immune-mediated survival in breast cancer. *OncoImmunology* **2018**, *7*, e1490854. [CrossRef]
27. Zhang, Y.; Asad, S.; Weber, Z.; Tallman, D.; Nock, W.; Wyse, M.; Bey, J.F.; Dean, K.L.; Adams, E.J.; Stockard, S.; et al. Genomic features of rapid versus late relapse in triple negative breast cancer. *BMC Cancer* **2021**, *21*, 568. [CrossRef]
28. Nishimura, R.; Osako, T.; Okumura, Y.; Nakano, M.; Otsuka, H.; Fujisue, M.; Arima, N. Triple Negative Breast Cancer: An Analysis of the Subtypes and the Effects of Menopausal Status on Invasive Breast Cancer. *J. Clin. Med.* **2022**, *11*, 2331. [CrossRef]
29. A Arafah, M.; Ouban, A.; Ameer, O.Z.; Quek, K.J. KI-67 LI Expression in Triple-Negative Breast Cancer Patients and Its Significance. *Breast Cancer: Basic Clin. Res.* **2021**, *15*, 11782234211016977. [CrossRef]
30. Inari, H.; Suganuma, N.; Kawachi, K.; Yoshida, T.; Yamanaka, T.; Nakamura, Y.; Yoshihara, M.; Nakayama, H.; Masudo, K.; Oshima, T.; et al. Clinicopathological and prognostic significance of Ki-67 immunohistochemical expression of distant metastatic lesions in patients with metastatic breast cancer. *Breast Cancer* **2017**, *24*, 748–755. [CrossRef]
31. Baumjohann, D.; Brossart, P. T follicular helper cells: Linking cancer immunotherapy and immune-related adverse events. *J. Immunother. Cancer* **2021**, *9*, e002588. [CrossRef]
32. Ma, Q.; Chen, Y.; Qin, Q.; Guo, F.; Wang, Y.-S.; Li, D. CXCL13 expression in mouse 4T1 breast cancer microenvironment elicits antitumor immune response by regulating immune cell infiltration. *Precis. Clin. Med.* **2021**, *4*, 155–167. [CrossRef]
33. Criscitiello, C.; Bayar, M.; Curigliano, G.; Symmans, F.; Desmedt, C.; Bonnefoi, H.; Sinn, B.; Pruneri, G.; Vicier, C.; Pierga, J.; et al. A gene signature to predict high tumor-infiltrating lymphocytes after neoadjuvant chemotherapy and outcome in patients with triple-negative breast cancer. *Ann. Oncol.* **2018**, *29*, 162–169. [CrossRef]
34. Cheriyath, V.; Kaur, J.; Davenport, A.; Khalel, A.; Chowdhury, N.; Gaddipati, L. G1P3 (IFI6), a mitochondrial localised antiapoptotic protein, promotes metastatic potential of breast cancer cells through mtROS. *Br. J. Cancer* **2018**, *119*, 52–64. [CrossRef]
35. Hollern, D.P.; Xu, N.; Thennavan, A.; Glodowski, C.; Garcia-Recio, S.; Mott, K.R.; He, X.; Garay, J.P.; Carey-Ewend, K.; Marron, D.; et al. B Cells and T Follicular Helper Cells Mediate Response to Checkpoint Inhibitors in High Mutation Burden Mouse Models of Breast Cancer. *Cell* **2019**, *179*, 1191–1206.e21. [CrossRef]
36. Mori, H.; Ouchida, R.; Hijikata, A.; Kitamura, H.; Ohara, O.; Li, Y.; Gao, X.; Yasui, A.; Lloyd, R.S.; Wang, J.-Y. Deficiency of the oxidative damage-specific DNA glycosylase NEIL1 leads to reduced germinal center B cell expansion. *DNA Repair.* **2009**, *8*, 1328–1332. [CrossRef]

37. Shinmura, K.; Kato, H.; Kawanishi, Y.; Igarashi, H.; Goto, M.; Tao, H.; Inoue, Y.; Nakamura, S.; Misawa, K.; Mineta, H.; et al. Abnormal Expressions of DNA Glycosylase Genes NEIL1, NEIL2, and NEIL3 Are Associated with Somatic Mutation Loads in Human Cancer. *Oxid. Med. Cell. Longev.* **2016**, *2016*, 1546392. [CrossRef]
38. Yeong, J.; Lim, J.C.T.; Lee, B.; Li, H.; Chia, N.; Ong, C.C.H.; Lye, W.K.; Putti, T.C.; Dent, R.; Lim, E.; et al. High Densities of Tumor-Associated Plasma Cells Predict Improved Prognosis in Triple Negative Breast Cancer. *Front. Immunol.* **2018**, *9*, 1209. [CrossRef]
39. Pelegrina, L.T.; Lombardi, M.G.; Fiszman, G.L.; Azar, M.E.; Morgado, C.C.; Sales, M.E. Immunoglobulin G from Breast Cancer Patients Regulates MCF-7 Cells Migration and MMP-9 Activity by Stimulating Muscarinic Acetylcholine Receptors. *J. Clin. Immunol.* **2012**, *33*, 427–435. [CrossRef]
40. López-Otín, C.; Matrisian, L.M. Emerging roles of proteases in tumour suppression. *Nat. Rev. Cancer* **2007**, *7*, 800–808. [CrossRef]
41. Pellikainen, J.M.; Ropponen, K.M.; Kataja, V.V.; Kellokoski, J.K.; Eskelinen, M.J.; Kosma, V.-M. Expression of Matrix Metalloproteinase (MMP)-2 and MMP-9 in Breast Cancer with a Special Reference to Activator Protein-2, HER2, and Prognosis. *Clin. Cancer Res.* **2004**, *10*, 7621–7628. [CrossRef]
42. Coussens, L.M.; Fingleton, B.; Matrisian, L.M. Matrix Metalloproteinase Inhibitors and Cancer—Trials and Tribulations. *Science* **2002**, *295*, 2387–2392. [CrossRef]
43. Bendrik, C.; Robertson, J.; Gauldie, J.; Dabrosin, C. Gene Transfer of Matrix Metalloproteinase-9 Induces Tumor Regression of Breast Cancer In Vivo. *Cancer Res.* **2008**, *68*, 3405–3412. [CrossRef]
44. Leifler, K.S.; Svensson, S.; Abrahamsson, A.; Bendrik, C.; Robertson, J.; Gauldie, J.; Olsson, A.-K.; Dabrosin, C. Inflammation Induced by MMP-9 Enhances Tumor Regression of Experimental Breast Cancer. *J. Immunol.* **2013**, *190*, 4420–4430. [CrossRef]
45. Sun, X.; Glynn, D.J.; Hodson, L.J.; Huo, C.; Britt, K.; Thompson, E.W.; Woolford, L.; Evdokiou, A.; Pollard, J.W.; Robertson, S.A.; et al. CCL2-driven inflammation increases mammary gland stromal density and cancer susceptibility in a transgenic mouse model. *Breast Cancer Res. BCR* **2017**, *19*, 4. [CrossRef]
46. Zheng, J.; Yang, M.; Shao, J.; Miao, Y.; Han, J.; Du, J. Chemokine receptor CX3CR1 contributes to macrophage survival in tumor metastasis. *Mol. Cancer* **2013**, *12*, 141. [CrossRef]
47. Cervantes-Badillo, M.G.; Paredes-Villa, A.; Gómez-Romero, V.; Cervantes-Roldán, R.; Arias-Romero, L.E.; Villamar-Cruz, O.; González-Montiel, M.; Barrios-García, T.; Cabrera-Quintero, A.J.; Rodríguez-Gómez, G.; et al. IFI27/ISG12 Downregulates Estrogen Receptor α Transactivation by Facilitating Its Interaction With CRM1/XPO1 in Breast Cancer Cells. *Front. Endocrinol.* **2020**, *11*, 568375. Available online: https://www.frontiersin.org/articles/10.3389/fendo.2020.568375 (accessed on 27 September 2022). [CrossRef]
48. Tulotta, C.; Lefley, D.V.; Moore, C.K.; Amariutei, A.E.; Spicer-Hadlington, A.R.; Quayle, L.A.; Hughes, R.O.; Ahmed, K.; Cookson, V.; Evans, C.A.; et al. IL-1B drives opposing responses in primary tumours and bone metastases; harnessing combination therapies to improve outcome in breast cancer. *NPJ Breast Cancer* **2021**, *7*, 95. [CrossRef]
49. Mizuno, M.; Khaledian, B.; Maeda, M.; Hayashi, T.; Mizuno, S.; Munetsuna, E.; Watanabe, T.; Kono, S.; Okada, S.; Suzuki, M.; et al. Adipsin-Dependent Secretion of Hepatocyte Growth Factor Regulates the Adipocyte-Cancer Stem Cell Interaction. *Cancers* **2021**, *13*, 4238. [CrossRef]
50. Liu, Z.; Gao, Z.; Li, B.; Li, J.; Ou, Y.; Yu, X.; Zhang, Z.; Liu, S.; Fu, X.; Jin, H.; et al. Lipid-associated macrophages in the tumor-adipose microenvironment facilitate breast cancer progression. *OncoImmunology* **2022**, *11*, 2085432. [CrossRef]
51. Howard, E.; Hurrell, B.P.; Helou, D.G.; Quach, C.; Painter, J.D.; Shafiei-Jahani, P.; Fung, M.; Gill, P.S.; Soroosh, P.; Sharpe, A.H.; et al. PD-1 Blockade on Tumor Microenvironment-Resident ILC2s Promotes TNF-α Production and Restricts Progression of Metastatic Melanoma. *Front. Immunol.* **2021**, *12*, 733136. Available online: https://www.frontiersin.org/articles/10.3389/fimmu.2021.733136 (accessed on 29 September 2022). [CrossRef]
52. Halim, T.Y.F.; Rana, B.M.J.; Walker, J.A.; Kerscher, B.; Knolle, M.D.; Jolin, H.E.; Serrao, E.M.; Haim-Vilmovsky, L.; Teichmann, S.A.; Rodewald, H.R.; et al. Tissue-Restricted Adaptive Type 2 Immunity Is Orchestrated by Expression of the Costimulatory Molecule OX40L on Group 2 Innate Lymphoid Cells. *Immunity* **2018**, *48*, 1195–1207.e6. [CrossRef]
53. Grisaru-Tal, S.; Itan, M.; Klion, A.D.; Munitz, A. A new dawn for eosinophils in the tumour microenvironment. *Nat. Rev. Cancer* **2020**, *20*, 594–607. [CrossRef]
54. Carretero, R.; Sektioglu, I.M.; Garbi, N.; Salgado, O.C.; Beckhove, P.; Hämmerling, G.J. Eosinophils orchestrate cancer rejection by normalizing tumor vessels and enhancing infiltration of CD8+ T cells. *Nat. Immunol.* **2015**, *16*, 609–617. [CrossRef]
55. Vienne, M.; Etiennot, M.; Escalière, B.; Galluso, J.; Spinelli, L.; Guia, S.; Fenis, A.; Vivier, E.; Kerdiles, Y.M. Type 1 Innate Lymphoid Cells Limit the Antitumoral Immune Response. *Front. Immunol.* **2021**, *12*, 768989. Available online: https://www.frontiersin.org/articles/10.3389/fimmu.2021.768989 (accessed on 29 September 2022). [CrossRef]
56. Chen, Q.; Massagué, J. Molecular Pathways: VCAM-1 as a Potential Therapeutic Target in Metastasis. *Clin. Cancer Res. Off. J. Am. Assoc. Cancer Res.* **2012**, *18*, 5520–5525. [CrossRef]
57. Kalaora, S.; Nagler, A.; Wargo, J.A.; Samuels, Y. Mechanisms of immune activation and regulation: Lessons from melanoma. *Nat. Rev. Cancer* **2022**, *22*, 195–207. [CrossRef]
58. Salemme, V.; Centonze, G.; Cavallo, F.; Defilippi, P.; Conti, L. The Crosstalk Between Tumor Cells and the Immune Microenvironment in Breast Cancer: Implications for Immunotherapy. *Front. Oncol.* **2021**, *11*, 610303. [CrossRef]

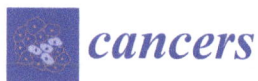

Article

A Multi-Center Clinical Study to Harvest and Characterize Circulating Tumor Cells from Patients with Metastatic Breast Cancer Using the Parsortix® PC1 System

Evan N. Cohen [1,†], Gitanjali Jayachandran [1,†], Richard G. Moore [2], Massimo Cristofanilli [3], Julie E. Lang [4], Joseph D. Khoury [5], Michael F. Press [5], Kyu Kwang Kim [2], Negar Khazan [2], Qiang Zhang [3], Youbin Zhang [3], Pushpinder Kaur [4], Roberta Guzman [5], Michael C. Miller [6], James M. Reuben [1,*] and Naoto T. Ueno [7,*]

[1] Department of Hematopathology Research, Division of Pathology and Laboratory Medicine, The University of Texas MD Anderson Cancer Center, Houston, TX 77030, USA
[2] Division of Gynecologic Oncology, Department of Obstetrics and Gynecology, Wilmot Cancer Institute, University of Rochester Medical Center, Rochester, NY 14620, USA
[3] Department of Medicine-Hematology and Oncology, Robert H Lurie Comprehensive Cancer Center, Feinberg School of Medicine, Northwestern University, Chicago, IL 60611, USA
[4] USC Breast Cancer Program, Keck School of Medicine, Norris Comprehensive Cancer Center, University of Southern California, Los Angeles, CA 90033, USA
[5] Department of Pathology, Breast Cancer Analysis Laboratory, Keck School of Medicine, Norris Comprehensive Cancer Center, University of Southern California, Los Angeles, CA 90033, USA
[6] ANGLE Clinical Studies, ANGLE Europe Limited, Guildford, Surrey GU2 7AF, UK
[7] Department of Breast Medical Oncology, The University of Texas MD Anderson Cancer Center, Houston, TX 77030, USA
* Correspondence: jreuben@mdanderson.org (J.M.R.); nueno@mdanderson.org (N.T.U.)
† These authors contributed equally to this work.

Citation: Cohen, E.N.; Jayachandran, G.; Moore, R.G.; Cristofanilli, M.; Lang, J.E.; Khoury, J.D.; Press, M.F.; Kim, K.K.; Khazan, N.; Zhang, Q.; et al. A Multi-Center Clinical Study to Harvest and Characterize Circulating Tumor Cells from Patients with Metastatic Breast Cancer Using the Parsortix® PC1 System. *Cancers* 2022, *14*, 5238. https://doi.org/10.3390/cancers14215238

Academic Editor: Emilie Mamessier-Birnbaum

Received: 23 September 2022
Accepted: 20 October 2022
Published: 26 October 2022

Publisher's Note: MDPI stays neutral with regard to jurisdictional claims in published maps and institutional affiliations.

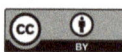

Copyright: © 2022 by the authors. Licensee MDPI, Basel, Switzerland. This article is an open access article distributed under the terms and conditions of the Creative Commons Attribution (CC BY) license (https://creativecommons.org/licenses/by/4.0/).

Simple Summary: There is a great need to understand the cellular and molecular characteristics of cancer when access to the tumor is limited. Circulating tumor cells (CTCs) captured from the blood of cancer patients may serve as a surrogate source of tumor material. However, the only FDA-cleared CTC assay has been limited to counting CTC in blood and and lack further characterization of the CTCs. In this study, we tested the Parsortix® PC1 System that captures and harvests a wide range of CTCs from peripheral blood that are amenable for further evaluation. The device was assessed in a large, multicenter clinical trial including patients with metastatic breast cancer and healthy volunteers, with enriched CTC evaluated by 4 downstream techniques commonly available in clinical laboratories. The data generated from this study was used to support FDA clearance for the Parsortix System.

Abstract: Circulating tumor cells (CTCs) captured from the blood of cancer patients may serve as a surrogate source of tumor material that can be obtained via a venipuncture (also known as a liquid biopsy) and used to better understand tumor characteristics. However, the only FDA-cleared CTC assay has been limited to the enumeration of surface marker–defined cells and not further characterization of the CTCs. In this study, we tested the ability of a semi-automated device capable of capturing and harvesting CTCs from peripheral blood based on cell size and deformability, agnostic of cell-surface markers (the Parsortix® PC1 System), to yield CTCs for evaluation by downstream techniques commonly available in clinical laboratories. The data generated from this study were used to support a De Novo request (DEN200062) for the classification of this device, which the FDA recently granted. As part of a multicenter clinical trial, peripheral blood samples from 216 patients with metastatic breast cancer (MBC) and 205 healthy volunteers were subjected to CTC enrichment. A board-certified pathologist enumerated the CTCs from each participant by cytologic evaluation of Wright-Giemsa–stained slides. As proof of principle, cells harvested from a concurrent parallel sample provided by each participant were evaluated using one of three additional evaluation techniques: molecular profiling by qRT-PCR, RNA sequencing, or cytogenetic analysis of HER2 amplification by FISH. The study demonstrated that the Parsortix® PC1 System can effectively capture and harvest

CTCs from the peripheral blood of MBC patients and that the harvested cells can be evaluated using orthogonal methodologies such as gene expression and/or Fluorescence In Situ Hybridization (FISH).

Keywords: circulating tumor cells; neoplastic cells; circulating; neoplasms/diagnosis; circulating/pathology; biopsy; breast neoplasms/pathology; biomarkers; tumor; blood; liquid biopsy

1. Introduction

Circulating tumor cells (CTCs) are carcinoma cells which migrate through the intracellular matrix, actively enter the circulation through endothelial cells, presumably of capillaries and venules, and are disseminated through the bloodstream. Some CTCs survive to attach and penetrate the endothelial cells of capillaries and venules in distant organs, thereby forming metastases in these distant organs. Hence, CTCs are characteristically found in the blood of patients with metastases. The potential of a liquid biopsy to procure tumor cells before and during treatment in a non-invasive fashion has generated substantial interest in its use in oncology research and clinical practice. However, isolating CTCs from blood is inherently challenging, which has limited the use of CTCs in the clinical setting [1].

CTCs are usually rare, representing a minuscule fraction of the cells present in a blood sample. Consequently, the number of CTCs isolated from a single-tube blood draw (5–10 mL of peripheral blood) is typically very low, frequently being from 1 to 15 cells. Nonetheless, these cells provide valuable data: several lines of evidence have confirmed that the detection of CTCs represents an innovative and reliable tool to predict disease progression and overall survival in patients with metastatic breast cancer (MBC) [2–7]. Furthermore, the enumeration of CTCs at different time points during treatment is considered a reliable surrogate marker of treatment response and a potential alternative form of non-invasive monitoring of response to therapy [5–7].

Many technologies have been developed to isolate, enumerate, and characterize CTCs [1,8–10]. Of these, the CELLSEARCH® System (Menarini-Silicon Biosystems, Huntingdon Valley, PA, USA) is the only CTC device cleared by the U.S. Food and Drug Administration (FDA). The CELLSEARCH® System was cleared specifically for the enumeration of CTCs from the blood of patients with metastatic breast, colorectal, and prostate cancer [11].

The CELLSEARCH® System captures CTCs based on immune affinity using antibodies specific to epithelial cell adhesion molecule (EpCAM). This cell-surface protein is expressed by many CTC subsets but is neither specific to CTCs nor is it universally expressed by all CTCs. Antibodies against surface EpCAM are routinely used to capture CTCs from blood, but such an approach is inherently limited to tumor cells with epithelial differentiation.

Cancer development frequently involves a transition of cells from an epithelial phenotype to a mesenchymal phenotype (a process referred to as epithelial-to-mesenchymal transition, or EMT), which results in the downregulation of EpCAM expression [12,13] and is associated with tumor-initiating potential [14,15]. During this switch to EMT, epithelial cells undergo upregulation of mesenchymal gene expression patterns and downregulation of epithelial genes. Furthermore, epithelial cells lose the ability to form streamlined cell–cell connections and cell polarity due to the restructuring of their cytoskeleton. Consequently, individual cells gain increased motility potential and an invasive phenotype [16]. EpCAM-based methods, therefore, fail to efficiently capture mesenchymal cells, leading to the selective isolation of CTC phenotypes that may not be representative of most cells being shed from a tumor that have the ability to establish themselves and grow at a distal site. In addition, not all epithelial cancer cells express EpCAM [17].

Antibody-based capture methods may also impact further characterization, such as gene expression analyses [18]. As gene expression, by nature, reflects external signals received by cells and consequent signaling pathways within them, the interaction of capture antibodies with the cell surface may alter gene expression data obtained from CTCs captured using immune-affinity enrichment methods. Altogether, these limitations underscore an unmet need for the agnostic enrichment of intact CTCs that can be used in clinically meaningful downstream analyses.

The Parsortix® PC1 System is a semi-automated device based on based microfluidic technology that enables the capture and harvest of rare cells (e.g., CTCs) from peripheral blood based on cell size and deformability [19–25]. It addresses several issues encountered with current CTC capture technologies because it does not use antibodies or other cell-surface affinity agents to capture the target cells. The isolation/capture mechanism employed by the system is a purely physical method rather than a chemical or biological one, making it epitope independent and consequently agnostic to cellular phenotypes [21–23] and able to capture cells with mesenchymal features.

This multi-center clinical study, entitled "Harvest of Circulating Tumor Cells (CTCs) from Patients with Metastatic Breast Cancer (MBC) Using the Parsortix® PC1 System" (the ANG-002 HOMING study; ClinicalTrials.gov identifier: NCT03427450), was designed and conducted to demonstrate that the Parsortix® PC1 System can capture and harvest CTCs from the peripheral blood of patients with MBC and that the CTCs harvested by the system can be used for subsequent downstream evaluation. Cytology evaluation, quantitative polymerase chain reaction (PCR), fluorescence in situ hybridization (FISH), and RNA-seq were chosen as representative downstream evaluation methods, covering a range of molecular, histopathological, and cytomorphological techniques currently used in clinical laboratories. The results from the HOMING study demonstrated that CTCs can indeed be harvested from the peripheral blood of patients with MBC and utilized in subsequent downstream analysis methods. The data generated under this study were included in a De Novo request for classification of the Parsortix® PC1 System (DEN200062) as a Class II prescription device, and the FDA granted the request on 24 May 2022 (https://www.accessdata.fda.gov/cdrh_docs/pdf20/DEN200062.pdf, accessed on 20 October 2022).

2. Materials and Methods

2.1. Ethical Conduct of the Study

The ANG-002 HOMING study was an IRB-approved prospective clinical trial registered with ClinicalTrials.gov (identifier: NCT03427450) and sponsored by ANGLE Europe Limited (Guildford, UK), the manufacturer of the Parsortix® PC1 System. The study involved the collection of whole-blood samples from patients with MBC (either women with newly diagnosed MBC who were about to start a new line of therapy of any type to treat and/or manage their disease or those with currently progressive or recurrent MBC) as well as from a control population of healthy female volunteers (HVs) consisting of women who self-declared no prior/current history of cancer and no known history of breast disease. All study participants provided informed consent before participation in the study. All laboratory testing was performed by operators blinded to the clinical status of the participants.

Participants were enrolled, and samples were collected and processed at four institutions: The University of Texas MD Anderson Cancer Center, Houston, TX, USA; University of Southern California, Los Angeles, CA, USA; University of Rochester Medical Center, Rochester, NY, USA; and Northwestern University, Chicago, IL, USA. The study was conducted with the approval of each institution's institutional review board and in accordance with the Declaration of Helsinki. A study-specific online database was designed, constructed, and maintained using the University of Rochester Medical Center's REDCap system [26,27].

2.2. Blood Collection and Processing

Each participant provided between ~7 mL and 23 mL of whole blood collected specifically for this study into one 3 mL K_2EDTA tube followed by two 10 mL K_2EDTA tubes at a single time point. For patients with MBC, blood was collected before the initiation of their new therapy and a minimum of 7 days after the last administration of any previous cytotoxic treatment, either from venipuncture or through an existing port. For patients continuing an existing oral hormonal and/or targeted immunotherapy in addition to starting a new treatment, blood was drawn before the next administration of their oral hormonal therapy and/or immunotherapy and before the initiation of their new therapy treatment. For HVs, blood was collected via venipuncture on the day of study.

For the capture of CTCs, all samples were processed using the Parsortix® PC1 System within 8 h of collection. First, the blood volume in each of the K_2EDTA tubes was estimated using an engineering ruler. The initial portion of blood collected into the 3 mL K_2EDTA tube immediately following the venipuncture or the port flushing was used for a complete blood count with leukocyte differential testing. For the two 10 mL K_2EDTA tubes, a minimum combined volume of $\geq$5 mL of blood was required for processing using the Parsortix® PC1 System equipped with a Parsortix GEN3D6.5 Cell Separation Cassette. If both tubes contained a combined total of <5 mL of blood, the participant was considered non-evaluable, and the blood was discarded. If only one of the 10 mL K_2EDTA tubes contained $\geq$5 mL of blood, then only the blood in that tube was processed for the primary cytological evaluation. If both tubes had <5 mL of blood, but the combined volume of blood in both tubes was $\geq$5 mL, then the blood from the two tubes was combined in a 10 mL K_2EDTA tube into $\geq$5 mL of blood that was processed for the primary cytological evaluation. If both 10 mL K_2EDTA tubes had $\geq$5 mL of blood, then the tube with the higher volume of blood was processed for the primary cytological evaluation, and the other tube was processed for one of the exploratory evaluations (qPCR, FISH, or RNA-seq).

Information about samples was blinded from the processors, and no follow-up information was collected for any participants. The population of cells captured from each blood sample by the Parsortix® PC1 System was harvested directly from the cell separation cassettes (each harvest consisting of a total volume of 210 µL of phosphate-buffered saline) into collection vessels and used for downstream processing and characterization.

2.3. Downstream Characterization

2.3.1. Primary Evaluation

For all participants, the cells harvested from the 10 mL K_2EDTA tube containing the larger volume of blood were subjected to cytomorphological evaluation by a qualified pathologist (JDK) to determine the presence and number of observable CTCs.

Cytology Processing

Following enrichment, cells were harvested into a 1.5 mL microfuge tube containing 60 µL of fetal bovine serum (FBS). The harvested cells suspended in FBS were pipetted into a Cytospin 4 Cytofunnel assembly (ThermoFisher Scientific, Waltham, MA, USA) containing a positively charged glass Cytoslide (ThermoFisher Scientific). The slide assembly was cytocentrifuged at 800 rpm for 3 min on low acceleration, and the slide was removed from the assembly and allowed to air-dry at room temperature for 1 min. The air-dried slide was then submersed in 100% methanol for 1 min, removed, gently tapped at the edge on a paper towel to remove any excess methanol, and allowed to air-dry at room temperature for 30 min. The fixed slides were stored at room temperature until shipment weekly to the designated central testing laboratory located at the MD Anderson Cancer Center.

At the laboratory, the slides underwent Wright-Giemsa staining on an automated stainer, and examination by a qualified pathologist (JDK) with expertise in blood evaluation and cytopathology who identified and enumerated CTCs using conventional cytomorphological criteria of malignancy, which included: increased nuclear-to-cytoplasmic ratio, cellular pleomorphism, large size relative to white blood cells, irregular nuclear membrane, chromatin structure, nuclear hyperchromasia, cytoplasmic vacuoles, cellular aggregates ($\geq$2 cells). The stained slides were evaluated by light microscopy, and the cells that had been cytomorphologically identified as CTCs by the qualified pathologist were photographed, identified, and counted. Cells without definite features of malignancy but distinct from usual peripheral blood–formed elements (e.g., neutrophils, immature granulocytic precursors, monocytes, nucleated red blood cells) were not counted as CTCs. Naked nuclei or cell fragments were not evaluated. Samples in which technical artifacts caused substantial deformation of peripheral blood elements to an extent that compromised their morphological evaluation were considered unsatisfactory.

2.3.2. Exploratory Evaluations

For participants for whom both 10 mL K_2EDTA tubes contained ≥ 5 mL of blood, the cells harvested from the second tube were subjected to one of the following exploratory evaluations.

Gene Expression Evaluation by qRT-PCR Processing

Cells captured in the cassette were harvested directly into a 2.0 mL microfuge tube and centrifuged at ~400× g for 5 min at 4 °C, and as much of the supernatant as possible was removed without disturbing the cell pellet. The cell pellet was resuspended in 320 µL of Qiagen buffer RLT containing 1% 2-mercaptoethanol. Lysates were stored at −80 °C until batch shipment to the designated central qPCR testing laboratory at The MD Anderson Cancer Center for gene expression analysis using quantitative reverse-transcriptase real-time PCR (qRT-PCR). Each lysate was evaluated for expression of the following genes using hydrolysis (TaqMan) probes (Bio-Rad Laboratories, Hercules, CA, USA): GAPDH and B2M (housekeeping genes), GYPA (a nucleated red blood cell marker), PTPRC (a white blood cell marker), EpCAM and KRT19 (epithelial cell markers), ERBB2 (a breast tumor marker), and TWIST1 and SNAI2 (mesenchymal cell markers). Each gene was analyzed in triplicate for every sample (including samples from patients, healthy volunteers, positive and negative controls), and 40 cycles of PCR were performed. PCR thermocycling and data acquisition were performed using the appropriate instrumentation and software, which automatically set the cycle threshold (Ct). The average of the three replicate Ct values for each gene target for each sample and for the positive and negative controls were used for the evaluations presented in this report. For all instances where a gene was undetectable after 40 cycles of PCR, a Ct value of 40.0 was assigned for analysis purposes. Aliquots of nuclease-free water were used as negative controls for the assay. The SUM149 triple-negative breast cancer cell line was selected as a positive control since it exhibits a partial EMT phenotype. Aliquots of SUM149 cell lysate were used as positive controls. They were expected to have positive expression for GAPDH, B2M, KRT19, EpCAM, ERBB2, TWIST1, and SNAI2 while lacking expression of the white blood cell marker PTPRC and the nucleated red blood cell marker GYPA. Expression results are shown as 40-Ct values so that increased values reflect increased expression, and undetectable values are represented as 0. Normalization was not used so that gene expression can be interpreted as expression per tube of blood since the number of captured CTCs is variable.

RNA-seq Processing

An aliquot of 200 µL of whole blood from the 10 mL K_2EDTA tube was transferred directly into a 1.5 mL microfuge tube containing 1 mL of RNAlater RNA Stabilization Solution before processing of the blood sample on the Parsortix® PC1 System. The remaining blood was processed on the Parsortix® PC1 System, and the cells captured in the cassette were harvested directly into a 0.2 mL PCR tube. The harvest was centrifuged at ~400× g for 5 min at room temperature, and as much of the supernatant as possible was removed without disturbing the cell pellet. The cell pellet was resuspended in 10 µL of Agilent SideStep lysis and stabilization buffer. Both lysates (i.e., the aliquot of whole blood and the harvest) were stored at −80 °C until shipment to the designated central RNA-seq testing laboratory at the University of Southern California. The RNA-seq laboratory isolated RNA from the whole blood lysates using Ambion RiboPure blood kits for RNA. The cDNA generated was amplified and purified using 50 ng of the purified RNA obtained from each of the whole blood lysates and 2 µL from each harvest lysates using NuGEN Trio RNA-Seq kits. cDNA libraries were then prepared, amplified, refined, and filtered for each sample using NuGEN Trio RNA-seq kits. The quantity and quality of each library preparation were assessed using DNA quantitation by a Qubit fluorometer. DNA fragment size distribution was determined using an Agilent 2100 Bioanalyzer. Only the cDNA libraries from the Parsortix® harvest samples (and not the whole blood aliquots) were evaluated as a part of this report. The cDNA libraries generated from the harvest samples were sequenced using an Illumina HiSeq 2500 at the University of Southern California Genomics Core with 2×125 bp paired-end reads. Data analysis was conducted by an experienced bioinformatician (DC) to determine the expression patterns of breast cancer–related genes.

The RNA-seq method described above was validated in whole-transcriptome profiling studies in CTC from patients with non-metastatic breast cancer (stage II-III). These studies' procedures and results were previously reported [28,29], and the results demonstrated that CTCs from patients with MBC could be used to generate cDNA libraries of sufficient quantity and quality that enable whole-genome sequencing.

Salmon 1.5.0 mapped the HV and MBC Parsortix® PC1 harvest sequencing data against the reference transcriptome V37 from Gencode [30]. Quantification output from Salmon is reported in transcripts per kilobase million (TPM), computed by dividing read counts by the length of each gene in kilobases to obtain reads per kilobase (RPK). All the RPK values in a sample are summed, and the summation is divided by 1,000,000 to provide a "per million" scaling factor. The RPK values are divided by the per million scaling factors to obtain the TPM value. The sum of all TPM values is the same in each sample, making it easier to compare the proportion of reads mapped to a gene in each sample.

In contrast, with reads per kilobase million (RPKM) and fragments per kilobase million (FPKM), the sum of the normalized reads in each sample may be different, making it harder to compare models directly. In a second analysis, a listing of all unmapped reads (i.e., reads that did not map to the transcriptome) from the Salmon analysis was tabulated for each sample. Magic-BLAST 1.5.0 was used to compare 100,000 randomly sampled reads from each of the unmapped reads files to the genome ver GRCh38 from Gencode, the transcriptome V37 from Gencode, and a file with all rDNA sequences downloaded from GenBank. The purpose was to determine whether the unmapped reads from Salmon analysis map better to the genome or the rDNA, instead of the transcriptome, which would support gDNA contamination. A result can contain more than 100,000 entries because a read can map to more than one genomic feature in the reference.

HER2 FISH Processing

Cells captured in the cassette were harvested directly into a 1.5 mL microfuge tube containing 60 µL of FBS. The harvested cells suspended in FBS were pipetted into a Cytospin 4 Cytofunnel assembly with a positively charged glass Cytoslide. The slide assembly was cytocentrifuged at 800 rpm for 3 min on low acceleration, and the slide was removed from the body and allowed to air-dry at room temperature for 1 min. The air-dried slide was then submersed in 100% methanol for 15 min, removed, gently tapped at the edge on a paper towel to remove any excess methanol, and allowed to air-dry at room temperature for 30 min. The fixed slides were stored at ≤ -20 °C until shipment to the designated central HER2 FISH testing laboratory at the University of Southern California for processing, as described elsewhere [31–33], using commercially available HER2 FISH reagents (Abbott PathVysion HER2 DNA Probes [PN 30-171060/1800], DAPI II Counterstain [PN 30-804861/8100], NP-40 [PN 30-804820/8100], 20X SSC [PN 805850], and Vysis FISH Pretreatment Reagent Kits [PN 32-801270]) and evaluated by a board-certified pathologist (MFP). The pathologist determined the presence or absence of cells showing human epidermal growth factor receptor 2 (HER2/ERBB2) gene amplification. Criteria for evaluating CTCs for HER2 gene amplification status by FISH involved an assessment of the nuclear morphology to distinguish tumor cells from normal leukocytes in the slide preparations, followed by an evaluation of the HER2 gene copy number and chromosome 17 centromere (CEP17) copy number in the tumor cells. The criteria used in distinguishing tumor cells from white blood cells are similar to the requirements described for the cytological evaluation of the peripheral blood cells with the Wright-Giemsa stain. These criteria of malignancy included an increased nucleus size, nuclear pleomorphism, increased size relative to white blood cells, irregular nuclear membranes, increased nuclear DAPI staining, uneven distribution of atomic chromatin (heterochromatin and euchromatin), and aggregation of multiple, large cells. Because the CTCs contained intact tumor cell nuclei, not 4-micron histology tissue sections through tumor cell nuclei, the average chromosome 17 number was considered a reflection of overall DNA ploidy status as well as chromosome 17 aneusomy. A sample was considered HER2-amplified if the HER2/CEP17 ratio was greater than 2 and HER2 gene copies were present in groups as observed in human breast cancer cell lines known to have HER2 gene amplification with HER2/ERBB2 gene copies arranged as aggregates in homogeneous staining regions [34] CTCs with increased HER2 gene copy number greater than 4 but also paired with individual chromosome 17 centromeres, as observed in human breast cancer cell lines that lack HER2 gene amplification and lack HER2 mRNA/protein overexpression, were evaluated as HER2-not-amplified.

3. Results and Discussion

3.1. Patient Characteristics

A flow chart of participants enrolled in the ANG-002 HOMING study is shown in Figure 1. A total of 216 patients with metastatic breast cancer and 205 female healthy volunteers were enrolled at the four clinical study sites between April 2018 and February 2019. Nine (4.2%) of the patients with MBC and one (0.5%) of the HVs enrolled were ineligible for the study, leaving 207 eligible patients with MBC and 204 eligible HVs that were evaluable for one or more of the study endpoints. The HVs tended to be younger, healthier, and more racially diverse than the patients with MBC (Table 1).

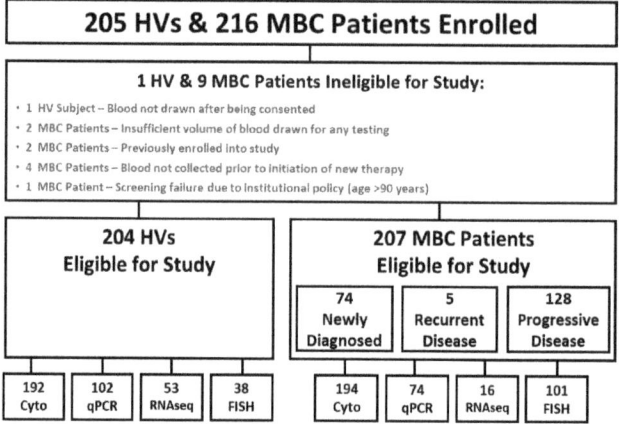

Figure 1. Study enrollment, eligibility, and evaluation. HV, healthy volunteer; MBC, metastatic breast cancer; Cyto, cytology evaluation; qPCR, quantitative polymerase chain reaction; FISH, fluorescence in situ hybridization.

Table 1. Summary of eligible MBC patients and HVs demographics and clinical characteristics.

Parameter and Categories	Eligible HV Subjects with Evaluable Results	Eligible MBC Patients with Evaluable Results	Eligible MBC Patients with Evaluable Results	
			Newly Diagnosed	Progression /Recurring
No. of eligible participants	204	207	74 (35.7%)	133 (64.3%)

Table 1. Cont.

Parameter and Categories	Eligible HV Subjects with Evaluable Results	Eligible MBC Patients with Evaluable Results	Eligible MBC Patients with Evaluable Results Newly Diagnosed	Eligible MBC Patients with Evaluable Results Progression /Recurring
Age at the time of the blood collection				
<57 years old	170 (83.3%)	103 (49.8%)	37 (50.0%)	66 (49.6%)
≥57 years old	34 (16.7%)	104 (50.2%)	37 (50.0%)	67 (50.4%)
Fisher exact p-value	<0.001		1.000	
Blood collection method				
Venipuncture	204 (100.0%)	171 (82.6%)	70 (94.6%)	101 (75.9%)
Port	0 (0.0%)	36 (17.4%)	4 (5.4%)	32 (24.1%)
Fisher exact p-value	<0.001		<0.001	
Menopausal status				
Pre-menopausal	130 (63.7%)	36 (17.4%)	15 (20.3%)	21 (15.8%)
Post-menopausal	53 (26.0%)	158 (76.3%)	50 (67.6%)	108 (81.2%)
Unknown	21 (10.3%)	13 (6.3%)	9 (12.2%)	4 (3.0%)
Fisher exact p-value *	<0.001		0.328	
Race/ethnicity				
White	109 (53.4%)	151 (72.9%)	55 (74.3%)	96 (72.2%)
Black	20 (9.8%)	22 (10.6%)	8 (10.8%)	14 (10.5%)
Hispanic	40 (19.6%)	21 (10.1%)	8 (10.8%)	13 (9.8%)
Other/unknown	35 (17.2%)	13 (6.3%)	3 (4.1%)	10 (7.5%)
Fisher exact p-value	<0.001		0.826	
Previous history of cancer?				
Yes	0 (0.0%)	15 (7.2%)	5 (6.8%)	10 (7.5%)
No	204 (100.0%)	192 (92.8%)	69 (93.2%)	123 (92.5%)
Fisher exact p-value	<0.001		1.000	
Breast cancer ER status				
Positive	—	160 (77.3%)	55 (74.3%)	105 (78.9%)
Negative	—	45 (21.7%)	18 (24.3%)	27 (20.3%)
Unknown	—	2 (1.0%)	1 (1.4%)	1 (0.8%)
Fisher exact p-value *	—		0.487	
Breast cancer PR status				
Positive	—	127 (61.4%)	44 (59.5%)	83 (62.4%)
Negative	—	73 (35.3%)	27 (36.5%)	46 (34.6%)
Unknown	—	7 (3.4%)	3 (4.1%)	4 (3.0%)
Fisher exact p-value *	—		0.761	
Breast cancer HR status				
Positive	—	39 (79.7%)	57 (77.0%)	108 (81.2%)
Negative	—	165 (18.8%)	16 (21.6%)	23 (17.3%)
Unknown	—	3 (1.4%)	1 (1.4%)	2 (1.5%)
Fisher exact p-value *	—		0.448	

Table 1. Cont.

Parameter and Categories	Eligible HV Subjects with Evaluable Results	Eligible MBC Patients with Evaluable Results	Eligible MBC Patients with Evaluable Results Newly Diagnosed	Eligible MBC Patients with Evaluable Results Progression/Recurring
Breast cancer HER2-Neu status				
Negative	—	165 (79.7%)	66 (89.2%)	99 (74.4%)
Positive	—	27 (13.0%)	4 (5.4%)	23 (17.3%)
Equivocal	—	8 (3.9%)	1 (1.4%)	7 (5.3%)
Unknown	—	7 (3.4%)	3 (4.1%)	4 (3.0%)
Fisher exact p-value *	—		0.014	
Breast cancer TNBC status				
TNBC	—	33 (15.9%)	54 (50.5%)	98 (73.7%)
Non-TNBC	—	152 (73.4%)	13 (12.1%)	20 (15.0%)
Unknown	—	22 (10.6%)	7 (6.5%)	15 (11.3%)
Fisher exact p-value *	—		0.675	
Metastatic disease status determined by (more than one may apply)				Fisher exact p-value **
Imaging	—	198 (95.7%)	70 (94.6%)	128 (96.2%)	0.724
Rising tumor markers	—	5 (2.4%)	2 (2.7%)	3 (2.3%)	1.000
Physical signs and symptoms	—	17 (8.2%)	8 (10.8%)	9 (6.8%)	0.306
Physician determination	—	4 (1.9%)	1 (1.4%)	3 (2.3%)	1.000
Other (primarily biopsy)	—	62 (30.0%)	49 (66.2%)	13 (9.8%)	0.000
Sites of metastasis (more than one may apply)				Fisher exact p-value **
Abdomen	—	6 (2.9%)	3 (4.1%)	3 (2.3%)	0.669
Adrenal gland	—	3 (1.4%)	0 (0.0%)	3 (2.3%)	0.554
Ascites	—	1 (0.5%)	1 (1.4%)	0 (0.0%)	0.357
Bone	—	139 (67.1%)	42 (56.8%)	97 (72.9%)	0.021
Brain	—	29 (14%)	5 (6.8%)	24 (18.0%)	0.035
Chest wall	—	16 (7.7%)	4 (5.4%)	12 (9.0%)	0.425
Liver	—	80 (38.6%)	10 (13.5%)	70 (52.6%)	0.000
Lung	—	77 (37.2%)	23 (31.1%)	54 (40.6%)	0.181
Lymph nodes	—	107 (51.7%)	33 (44.6%)	74 (55.6%)	0.148
Other site(s)	—	33 (15.9%)	9 (12.2%)	24 (18.0%)	0.325

* Comparisons do not include the "Unknown" category. MBC, metastatic breast cancer; HV, healthy volunteer; TNBC, triple-negative breast cancer; ER, estrogen receptor; PR, progesterone receptor; HR, hormone receptor. ** Fisher exact p-value for comparison between MBC patients with newly diagnosed disease and those with progression/recurring disease.

As enrollment was open to any patient with MBC starting a new line of therapy, the patient population was split between those with newly diagnosed metastatic disease and others with progressive or recurrent disease at the time of the sample collection. Patient characteristics between these two cohorts were generally well-balanced. Overall, 27 (13.0%) of the patients with MBC had HER2-positive tumors (as determined from their medical records using the available HER2 IHC and/or FISH testing results on their primary and/or metastatic tumor tissue); only 4 (5.4%) of patients with newly diagnosed MBC had HER2-positive tumors, in contrast to 23 (17.3%, $p = 0.014$) of the patients with MBC with progressive and/or recurrent disease (Table 1). Despite these differences, the MBC patients enrolled in the ANG-002 study were representative of patients with MBC that would be seen in the general population [35].

3.2. Cytology Evaluation

To enumerate CTCs agnostic to protein expression bias, we used standard cytology techniques to identify cells based on longstanding morphologic features associated with malignancy. In validation studies, the cytocentrifugation (cytospin) method used to prepare slides for cytology and FISH evaluation showed significant cell loss for three cell lines (Figure S1). These results indicated that 37–51% of the cells harvested by the Parsortix® PC1 System were lost due to the cytology slide preparation method and/or the Wright-Giemsa staining procedure (compared to harvesting the cells directly into 96-well plates).

For the identification and enumeration of CTCs, the cells harvested from blood samples were fixed, Wright-Giemsa stained, and reviewed by a single pathologist; the resulting CTC prevalence rates in HVs and patients with MBC are shown in (Table 2). A flow diagram of the eligible subjects with evaluable cytology slides is shown in Figure 2a. In the 204 eligible HVs and 207 eligible patients with MBC, 12 (5.9%) and 13 (6.3%), respectively, did not produce evaluable slides for cytology examination, leaving a total of 192 HVs and 194 patients with MBC with evaluable Wright-Giemsa-stained cytology slides.

Table 2. CTC prevalence rates from initial cytopathology review in MBC patients and HVs by demographic and clinical characteristics.

Parameter and Categories	Eligible HV Subjects and MBC Patients with Evaluable Cytology Slides										
	All Eligible and Evaluable HV Subjects			All Eligible and Evaluable MBC Patients			Newly Diagnosed MBC Patients			Progression/Recurring MBC Patients	
	N	≥1 CTC	≥5 CTC	N	≥1 CTC	≥5 CTC	N	≥1 CTC	≥5 CTC	N	≥1 CTC	≥5 CTC
All participants	192	19 (9.9%)	2 (1.0%)	194	94 (48.5%)	44 (22.7%)	69	23 (33.3%)	9 (13.0%)	125	71 (56.8%)	35 (28.0%)
Age at the time of the blood collection												
<57 Years Old	159	15 (9.4%)	1 (0.6%)	96	41 (42.7%)	17 (17.7%)	33	6 (18.2%)	3 (9.1%)	63	35 (55.6%)	14 (22.2%)
≥57 Years Old	33	4 (12.1%)	1 (3.0%)	98	53 (54.1%)	27 (27.6%)	36	17 (47.2%)	6 (16.7%)	62	36 (58.1%)	21 (33.9%)
Fisher exact test p-value		0.748	0.315		0.117	0.123		0.012	0.481		0.857	0.167
Blood collection method												
via Venipuncture	192	19 (9.9%)	2 (1.0%)	159	61 (38.4%)	22 (13.8%)	65	19 (29.2%)	7 (10.8%)	94	42 (44.7%)	15 (16.0%)
via Port	0	0 (0.0%)	0 (0.0%)	35	33 (94.3%)	22 (62.9%)	4	4 (100.0%)	2 (50.0%)	31	29 (93.5%)	20 (64.5%)
Fisher exact test p-value		—	—		<0.001	<0.001		0.010	0.080		<0.001	<0.001
Menopausal status												
Pre-Menopausal	124	12 (9.7%)	1 (0.8%)	34	14 (41.2%)	7 (20.6%)	14	2 (14.3%)	1 (7.1%)	20	12 (60.0%)	6 (30.0%)
Post-Menopausal	51	5 (9.8%)	1 (2.0%)	147	75 (51.0%)	35 (23.8%)	46	19 (41.3%)	8 (17.4%)	101	56 (55.4%)	27 (26.7%)
Unknown	17	2 (11.8%)	0 (0.0%)	13	5 (38.5%)	2 (15.4%)	9	2 (22.2%)	0 (0.0%)	4	3 (75.0%)	2 (50.0%)
Fisher exact test p-value		1.000	0.499		0.344	0.832		0.108	0.671		0.808	0.787
Race/ethnicity												
White	102	7 (6.9%)	1 (1.0%)	141	71 (50.4%)	31 (22.0%)	51	19 (37.3%)	7 (13.7%)	90	52 (57.8%)	24 (26.7%)
Black	20	5 (25.0%)	0 (0.0%)	21	13 (61.9%)	9 (42.9%)	7	2 (28.6%)	2 (28.6%)	14	11 (78.6%)	7 (50.0%)
Hispanic	37	4 (10.8%)	1 (2.7%)	21	4 (19.0%)	1 (4.8%)	8	2 (25.0%)	0 (0.0%)	13	2 (15.4%)	1 (7.7%)
Other/Unknown	33	3 (9.1%)	0 (0.0%)	11	6 (54.5%)	3 (27.3%)	3	0 (0.0%)	0 (0.0%)	8	6 (75.0%)	3 (37.5%)
Fisher exact test p-value		0.114	0.719		0.022	0.026		0.740	0.388		0.004	0.084

Table 2. Cont.

Parameter and Categories		All Eligible and Evaluable HV Subjects		Eligible HV Subjects and MBC Patients with Evaluable Cytology Slides							
				All Eligible and Evaluable MBC Patients			Newly Diagnosed MBC Patients			Progression/Recurring MBC Patients		
	N	≥1 CTC	≥5 CTC	N	≥1 CTC	≥5 CTC	N	≥1 CTC	≥5 CTC	N	≥1 CTC	≥5 CTC
Breast cancer ER status												
Positive	0	0 (0.0%)	0 (0.0%)	151	70 (46.4%)	35 (23.2%)	52	18 (34.6%)	7 (13.5%)	99	52 (52.5%)	28 (28.3%)
Negative	0	0 (0.0%)	0 (0.0%)	42	24 (57.1%)	9 (21.4%)	16	5 (31.3%)	2 (12.5%)	26	19 (73.1%)	7 (26.9%)
Fisher's Exact Test p-value		—	—		0.227	1.000		1.000	1.000		0.076	1.000
Breast Cancer PR Status												
Positive	0	0 (0.0%)	0 (0.0%)	121	57 (47.1%)	26 (21.5%)	42	13 (31.0%)	6 (14.3%)	79	44 (55.7%)	20 (25.3%)
Negative	0	0 (0.0%)	0 (0.0%)	67	33 (49.3%)	15 (22.4%)	24	9 (37.5%)	3 (12.5%)	43	24 (55.8%)	12 (27.9%)
Unknown	0	0 (0.0%)	0 (0.0%)	6	4 (66.7%)	3 (50.0%)	3	1 (33.3%)	0 (0.0%)	3	3 (100.0%)	3 (100.0%)
Fisher exact test p-value		—	—		0.879	1.000		0.599	1.000		1.000	0.830
Breast cancer HER2-Neu status												
Negative	0	0 (0.0%)	0 (0.0%)	156	70 (44.9%)	33 (21.2%)	62	21 (33.9%)	8 (12.9%)	94	49 (52.1%)	25 (26.6%)
Positive	0	0 (0.0%)	0 (0.0%)	24	17 (70.8%)	8 (33.3%)	3	1 (33.3%)	1 (33.3%)	21	16 (76.2%)	7 (33.3%)
Equivocal	0	0 (0.0%)	0 (0.0%)	8	4 (50.0%)	2 (25.0%)	1	1 (100.0%)	0 (0.0%)	7	3 (42.9%)	2 (28.6%)
Unknown	0	0 (0.0%)	0 (0.0%)	6	3 (50.0%)	1 (16.7%)	3	0 (0.0%)	0 (0.0%)	3	3 (100.0%)	1 (33.3%)
Fisher exact test p-value		—	—		0.061	0.378		0.533	0.452		0.098	0.809
Breast cancer TNBC status												
Non-TNBC	0	0 (0.0%)	0 (0.0%)	143	66 (46.2%)	33 (23.1%)	51	17 (33.3%)	7 (13.7%)	92	49 (64.1%)	26 (28.3%)
TNBC	0	0 (0.0%)	0 (0.0%)	31	19 (61.3%)	6 (19.4%)	12	5 (4.2%)	2 (16.7%)	19	14 (73.7%)	4 (21.0%)
Unknown	0	0 (0.0%)	0 (0.0%)	20	9 (45.0%)	5 (25.0%)	6	1 (16.7%)	0 (0.0%)	14	8 (57.1%)	5 (35.7%)
Fisher exact test p-value		—	—		0.4499	0.6523		0.5859	0.1019		0.6209	0.5195
Sites of metastasis (more than one may apply)												
Abdomen	0	0 (0.0%)	0 (0.0%)	6	3 (50.0%)	2 (33.3%)	3	1 (33.3%)	1 (33.3%)	3	2 (66.7%)	1 (33.3%)
Adrenal gland	0	0 (0.0%)	0 (0.0%)	3	2 (66.7%)	1 (33.3%)	0	0 (0.0%)	0 (0.0%)	3	2 (66.7%)	1 (33.3%)
Ascites	0	0 (0.0%)	0 (0.0%)	1	0 (0.0%)	0 (0.0%)	1	0 (0.0%)	0 (0.0%)	0	0 (0.0%)	0 (0.0%)
Bone	0	0 (0.0%)	0 (0.0%)	132	72 (54.5%)	40 (30.3%)	39	14 (35.9%)	9 (23.1%)	93	58 (62.4%)	31 (33.3%)
Brain	0	0 (0.0%)	0 (0.0%)	26	17 (65.4%)	9 (34.6%)	4	2 (50.0%)	1 (25.0%)	22	15 (68.2%)	8 (36.4%)
Chest wall	0	0 (0.0%)	0 (0.0%)	16	11 (68.8%)	4 (25.0%)	4	3 (75.0%)	2 (50.0%)	12	8 (66.7%)	2 (16.7%)
Kidney	0	0 (0.0%)	0 (0.0%)	0	0 (0.0%)	0 (0.0%)	0	0 (0.0%)	0 (0.0%)	0	0 (0.0%)	0 (0.0%)
Liver	0	0 (0.0%)	0 (0.0%)	73	41 (56.2%)	19 (26.0%)	9	2 (22.2%)	2 (22.2%)	64	39 (60.9%)	17 (26.6%)
Lung	0	0 (0.0%)	0 (0.0%)	70	35 (50.0%)	19 (27.1%)	22	6 (27.3%)	1 (4.5%)	48	29 (60.4%)	18 (37.5%)
Lymph nodes	0	0 (0.0%)	0 (0.0%)	101	48 (47.5%)	19 (18.8%)	31	10 (32.3%)	3 (9.7%)	70	38 (54.3%)	16 (22.9%)
Other site(s)	0	0 (0.0%)	0 (0.0%)	33	15 (45.5%)	4 (12.1%)	9	4 (44.4%)	1 (11.1%)	24	11 (45.8%)	3 (12.5%)

MBC, metastatic breast cancer; HV, healthy volunteer; TNBC, triple-negative breast cancer; ER, estrogen receptor; PR, progesterone receptor; HR, hormone receptor.

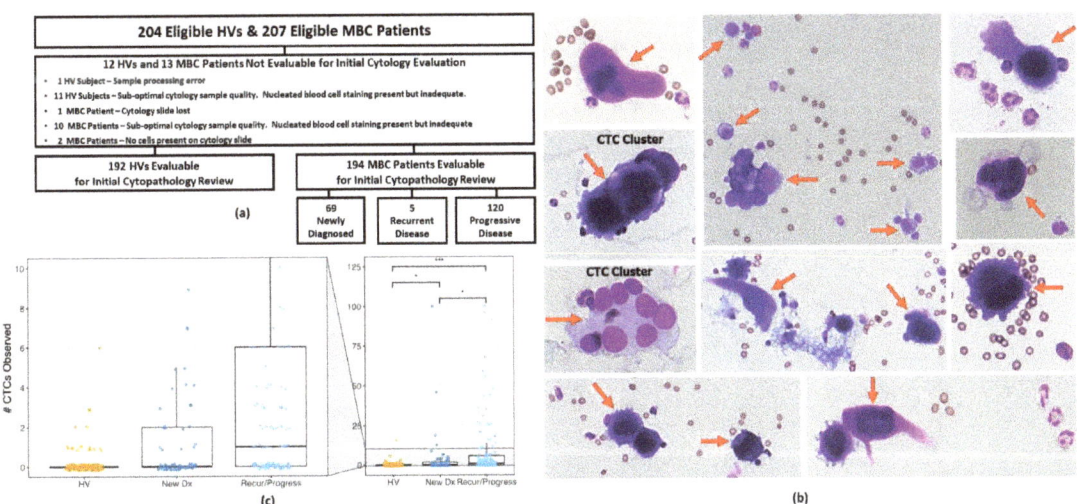

Figure 2. (**a**) Flow diagram for cytopathology evaluation in 207 eligible MBC patients. (**b**) Representative images of cells classified as CTCs (red arrows) from MBC patients that were harvested by the Parsortix PC1 system and deposited onto cytology slides by cytocentrifugation (images not to same scale) and Wright-Giemsa stained. (**c**) CTC numbers from the review of evaluable Wright-Giemsa-stained cytology slides. CTC, circulating tumor cell; HV, healthy volunteer; MBC, metastatic breast cancer. * $p < 0.05$, *** $p < 0.001$.

Examples of the Wright-Giemsa-stained CTCs are shown in Figure 2b, including harvested CTC clusters. Among the 194 patients with MBC with evaluable results, 94 (48.5%, 95% CI 41.5–55.4%) had one or more cells classified as CTCs, whereas 100 (51.5%, 95% CI 44.6–58.5%) had no cells classified as CTCs (Tables 2 and 3, Figure 2c). Among the 192 HVs that had evaluable results, 173 (90.1%, 95% CI 85.1–93.6%) had no cells classified as CTCs, whereas 19 (9.9%, 95% CI 6.4–14.9%) had one or more cells classified as CTCs, representing a significantly lower rate of CTC detection compared to that of the patients with MBC (Fisher exact test $p < 0.001$, Table 3).

Table 3. Summary of CTCs from review of evaluable Wright-Giemsa stained cytology slides from 192 HV subjects and 194 MBC patients.

No. of CTCs Observed	Cytopathology Review Results: Eligible HV Subjects and MBC Patients with Adequate Cytology Slides (% [95% CI])					
	Evaluable HV Subjects	Evaluable MBC Patients	Fisher Exact p-Value	Newly Diagnosed MBC Patients	Recurring/Progressing MBC Patients	Fisher Exact p-Value
0 CTC	173 (90.1% [85.1–93.6%])	100 (51.5% [44.6–58.5%])	—	46 (66.7% [54.9–76.6%])	54 (43.2% [34.8–52.0%])	—
≥1 CTC	19 (9.9% [6.4–14.9%])	94 (48.5% [41.5–55.4%])	<0.001	23 (33.3% [23.4–45.1%])	71 (56.8% [48.0–65.2%])	0.003
≥2 CTC	6 (3.1% [1.4–6.6%])	77 (39.7% [33.1–46.7%])	<0.001	18 (26.1% [17.2–37.5%])	59 (47.2% [38.7–55.9%])	0.006
≥3 CTC	4 (2.1% [0.8–5.2%])	63 (32.5% [26.3–39.4%])	<0.001	14 (20.3% [12.5–31.2%])	49 (39.2% [31.1–48.0%])	0.010
≥4 CTC	2 (1.0% [0.3–3.7%])	53 (27.3% [21.5–34.0%])	<0.001	12 (17.4% [10.2–28.0%])	41 (32.8% [25.2–41.4%])	0.028
≥5 CTC	2 (1.0% [0.3–3.7%])	44 (22.7% [17.3–29.1%])	<0.001	9 (13.0% [7.0–23.0%])	35 (28.0% [20.9–36.4%])	0.020

Table 3. *Cont.*

No. of CTCs Observed	Cytopathology Review Results: Eligible HV Subjects and MBC Patients with Adequate Cytology Slides (% [95% CI])					
	Evaluable HV Subjects	Evaluable MBC Patients	Fisher Exact *p*-Value	Newly Diagnosed MBC Patients	Recurring/Progressing MBC Patients	Fisher Exact *p*-Value
≥10 CTC	1 (0.5% [0.1–2.9%])	30 (15.5% [11.0–21.2%])	<0.001	4 (5.8% [2.3–14.0%])	26 (20.8% [14.6–28.7%])	0.006
TOTAL N	192	194		69	125	

HV, healthy volunteer; MBC, metastatic breast cancer.

A significantly larger proportion of patients with MBC with recurring or progressive metastatic disease were found to have one or more CTCs compared to those with newly diagnosed metastatic disease (Table 3), which is consistent with what has been reported in the literature on CTCs in metastatic breast cancer [36]. Furthermore, CTC counts were significantly higher in patients with recurring/progressive disease ($p = 0.019$, Figure 2c).

Table 2 further summarizes the proportions of HVs and patients with MBC with CTCs observed on their cytology slides according to various demographic and clinical subgroups. Interestingly, among women with newly diagnosed MBC, approximately twice as many who were ≥ 57 years old (i.e., post-menopausal women) were observed to have CTCs compared to those who were < 57 years old (47.2% vs. 18.2%, respectively, $p = 0.012$).

There is also some evidence that the sample collection method had an impact on the CTC counts. A significantly larger proportion of the patients with MBC whose blood was drawn via a central port were observed to have CTCs compared with the patients whose blood was drawn via venipuncture (≥1 CTC: 94.3% vs. 38.4%, respectively, Fisher exact test $p < 0.001$, ≥5 CTCs: 62.9% vs. 13.8%, respectively, Fisher exact test $p < 0.001$, Table 2). This may be due to technical or procedural differences, volume, anatomic collection location, or patient population (a larger percentage of patients with progressive or recurrent disease had their blood samples collected via an installed port; Table 1). Previous reports have also shown that CTC levels can vary by anatomical location of cancer [37,38]. Additionally, peripheral blood drawn from antecubital veins has likely circulated through both lung and peripheral capillaries after egressing from tumors (from either primary, i.e., breast, or metastatic sites). In contrast, some blood from a central port comes directly from the tumor without first filtering through additional capillary beds. The Parsortix® PC1 System enriches for cells that cannot pass through the ~6.5-µm critical gap of the separation cassette at 99 millibars of pressure (roughly equivalent to typical diastolic blood pressure); these same cells may likewise be unable to traverse the microcirculation of a capillary lumen. Another possible explanation for this observation is that patients with MBC with a central port indwelling usually receive intravenous treatments such as chemotherapy and thus may have a more aggressive disease compared to the wider population of patients with MBC. Progressive disease was noted in 31 (88.6%) of the 35 patients who had blood drawn from a central port and in only 94 (59.1%) of the 159 patients who had blood drawn via venipuncture (Fisher exact test $p = 0.001$, Table 2). Consequently, this subset of patients with MBC (i.e., those with a central port installed experiencing disease progression) is a specific population that would likely benefit from CTC evaluation.

In summary, cytologic evaluation showed that 48.5% (95% CI 41.5–55.4%) of all patients with MBC with evaluable staining results had one or more CTCs identified. Even though cytocentrifugation is a widely used method for depositing cells onto cytology slides and recent studies have shown that Parsortix-harvested cells deposited onto cytology slides via cytocentrifugation have effectively preserved cellular morphology [39], it is essential to note that this method caused significant loss (~57% on average) of the cells present in the Parsortix® PC1 System harvests. Given this large observed cell loss, it is possible that a larger proportion of patients with MBC had CTCs present in their harvests, but these cells were simply not retained on the cytology slides. Alternative techniques to place cells on microscope slides without using the cytocentrifugation methods are under development. However, other downstream analysis techniques, such as gene expression analysis, may be able to utilize cells captured and harvested directly into a container without loss of the harvested cells potentially caused by subsequent manipulations of the harvested material.

3.3. Gene Expression by qRT-PCR

As described above, CTCs harvested directly for gene expression may serve as more effective biomarkers of CTCs. Although still subject to variation, gene expression analysis is relatively less subjective than image analysis and does not require deposition of the cells onto a slide. A subset of enrolled patients had a second blood tube processed by the Parsortix® PC1 System, and the cells harvested were subjected to gene expression analysis by qRT-PCR (as described in this section) or RNA-seq (as described in the next section). The qRT-PCR assay used to evaluate gene markers for epithelial, mesenchymal and breast cancer cells was shown to be reliable and reproducible [40] and was able to detect a single epithelial cell that expressed *KRT19*, a single epithelial cell that expressed *ERRB2*, 10 cells that expressed *EPCAM*, or approximately 25–50 mesenchymal cells that expressed *SNAI2* and/or *TWIST1* (data not shown).

Figure 3a provides the flow chart for the 77 eligible patients with MBC and 105 eligible HVs where the second blood sample was used for qPCR regarding their eligibility for this exploratory evaluation. Only one of the lysates from the 75 patients with MBC and two lysates from the 104 HVs who had a sufficient volume of blood for processing failed to produce a reliable PCR readout (as determined by the lack of positive signal for the housekeeping genes), leaving a total of 74 patients with MBC and 102 HVs with evaluable qPCR results.

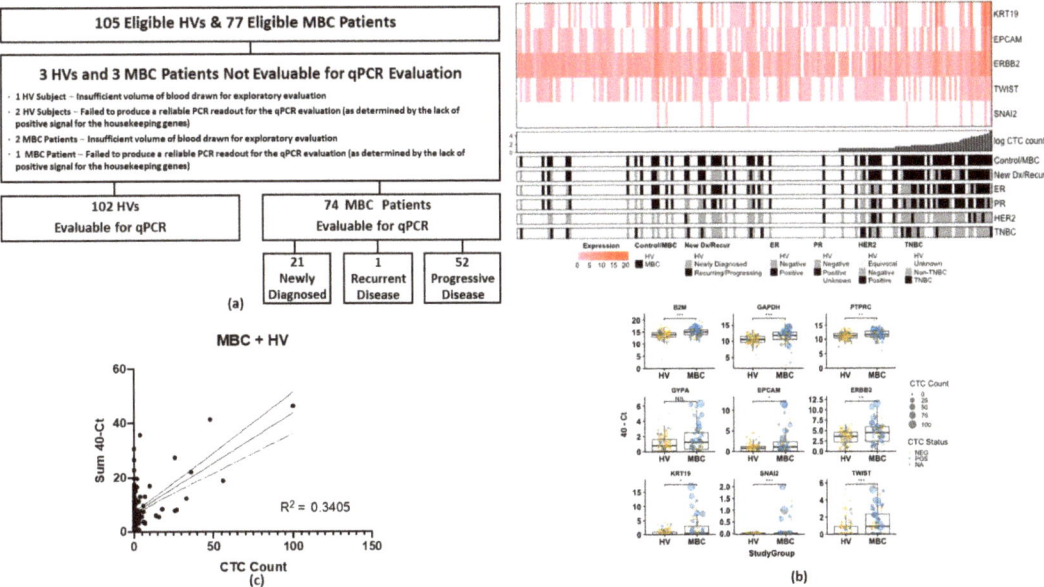

Figure 3. (a) Flow diagram for qPCR evaluation in eligible HV and MBC patients. (b) CTC count correlates with total CTC-related gene expression (40-Sum of KRT19, EPCAM, ERBB2, TWIST, and SNAI2 Ct values). Heat map and scatter plots of CTC gene expression show correlation of gene expression with the number of CTCs observed (c) Sum CTC related genes expression = 0.3701 ∗ CTC count + 6.771; R square = 0.3405, slope significantly different from zero ($p < 0.0001$). HV, healthy volunteer; MBC, metastatic breast cancer; qPCR, quantitative polymerase chain reaction. NS = $p \geq 0.05$, * $p < 0.05$, ** $p < 0.01$, *** $p < 0.001$.

CTC gene expression from the qPCR evaluation and the corresponding enumeration from the cytology evaluation are summarized in Table 4. A total of 18 negative controls (nuclease-free water) and 18 positive controls (SUM149 cell lysate) were compared with the patient and HV samples. Using a Ct threshold of ≤35.0 for each of the genes to define positivity, none of the negative controls were positive for any of the genes, and 100% of the positive controls were positive for all of the genes (except the *GYPA* and *PTPRC* genes, as expected). In both the patients with MBC and HVs, 100% were positive for one or both of the housekeeping genes, 100% were positive for *PTPRC* (indicating the presence of white blood cells in all of the harvests), and <7% were positive for *GYPA* (indicating a low incidence of red blood cell contamination). As shown in Table 4, 52.7% of the patients with MBC were positive (Ct value ≤ 35.0) for at least one of the CTC-related genes (*KRT19*, *EPCAM*, *ERBB2*, *TWIST1*, and/or *SNAI2*), whereas only 19.6% of the HVs were positive for at least one of the CTC-related genes. Optimizing the Ct thresholds for each gene based on expression in the HVs increased the specificity of CTC genes at the expense of sensitivity (Table S1).

Table 4. Proportions of HV subjects and MBC patients with positive gene expression using a Ct value threshold of ≤35.0 for each gene to determine positivity and comparisons to numbers of CTCs observed on Wright-Giemsa-stained slides during cytopathology review.

Group *	N	GAPDH	B2M	GYPA	PTPRC	KRT19	EpCAM	ERBB2	TWIST1	SNAI2	KRT19, EpCAM, ERBB2, TWIST &/or SNAI2	KRT19, EpCAM, TWIST &/or SNAI2
Negative Controls	18	0.0%	0.0%	0.0%	0.0%	0.0%	0.0%	0.0%	0.0%	0.0%	0.0%	0.0%
Positive Controls	18	100.0%	100.0%	5.6%	16.7%	100.0%	100.0%	100.0%	100.0%	100.0%	100.0%	100.0%
All HVs	102	99.0%	100.0%	2.0%	100.0%	0.0%	1.0%	19.6%	1.0%	0.0%	19.6%	1.0%
with a CTC count	99 (97.1%)	100.0%	100.0%	2.0%	100.0%	0.0%	1.0%	20.2%	1.0%	0.0%	20.2%	1.0%
with 0 CTC	83 (83.8%)	100.0%	100.0%	2.4%	100.0%	0.0%	1.2%	21.7%	1.2%	0.0%	21.7%	1.2%
with 1 CTC	11 (11.1%)	100.0%	100.0%	0.0%	100.0%	0.0%	0.0%	18.2%	0.0%	0.0%	18.2%	0.0%
with 2–4 CTCs	3 (3.1%)	100.0%	100.0%	0.0%	100.0%	0.0%	0.0%	0.0%	0.0%	0.0%	0.0%	0.0%
with 5–9 CTCs	1 (1.0%)	100.0%	100.0%	0.0%	100.0%	0.0%	0.0%	0.0%	0.0%	0.0%	0.0%	0.0%
with ≥10 CTCs	1 (1.0%)	100.0%	100.0%	0.0%	100.0%	0.0%	0.0%	0.0%	0.0%	0.0%	0.0%	0.0%
All MBC patients	74	98.6%	100.0%	5.4%	100.0%	21.6%	13.5%	47.3%	5.4%	0.0%	52.7%	24.3%
with a CTC count	71 (95.9%)	98.6%	100.0%	5.6%	100.0%	22.5%	14.1%	47.9%	5.6%	0.0%	53.5%	25.4%
with 0 CTC	31 (43.7%)	100.0%	100.0%	3.2%	100.0%	22.6%	9.7%	48.4%	6.5%	0.0%	54.8%	25.8%
with 1 CTC	10 (14.1%)	100.0%	100.0%	0.0%	100.0%	0.0%	0.0%	30.0%	0.0%	0.0%	30.0%	0.0%
with 2–4 CTCs	14 (19.7%)	92.9%	100.0%	0.0%	100.0%	28.6%	21.4%	42.9%	7.1%	0.0%	57.1%	35.7%
with 5–9 CTCs	5 (7.0%)	100.0%	100.0%	0.0%	100.0%	0.0%	0.0%	40.0%	0.0%	0.0%	40.0%	0.0%
with ≥10 CTCs	11 (15.5%)	100.0%	100.0%	27.3%	100.0%	45.5%	36.4%	72.7%	9.1%	0.0%	72.7%	45.5%
All newly diagnosed MBC patients	21	100.0%	100.0%	9.5%	100.0%	23.8%	9.5%	66.7%	14.3%	0.0%	71.4%	28.6%
with a CTC count	20 (95.2%)	100.0%	100.0%	10.0%	100.0%	25.0%	10.0%	65.0%	15.0%	0.0%	70.0%	30.0%
with 0 CTC	12 (60.0%)	100.0%	100.0%	8.3%	100.0%	33.3%	8.3%	66.7%	16.7%	0.0%	75.0%	41.7%
with 1 CTC	2 (10.0%)	100.0%	100.0%	0.0%	100.0%	0.0%	0.0%	50.0%	0.0%	0.0%	50.0%	0.0%
with 2–4 CTCs	3 (15.0%)	100.0%	100.0%	0.0%	100.0%	0.0%	0.0%	66.7%	0.0%	0.0%	66.7%	0.0%
with 5–9 CTCs	2 (10.0%)	100.0%	100.0%	0.0%	100.0%	0.0%	0.0%	50.0%	0.0%	0.0%	50.0%	0.0%
with ≥10 CTCs	1 (5.0%)	100.0%	100.0%	100.0%	100.0%	100.0%	100.0%	100.0%	0.0%	0.0%	100.0%	100.0%

Table 4. Cont.

Group *	N	GAPDH	B2M	GYPA	PTPRC	KRT19	EpCAM	ERBB2	TWIST1	SNAI2	KRT19, EpCAM, ERBB2, TWIST &/or SNAI2	KRT19, EpCAM, TWIST &/or SNAI2
All recurrent/progressive MBC patients	53	98.1%	100.0%	3.8%	100.0%	20.8%	15.1%	39.6%	1.9%	0.0%	45.3%	22.6%
MBC patients with CTC count	51 (96.2%)	98.0%	100.0%	3.9%	100.0%	21.6%	15.7%	41.2%	2.0%	0.0%	47.1%	23.5%
with 0 CTC	19 (37.2%)	100.0%	100.0%	0.0%	100.0%	15.8%	10.5%	36.8%	0.0%	0.0%	42.1%	15.8%
with 1 CTC	8 (15.7%)	100.0%	100.0%	0.0%	100.0%	0.0%	0.0%	25.0%	0.0%	0.0%	25.0%	0.0%
with 2–4 CTCs	11 (21.6%)	90.9%	100.0%	0.0%	100.0%	36.4%	27.3%	36.4%	9.1%	0.0%	54.5%	45.5%
with 5–9 CTCs	3 (5.9%)	100.0%	100.0%	0.0%	100.0%	0.0%	0.0%	33.3%	0.0%	0.0%	33.3%	0.0%
with ≥10 CTCs	10 (19.6%)	100.0%	100.0%	20.0%	100.0%	40.0%	30.0%	70.0%	0.0%	0.0%	70.0%	40.0%

HV, healthy volunteer; MBC, metastatic breast cancer. * CTC count and gene expression are from separate, parallel blood tubes.

As shown in Figure 3b, control genes, including *GAPDH*, *B2M*, and *PTPRC* (CD45), were elevated in the samples from the MBC patients, suggesting both putative CTCs and white blood cells have a higher capture rate in samples from patients with MBC compared to samples from HVs. In the patients with MBC and HVs, respectively, 21.6% vs. 0% were positive for KRT19, 13.5% vs. 1.0% were positive for *EPCAM*, 47.3% vs. 19.6% were positive for ERBB2 (indicating a level of background expression for this gene), 5.4% vs. 1.0% were positive for TWIST1, and none were positive for SNAI2 (Table 4). Looking at the combined expression of only the KRT19, *EPCAM*, *TWIST1*, and/or *SNAI2* genes, only 1.0% of the HVs compared to 24.3% of the patients with MBC were positive for one or more of those cancer cell–related genes (Fisher exact test $p < 0.001$) (Table 4).

When compared to the number of CTCs identified using a cytomorphological review of the Wright-Giemsa stained cytology slides, the sum total expression of CTC-related genes (40-Ct of KRT19, *EPCAM*, ERBB2, *TWIST1*, and *SNAI2*) showed a general correlation with CTC enumeration, particularly at higher CTC burdens ($R^2 = 0.3405$, Pearson' rho = 0.569, $p < 0.001$, Spearman's rho [less influenced by outliers] = 0.159, $p = 0.034$, Figure 3b,c). The discrepancy at lower CTC counts may reflect the utility of gene expression when morphology may be hard to distinguish or may reflect differences between parallel blood tubes (e.g., significant loss of harvested cells on the cytology slides due to cytocentrifugation slide preparation method). Furthermore, as seen in Table 4, only 1 (1.2%) of the 83 HVs with 0 CTCs identified on their cytology slides and none (0%) of the 16 HVs with ≥1 CTC identified on their cytology slides were positive for the combination of *KRT19*, *EPCAM*, *TWIST1*, and/or *SNAI2*, in contrast to 8 (25.8%) of the 31 patients with MBC with 0 CTCs identified on their cytology slides and 9 (22.5%) of the 40 patients with MBC with ≥1 CTC identified on their cytology slides (Table 4). This suggests that the orthogonal measures of morphology and gene expression could help increase detection specificity.

As seen in Figure 3b, samples enriched from patients with MBC had significantly elevated expression of *EPCAM* (Mann–Whitney U $p = 0.016$), ERBB2 ($p = 0.0025$), KRT19 ($p = 0.049$), and the mesenchymal cell–related genes SNAI2 ($p < 0.001$) and TWIST1 ($p < 0.001$). Interestingly, when no CTCs were detected on the paired cytology slide, there was no difference in *EPCAM* or *KRT19* expression between patients with MBC and HVs, but ERBB2, SNAI2, and TWIST1 remained elevated in the patient samples (Figure S2). Furthermore, samples from patients with MBC had elevated housekeeping control genes *B2M* and *GAPDH* independent of the detection of CTCs. In contrast, the white blood cell and red blood cell control genes *PTPRC* and *GYPA* were not elevated (Figure S2). Together, these results suggest that CTCs with mesenchymal features are less likely to be detected visually (or are more easily lost during the cytocentrifugation slide preparation method) and that adding the molecular characterization aided in their detection.

Comparing samples from patients with newly diagnosed MBC and patients with recurrent or progressive MBC, there were no significant differences in total CTC gene expression (Figure 4a), in contrast to the stark differences in CTC counts between patients with MBC and HVs. However, compared to the HVs, *EPCAM*, *KRT19*, and *TWIST1* were significantly higher in patients with progressive/recurrent MBC (but not in newly diagnosed MBC); only *ERBB2* and *SNAI2* were elevated in both patient cohorts (Figure S3). This may be due to the relatively smaller sample size of patients in the newly diagnosed MBC patient cohort.

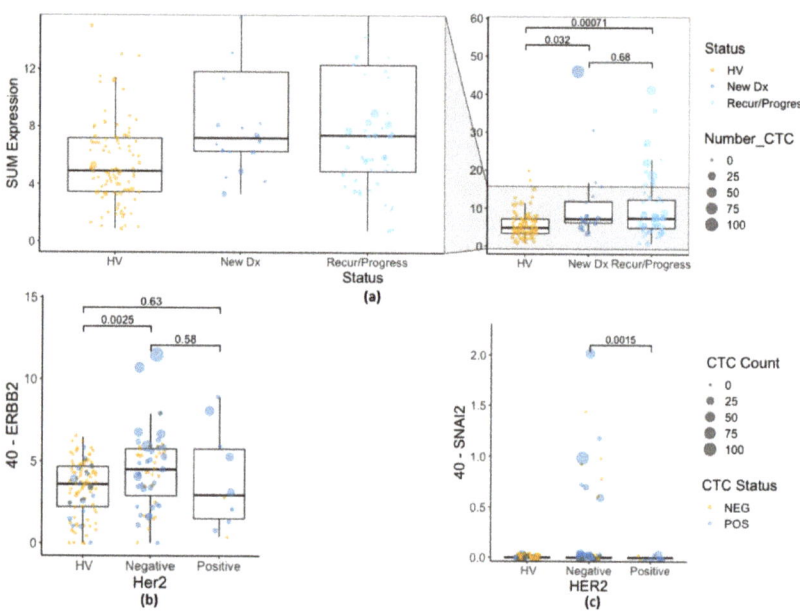

Figure 4. (a) Sum of CTC-related gene expression (40-Sum of EPCAM, KRT19, ERBB2, SNAI2, and TWIST Ct values) in HV, newly diagnosed MBC, and MBC with recurrence or progression. (b) ERBB2 expression in CTC-enriched samples by tissue HER2 status. (c) SNAI2 expression in CTC-enriched samples by tissue HER2 status. CTC, circulating tumor cell; HV, healthy volunteer; MBC, metastatic breast cancer.

Patients with HER2-positive tumor tissue would be expected to have CTCs with elevated expression of *ERBB2* (the gene product for the HER2 protein). However, there was no significant difference in the *ERBB2* expression by enriched CTCs in patients with HER2-positive tumors compared to those with HER2-negative tumors, with the caveat that there were very few patients with HER2-positive MBC disease (40-Ct = 3.87 for patients with HER2-positive tumors vs. 40-Ct = 4.44 for patients with HER2-negative tumors, Wilcoxon signed rank test $p = 0.4$, Student's t-test $p = 0.5823$, Figure 4b). Likewise, among the patients with MBC with detectable CTCs on their cytology slide, qPCR expression of *ERBB2* was nearly identical between HER2 groups (40-Ct = 4.44 for patients with HER2-positive tumors vs. 40-Ct = 4.53 for patients with HER2-negative tumors, Student's t-test $p = 0.936$). However, in this study, all of the patients with MBC with HER2-positive tumors had recurring or progressing diseases at the time; none of the patients with HER2-positive tumors were newly diagnosed. Patients with MBC with HER2-negative tumors (who consequently did not receive HER2-targeted therapy) had higher expression of ERBB2 than HVs ($p = 0.0025$), whereas MBC patients with HER2-positive tumors did not ($p = 0.63$) (Figure 4b).

Furthermore, only patients with MBC with HER2-negative tumor tissue expressed SNAI2, although this difference was not statistically significant. Eleven patients with MBC with HER2-negative tumors showed expression of *SNAI2* by qPCR, while no patients with MBC with HER2-positive tumors and no HVs showed *SNAI2* expression (Fisher exact test p = 0.3455); average *SNAI2* expression was higher in the HER2-negative cohort (Figure 4c). Others have noted that HER2 expression can drive EMT [41–46], including EMT in CTCs [47], and can predict the presence of CTCs [48]. All the patients with MBC with HER2-positive tumor tissue in the current study were enrolled with progressive and/or recurrent disease.

There were no other significant differences in expression levels of the CTC-related genes between various breast cancer subtypes (estrogen receptor-positive, progesterone receptor positive, HER2-positive, triple-negative). However, some weak trends were observed (Figure 3c, sorted by CTC count, and Figure S4, hierarchical clustering by gene expression). High gene expression was generally associated with high CTC counts on the corresponding cytology slide. CTC gene expression in patients with triple-negative breast cancer was dispersed but tended to cluster with higher expression (Figure S4).

As described above, samples collected via a port had a much higher CTC count by cytology review. However, molecular profiling (Figure S5) showed only a slight trend for higher expression of CTC genes. Only the white blood cell marker *PTPRC* (CD45) was significantly higher in samples from patients with MBC collected via the port. These results suggest that the decrease in CTC counts by cytology review could be partially due to sample quality related to the slide preparation method since the morphology is lost to a greater extent compared to the gene expression.

These results demonstrated that the cells harvested from the peripheral blood of patients with MBC by the Parsortix® PC1 System could be analyzed with a qPCR method to evaluate the expression of genes using standard molecular techniques currently used in many clinical and/or research laboratory settings.

3.4. Combining Gene Expression Results with CTC Counts Reduces Classification Uncertainty

Among the 176 samples evaluated for gene expression and CTC enumeration, there were no HVs that had both >1 observed CTC and expression of any CTC-related genes (excluding ERBB2) below a standard Ct threshold of 35.0. At the same time, 17 patients with MBC met both criteria (Figure S6, Node 6, far-right). Furthermore, only 15 of the 74 patients with MBC (20.3%) had both no observed CTCs and no expression of any CTC-related genes (Figure S6, Node 7, far-left). Additionally, 8 (10.6%) patients with MBC that had no CTCs detected by cytology were positive for at least 1 CTC-related gene, suggesting an increased sensitivity due to the inclusion of gene expression compared to the use of CTC counts alone.

3.5. RNA-Sequencing

For unbiased evaluation of gene expression, RNA-seq was performed using cDNA prepared from RNA isolated from the CTC harvests of a subset of HVs and a small number of patients with MBC. Figure 5a provides the flow chart for the 18 eligible patients with MBC and 59 HVs whose second blood sample was intended to be used for the RNA-seq evaluation. A total of 53 HVs and 16 patients with MBC were evaluable for the analysis. The data contained a significant percentage of genomic DNA or other non-mRNA materials, representing approximately 90% of the sequenced reads. However, there were no significant differences (Student's t-test) in the observed transcriptome reads, total reads, or percentage mapped to the transcriptome between the Parsortix® PC1 System harvests obtained from the HVs and the patients with MBC. There was minimal non-human and ribosomal contamination. To assess the quality of the sequencing, a quality score (Q-score), which is a prediction of the probability of an error in base calling, was used. A high Q-score implies that a base call is more reliable and less likely to be incorrect, where $Q = -10 \log 10$ (e). For example, for base calls with a quality score of Q30, one base call in 1000 is predicted to be incorrect. The Q30 values for the sequencing data from the 53 HVs and 16 patients with MBC were all more than 90%, and the coverages (the rate of sequencing reads covering the reference genome cDNA sequence) were of a sufficient level in all samples. The transcriptome mapping results were consistent across all samples, so differential gene expression comparison was possible.

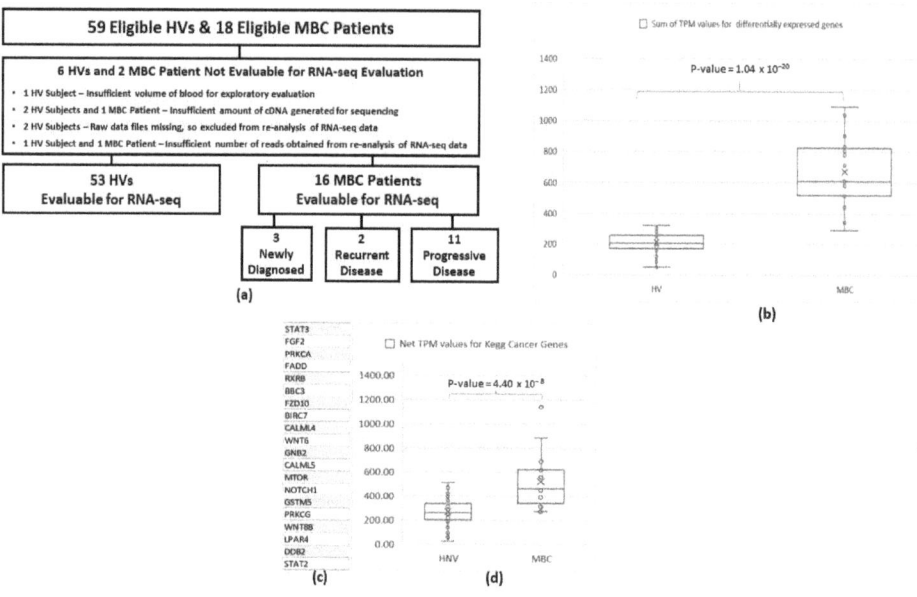

Figure 5. (**a**) Flow diagram for RNA-seq evaluation in eligible HV and MBC patients. (**b**) Sum of TPM values for all genes differentially expressed ($p < 0.001$) between Parsortix PC1 harvests obtained from HV comparators and MBC patients. (**c**) Genes from the KEGG Cancer Pathway were differentially expressed between the HV and MBC harvests ($p < 0.05$) (**d**). Net TPM score of these 20 genes for HV and MBC samples. CTC, circulating tumor cell; HV, healthy volunteer; MBC, metastatic breast cancer.

TPM-normalized expression values per gene were generated for all samples. A total of 200 genes were found to be differentially expressed between HVs and patients with MBC with $p < 0.005$ (Student's t-test), 424 genes were differentially expressed with $p < 0.01$, and 2570 genes were differentially expressed with $p < 0.05$. Figure 5b plots the sum of the TPM values from each sample for the differentially expressed genes between the HVs and patients with MBC with individual p-values of <0.001. The two groups are well differentiated by this set of genes, with a p-value of <0.0001 (Student's t-test).

The expression of genes in the harvests from the Parsortix® PC1 System known to be associated with the KEGG Pathways in cancer (https://www.kegg.jp, accessed on 20 October 2022) was examined for differential expression between the HVs and patients with MBC. Figure 5c lists the genes in the KEGG cancer pathways set that were determined to be differentially expressed between the HVs and patients with MBC with p-values of <0.05 (Student's t-test). For illustrative purposes, a simple combination of the TPM values for these genes (net TPM score equals the sum of TPM for upregulated genes minus the sum of TPM values for downregulated genes) was calculated for each sample. Figure 5d illustrates the net TPM values derived from the 20 KEGG cancer pathway genes with p-values of <0.05 (Student's t-test) for each of the HV and MBC samples. Significant discrimination was observed between the groups (Student's t-test $p < 0.0001$). Since cancer signaling pathways were significantly enriched in the samples from the MBC patients compared to those from the HVs, this result suggests that the population of cells captured and harvested from the peripheral blood of patients with MBC processed by the Parsortix® PC1 System does contain cancer cells.

Further examples are illustrated in Figures S7–S9, where harvests from various subgroups of patients with MBC are compared. Genes from the KEGG cancer pathway list were examined for differential expression between the identified groups. A net TPM score was generated for each sample using the genes that exhibited individual p-values of <0.05. Figure S7 lists the relevant genes and illustrates discrimination based on grouping patients by tissue HER2 status. Figure S8 provides a list of genes that appear to be associated with metastases to the lymph nodes. Figure S9 identifies a different gene expression profile potentially reflecting the presence of bone metastases.

The RNA-seq data confirm that the cells harvested by the Parsortix® PC1 System from the peripheral blood of patients with MBC (and HVs) can be used to generate RNA-seq data that directly reflect cancer-associated gene expression patterns. This was demonstrated despite contaminating genomic DNA, illustrating the further potential to be realized with alternative RNA-seq sample preparation protocols.

3.6. HER2 FISH

HER2 is an important diagnostic component of breast cancer management and is typically evaluable at the single-cell level. Therefore, one of our exploratory evaluations involved interrogating the HER2 amplification status in the population of cells harvested from a subset of the HVs and patients with MBC using the Parsortix® PC1 System.

Figure 6a provides the flow chart for the 40 eligible HVs and 112 patients with MBC, collected at The MD Anderson Cancer Center, University of Rochester Medical Center, and Northwestern University, whose second blood sample was intended to be used for the HER2 FISH evaluation. A total of 38 (95.0%) of the 40 eligible HVs and 101 (90.2%) of the 112 eligible patients with MBC had evaluable HER2 FISH-stained cytology slides; 5 (13.2%) of the 38 evaluable HVs and 28 (27.7%) of the 101 evaluable patients with MBC had one or more CTCs identified on their HER2 FISH-stained cytology slides (Table S2).

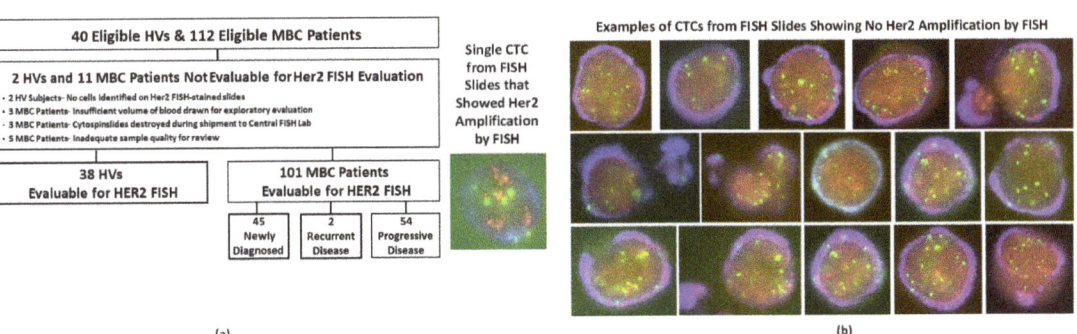

Figure 6. (a) Flow diagram for HER2 FISH evaluation in eligible MBC patients. (b) Example images of HER2 FISH-stained CTCs from MBC patients that were harvested by the Parsortix PC1 system and deposited onto cytology slides (images not to scale). CTC, circulating tumor cell; HV, healthy volunteer; MBC, metastatic breast cancer; FISH, fluorescence in situ hybridization.

Figure 6b provides example images of the CTCs identified on the HER2 FISH slides of patients with MBC, including the single CTC from a newly diagnosed patient with HER2-positive MBC that demonstrated HER2 amplification. The single sample showing HER2 amplification represents 33.3% of the patients with MBC who had HER2-positive disease and had CTCs identified on their HER2 FISH slides (Table 5). Approximately 83% of the patients with MBC had estrogen receptor–positive and/or progesterone receptor–positive disease, and only 9.9% had HER2-positive breast cancer, which is lower than the proportion generally described in the literature (~20%). Therefore, although a reasonable number of samples were tested for HER2 status by FISH, only a minimal number were expected to have HER2 amplification. It should be noted that a strict definition of HER2 FISH positivity was used for this study, permitting resolution of all CTCs into either "HER2-amplified" or "HER2-not-amplified" status, as described previously in large cohorts of breast cancer patients and patients screened for entry to large clinical trials [31–33].

Table 5. Results from evaluation of Parsortix harvests using HER2 FISH. The number and proportion of samples with CTCs identified on the FISH slide and the number and proportion of samples showing CTCs with HER2 amplification in the HV subjects and MBC patients by their tissue HER2 status.

Parameter and Categories	HVs	MBC Patients by Tissue HER2 Status			
		Unknown	Equivocal	Negative	Positive
n	38	3	4	84	10
No. with CTC identified	5 (13.2%)	0 (0.0%)	2 (50.0%)	23 (27.4%)	3 (30.0%)
No. with HER2 amplified in CTC	0 of 5 (0%)	-	0 of 2 (0%)	0 of 23 (0%)	1 of 3 (33.3%)

FISH, fluorescence in situ hybridization; HV, healthy volunteer; MBC, metastatic breast cancer.

These results demonstrated that the Parsortix® PC1 System can capture and harvest CTCs from the peripheral blood of patients with MBC and that the population of cells harvested can be effectively evaluated using a commercially available HER2 FISH assay and reagents.

4. Study Limitations

The open platform of the Parsortix system allows for multiple downstream analyses. However, this openness may limit immediate introduction to clinical environments as it requires additional technology, personnel, and equipment out of the box. It was difficult to comprehensively demonstrate all potential downstream evaluation methods that a user could employ to evaluate the cells harvested by the Parsortix® PC1 System from the peripheral blood of patients with MBC. In this study, we focused on cytology evaluation, qPCR, FISH, and RNA-seq as examples of downstream analysis methods. These four methods cover a range of cytology and molecular techniques currently used in clinical laboratories and many FDA-cleared tests, including protein, RNA, and DNA analysis techniques.

We recognize that the study is limited by a lack of additional alternative downstream analyses, such as interrogation for mutations. Still, the study design and amount of testing that could be done for each subject were limited by the volume of blood that we could safely and ethically draw from the patients with MBC. In addition, the cytology evaluation method used to identify CTCs was based solely on morphological characteristics and, therefore, more subjective than an immunofluorescence staining assay. Additionally, the slide preparation method for the cytology and FISH analyses proved to have a high cell loss, with 37–51% of the harvested cells not being deposited on the slides. This most likely resulted in underestimation of the number of CTCs in the blood samples. However, a correction factor would not be practical for the high number of samples with no CTCs observed, as the cell loss caused by the cytology slide preparation method was highly variable. However, we used cytocentrifugation (also known as cytospin) because it is a routine procedure performed in pathology laboratory practice and readily available to most laboratories. In addition to the cell loss caused by the cytology slide preparation method, the degree of subjectivity around the cytomorphological interpretation/identification of CTCs is another study limitation. CTC-specific markers (such as pan-cytokeratin), in addition to the Wright-Giemsa staining, to assess the phenotype of the atypical, non-normal, and malignant cells identified on the CTC slides may have provided additional evidence that the malignant cells indeed were CTCs. However, the morphological scoring of CTCs has more clinical value and avoids the use of potentially poor-performing antibodies. Future efforts to establish diagnostic criteria for morphologic CTC evaluation are needed in conjunction with broader adoption of the Parsortix® PC1 System in clinical practice.

The study specified that a minimum volume of blood needed to be available (≥ 5 mL) for the processing of each sample instead of specifying that an exact volume of blood be used for each sample (e.g., 7.5 mL or 8 mL). However, the use of varying volumes of blood for each sample makes it impossible to directly compare results between samples that used different volumes of blood. Furthermore, there is known variability in the numbers of cells present between different tubes of blood taken from the same patient (tube-to-tube variability).

No FDA-cleared orthogonal method was tested to demonstrate the equivalency of the Parsortix® PC1 System for the capture and harvest of CTCs. The FDA-cleared CELLSEARCH® System was not deemed suitable for inclusion as a reference method because its technological operating characteristics are fundamentally different. The CELLSEARCH® System enriches CTCs based on immunoaffinity to EpCAM, magnetically immobilizes the cells inside a visualization chamber, stains the captured cells with DAPI and anti-EpCAM and anti-CD45 antibodies, captures fluorescent images of the stained cells, and presents the digitized images to a user for identification of CTCs. In contrast, the Parsortix® PC1 System uses microfluidics to enrich cells based on their size and deformability, and it allows the cells captured by the microfluidic device to be harvested into a small buffer volume for further evaluation. The Parsortix PC1 System may have an advantage over the CELL-SEARCH System in detecting mesenchymal CTCs, but CTCs can be epithelial, mesenchymal, or hybrid. Furthermore, the clinical significance of the amount and type of CTC on therapeutic efficacy in MBC as well as primary breast cancer is still unknown. It remains to be seen how the CTCs detected in the current study will affect the clinical outcome of MBC patients.

Follow-up studies will be required to demonstrate the clinical utility of CTC enrichment in patients with MBC using the Parsortix® PC1 System in combination with analytically validated subsequent downstream analysis methods for molecular characteristics. This study was designed only to test the enrichment platform, and thus, the samples obtained were de-identified, and no follow-up clinical data was collected.

Overall, the results of this study showed that the population of cells harvested by the Parsortix® PC1 System from the peripheral blood of patients with MBC could be evaluated using currently available laboratory methods for the identification and characterization of CTCs. As CTCs are obtained from peripheral blood (i.e., a liquid biopsy), additional samples can easily be obtained with minimal impact if there is a processing error and/or no CTCs are present in the population of cells harvested or if additional blood volume is deemed necessary to meet downstream assay performance requirements.

5. Conclusions

The HOMING Study "Harvest of CTCs from Patients with MBC using the Parsortix® System" was a multi-center, prospective, blinded study that enrolled over 200 evaluable healthy volunteers and 200 patients with MBC at four US-based clinical sites to demonstrate the ability of the system to enrich CTC for subsequent downstream analysis. The data here showed that cells harvested from the peripheral blood of the eligible HVs and patients with MBC using the Parsortix® PC1 System can be successfully evaluated using cytology (i.e., Wright-Giemsa staining), qRT-PCR, RNA-sequencing, and FISH. The data generated from this study were used to support a De Novo request for classification of the Parsortix® PC1 system (DEN200062) as a Class II prescription device that was granted by the FDA on 24 May 2022 (https://www.accessdata.fda.gov/cdrh_docs/pdf20/DEN200062.pdf, accessed on 20 October 2022).

Supplementary Materials: The following supporting information can be downloaded at: https://www.mdpi.com/article/10.3390/cancers14215238/s1, Figure S1: Comparison of linearity, Figure S2: Gene expression in samples with and without detected CTCs in corresponding cytology slides, Figure S3: CTC-related gene expression in newly diagnosed and recurrent/progressive metastatic breast cancer (MBC), Figure S4: CTC count and CTC-related gene expression hierarchical clustering, Figure S5: Trend for higher CTC-related gene expression from samples collected from a port, Figure S6: Decision Tree, Figure S7: Genes from the KEGG Cancer for HER Primary Tumors, Figure S8: Genes from the KEGG Cancer for LN Positive MBC, Figure S9: Genes from the KEGG Cancer for Bone Metastasis MBC, Table S1: Proportions of healthy volunteers and MBC patients with positive gene expression, Table S2: Summary of CTC counts on HER2.

Author Contributions: Conceptualization, E.N.C., G.J., R.G.M., M.C., J.E.L., J.D.K., M.F.P., M.C.M., J.M.R. and N.T.U.; methodology, E.N.C., G.J., J.E.L., J.D.K., M.F.P., M.C.M. and J.M.R.; formal analysis, E.N.C., G.J., J.D.K., M.C.M. and J.M.R.; investigation, R.G.M., M.C., J.E.L., J.D.K., M.F.P. and N.T.U.; data curation, J.D.K., M.F.P., K.K.K., N.K., Q.Z., Y.Z., P.K., R.G. and M.C.M.; writing—original draft preparation, E.N.C., G.J., M.C.M. and J.M.R.; writing—review and editing, E.N.C., G.J., R.G.M., M.C., J.E.L., J.D.K., M.F.P., M.C.M., J.M.R. and N.T.U.; project administration, M.C.M. All authors have read and agreed to the published version of the manuscript.

Funding: This study was supported by ANGLE Europe Limited. M.F. Press was supported by grants from the Breast Cancer Research Program (BCRF-20, 21, 22-132), Tower Cancer Research Program (Grant Number 006886-0001), Miriam and Sheldon G. Adelson Medical Research Program, and a gift from Richard Balch.

Institutional Review Board Statement: Study ANG-002 was conducted in accordance with the Declaration of Helsinki, and approved by the Institutional Review Board of The University of Texas MD Anderson Cancer Center (PA17-1047 approved November 28, 2017) and the Institutional Review Board (IRB) or Independent Ethics Committee (IEC) for each of the 4 participating sites (full list can be found at https://clinicaltrials.gov/ct2/show/NCT03427450, accessed 20 October 2022).

Informed Consent Statement: Informed consent was obtained from all subjects involved in the study.

Data Availability Statement: The data can be shared up on request.

Acknowledgments: The authors would like to acknowledge and thank all of the women who participated in the clinical study and provided their clinical samples, as well as the following individuals at each of the clinical study sites for their contributions to the conduct of the study, processing of the clinical samples, and evaluation of the results: MD Anderson Cancer Center (Houston, TX): Sausan Abouharb, Angela Alexander, Heather B McBride, Franklin D Alvarez, Carlos Barcenas, Daniel Booser, Mariana Chavez MacGregor, Senthil Damodaran, Min Fu, Nuhad Ibrahim, Kai Megumi, Meghan Karuturi, Kimberly Koenig, Rachel Layman, Bora Lim, Jennifer Litton, Angela Marx, Rashmi Murthy, Charla Parker, Phillip R Peabody, David Parker, Phillip R Peabody, David Ramirez, LaToya Samuel, Maryanne E Sapon, Huiming Sun, Parijatham Thomas, Debasish Tripathy, Vincent Valero, Jie Willey, Anita Woods; University of Rochester Cancer Center (Rochester, NY): Erin Bodekor, Robin Boerman, Erika Bronk, Erica Burgeson, Jennifer Cocking, Kathryn Corcoran, Lauren Curran, Ajay Dhakal, Jacqueline Doucette, Laura Eckert-Davis, Ashley Essom, Rachel Farkas, Kristina Galton, Jessica Gooch, Holly Greiner, Amy Hayes, Alissa Huston, Amber Johnson, Dina Johnson, Barbara Kavinsky, Anne Keefer, Jennifer Knaak, Susan Koomen, Jacqueline Lenhard, Peter MacDowell, Allison Magnuson, Chelsea Marsh, Philip J Meacham, Michelle Miller, Laura Mitchell, Ildiko Nagy, Farishta Nezomuddin, Anne Olzinksi-Kunze, Stasia Ortu, Kelvin Peek, Peter Prieto, Christine Quinn, Crystal Regis, Amy Rovitelli, Mary Sears, Michelle Shayne, Umayal Sivagnanalingam, Kristin Skinner, Sarah Strause, Deborah Street, Cody Tallett, Brian Yirinec; University of Southern California (Los Angeles, CA): Richa Aggarwal, Sibley Bardales, Daniel Campo, Amab Basu, Margie Carranza, America Casillas-Lopez, Yvonne Chairez, Victor Chiu, Aniska D'Souza, Simon Davenport, Grace Facio, Lilia Frausto, Umair Ghani, John Greco, Erwin Grussie, John Y Hu, Irene Kang, Jasleen Khanuja, Nara Lee, Grace Li, Ming Li, Janice Lu, Yi-Tsung Lu, Aaron Mejia, Gangothri Namasivayam, Maria Nelson, Caitlin O'Neill, Ravi Patel, Tania Porras, Nathan Punwani, Lusine Raddatz, Pauline Reonisto, Shirley Sain, Naomi Schechter, Stephen Sener, Anson Snow, Jacob Thomas, Varsha Tulpule, Rebecca Umayam, Ivonne Villalobos Press, Kristy Watkins, Kristopher Wentzel, Bin Xie, Yue Zhu; Northwestern University (Chicago, IL): Madonna Breganio, Sarah Craig, Rebecca Curry-Edwards, Tara Dedic, Carmen Diaz, Lisa Flaum, William Gradishar, Leeaht Gross, Levon Guzman, Katy Kerby, Kelly Kindy, Marissa Malaret, Ellen Malone, Adrianna Rodriguez, Ami Shah, Marian Tentler, Regina Uthe, Amy Youngkin; ANGLE Europe Limited (Study Sponsor): Khalil Al-bacha Hjazi, Martin Cooke, Andrew Newland, Anne-Sophie Pailhes-Jimenez, Peggy Robinson, Paul Smith, Amy Templeman, Christopher Wagner. The manuscript was edited by Sarah Bronson, ELS, of the Research Medical Library in The University of Texas MD Anderson Cancer Center.

Conflicts of Interest: The authors ENC, GJ, KKK, NK, QZ, YZ, PK and RG declare no conflict of interest. RGM reports consulting fees from Fujirebio Diagnostics; MC reports AstraZeneca (Consulting Fees (e.g., advisory boards), Contracted Research) Celcuity (Consulting Fees (e.g., advisory boards)) Eli Lilly (Consulting Fees (e.g., advisory boards), Contracted Research, Fees for Non-CMEServices Received Directly from Commercial Interest or their Agents (e.g., speakers' bureaus)) Ellipses

(Consulting Fees (e.g., advisory boards)) Foundation Medicine (Fees for Non-CME Services Received Directly from Commercial Interest or their Agents (e.g., speakers' bureaus)) Guardant (Fees for Non-CME Services Received Directly from Commercial Interest or their Agents (e.g., speakers' bureaus)) Menarini (Consulting Fees (e.g., advisory boards)) Olaris (Consulting Fees (e.g., advisory boards)) Pfizer (Contracted Research, Fees for Non-CME Services Received Directly from Commercial Interest or their Agents (e.g., speakers' bureaus)) Semonix (Consulting Fees (e.g., advisory boards)); JEL reports grant from ANGLE (Contracted Research); JDK reports Angle, plc (Consulting Fees (e.g., advisory boards), Contracted Research); MFP reports AstraZeneca (Consulting Fees (e.g., advisory boards)) Biocartis SA (Consulting Fees (e.g., advisory boards)) CEPHEID (Consulting Fees (e.g., advisory boards)) Eli Lilly & Company (Consulting Fees (e.g., advisory boards)) Lilly USA, LLC (Consulting Fees (e.g., advisory boards)) Merck & Co. (Consulting Fees (e.g., advisory boards)) Puma Biotechnology (Consulting Fees (e.g., advisory boards)) TORL BIOTHERAPEUTICS LLC (Ownership Interest (stocks, stock options, patent or other intellectual property or other ownership interest excluding diversified mutual funds)) Zymeworks Inc. (Consulting Fees (e.g., advisory boards)); MCM reports ANGLE plc (Full-time employee, Ownership Interest (stocks, stock options, patent or other intellectual property or other ownership interest excluding diversified mutual funds)); JMR reports Angle plc (Consulting Fees (e.g., advisory boards), Contracted Research); NTU reports Angle plc (Contracted Research) AnHeart Therapeutics Inc. (Consulting Fees (e.g., advisory boards)) AstraZeneca Pharmaceutical (Consulting Fees (e.g., advisory boards)) Carisma Therapeutics, Inc. (Consulting Fees (e.g., advisory boards), Contracted Research) CARNA Biosciences, Inc. (Consulting Fees (e.g., advisory boards)) ChemDiv, Inc. (Consulting Fees (e.g., advisory boards), Contracted Research) Chugai Pharmaceutical (Consulting Fees (e.g., advisory boards)) Daiichi Sankyo, Inc. (Consulting Fees (e.g., advisory boards), Contracted Research) DualityBio (Consulting Fees (e.g., advisory boards), Contracted Research) DynaMed (Consulting Fees (e.g., advisory boards)) Eisai Medical Research Inc (Consulting Fees (e.g., advisory boards), Contracted Research) Epic Science (Contracted Research) Gilead Sciences, Inc. (Consulting Fees (e.g., advisory boards), Contracted Research) Kechow Pharma (Consulting Fees (e.g., advisory boards)) Kirilys Therapeutics, Inc. (Consulting Fees (e.g., advisory boards)) Kyowa Hakko Kirin Co., Ltd. (Speaker) LARVOL (Consulting Fees (e.g., advisory boards)) Merck Co. (Contracted Research) OBI Pharma Inc. (Contracted Research) OncoCyte Co. (Consulting Fees (e.g., advisory boards)) Oncolys BioPharma Inc. (Contracted Research) Ourotech, Inc., DBA Pear Bio (Royalty) Peptilogics, Inc. (Consulting Fees (e.g., advisory boards)) Pfizer Inc. (Consulting Fees (e.g., advisory boards), Contracted Research) Phoenix Molecular Designs (Consulting Fees (e.g., advisory boards)) Preferred Medicine, Inc. (Consulting Fees (e.g., advisory boards), Contracted Research) Rakuten Medical, Inc. (Consulting Fees (e.g., advisory boards)) Sumitomo Dainippon Pharma, Inc. (Contracted Research) Sysmex Co. Ltd. (Consulting Fees (e.g., advisory boards)) Takeda Pharmaceuticals, Ltd. (Consulting Fees (e.g., advisory boards)) Unitech Medical, Inc. (Consulting Fees (e.g., advisory boards)). MCM, a full-time employee of ANGLE North America, Inc., a subsidiary of ANGLE plc, and was involved in the design of the study, the analysis and interpretation of the data, the decision to publish the results, and in the writing of the manuscript. The information and results reported in the manuscript, as well as their interpretations, are based on generally accepted scientific principals and methods and as such were not inappropriately influenced by the commercial interest of the funder (ANGLE Europe Limited).

References

1. Hong, B.; Zu, Y. Detecting circulating tumor cells: Current challenges and new trends. *Theranostics* **2013**, *3*, 377–394. [CrossRef] [PubMed]
2. Cristofanilli, M.; Hayes, D.F.; Budd, G.T.; Ellis, M.J.; Stopeck, A.; Reuben, J.M.; Doyle, G.V.; Matera, J.; Allard, W.J.; Miller, M.C.; et al. Circulating tumor cells: A novel prognostic factor for newly diagnosed metastatic breast cancer. *J. Clin. Oncol.* **2005**, *23*, 1420–1430. [CrossRef] [PubMed]
3. Dawood, S.; Broglio, K.; Valero, V.; Reuben, J.; Handy, B.; Islam, R.; Jackson, S.; Hortobagyi, G.N.; Fritsche, H.; Cristofanilli, M. Circulating tumor cells in metastatic breast cancer: From prognostic stratification to modification of the staging system? *Cancer* **2008**, *113*, 2422–2430. [CrossRef] [PubMed]
4. Hayes, D.F.; Cristofanilli, M.; Budd, G.T.; Ellis, M.J.; Stopeck, A.; Miller, M.C.; Matera, J.; Allard, W.J.; Doyle, G.V.; Terstappen, L.W. Circulating tumor cells at each follow-up time point during therapy of metastatic breast cancer patients predict progression-free and overall survival. *Clin. Cancer Res.* **2006**, *12*, 4218–4224. [CrossRef] [PubMed]
5. Budd, G.T.; Cristofanilli, M.; Ellis, M.J.; Stopeck, A.; Borden, E.; Miller, M.C.; Matera, J.; Repollet, M.; Doyle, G.V.; Terstappen, L.W.; et al. Circulating tumor cells versus imaging–predicting overall survival in metastatic breast cancer. *Clin. Cancer Res.* **2006**, *12*, 6403–6409. [CrossRef] [PubMed]

6. Liu, M.C.; Shields, P.G.; Warren, R.D.; Cohen, P.; Wilkinson, M.; Ottaviano, Y.L.; Rao, S.B.; Eng-Wong, J.; Seillier-Moiseiwitsch, F.; Noone, A.M.; et al. Circulating tumor cells: A useful predictor of treatment efficacy in metastatic breast cancer. *J. Clin. Oncol.* **2009**, *27*, 5153–5159. [CrossRef] [PubMed]
7. Hayes, D.F.; Smerage, J. Is there a role for circulating tumor cells in the management of breast cancer? *Clin. Cancer Res.* **2008**, *14*, 3646–3650. [CrossRef] [PubMed]
8. Pantel, K.; Alix-Panabieres, C. Real-time liquid biopsy in cancer patients: Fact or fiction? *Cancer Res.* **2013**, *73*, 6384–6388. [CrossRef] [PubMed]
9. Alunni-Fabbroni, M.; Sandri, M.T. Circulating tumour cells in clinical practice: Methods of detection and possible characterization. *Methods* **2010**, *50*, 289–297. [CrossRef] [PubMed]
10. Allard, W.J.; Matera, J.; Miller, M.C.; Repollet, M.; Connelly, M.C.; Rao, C.; Tibbe, A.G.; Uhr, J.W.; Terstappen, L.W. Tumor cells circulate in the peripheral blood of all major carcinomas but not in healthy subjects or patients with nonmalignant diseases. *Clin. Cancer Res.* **2004**, *10*, 6897–6904. [CrossRef] [PubMed]
11. Cristofanilli, M.; Budd, G.T.; Ellis, M.J.; Stopeck, A.; Matera, J.; Miller, M.C.; Reuben, J.M.; Doyle, G.V.; Allard, W.J.; Terstappen, L.W.; et al. Circulating tumor cells, disease progression, and survival in metastatic breast cancer. *N. Engl. J. Med.* **2004**, *351*, 781–791. [CrossRef] [PubMed]
12. Zhang, Z.; Wuethrich, A.; Wang, J.; Korbie, D.; Lin, L.L.; Trau, M. Dynamic Monitoring of EMT in CTCs as an Indicator of Cancer Metastasis. *Anal. Chem.* **2021**, *93*, 16787–16795. [CrossRef] [PubMed]
13. Sankpal, N.V.; Fleming, T.P.; Sharma, P.K.; Wiedner, H.J.; Gillanders, W.E. A double-negative feedback loop between EpCAM and ERK contributes to the regulation of epithelial-mesenchymal transition in cancer. *Oncogene* **2017**, *36*, 3706–3717. [CrossRef] [PubMed]
14. Yang, J.; Mani, S.A.; Donaher, J.L.; Ramaswamy, S.; Itzykson, R.A.; Come, C.; Savagner, P.; Gitelman, I.; Richardson, A.; Weinberg, R.A. Twist, a master regulator of morphogenesis, plays an essential role in tumor metastasis. *Cell* **2004**, *117*, 927–939. [CrossRef] [PubMed]
15. Mani, S.A.; Guo, W.; Liao, M.J.; Eaton, E.N.; Ayyanan, A.; Zhou, A.Y.; Brooks, M.; Reinhard, F.; Zhang, C.C.; Shipitsin, M.; et al. The epithelial-mesenchymal transition generates cells with properties of stem cells. *Cell* **2008**, *133*, 704–715. [CrossRef] [PubMed]
16. Hollier, B.G.; Evans, K.; Mani, S.A. The epithelial-to-mesenchymal transition and cancer stem cells: A coalition against cancer therapies. *J. Mammary Gland. Biol. Neoplasia* **2009**, *14*, 29–43. [CrossRef] [PubMed]
17. Chudziak, J.; Burt, D.J.; Mohan, S.; Rothwell, D.G.; Mesquita, B.; Antonello, J.; Dalby, S.; Ayub, M.; Priest, L.; Carter, L.; et al. Clinical evaluation of a novel microfluidic device for epitope-independent enrichment of circulating tumour cells in patients with small cell lung cancer. *Analyst* **2016**, *141*, 669–678. [CrossRef] [PubMed]
18. Yap, K.; Cohen, E.N.; Reuben, J.M.; Khoury, J.D. Circulating Tumor Cells: State-of-the-art Update on Technologies and Clinical Applications. *Curr. Hematol. Malig. Rep.* **2019**, *14*, 353–357. [CrossRef] [PubMed]
19. Hvichia, G.E.; Parveen, Z.; Wagner, C.; Janning, M.; Quidde, J.; Stein, A.; Muller, V.; Loges, S.; Neves, R.P.; Stoecklein, N.H.; et al. A novel microfluidic platform for size and deformability based separation and the subsequent molecular characterization of viable circulating tumor cells. *Int. J. Cancer* **2016**, *138*, 2894–2904. [CrossRef] [PubMed]
20. Lampignano, R.; Yang, L.; Neumann, M.H.D.; Franken, A.; Fehm, T.; Niederacher, D.; Neubauer, H. A Novel Workflow to Enrich and Isolate Patient-Matched EpCAM(high) and EpCAM(low/negative) CTCs Enables the Comparative Characterization of the PIK3CA Status in Metastatic Breast Cancer. *Int. J. Mol. Sci.* **2017**, *18*, 1885. [CrossRef] [PubMed]
21. Miller, M.C.; Robinson, P.S.; Wagner, C.; O'Shannessy, D.J. The Parsortix Cell Separation System-A versatile liquid biopsy platform. *Cytom. Part A* **2018**, *93*, 1234–1239. [CrossRef] [PubMed]
22. Gorges, T.M.; Kuske, A.; Rock, K.; Mauermann, O.; Muller, V.; Peine, S.; Verpoort, K.; Novosadova, V.; Kubista, M.; Riethdorf, S.; et al. Accession of Tumor Heterogeneity by Multiplex Transcriptome Profiling of Single Circulating Tumor Cells. *Clin. Chem.* **2016**, *62*, 1504–1515. [CrossRef] [PubMed]
23. Xu, L.; Mao, X.; Guo, T.; Chan, P.Y.; Shaw, G.; Hines, J.; Stankiewicz, E.; Wang, Y.; Oliver, R.T.D.; Ahmad, A.S.; et al. The Novel Association of Circulating Tumor Cells and Circulating Megakaryocytes with Prostate Cancer Prognosis. *Clin. Cancer Res.* **2017**, *23*, 5112–5122. [CrossRef] [PubMed]
24. Maertens, Y.; Humberg, V.; Erlmeier, F.; Steffens, S.; Steinestel, J.; Bogemann, M.; Schrader, A.J.; Bernemann, C. Comparison of isolation platforms for detection of circulating renal cell carcinoma cells. *Oncotarget* **2017**, *8*, 87710–87717. [CrossRef] [PubMed]
25. Obermayr, E.; Maritschnegg, E.; Agreiter, C.; Pecha, N.; Speiser, P.; Helmy-Bader, S.; Danzinger, S.; Krainer, M.; Singer, C.; Zeillinger, R. Efficient leukocyte depletion by a novel microfluidic platform enables the molecular detection and characterization of circulating tumor cells. *Oncotarget* **2018**, *9*, 812–823. [CrossRef] [PubMed]
26. Harris, P.A.; Taylor, R.; Thielke, R.; Payne, J.; Gonzalez, N.; Conde, J.G. Research electronic data capture (REDCap)—A metadata-driven methodology and workflow process for providing translational research informatics support. *J. Biomed. Inform.* **2009**, *42*, 377–381. [CrossRef] [PubMed]
27. Harris, P.A.; Taylor, R.; Minor, B.L.; Elliott, V.; Fernandez, M.; O'Neal, L.; McLeod, L.; Delacqua, G.; Delacqua, F.; Kirby, J.; et al. The REDCap consortium: Building an international community of software platform partners. *J. Biomed. Inform.* **2019**, *95*, 103208. [CrossRef] [PubMed]
28. Lang, J.E.; Ring, A.; Porras, T.; Kaur, P.; Forte, V.A.; Mineyev, N.; Tripathy, D.; Press, M.F.; Campo, D. RNA-Seq of Circulating Tumor Cells in Stage II-III Breast Cancer. *Ann. Surg. Oncol.* **2018**, *25*, 2261–2270. [CrossRef] [PubMed]

29. Kaur, P.; Campo, D.; Porras, T.B.; Ring, A.; Lu, J.; Chairez, Y.; Su, Y.; Kang, I.; Lang, J.E. A Pilot Study for the Feasibility of Exome-Sequencing in Circulating Tumor Cells Versus Single Metastatic Biopsies in Breast Cancer. *Int. J. Mol. Sci.* **2020**, *21*, 4826. [CrossRef] [PubMed]
30. Patro, R.; Duggal, G.; Love, M.I.; Irizarry, R.A.; Kingsford, C. Salmon provides fast and bias-aware quantification of transcript expression. *Nat. Methods* **2017**, *14*, 417–419. [CrossRef] [PubMed]
31. Press, M.F.; Villalobos, I.; Santiago, A.; Guzman, R.; Cervantes, M.; Gasparyan, A.; Campeau, A.; Ma, Y.; Tsao-Wei, D.D.; Groshen, S. Assessing the New American Society of Clinical Oncology/College of American Pathologists Guidelines for HER2 Testing by Fluorescence In Situ Hybridization: Experience of an Academic Consultation Practice. *Arch. Pathol. Lab. Med.* **2016**, *140*, 1250–1258. [CrossRef] [PubMed]
32. Press, M.F.; Sauter, G.; Buyse, M.; Fourmanoir, H.; Quinaux, E.; Tsao-Wei, D.D.; Eiermann, W.; Robert, N.; Pienkowski, T.; Crown, J.; et al. HER2 Gene Amplification Testing by Fluorescent In Situ Hybridization (FISH): Comparison of the ASCO-College of American Pathologists Guidelines With FISH Scores Used for Enrollment in Breast Cancer International Research Group Clinical Trials. *J. Clin. Oncol.* **2016**, *34*, 3518–3528. [CrossRef] [PubMed]
33. Press, M.F.; Seoane, J.A.; Curtis, C.; Quinaux, E.; Guzman, R.; Sauter, G.; Eiermann, W.; Mackey, J.R.; Robert, N.; Pienkowski, T.; et al. Assessment of ERBB2/HER2 Status in HER2-Equivocal Breast Cancers by FISH and 2013/2014 ASCO-CAP Guidelines. *JAMA Oncol.* **2019**, *5*, 366–375. [CrossRef] [PubMed]
34. Press, M.F.; Sauter, G.; Buyse, M.; Bernstein, L.; Guzman, R.; Santiago, A.; Villalobos, I.E.; Eiermann, W.; Pienkowski, T.; Martin, M.; et al. Alteration of topoisomerase II-alpha gene in human breast cancer: Association with responsiveness to anthracycline-based chemotherapy. *J. Clin. Oncol.* **2011**, *29*, 859–867. [CrossRef] [PubMed]
35. Howlader, N.; Altekruse, S.F.; Li, C.I.; Chen, V.W.; Clarke, C.A.; Ries, L.A.; Cronin, K.A. US incidence of breast cancer subtypes defined by joint hormone receptor and HER2 status. *J. Natl. Cancer Inst.* **2014**, *106*. [CrossRef] [PubMed]
36. Bidard, F.C.; Peeters, D.J.; Fehm, T.; Nole, F.; Gisbert-Criado, R.; Mavroudis, D.; Grisanti, S.; Generali, D.; Garcia-Saenz, J.A.; Stebbing, J.; et al. Clinical validity of circulating tumour cells in patients with metastatic breast cancer: A pooled analysis of individual patient data. *Lancet Oncol.* **2014**, *15*, 406–414. [CrossRef] [PubMed]
37. Sun, Y.F.; Guo, W.; Xu, Y.; Shi, Y.H.; Gong, Z.J.; Ji, Y.; Du, M.; Zhang, X.; Hu, B.; Huang, A.; et al. Circulating Tumor Cells from Different Vascular Sites Exhibit Spatial Heterogeneity in Epithelial and Mesenchymal Composition and Distinct Clinical Significance in Hepatocellular Carcinoma. *Clin. Cancer Res.* **2018**, *24*, 547–559. [CrossRef] [PubMed]
38. Terai, M.; Mu, Z.; Eschelman, D.J.; Gonsalves, C.F.; Kageyama, K.; Chervoneva, I.; Orloff, M.; Weight, R.; Mastrangelo, M.J.; Cristofanilli, M.; et al. Arterial Blood, Rather Than Venous Blood, is a Better Source for Circulating Melanoma Cells. *EBioMedicine* **2015**, *2*, 1821–1826. [CrossRef] [PubMed]
39. Jesenko, T.; Modic, Z.; Kuhar, C.G.; Cemazar, M.; Matkovic, U.; Miceska, S.; Varl, J.; Kuhar, A.; Kloboves-Prevodnik, V. Morphological features of breast cancer circulating tumor cells in blood after physical and biological type of isolation. *Radiol. Oncol.* **2021**, *55*, 292–304. [CrossRef] [PubMed]
40. Cohen, E.N.; Jayachandran, G.; Hardy, M.R.; Venkata Subramanian, A.M.; Meng, X.; Reuben, J.M. Antigen-agnostic microfluidics-based circulating tumor cell enrichment and downstream molecular characterization. *PLoS ONE* **2020**, *15*, e0241123. [CrossRef] [PubMed]
41. Ingthorsson, S.; Andersen, K.; Hilmarsdottir, B.; Maelandsmo, G.M.; Magnusson, M.K.; Gudjonsson, T. HER2 induced EMT and tumorigenicity in breast epithelial progenitor cells is inhibited by coexpression of EGFR. *Oncogene* **2016**, *35*, 4244–4255. [CrossRef] [PubMed]
42. Gupta, P.; Srivastava, S.K. HER2 mediated de novo production of TGFbeta leads to SNAIL driven epithelial-to-mesenchymal transition and metastasis of breast cancer. *Mol. Oncol.* **2014**, *8*, 1532–1547. [CrossRef] [PubMed]
43. Jenndahl, L.E.; Isakson, P.; Baeckstrom, D. c-erbB2-induced epithelial-mesenchymal transition in mammary epithelial cells is suppressed by cell-cell contact and initiated prior to E-cadherin downregulation. *Int. J. Oncol.* **2005**, *27*, 439–448. [CrossRef] [PubMed]
44. D'Souza, B.; Berdichevsky, F.; Kyprianou, N.; Taylor-Papadimitriou, J. Collagen-induced morphogenesis and expression of the alpha 2-integrin subunit is inhibited in c-erbB2-transfected human mammary epithelial cells. *Oncogene* **1993**, *8*, 1797–1806. [PubMed]
45. D'Souza, B.; Taylor-Papadimitriou, J. Overexpression of ERBB2 in human mammary epithelial cells signals inhibition of transcription of the E-cadherin gene. *Proc. Natl. Acad. Sci. USA* **1994**, *91*, 7202–7206. [CrossRef] [PubMed]
46. Khoury, H.; Dankort, D.L.; Sadekova, S.; Naujokas, M.A.; Muller, W.J.; Park, M. Distinct tyrosine autophosphorylation sites mediate induction of epithelial mesenchymal like transition by an activated ErbB-2/Neu receptor. *Oncogene* **2001**, *20*, 788–799. [CrossRef] [PubMed]
47. Giordano, A.; Gao, H.; Anfossi, S.; Cohen, E.; Mego, M.; Lee, B.N.; Tin, S.; De Laurentiis, M.; Parker, C.A.; Alvarez, R.H.; et al. Epithelial-mesenchymal transition and stem cell markers in patients with HER2-positive metastatic breast cancer. *Mol. Cancer Ther.* **2012**, *11*, 2526–2534. [CrossRef] [PubMed]
48. Lang, J.E.; Mosalpuria, K.; Cristofanilli, M.; Krishnamurthy, S.; Reuben, J.; Singh, B.; Bedrosian, I.; Meric-Bernstam, F.; Lucci, A. HER2 status predicts the presence of circulating tumor cells in patients with operable breast cancer. *Breast Cancer Res. Treat.* **2009**, *113*, 501–507. [CrossRef] [PubMed]

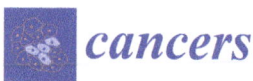

Article

HER2-Low Status Does Not Affect Survival Outcomes of Patients with Metastatic Breast Cancer (MBC) Undergoing First-Line Treatment with Endocrine Therapy plus Palbociclib: Results of a Multicenter, Retrospective Cohort Study

Francesca Carlino [1,2,*], Anna Diana [3], Anna Ventriglia [1], Antonio Piccolo [1], Carmela Mocerino [4], Ferdinando Riccardi [4], Domenico Bilancia [5], Francesco Giotta [6], Giulio Antoniol [7], Vincenzo Famiglietti [1], Salvatore Feliciano [2], Rodolfo Cangiano [8], Lorenzo Lobianco [1], Benedetta Pellegrino [9], Ferdinando De Vita [1], Fortunato Ciardiello [1] and Michele Orditura [1]

1. Department of Precision Medicine, Division of Medical Oncology, University of Campania Luigi Vanvitelli, 80131 Naples, Italy
2. Medical Oncology Unit, Ospedale Ave Gratia Plena, San Felice a Cancello, 81027 Caserta, Italy
3. Medical Oncology Unit, Ospedale del Mare, 80147 Naples, Italy
4. Medical Oncology Unit, Ospedale Cardarelli, 80131 Naples, Italy
5. Operating Unit, Medical Oncology, Hospital "Azienda Ospedaliera S. Carlo", 85100 Potenza, Italy
6. Medical Oncology Unit, IRCCS-Istituto Tumori "Giovanni Paolo II", 70124 Bari, Italy
7. Département de Génie Informatique et Génie Logiciel, 2500 Chemin de Ecole Polytechnique de Montréal, Montreal, QC H3T 1J4, Canada
8. Medical Oncology Unit, Ospedale Ave Gratia Plena, Piedimonte Matese, 81016 Caserta, Italy
9. Medical Oncology and Breast Unit, University Hospital of Parma, 43126 Parma, Italy
* Correspondence: francesca91carlino@gmail.com or francesca.carlino@unicampania.it

Citation: Carlino, F.; Diana, A.; Ventriglia, A.; Piccolo, A.; Mocerino, C.; Riccardi, F.; Bilancia, D.; Giotta, F.; Antoniol, G.; Famiglietti, V.; et al. HER2-Low Status Does Not Affect Survival Outcomes of Patients with Metastatic Breast Cancer (MBC) Undergoing First-Line Treatment with Endocrine Therapy plus Palbociclib: Results of a Multicenter, Retrospective Cohort Study. *Cancers* 2022, *14*, 4981. https://doi.org/10.3390/cancers14204981

Academic Editor: Javier Cortes

Received: 18 September 2022
Accepted: 7 October 2022
Published: 11 October 2022

Publisher's Note: MDPI stays neutral with regard to jurisdictional claims in published maps and institutional affiliations.

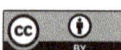

Copyright: © 2022 by the authors. Licensee MDPI, Basel, Switzerland. This article is an open access article distributed under the terms and conditions of the Creative Commons Attribution (CC BY) license (https://creativecommons.org/licenses/by/4.0/).

Simple Summary: Breast cancers (BCs) with a HER2 immunohistochemical score of 1+ or 2+ with negative in situ hybridization are referred as HER2-low BCs. The knowledge about the biological and clinical characteristics of HER2-low BCs is still limited and controversial. Despite that new anti-HER2 antibody-drug conjugates (ADCs) have demonstrated significant activity in HER2-low BCs, no anti-HER2 agents are currently approved for this subgroup in Europe. Therefore, treatment for HER2-low BCs is determined by HR expression status. In this study, we aimed to investigate the prognostic significance of HER2-low status in HR+/HER2 negative (HER2-) metastatic BC (MBC) patients treated with endocrine therapy (ET) plus palbociclib as first line. HR+ MBC patients with HER2-low tumors who received first-line treatment with ET plus palbociclib show similar survival outcomes compared to those HER2-0 disease.

Abstract: Background: Approximately 45–50% of breast cancers (BCs) have a HER2 immunohistochemical score of 1+ or 2+ with negative in situ hybridization, defining the "HER2-low BC" subtype. No anti-HER2 agents are currently approved for this subgroup in Europe, where treatment is still determined by HR expression status. In this study, we investigated the prognostic significance of HER2-low status in HR+/HER2- metastatic BC (MBC) patients treated with endocrine therapy (ET) plus palbociclib as first line. Methods: We conducted a retrospective study including 252 consecutive HR+/HER2- MBC patients who received first-line ET plus palbociclib at six Italian Oncology Units between March 2016 and June 2021. The chi-square test was used to assess differences in the distribution of clinical and pathological variables between the HER-0 and HER2-low subgroups. Survival outcomes, progression-free survival (PFS) and overall survival (OS), were calculated by the Kaplan–Meier method, and the log-rank test was performed to estimate the differences between the curves. Results: A total of 165 patients were included in the analysis: 94 (57%) and 71 (43%) patients had HER2-0 and HER2-low disease, respectively. The median age at treatment start was 64 years. No correlation between patients and tumor characteristics and HER2 status was found. Median PFS (mPFS) for the entire study cohort was 20 months (95% CI,18–25 months), while median OS (mOS) was not reached at the time of analysis. No statistically significant differences, in terms of PFS

(p = 0.20) and OS (p = 0.1), were observed between HER2-low and HER2-0 subgroups. Conclusions: In our analysis, HR+ MBC patients with low HER2 expression who received first-line treatment with ET plus Palbociclib reported no statistically different survival outcomes compared to HER2-0 patients. Further prospective studies are needed to confirm the clinical role of HER2 expression level.

Keywords: breast cancer; cyclin-dependent kinase inhibitor 4 and 6; HER2-low; palbociclib

1. Introduction

Breast cancer (BC) is the most common malignancy and the leading cause of cancer morbidity among women worldwide [1]. BC presents a wide spectrum of heterogeneity in terms of gene expression, immunophenotypic features, response to treatment and clinical outcomes [2]. In daily clinical practice, therapeutic choice is still driven by the human epidermal growth factor receptor 2 (HER2) and hormone-receptor (HR) status, since gene expression profiling is not routinely available. Although tumors harboring HER2 positivity are characterized by a more aggressive behavior and poorer prognosis than other subtypes, the development of several anti-HER2 targeted agents has dramatically improved the survival outcomes of HER2 positive (HER2+) BC patients, both in early and advanced settings [3–8]. According to the dichotomic classification proposed by the 2018 American Society of Clinical Oncology (ASCO)/College of American Pathologists (CAP) guidelines, about 80% of breast tumors, lacking HER2 protein overexpression, are classified as HER2 negative (HER2-); within them, approximately 45–55% are characterized by HER2 immuno-histochemistry (IHC) assay score of 1+ or 2+ with negative in situ hybridization (ISH), referred to as HER2-low BC [9,10]. In recent years, several studies have demonstrated the activity of the new anti-HER2 antibody-drug conjugates (ADCs) in both HER2+ and HER2-low BCs, leading researchers to shed new light on the latter type of tumors and to investigate whether they may represent a distinct subtype with specific behavior and prognosis [11]. The knowledge on the biological and clinical features of HER2-low BC is still limited and controversial [12]. Likewise, published studies evaluating the prognostic value of HER2-low expression have reported inconsistent and mixed results depending on disease stage and HR status (early vs. advanced, HR positive vs. triple negative breast cancer) [13–18]. Although ADCs have demonstrated to improve clinical outcomes of HER2-low tumors, this innovative strategy is not available yet in clinical practice for this subset of BC patients; therefore, the treatment choice is guided by HR expression status [7,8,19]. In detail, the combination of endocrine therapy (ET) plus cyclin-dependent kinase 4 and 6 inhibitors (CDK4/6i), palbociclib, ribociclib and abemaciclib, represents the mainstay of treatment for patients with HR+/HER2- metastatic disease, while for triple negative tumors, chemotherapy is still the standard of care, although promising drugs are emerging as novel therapeutic weapons. The advent of CDK4/6i has significantly changed the treatment paradigm with an impressive improvement in life expectancy for HR+/HER2- locally advanced or metastatic BC (MBC) patients. Despite this indisputable success, the knowledge of resistance mechanisms and the identification of potential biomarkers still represent an unmet clinical need. To this aim, several retrospective and prospective biomarker studies have been conducted [20]. Exploratory analyses of PALOMA-2 and 3 and MONALEESA trials have suggested a possible correlation between intrinsic subtypes and survival outcomes of MBC patients treated with CDK4/6i in addition to ET [21–24]. Furthermore, the bidirectional crosstalk between the HER and HR pathways as mechanisms of endocrine resistance could indicate a potential effect of low HER2 expression on CDK4/6i efficacy [25].

Recently, based on this assumption, Bao et al. conducted a retrospective analysis in patients treated with ET plus CDK4/6i, demonstrating a worse PFS in the HER2-low cohort compared to the HER2-0 subgroup [26]. These findings have led to further retrospective and subgroup analyses, which have reported opposite results [27]. Since this topic has raised a great deal of interest, in the present study, we evaluated the prognostic value of

HER2 expression in a retrospective series of HR+/HER2- MBC patients treated with ET plus palbociclib as first line therapy.

2. Materials and Methods

2.1. Study Population

Data from 252 consecutive HR+/HER2- MBC patients who started treatment with palbociclib plus ET (aromatase inhibitors or fulvestrant) as first line treatment between March 2016 and June 2021 at six Medical Oncology Units were registered in a comprehensive database. We excluded patients for whom the date of diagnosis or metastatic relapse was unknown or in cases for whom HR and HER2 status or treatments were not documented. A total of 165 patients with HR+/HER2- MBC treated with ET plus palbociclib were eligible for the final analysis. Medical and pathology reports were reviewed for the following clinicopathological characteristics: age, histological type, tumor size, nodal involvement, grade of differentiation, HR and HER2 expression status, Ki67 index, type of treatments, date of diagnosis, date of relapse, and sites of metastases. A radiological assessment with total body computed tomography (CT) was performed at intervals of 3–4 months as recommended by guidelines and evaluated according to the criteria of Response Evaluation Criteria in Solid tumors (RECIST) 1.1.

This study was approved by the University of Campania Luigi Vanvitelli Ethic Committee (ID number: 15.03-20220005385*, 17 February 2022). All patients signed written informed consent form.

2.2. Definitions of Biomarker (ER, PR, Ki67 and HER 2)

Estrogen receptor (ER), progesterone receptor (PR) and Ki67 were assessed by IHC, and HER2 was assessed by IHC and/or ISH in primary tumor sample. When available, biomarkers obtained from the latest biopsy specimen were also collected. Biomarker positivity was detected and quantified as the percentage between immune-positive tumor cells and the total number of tumor cells and classified according to the St. Gallen and ASCO-CAP guidelines [28–30]. In particular, tumors were considered ER positive and/or PR positive when $\geq 1\%$ of tumor cells demonstrate positive nuclear staining by IHC. Ki67 and PR were analyzed both as continuous and dichotomized variables (high vs. low). The cutoff for both variables was set at $\geq 20\%$ and $<20\%$ of positively stained cells, for high and low, respectively [31,32]. HER2 was assessed using the HercepTest (DAKO Corporation), which uses the 0–3+ recommended scale to measure the percentage of immunoreactive neoplastic cells defined according to the intensity and completeness of membrane staining. A score of 3+ was considered HER2 positive. In cases of equivocal HER2 immunostaining (2+), ISH methodologies were applied [33]. Among HER2-negative tumors, HER2-low is referred to those with IHC score 1+ or 2+ and negative results on ISH [9]. There was no central review of biomarkers, but the pathological evaluations were performed by accredited anatomic pathology units, which ensure high rigor in methods and procedures in line with the best international standards.

2.3. Statistical Analysis

The primary study aim was to evaluate the survival outcomes, progression-free survival (PFS) and overall survival (OS) in a real-life cohort of HR+/HER2- BC patients who received ET (AI or fulvestrant) plus palbociclib as first line for metastatic disease categorized according to HER2 expression status as follows: HR+/HER2-0 or HR+/HER2-low. For descriptive analysis, percentages were used for categorical variables, and medians and ranges were used for continuous variables. PFS was the time from the beginning of treatment until disease progression or worsening. OS was defined as the time from treatment start to death from any cause. Patients who were alive at the last follow-up without recurrence or lost during follow-up and patients who had died without recurrence were censored at the date of the last recorded visit and the date of death, respectively. The median follow-up period was evaluated by the reverse Kaplan–Meier (KM) method. Chi square test was used to assess the differences in the distribution of clinical and pathological variables between the HER-0 and HER2-low subgroups. The survival curves were created using the KM method. The log-rank test was used to compare the differences among the curves [34]. Unadjusted hazard ratios (HRs) and univariate PFS probabilities were calculated using simple Cox proportional hazard regression models. Adjusted HRs for HER2 status were estimated by multivariate regression analysis with factors found to be statistically significantly associated with PFS in the univariate analyses using a p value threshold of 0.05. Similar analyses were performed for OS. All statistical analyses were performed using the R statistical computing environment release 4.1.2 on an Apple MacBook Pro M1 Max. In all computations, significance was assigned at p value of less than 0.05.

3. Results

3.1. Patients and Tumor Characteristics

A total of 165 patients were included in the analysis of who 94 (57%) had HER2-0 and 71 (43%) had HER2-low disease. Median age at treatment start was 64 years (34–88 years). Ductal carcinoma was the most common histological type found in 138 tumors (more than 83%); 112 (68%) and 131 (79%) cases displayed high ($\geq$20%) Ki67 and PR levels, respectively. The majority of patients (64%, n = 106) had recurrent disease, while 59 patients (36%) presented with de novo metastatic breast cancer. Adjuvant ET was administered to 102 (62%) patients according to international guidelines. Among the 63 (38%) patients who did not receive adjuvant endocrine therapy, 59 were de novo metastatic and 4 relapsed during adjuvant chemotherapy. Regarding metastatic tumor burden, 63 (38%) and 102 (62%) patients had visceral and non-visceral disease, respectively. About two-thirds of the entire study cohort (112 patients) was AI sensitive (represented by patients who never received AI in early BC stage, or those who relapsed $\geq$12 months after completing adjuvant AI-based ET, or those who have been diagnosed with de novo stage IV BC), while 32% (53 patients) was AI-resistant (including patients who have been relapsed during adjuvant AI, or <12 months after its completion). Palbociclib was prescribed in combination with aromatase inhibitors or fulvestrant for AI-sensitive and AI-resistant patients, respectively. Key patient characteristics are presented in Table 1. No correlation between patients and tumor characteristics and HER2 status was found.

Table 1. Association of HER2 status with clinical and pathological characteristics and the derived Chi square test p value.

Characteristics	HER2-0 (94)	HER2-Low (71)	p Value
Age, years			
<65	50 (53%)	40 (56%)	0.80
$\geq$65	44 (47%)	31 (44%)	
Ki67 index %			
High $\geq$ 20%	59 (63%)	53 (75%)	0.14
Low < 20%	35 (37%)	18 (25%)	
Progesterone Receptor			
Low < 20%	16 (17%)	18 (25%)	0.26
High $\geq$ 20%	78 (83%)	53 (75%)	
Estrogen Receptor			
Low (1–9%)	1	1	0.88
Moderate (10–49%)	6	6	
High (50–95%)	87	64	

Table 1. Cont.

Characteristics	HER2-0 (94)	HER2-Low (71)	p Value
Grading			
Grade 1	12	4	0.32
Grade 2	50	43	
Grade 3	32	24	
Adjuvant Endocrine Therapy			
Tamoxifene	12 (20%)	13 (31%)	0.58
AI	40 (66,7%)	24 (57.1%)	
Tam + AI	8 (13.3%)	5 (11.9%)	
Not done	34 (36.2%)	29 (40.8%)	
Histologic type			
Ductal	78 (83%)	60 (85%)	0.90
Lobular	16 (17%)	11 (15%)	
Site of metastases			
Visceral	35 (37%)	28 (39%)	0.89
Non visceral	59 (63%)	43 (61%)	
AI sensitivity			
AI sensitive	59 (63%)	53 (75%)	0.15
AI resistant	35 (37%)	18 (25%)	
M status at diagnosis			
M0	61 (66%)	45 (63%)	0.97
M1	33 (34%)	26 (37%)	

AI, aromatase inhibitors; Tam, tamoxifene.

3.2. Survival Analysis

The median follow-up was 31 months (27.4–34.1 months) using 31 January 2022 as the data cut off. During this timeframe, progression of disease was registered in 105 patients (64%), of who 58 (55%) and 47 (45%) with HER2-0 and HER2-low tumors, respectively. Death for any cause occurred in 40 (38%) patients including 19 and 21 patients with HER2-0 and HER2-low tumors, respectively. The median PFS (mPFS) for the entire study cohort was 20 months (95% CI, 18–25 months). More than half of the study population was still alive at the time of the analysis; thus, median OS (mOS) could not be computed. Disease outcomes, in terms of PFS and OS, were compared between HER2-0 and HER2-low patients. No statistically significant differences, for each survival variable, were observed between the two subgroups. The mPFS for HER2-low was 19 months (95% CI, 14–21 months) compared with 23 months (95%CI, 18–27 months) for HER2-zero tumors ($p = 0.20$). Although median OS was not reached, the survival probabilities at 24, 36 and 48 months for HER2-0 and HER2-low patients were 86% and 80%, 76% and 60%, 62% and 51%, respectively ($p = 0.1$). (Table 2).

Table 2. Survival probability at 24, 36 and 48 months.

Months	Entire Population		Her2-0		Her2-Low	
	Survival Probability	95% CI	Survival Probability	95% CI	Survival Probability	95% CI
24	83%	77–88	86%	78–94	80%	70–80
36	69%	60–78	76%	65–87	60%	45–75
48	59%	47–70	62%	45–80	51%	34–69

CI, confidence interval.

Kaplan–Meier curves for PFS and OS are shown in Figure 1.

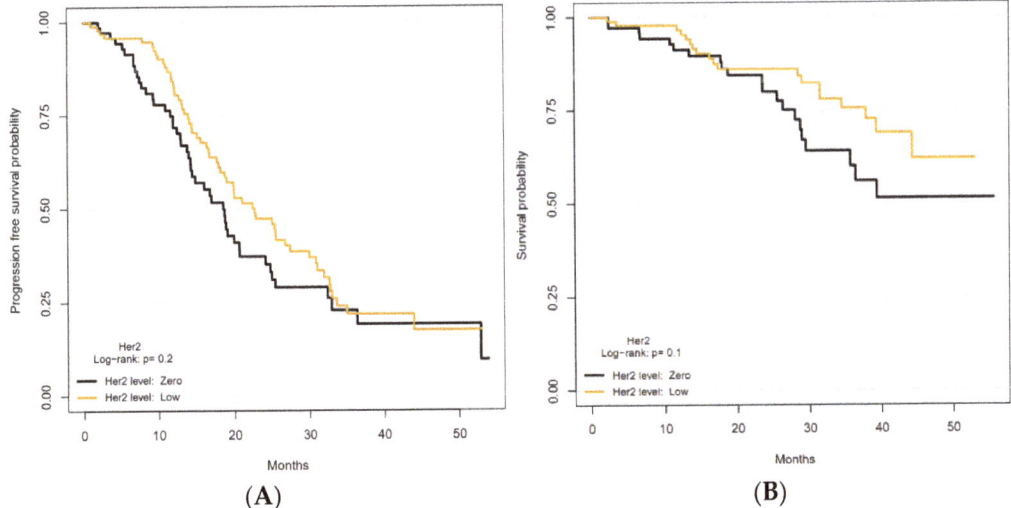

Figure 1. Kaplan–Meier curves demonstrating (**A**) progression-free survival, and (**B**) overall survival, according to HER2 status.

In the univariate analysis for PFS, visceral disease and AI resistance were significantly associated with shorter PFS ($p = 0.0041$ and $p = 0.05$, respectively) while HER2-low expression seemed to be related to slightly, but not statistically significant, worse PFS ($p = 0.18$).

Results from multivariate Cox proportional hazard models, confirmed that AI resistance and visceral disease were significantly associated with poorer outcome (HR: 1.64; 95% CI, 1.09–2.45; $p = 0.016$ and HR: 1.92; 95% CI, 1.28–2.87; $p = 0.001$) (Table 3).

Table 3. Prognostic variables for progression free survival in univariate analysis and multivariate analysis.

Variables	Univariate Analysis		Multivariate Analysis	
	HR (95% CI for HR)	*p* Value	HR (95% CI for HR)	*p* Value
HER2-0 vs. HER2-low	0.77 (0.52–1.1)	0.18		
PR < 20% vs. PR ≥ 20%	1.5 (0.93–2.3)	0.096		
M1 vs. M0	1.1 (0.71–1.6)	0.77		
Ki67 < 20% vs. Ki67 ≥ 20%	1 (0.69–1.6)	0.85		
Age ≥ 65 years vs. <65 years	1.2 (0.79–1.7)	0.45		
AI-resistant vs. AI-Sensitive	1.5 (1–2.2)	**0.05**	**1.64 (1.09–2.45)**	**0.016**
Visceral vs. non-visceral disease	1.8 (1.2–2.7)	**0.0041**	**1.92 (1.28–2.87)**	**0.001**

HR, hazard ratio; CI, confidence interval; PR, progesterone receptor; AI, aromatase inhibitor. Significant values are indicated in bold.

Univariate analysis for OS revealed that low PR value and visceral disease were clinical parameters significantly associated with a worse OS. The multivariable analysis confirmed that low PR levels and visceral disease were independently associated with shorter OS (HR: 2.43; 95% CI, 1.24–4.74; $p < 0.001$ and HR: 4.19; 95% CI, 2.17–8.08, $p < 0.001$) (Table 4).

Table 4. Prognostic variables for overall survival in univariate and multivariate analysis.

Variables	Univariate Analysis		Multivariate Analysis	
	HR (95% CI for HR)	p Value	HR (95% CI for HR)	p Value
HER2 0 vs. HER2 low	0.62 (0.32–1.16)	0.13		
PR < 20% vs. PR ≥ 20%	2.4 (1.2–4.6)	**0.011**	2.43 (1.24–4.74)	**<0.001**
M1 vs. M0	1.29 (0.69–2.41)	0.42		
Ki67 < 20% vs. Ki67 ≥ 20%	0.75 (0.37–1.52)	0.44		
Age ≥ 65 vs. <65	1.24 (0.66–2.33)	0.48		
AI-resistant vs. AI-sensitive	0.95 (0.48–1.87)	0.89		
Visceral vs. non-visceral disease	4.12 (2.14–7.95)	**<0.001**	4.19 (2.17–8.08)	**<0.001**

HR, hazard ratio; CI, confidence interval; PR, progesterone receptor; AI, aromatase inhibitor. Significant values are indicated in bold.

4. Discussion

In HR+/HER2- MBC, CDK4/6i are now considered the standard of care, in combination with ET, as first- or second-line systemic treatment for both endocrine-sensitive and endocrine-resistant patients because of meaningful improvement in clinical outcomes [35–40]. Despite the excellent results reported in the randomized trials, in clinical practice, a wide heterogeneity in treatment response is observed between patients due to primary or acquired resistance. In our study population, the median PFS was 20 months, and although the direct comparison of clinical outcomes data between real world and randomized trials is not statistically appropriate, the shorter PFS of CDK4/6i in clinical practice suggests that a proper patients' selection might be a determinant for treatment efficacy. Therefore, in the absence of validated biomarkers, key questions about their optimal use still remain open, including whether all patients with HR+ MBC should receive a CDK4/6i. Mechanisms of resistance to these agents are multifactorial, but biomarkers with the ability to recognize early relapsers, or to predict the beneficial effect of CDK4/6i, are still to be identified. In order to address this issue, several genomic and retrospective analyses have been performed, and many others are still ongoing. In particular, research efforts are focusing on circulating biomarkers, given their many advantages in terms of ease of application and reproducibility at different time points that can capture spatial and temporal heterogeneity [41,42]. Retrospective analyses of large, randomized trials, PALOMA-2 and 3 and MONALEESA, have suggested a correlation between intrinsic subtype and efficacy of palbociclib and ribociclib in HR+/HER2- ABC treated with endocrine-based strategies. In particular, a joint retrospective analysis of PALOMA-2 and PALOMA-3 clinical trials showed an absolute advantage of palbociclib in Luminal A and Luminal B tumors defined using The EdgeSeq Oncology Biomarker Panel on the collected FFPE samples [43]. In the retrospective exploratory analysis of MONALEESA trials, evaluating clinical outcomes of intrinsic subtypes defined using NanoString technologies, all breast cancers, except those with basal-like genomic features, gained a consistent advantage in terms of PFS and OS with ribociclib [22]. Based on these findings, we hypothesized that the surrogate BC subtype, mirroring specific IHC features and clinical behaviors, could also have particular influence on survival outcomes in a metastatic setting. In this context, HER2-low BC is emerging as a potential distinct entity among the heterogenous population of HER2-tumors, comprising a non-negligible proportion of HR+ BC. Some reports in early stage settings showed that patients with HER2-low expression were more often associated with worse clinical features such as lymph node positive, poorly differentiated tumor grading and higher proliferation index [13,16]. As a result of these differences in tumor characteristics, a probable effect of HER2-low expression on clinical outcomes has been hypothesized. Studies focused on the prognostic value of HER2 expression level are limited, and the available results are controversial, highly depending on HR status and disease setting [12,13,15,16]. In particular, some retrospective data support a possible negative prognostic impact of HER2-low status in early settings, since higher pCR rates were registered among HER-0 patients treated with neoadjuvant chemotherapy [14–16]. However, data extrapolated from early stage cannot be translated to the metastatic setting due to the different genetic backgrounds that influence the clinical validity of the prognostic factors in these two contexts. In particular, an exploratory OS analysis including 1304 patients with ABC extrapolated from two datasets did not demonstrate statistically significant survival differences between the HER2-low and HER2-0 groups ($p = 0.787$) regardless of HR status [13]. Similar conclusions were drawn by Agostinetto and colleagues who compared survival outcomes between HER2-low and non-HER-low BC [12]. The Austrian Study Group of Medical Tumor Therapy (AGMT) analyzed data of 1729 patients, derived from a comprehensive metastatic BC registry including a widely heterogeneous population unselected for HR status, type or line of treatment showing that low HER2- expression has no impact on prognosis of metastatic BC [44]. Similarly, the analysis of data collected in the PRAEGNANT registry did not demonstrate the validity of a low level of HER2 to discriminate different prognostic groups among ABC patients with either HR+ or TNBC [45]. A recent retrospective analysis focused on 106 women with ABC treated with palbociclib or ribociclib plus ET as first or second line showed a potential impact of low HER2 expression on survival outcomes. This specific biological behavior could be driven by a bidirectional crosstalk between the ER and the HER2/HER3 axis, leading to ET resistance mechanisms [25]. Subsequently, Tarantino et al. performed a subgroup analysis including only patients receiving first-line ET (AI or fulvestrant) plus a CDK4/6 inhibitor (palbociclib, ribociclib or abemaciclib), demonstrating that treatment outcome (PFS1) was not influenced by HER2- expression [27]. The unresolved "dilemma" of the prognostic value of HER2- expression prompted our research to investigate whether HER2 expression in metastatic HR-positive, HER2-negative disease could have an impact on clinical outcomes of patients treated with ET plus palbociclib as first line. In the present study, including only patients with HR+ MBC, HER2-low expression was found in 43% of the participants, in line with other large studies that reported rates ranging from 31% to 64% [46,47]. In our study cohort, the survival analyses revealed a mPFS of 19 and 23 months in HER2-low and HER2-0, respectively, and the survival probabilities at 24, 36 and 48 months were slightly better for HER2-0 in respect to HER2-low. These differences in survival outcomes, although too small to draw conclusions, could be attributed to a higher likelihood of developing endocrine resistance in patients with lower HER2 expression. Overall, these results are intriguing, but we are aware that our data should be interpreted with caution and cannot be generalized due to the retrospective nature of the design and small sample size examined. Overall, these data highlight the high prevalence of this subtype, strengthening that the prognostic value of HER2-low should be reconsidered and further investigated in light of new potential treatment strategies. In this context, a new generation of anti-HER2 agents, represented by ADCs, have recently proven clinical activity with an acceptable safety profile in HER2-low disease [11,48]. Based on DESTINY-Breast04 results, trastuzumab deruxtecan (T-DXd), an ADC in which the trastuzumab antitumor properties are associated with a potent cytotoxic payload, was approved in the United States as the first HER2-directed therapy for patients with HER2-low MBC. Since signaling interactions between ER and HER family receptors are well-known endocrine resistance mechanisms, co-targeting of the HER2 and ER pathways with T-DXd and ET (anastrazole or fulvestrant), respectively, is being investigated in the phase IB DESTINY-Breast08 [49]. In this direction, zenocutuzumab, a HER2-HER3 bispecific antibody combined with ET, has demonstrated encouraging antitumor effects in xenograft models, opening the window to a new possible chemotherapy-free approach for patients with endocrine-resistant HER2-low BC [50]. Clearly, our study presents limitations that require attention and restrict the validity of the conclusions drawn. In addition to the above-mentioned limits (the small sample size, the retrospective design), technical issues related to the HER2 status evaluation method cannot be neglected. In particular, HER2 evaluation accuracy and reproducibility could be affected by no standardized pre-analytical and post-analytical processes and by the lack of a central confirmation of pathological assessment. Future studies might benefit from central assessment of HER2 to ensure standardized scoring within the low-level range, as well as from a molecular profile or an assessment by mRNA quantification to generate a more refined biomarker to define low HER2-expressing tumors.

5. Conclusions

In conclusion, our exploratory analysis suggests that low HER2 expression does not affect survival outcome in patients with MBC undergoing first-line treatment with ET plus palbociclib. Further prospective studies are needed to confirm the clinical implication of HER2 expression level, especially in view of the availability of new targeted agents and/or treatment combination strategies that could be incorporated into a therapeutic sequence.

Author Contributions: Conceptualization, F.C. (Francesca Carlino), A.D., S.F. and M.O.; Data curation, G.A., V.F., R.C., L.L. and B.P.; Methodology, F.C. (Francesca Carlino), A.D., A.P., C.M., G.A., V.F., R.C. and M.O.; Resources, F.C. (Francesca Carlino), A.V., A.P., C.M., D.B., F.G. and R.C.; Supervision, A.D., F.R., D.B., F.C. (Fortunato Ciardiello) and M.O.; Validation, A.V., F.R., F.G., B.P., F.D.V. and F.C. (Fortunato Ciardiello); Visualization, F.C. (Francesca Carlino), A.P., S.F., F.D.V. and F.C (Fortunato Ciardiello).; Writing—original draft, F.C. (Francesca Carlino) and A.D.; Writing—review and editing, F.C. (Francesca Carlino), A.D., L.L. and M.O. All authors have read and agreed to the published version of the manuscript.

Funding: This research received no external funding.

Institutional Review Board Statement: The study was conducted in accordance with the Declaration of Helsinki. This study was approved by the University of Campania Luigi Vanvitelli Ethic Committee (ID number: 15.03-20220005385*, 17 February 2022).

Informed Consent Statement: Informed consent was obtained from all subjects involved in the study.

Data Availability Statement: The data that support the findings of this study are available on request from the corresponding author.

Conflicts of Interest: The authors declare no conflict of interest.

References

1. Available online: https://www.cancer.gov/about-cancer/understanding/statistics (accessed on 27 August 2022).
2. Polyak, K. Breast cancer: Origins and evolution. *J. Clin. Investig.* **2007**, *117*, 3155–3163. [CrossRef] [PubMed]
3. Slamon, D.J.; Clark, G.M.; Wong, S.G.; Levin, W.J.; Ullrich, A.; McGuire, W.L. Human breast cancer: Correlation of relapse and survival with amplification of the HER-2/neu oncogene. *Science* **1987**, *235*, 177–182. [CrossRef]
4. Seshadri, R.; Firgaira, F.A.; Horsfall, D.J.; McCaul, K.; Setlur, V.; Kitchen, P. Clinical significance of HER-2/neu oncogene amplification in primary breast cancer. The South Australian Breast Cancer Study Group. *J. Clin. Oncol.* **1993**, *11*, 1936–1942. [CrossRef] [PubMed]
5. Pondé, N.; Brandão, M.; El-Hachem, G.; Werbrouck, E.; Piccart, M. Treatment of advanced HER2-positive breast cancer: 2018 and beyond. *Cancer Treat. Rev.* **2018**, *67*, 10–20. [CrossRef] [PubMed]
6. Riecke, K.; Witzel, I. Targeting the Human Epidermal Growth Factor Receptor Family in Breast Cancer beyond HER2. *Breast Care* **2020**, *15*, 579–585. [CrossRef]
7. Fehrenbacher, L.; Cecchini, R.S.; Geyer, C.E., Jr.; Rastogi, P.; Costantino, J.P.; Atkins, J.N.; Crown, J.P.; Polikoff, J.; Boileau, J.F.; Provencher, L.; et al. NSABP B-47/NRG Oncology Phase III Randomized Trial Comparing Adjuvant Chemotherapy with or Without Trastuzumab in High-Risk Invasive Breast Cancer Negative for HER2 by FISH and With IHC 1+ or 2+. *J. Clin. Oncol.* **2020**, *38*, 444–453. [CrossRef] [PubMed]
8. Gianni, L.; Lladó, A.; Bianchi, G.; Cortes, J.; Kellokumpu-Lehtinen, P.L.; Cameron, D.A.; Miles, D.; Salvagni, S.; Wardley, A.; Goeminne, J.C.; et al. Open-label, phase II, multicenter, randomized study of the efficacy and safety of two dose levels of Pertuzumab, a human epidermal growth factor receptor 2 dimerization inhibitor, in patients with human epidermal growth factor receptor 2-negative metastatic breast cancer. *J. Clin. Oncol.* **2010**, *28*, 1131–1137. [CrossRef] [PubMed]
9. Tarantino, P.; Hamilton, E.; Tolaney, S.M.; Cortes, J.; Morganti, S.; Ferraro, E.; Marra, A.; Viale, G.; Trapani, D.; Cardoso, F.; et al. HER2-Low Breast Cancer: Pathological and Clinical Landscape. *J. Clin. Oncol.* **2020**, *38*, 1951–1962. [CrossRef]
10. Marchiò, C.; Annaratone, L.; Marques, A.; Casorzo, L.; Berrino, E.; Sapino, A. Evolving concepts in HER2 evaluation in breast cancer: Heterogeneity, HER2-low carcinomas and beyond. *Semin. Cancer Biol.* **2021**, *72*, 123–135. [CrossRef]
11. Modi, S.; Jacot, W.; Yamashita, T.; Sohn, J.; Vidal, M.; Tokunaga, E.; Tsurutani, J.; Ueno, N.T.; Prat, A.; Chae, Y.S.; et al. Trastuzumab Deruxtecan in Previously Treated HER2-Low Advanced Breast Cancer. *N. Engl. J. Med.* **2022**, *387*, 9–20. [CrossRef] [PubMed]
12. Agostinetto, E.; Rediti, M.; Fimereli, D.; Debien, V.; Piccart, M.; Aftimos, P.; Sotiriou, C.; de Azambuja, E. HER2-Low Breast Cancer: Molecular Characteristics and Prognosis. *Cancers* **2021**, *13*, 2824. [CrossRef] [PubMed]

13. Schettini, F.; Chic, N.; Brasó-Maristany, F.; Paré, L.; Pascual, T.; Conte, B.; Martínez-Sáez, O.; Adamo, B.; Vidal, M.; Barnadas, E.; et al. Clinical, pathological, and PAM50 gene expression features of HER2-low breast cancer. *NPJ Breast Cancer* **2021**, *7*, 1. [CrossRef] [PubMed]
14. Denkert, C.; Seither, F.; Schneeweiss, A.; Link, T.; Blohmer, J.U.; Just, M.; Wimberger, P.; Forberger, A.; Tesch, H.; Jackisch, C.; et al. Clinical and molecular characteristics of HER2-low-positive breast cancer: Pooled analysis of individual patient data from four prospective, neoadjuvant clinical trials. *Lancet Oncol.* **2021**, *22*, 1151–1161. [CrossRef]
15. Rossi, V.; Sarotto, I.; Maggiorotto, F.; Berchialla, P.; Kubatzki, F.; Tomasi, N.; Redana, S.; Martinello, R.; Valabrega, G.; Aglietta, M.; et al. Moderate immunohistochemical expression of HER-2 (2+) without HER-2 gene amplification is a negative prognostic factor in early breast cancer. *Oncologist* **2012**, *17*, 1418–1425. [CrossRef] [PubMed]
16. Eggemann, H.; Ignatov, T.; Burger, E.; Kantelhardt, E.J.; Fettke, F.; Thomssen, C.; Costa, S.D.; Ignatov, A. Moderate HER2 expression as a prognostic factor in hormone receptor positive breast cancer. *Endocr. Relat. Cancer* **2015**, *22*, 725–733. [CrossRef] [PubMed]
17. Gilcrease, M.Z.; Woodward, W.A.; Nicolas, M.M.; Corley, L.J.; Fuller, G.N.; Esteva, F.J.; Tucker, S.L.; Buchholz, T.A. Even low-level HER2 expression may be associated with worse outcome in node-positive breast cancer. *Am. J. Surg. Pathol.* **2009**, *33*, 759–767. [CrossRef] [PubMed]
18. Poulakaki, N.; Makris, G.M.; Battista, M.J.; Böhm, D.; Petraki, K.; Bafaloukos, D.; Sergentanis, T.N.; Siristatidis, C.; Chrelias, C.; Papantoniou, N. Hormonal receptor status, Ki-67 and HER2 expression: Prognostic value in the recurrence of ductal carcinoma in situ of the breast? *Breast* **2016**, *25*, 57–61. [CrossRef]
19. Burris, H.A., 3rd; Rugo, H.S.; Vukelja, S.J.; Vogel, C.L.; Borson, R.A.; Limentani, S.; Tan-Chiu, E.; Krop, I.E.; Michaelson, R.A.; Girish, S.; et al. Phase II study of the antibody drug conjugate trastuzumab-DM1 for the treatment of human epidermal growth factor receptor 2 (HER2)-positive breast cancer after prior HER2-directed therapy. *J. Clin. Oncol.* **2011**, *29*, 398–405. [CrossRef] [PubMed]
20. Asghar, U.S.; Kanani, R.; Roylance, R.; Mittnacht, S. Systematic Review of Molecular Biomarkers Predictive of Resistance to CDK4/6 Inhibition in Metastatic Breast Cancer. *JCO Precis. Oncol.* **2022**, *6*, e2100002. [CrossRef]
21. Turner, N.C.; Liu, Y.; Zhu, Z.; Loi, S.; Colleoni, M.; Loibl, S.; DeMichele, A.; Harbeck, N.; André, F.; Bayar, M.A.; et al. Cyclin E1 Expression and Palbociclib Efficacy in Previously Treated Hormone Receptor-Positive Metastatic Breast Cancer. *J. Clin. Oncol.* **2019**, *37*, 1169–1178, Erratum in *J. Clin. Oncol.* **2019**, *37*, 2956. [CrossRef] [PubMed]
22. Prat, A.; Chaudhury, A.; Solovieff, N.; Paré, L.; Martinez, D.; Chic, N.; Martínez-Sáez, O.; Brasó-Maristany, F.; Lteif, A.; Taran, T.; et al. Correlative Biomarker Analysis of Intrinsic Subtypes and Efficacy Across the MONALEESA Phase III Studies. *J. Clin. Oncol.* **2021**, *39*, 1458–1467, Erratum in *J. Clin. Oncol.* **2021**, *39*, 3525. [CrossRef] [PubMed]
23. Finn, R.S.; Liu, Y.; Zhu, Z.; Martin, M.; Rugo, H.S.; Diéras, V.; Im, S.A.; Gelmon, K.A.; Harbeck, N.; Lu, D.R.; et al. Biomarker Analyses of Response to Cyclin-Dependent Kinase 4/6 Inhibition and Endocrine Therapy in Women with Treatment-Naïve Metastatic Breast Cancer. *Clin. Cancer Res.* **2020**, *26*, 110–121. [CrossRef] [PubMed]
24. Prat, A.; Parker, J.S. Standardized versus research-based PAM50 intrinsic subtyping of breast cancer. *Clin. Transl. Oncol.* **2020**, *22*, 953–955. [CrossRef] [PubMed]
25. Giuliano, M.; Trivedi, M.V.; Schiff, R. Bidirectional Crosstalk between the Estrogen Receptor and Human Epidermal Growth Factor Receptor 2 Signaling Pathways in Breast Cancer: Molecular Basis and Clinical Implications. *Breast Care* **2013**, *8*, 256–262. [CrossRef]
26. Bao, K.K.H.; Sutanto, L.; Tse, S.S.W.; Cheung, K.M.; Chan, J.C.H. The Association of ERBB2-Low Expression with the Efficacy of Cyclin-Dependent Kinase 4/6 Inhibitor in Hormone Receptor-Positive, ERBB2-Negative Metastatic Breast Cancer. *JAMA Netw. Open* **2021**, *4*, e2133132. [CrossRef]
27. Tarantino, P.; Gandini, S.; Nicolò, E.; Trillo, P.; Giugliano, F.; Zagami, P.; Vivanet, G.; Bellerba, F.; Trapani, D.; Marra, A.; et al. Evolution of low HER2 expression between early and advanced-stage breast cancer. *Eur. J. Cancer* **2022**, *163*, 35–43. [CrossRef]
28. Goldhirsch, A.; Wood, W.C.; Coates, A.S.; Gelber, R.D.; Thürlimann, B.; Senn, H.J. Strategies for subtypes—Dealing with the diversity of breast cancer: Highlights of the St. Gallen International Expert Consensus on the Primary Therapy of Early Breast Cancer 2011. *Ann. Oncol.* **2011**, *22*, 1736–1747. [CrossRef]
29. Coates, A.S.; Winer, E.P.; Goldhirsch, A.; Gelber, R.D.; Gnant, M.; Piccart-Gebhart, M.; Thürlimann, B.; Senn, H.J. Tailoring therapies—Improving the management of early breast cancer: St Gallen International Expert Consensus on the Primary Therapy of Early Breast Cancer 2015. *Ann. Oncol.* **2015**, *26*, 1533–1546. [CrossRef]
30. Allison, K.H.; Hammond, M.E.H.; Dowsett, M.; McKernin, S.E.; Carey, L.A.; Fitzgibbons, P.L.; Hayes, D.F.; Lakhani, S.R.; Chavez-MacGregor, M.; Perlmutter, J.; et al. Estrogen and Progesterone Receptor Testing in Breast Cancer: American Society of Clinical Oncology/College of American Pathologists Guideline Update. *Arch. Pathol. Lab. Med.* **2020**, *144*, 545–563. [CrossRef]
31. Goldhirsch, A.; Winer, E.P.; Coates, A.S.; Gelber, R.D.; Piccart-Gebhart, M.; Thürlimann, B.; Senn, H.J. Personalizing the treatment of women with early breast cancer: Highlights of the St Gallen International Expert Consensus on the Primary Therapy of Early Breast Cancer 2013. *Ann. Oncol.* **2013**, *24*, 2206–2223. [CrossRef]
32. Hammond, M.E.; Hayes, D.F.; Dowsett, M.; Allred, D.C.; Hagerty, K.L.; Badve, S.; Fitzgibbons, P.L.; Francis, G.; Goldstein, N.S.; Hayes, M.; et al. American Society of Clinical Oncology/College of American Pathologists guideline recommendations for immunohistochemical testing of estrogen and progesterone receptors in breast cancer (unabridged version). *Arch. Pathol. Lab. Med.* **2010**, *134*, e48–e72. [CrossRef] [PubMed]

33. Wolff, A.C.; Hammond, M.E.H.; Allison, K.H.; Harvey, B.E.; Mangu, P.B.; Bartlett, J.M.S.; Bilous, M.; Ellis, I.O.; Fitzgibbons, P.; Hanna, W.; et al. Human Epidermal Growth Factor Receptor 2 Testing in Breast Cancer: American Society of Clinical Oncology/College of American Pathologists Clinical Practice Guideline Focused Update. *J. Clin. Oncol.* **2018**, *36*, 2105–2122. [CrossRef]
34. Bewick, V.; Cheek, L.; Ball, J. Statistics review 12: Survival analysis. *Crit. Care* **2004**, *8*, 389–394. [CrossRef]
35. Hortobagyi, G.N.; Stemmer, S.M.; Burris, H.A.; Yap, Y.S.; Sonke, G.S.; Paluch-Shimon, S.; Campone, M.; Blackwell, K.L.; André, F.; Winer, E.P.; et al. Ribociclib as First-Line Therapy for HR-Positive, Advanced Breast Cancer. *N. Engl. J. Med.* **2016**, *375*, 1738–1748. [CrossRef]
36. Finn, R.S.; Martin, M.; Rugo, H.S.; Jones, S.; Im, S.A.; Gelmon, K.; Harbeck, N.; Lipatov, O.N.; Walshe, J.M.; Moulder, S.; et al. Palbociclib and Letrozole in Advanced Breast Cancer. *N. Engl. J. Med.* **2016**, *375*, 1925–1936. [CrossRef]
37. Goetz, M.P.; Toi, M.; Campone, M.; Sohn, J.; Paluch-Shimon, S.; Huober, J.; Park, I.H.; Trédan, O.; Chen, S.C.; Manso, L.; et al. MONARCH 3: Abemaciclib as Initial Therapy for Advanced Breast Cancer. *J. Clin. Oncol.* **2017**, *35*, 3638–3646. [CrossRef]
38. Sledge, G.W., Jr.; Toi, M.; Neven, P.; Sohn, J.; Inoue, K.; Pivot, X.; Burdaeva, O.; Okera, M.; Masuda, N.; Kaufman, P.A.; et al. MONARCH 2: Abemaciclib in Combination with Fulvestrant in Women With HR+/HER2- Advanced Breast Cancer Who Had Progressed While Receiving Endocrine Therapy. *J. Clin. Oncol.* **2017**, *35*, 2875–2884. [CrossRef]
39. Slamon, D.J.; Neven, P.; Chia, S.; Fasching, P.A.; De Laurentiis, M.; Im, S.A.; Petrakova, K.; Bianchi, G.V.; Esteva, F.J.; Martín, M.; et al. Phase III Randomized Study of Ribociclib and Fulvestrant in Hormone Receptor-Positive, Human Epidermal Growth Factor Receptor 2-Negative Advanced Breast Cancer: MONALEESA-3. *J. Clin. Oncol.* **2018**, *36*, 2465–2472. [CrossRef] [PubMed]
40. Cristofanilli, M.; Turner, N.C.; Bondarenko, I.; Ro, J.; Im, S.A.; Masuda, N.; Colleoni, M.; DeMichele, A.; Loi, S.; Verma, S.; et al. Fulvestrant plus palbociclib versus fulvestrant plus placebo for treatment of hormone-receptor-positive, HER2-negative metastatic breast cancer that progressed on previous endocrine therapy (PALOMA-3): Final analysis of the multicentre, double-blind, phase 3 randomised controlled trial. *Lancet Oncol.* **2016**, *17*, 425–439. [CrossRef] [PubMed]
41. Arpino, G.; Bianchini, G.; Malorni, L.; Zambelli, A.; Puglisi, F.; Del Mastro, L.; Colleoni, M.; Montemurro, F.; Bianchi, G.V.; Paris, I.; et al. Circulating tumor DNA (ctDNA) and serum thymidine kinase 1 activity (TKa) matched dynamics in patients (pts) with hormone receptor–positive (HR+), human epidermal growth factor 2–negative (HER2-) advanced breast cancer (ABC) treated in first-line (1L) with ribociclib (RIB) and letrozole (LET) in the BioItaLEE trial. *J. Clin. Oncol.* **2022**, *40* (Suppl. 16), 1012.
42. Watt, A.C.; Goel, S. Cellular mechanisms underlying response and resistance to CDK4/6 inhibitors in the treatment of hormone receptor-positive breast cancer. *Breast Cancer Res.* **2022**, *24*, 17. [CrossRef] [PubMed]
43. Finn, R.S.; Cristofanilli, M.; Ettl, J.; Gelmon, K.A.; Colleoni, M.; Giorgetti, C.; Gauthier, E.; Liu, Y.; Lu, D.R.; Zhang, Z.; et al. Treatment effect of palbociclib plus endocrine therapy by prognostic and intrinsic subtype and biomarker analysis in patients with bone-only disease: A joint analysis of PALOMA-2 and PALOMA-3 clinical trials. *Breast Cancer Res. Treat.* **2020**, *184*, 23–35. [CrossRef]
44. Gampenrieder, S.P.; Rinnerthaler, G.; Tinchon, C.; Petzer, A.; Balic, M.; Heibl, S.; Schmitt, C.; Zabernigg, A.F.; Egle, D.; Sandholzer, M.; et al. Landscape of HER2-low metastatic breast cancer (MBC): Results from the Austrian AGMT_MBC-Registry. *Breast Cancer Res.* **2021**, *23*, 112. [CrossRef] [PubMed]
45. Hein, A.; Hartkopf, A.D.; Emons, J.; Lux, M.P.; Volz, B.; Taran, F.A.; Overkamp, F.; Hadji, P.; Tesch, H.; Häberle, L.; et al. Prognostic effect of low-level HER2 expression in patients with clinically negative HER2 status. *Eur. J. Cancer* **2021**, *155*, 1–12. [CrossRef] [PubMed]
46. Won, H.S.; Ahn, J.; Kim, Y.; Kim, J.S.; Song, J.Y.; Kim, H.K.; Lee, J.; Park, H.K.; Kim, Y.S. Clinical significance of HER2-low expression in early breast cancer: A nationwide study from the Korean Breast Cancer Society. *Breast Cancer Res.* **2022**, *24*, 22. [CrossRef] [PubMed]
47. Horisawa, N.; Adachi, Y.; Takatsuka, D.; Nozawa, K.; Endo, Y.; Ozaki, Y.; Sugino, K.; Kataoka, A.; Kotani, H.; Yoshimura, A.; et al. The frequency of low HER2 expression in breast cancer and a comparison of prognosis between patients with HER2-low and HER2-negative breast cancer by HR status. *Breast Cancer* **2022**, *29*, 234–241. [CrossRef]
48. Banerji, U.; van Herpen, C.M.L.; Saura, C.; Thistlethwaite, F.; Lord, S.; Moreno, V.; Macpherson, I.R.; Boni, V.; Rolfo, C.; de Vries, E.G.E.; et al. Trastuzumab duocarmazine in locally advanced and metastatic solid tumours and HER2-expressing breast cancer: A phase 1 dose-escalation and dose-expansion study. *Lancet Oncol.* **2019**, *20*, 1124–1135. [CrossRef]
49. Jhaveri, K.; Hamilton, E.; Loi, S.; Schmid, P.; Darilay, A.; Gao, C.; Patel, G.; Wrona, M.; Andre, F. Abstract OT-03-05: Trastuzumab deruxtecan (T-DXd; DS-8201) in combination with other anticancer agents in patients with HER2-low metastatic breast cancer: A phase 1b, open-label, multicenter, dose-finding and dose-expansion study (DESTINY-Breast08). *Cancer Res.* **2021**, *81* (Suppl. S4), OT-03. [CrossRef]
50. Pistilli, B.; Wildiers, H.; Hamilton, E.P.; Ferreira, A.A.; Dalenc, F.; Vidal, M.; Gavilá, J.; Goncalves, A.; Murias, C.; Mouret-Reynier, M.A.; et al. Clinical activity of MCLA-128 (zenocutuzumab) in combination with endocrine therapy (ET) in ER+/HER2-low, non-amplified metastatic breast cancer (MBC) patients (pts) with ET-resistant disease who had progressed on a CDK4/6 inhibitor (CDK4/6i). *J. Clin. Oncol.* **2020**, *38* (Suppl. 15), 1037. [CrossRef]

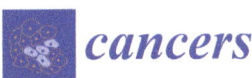

Article

Splicing Analysis of 16 *PALB2* ClinVar Variants by Minigene Assays: Identification of Six Likely Pathogenic Variants

Alberto Valenzuela-Palomo [1], Lara Sanoguera-Miralles [1], Elena Bueno-Martínez [1], Ada Esteban-Sánchez [2], Inés Llinares-Burguet [1], Alicia García-Álvarez [1], Pedro Pérez-Segura [2], Susana Gómez-Barrero [3], Miguel de la Hoya [2] and Eladio A. Velasco-Sampedro [1,*]

[1] Splicing and Genetic Susceptibility to Cancer, Unidad de Excelencia Instituto de Biología y Genética Molecular, Consejo Superior de Investigaciones Científicas (CSIC-UVa), 47003 Valladolid, Spain
[2] Molecular Oncology Laboratory, Hospital Clínico San Carlos, IdISSC (Instituto de Investigación Sanitaria del Hospital Clínico San Carlos), 28040 Madrid, Spain
[3] Facultad de Ciencias de la Salud, Universidad Alfonso X "El Sabio", Avda. de la Universidad 1, Villanueva de la Cañada, 28691 Madrid, Spain
* Correspondence: eavelsam@ibgm.uva.es

Simple Summary: *PALB2* pathogenic variants confer high risk of breast cancer. Here, we have analyzed the impact of *PALB2* variants on splicing, a gene expression step that removes introns to form the mature messenger RNA. This process is performed by the splicing machinery through the recognition of specific sequences, namely the 3′ and 5′ splice sites, which determine the exon ends. Variants at these sequences may trigger anomalous splicing and aberrant transcripts that may be associated with a disease. To test the impact of variants on splicing, we used a biotechnological tool called minigene, which replicates, at small-scale, the human gene of interest. Thus, we checked 16 *PALB2* variants at the intron/exon boundaries using the minigene mgPALB2_ex1-3. We found that twelve variants disrupted splicing, six of which could be classified as likely pathogenic. These results facilitate the clinical management of carrier patients and families since they may benefit from tailored prevention protocols and therapies.

Abstract: *PALB2* loss-of-function variants are associated with significant increased risk of breast cancer as well as other types of tumors. Likewise, splicing disruptions are a common mechanism of disease susceptibility. Indeed, we previously showed, by minigene assays, that 35 out of 42 *PALB2* variants impaired splicing. Taking advantage of one of these constructs (mgPALB2_ex1-3), we proceeded to analyze other variants at exons 1 to 3 reported at the ClinVar database. Thirty-one variants were bioinformatically analyzed with MaxEntScan and SpliceAI. Then, 16 variants were selected for subsequent RNA assays. We identified a total of 12 spliceogenic variants, 11 of which did not produce any trace of the expected minigene full-length transcript. Interestingly, variant c.49-1G > A mimicked previous outcomes in patient RNA (transcript ∆(E2p6)), supporting the reproducibility of the minigene approach. A total of eight variant-induced transcripts were characterized, three of which (∆(E1q17), ∆(E3p11), and ∆(E3)) were predicted to introduce a premature termination codon and to undergo nonsense-mediated decay, and five (▼(E1q9), ∆(E2p6), ∆(E2), ▼(E3q48)-a, and ▼(E3q48)-b) maintained the reading frame. According to an ACMG/AMP (American College of Medical Genetics and Genomics/Association for Molecular Pathology)-based classification scheme, which integrates mgPALB2 data, six *PALB2* variants were classified as pathogenic/likely pathogenic, five as VUS, and five as likely benign. Furthermore, five ±1,2 variants were catalogued as VUS because they produced significant proportions of in-frame transcripts of unknown impact on protein function.

Keywords: hereditary breast cancer; cancer susceptibility genes; *PALB2*; aberrant splicing; functional assay; minigenes; clinical interpretation

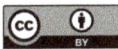

Citation: Valenzuela-Palomo, A.; Sanoguera-Miralles, L.; Bueno-Martínez, E.; Esteban-Sánchez, A.; Llinares-Burguet, I.; García-Álvarez, A.; Pérez-Segura, P.; Gómez-Barrero, S.; de la Hoya, M.; Velasco-Sampedro, E.A. Splicing Analysis of 16 *PALB2* ClinVar Variants by Minigene Assays: Identification of Six Likely Pathogenic Variants. *Cancers* 2022, 14, 4541. https://doi.org/10.3390/cancers14184541

Academic Editor: Christian Singer

Received: 5 August 2022
Accepted: 15 September 2022
Published: 19 September 2022

Publisher's Note: MDPI stays neutral with regard to jurisdictional claims in published maps and institutional affiliations.

Copyright: © 2022 by the authors. Licensee MDPI, Basel, Switzerland. This article is an open access article distributed under the terms and conditions of the Creative Commons Attribution (CC BY) license (https://creativecommons.org/licenses/by/4.0/).

1. Introduction

Hereditary breast cancer (BC) is a highly heterogenous genetic disease, in which more than 20 genes of the DNA repair pathway have been proposed as breast cancer susceptibility genes [1]. Historically, genetic testing was focused on the main BC genes *BRCA1* and *BRCA2* by different methods [2,3]. The development of next-generation sequencing (NGS) enabled the development of panels of cancer predisposing genes and the simultaneous sequencing of multiple genes, thus boosting efficiency and cost-effectiveness. Recently, two large-scale sequencing studies, which sequenced a panel of breast cancer genes in more than 170,000 women, refined the BC/OC genetic predisposition spectrum [4,5]. At least eight genes were found to be significantly associated with breast cancer risk: *BRCA1* (MIM#113705), *BRCA2* (MIM#600185), *ATM* (MIM#607585), *BARD1* (MIM #601593), *CHEK2* (MIM#604373), *PALB2* (MIM#610355), *RAD51C* (MIM#602774), and *RAD51D* (MIM#602954) [4–6]. Biallelic loss-of-function variants of *PALB2* (also known as *FANCN*) and other BC susceptibility genes, such as *BRCA2*, *RAD51C*, and *BRCA1*, cause Fanconi anemia [7], which is characterized by a high genomic instability and increased cancer predisposition.

The partner and localizer of BRCA2 (PALB2) interacts with BRCA1 and BRCA2 and is implicated in repair of double-strand DNA breaks by homologous recombination. While BRCA1 recruits PALB2 at the sites of DNA damage, PALB2 stabilizes BRCA2 during formation of the RAD51 nucleoprotein filament [8,9]. *PALB2* loss-of-function variants confer high risk of developing breast cancer (BC) as well as other types of cancers [10–12]. Two recent reports have shown that *PALB2* protein truncating variants are associated with a significantly increased risk of breast cancer (BC relative risk 3.83 and 5.02, respectively) and accounts for 9.5–10.1% of the protein truncating variants of the eight core BC genes mentioned above (0.39–0.56% of all BC cases) [4,5]. Furthermore, associations with estrogen-negative and triple-negative BC are even higher, with relative risks of 7.35 (4.25–12.72) and 10.36 (6.42–16.71), respectively [4]. Hence, *PALB2* belongs to the high-risk category of BC susceptibility genes together with *BRCA1* and *BRCA2*.

On the other hand, a deleterious effect on gene function cannot be assigned for a relevant proportion of variants detected in patients, the so-called variants of uncertain clinical significance (VUS) [13]. In the case of *PALB2*, VUS frequency is approximately four times greater than that of pathogenic variants [5]. Consequently, they represent a challenge in genetic counselling because cancer risk assessment in VUS carriers is only based on cancer family history [14]. Apart from protein translation, there are other gene expression steps that may be targeted by disease-causing variants, such as transcription, splicing, as well as other post-transcriptional mechanisms [15–18]. Functional studies of these processes provide key information for the clinical interpretation of VUS.

The splicing process Is controlled by a large collection of splicing factors and cis-acting sequences that include: the 5′ or donor (GT) and the 3′ or acceptor (AG) splice sites (5′SS and 3′SS, respectively), the polypyrimidine tract and the branch point, as well as exonic and intronic elements that promote (enhancers) or repress (silencers) exon recognition [19]. All these motifs may be targets of splicing-disrupting mutations (spliceogenic variants) so that an unexpectedly large fraction of variants can actually induce splicing anomalies [17, 20,21]. In fact, it was estimated that about 62% of pathogenic variants impair splicing [22]. Interestingly, several cancer susceptibility genes, such as *MLH1*, *MSH2*, and *PMS2*, are enriched in spliceogenic variants [23].

We have focused our efforts on the study of the impact of genetic variants on the splicing of the BC genes by minigene assays, by which we found a large proportion of spliceogenic variants [24]. We comprehensively analyzed by minigene assays several BC susceptibility genes, such as *BRCA2* [25], along with *RAD51C*, *RAD51D*, *PALB2*, and *ATM* within the framework of the European Project BRIDGES (Breast Cancer Risk after Diagnostic Gene Sequencing; https://bridges-research.eu/, accessed on 12 July 2022) [26–29].

In a recent work, we studied the *PALB2* gene and tested, in three different minigenes, 42 candidate BRIDGES variants [28], 35 of which disrupted splicing, with 23 of them being classified as pathogenic or likely pathogenic, demonstrating the usefulness of minigenes for RNA assays and clinical interpretation of variants. Moreover, these constructs are highly valuable since any other potentially spliceogenic variants of the gene of interest can be so assayed.

Taking advantage of the minigene mgPALB2_ex1-3, we selected 31 ClinVar splice-site variants located at exons 1–3 (https://www.ncbi.nlm.nih.gov/clinvar/, accessed on 3 August 2021) to carry out splicing assays of the potentially damaging variants.

2. Materials and Methods

2.1. Variant and Transcript Annotations

The analysis of the ClinVar data identified a total of 31 variants at exons 1, 2, and 3 and flanking intronic sequences located at the PALB2 5′ and 3′ splice sites (5′SS and 3′ SS, respectively), defined for the purpose of the present study as: (i) intron/exon (IVS −10 to −1/2 nt) boundaries (3′SS) and (ii) exon/intron (2 nt/IVS +1 to +6) boundaries (5′SS). Variants, transcripts and predicted protein products were described according to the Human Genome Variation Society (HGVS) guidelines (https://varnomen.hgvs.org/, accessed on 1 June 2022), using the Ensembl reference transcript ID ENSG00000083093 (Genbank NM_024675.4). We also annotated splicing events according to a former shortened description [30,31].

2.2. Bioinformatics: Databases and In Silico Studies

All the 31 PALB2 ClinVar splice-site variants at exons 1, 2, and 3 were analyzed with MaxEntScan (MES) http://hollywood.mit.edu/burgelab/maxent/Xmaxentscan_scoreseq.html, accessed on 3 August 2021) to identify potentially spliceogenic variants [32]. Candidate variants were analyzed under the following criteria [28]: (i) splice site disruption at the ±1,2 (AG/GT) positions and (ii) relevant MES score changes ($\geq 15\%$) [33,34]. All variants were further evaluated with the splice-site predictor SpliceAI (https://spliceailookup.broadinstitute.org/, accessed on 3 August 2021) [35]. SpliceAI outputs were helpful to predict putative splicing outcomes based on a "two score" approach (e.g., donor loss + acceptor loss predicts exon skipping, while donor loss + donor gain predicts a donor shift). SpliceAI parameters were as follows: genome version hg38; score type raw; max distance 10,000 nt; Illumina's pre-computed scores yes. Scores range 0–1 is interpreted as probability of impact on splicing with the following cutoffs: 0.2–0.49 (high recall), 0.5–0.79 (recommended), and >0.8 (high precision). SpliceAI was not herein used to filter out variants. On basis of the MES outcomes, we decided to carry out the subsequent splicing assays for 16 potentially spliceogenic variants.

2.3. Minigene Construction and Mutagenesis

The minigene mgPALB2_ex1–3 was built in the splicing vector pSAD as previously reported [28,36,37] (Figure 1a). In brief, this construct contains a 974 bp insert (final minigene size: 5068 bp) that includes exons 1 to 3. This construct has the special feature of a chimeric exon 1 composed of vector exon 1 and PALB2 exon 1 so that 5′SS variants of exon 1 can be tested [28].

The wild-type minigene was used as template to generate 16 DNA ClinVar variants by site-directed mutagenesis with the QuikChange Lightning Kit (Agilent, Santa Clara, CA, USA) (Table 1). All mutant constructs were confirmed by sequencing (Macrogen, Madrid, Spain).

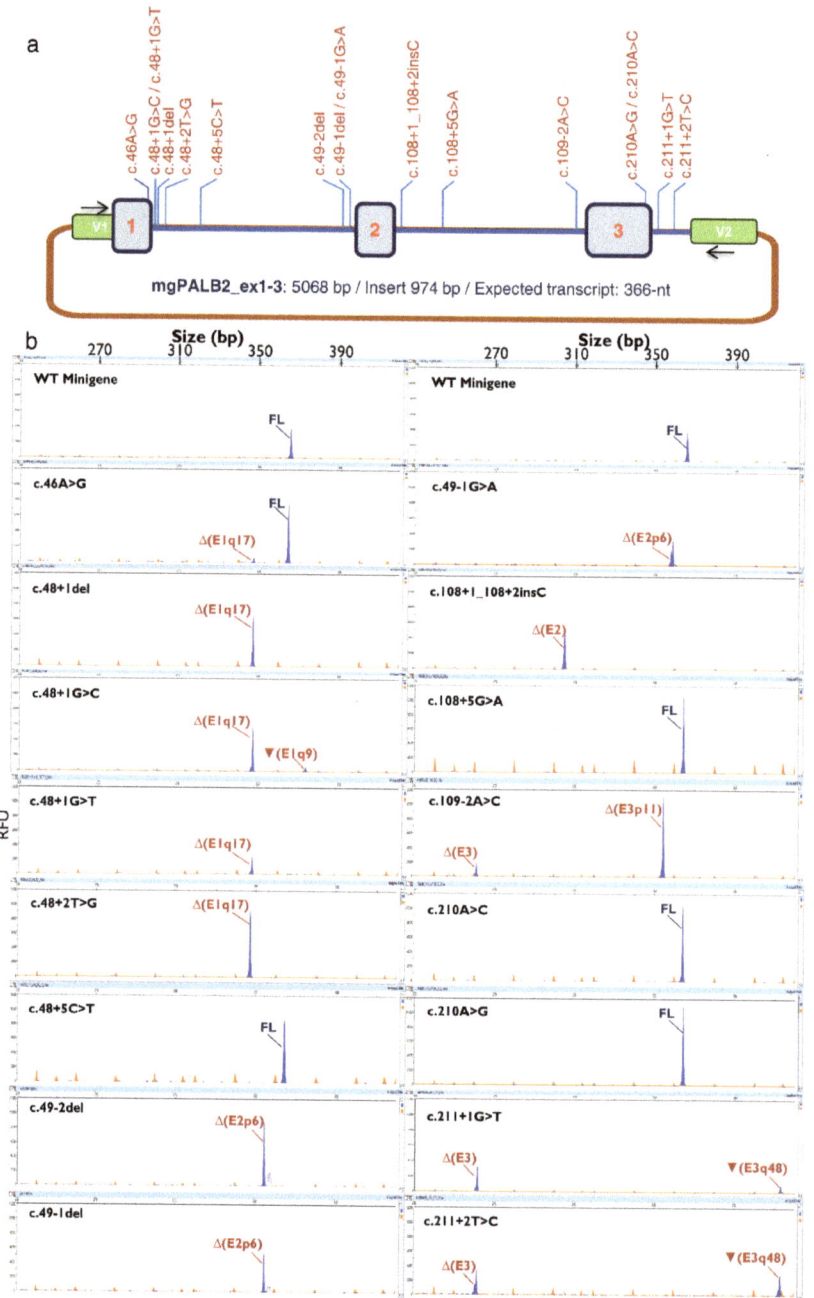

Figure 1. Minigene splicing assays of selected *PALB2* variants. (**a**) Map of variants in the minigene mgPALB2_ex1–3. V1 and V2 are the vector exons while variants are shown in red above the minigene construct (**b**) Fluorescent fragment analysis of 16 variants. The electropherogram of the wild-type minigene is shown on the top of each column. FAM-labelled products (blue peaks) were run together with LIZ-600 (orange peaks) as size standard (FL, minigene full-length transcript). The x-axis indicates size in bp (electropherograms on the top) and the y-axis represents relative fluorescence units (RFU).

Table 1. Mutagenesis primers of *PALB2* variants.

Variant	Exon/Intron	Primers (5′→3′)
c.46A > G	Ex1	CTGTGAGGAGAAGGAAGAGGTGCCGGGGGTGCGGGAAGGG
		CCCTTCCCGCACCCCCGGCACCTCTTCCTTCTCCTCACAG
c.48 + 1del	IVS1	AGCTGTGAGGAGAAGGAAAAGGGGCCGGGGGTGCGGGAAG
		CTTCCCGCACCCCCGGCCCCTTTTCCTTCTCCTCACAGCT
c.48 + 1G > C	IVS1	GCTGTGAGGAGAAGGAAAAGCTGCCGGGGGTGCGGGAAGG
		CCTTCCCGCACCCCCGGCAGCTTTTCCTTCTCCTCACAGC
c.48 + 1G > T	IVS1	TCAGCTGTGAGGAGAAGGAAAAGTTGCCGGGGGTGCGGGA
		TCCCGCACCCCCGGCAACTTTTCCTTCTCCTCACAGCTGA
c.48 + 2T > G	IVS1	CAGCTGTGAGGAGAAGGAAAAGTGCCGGGGGTGCGGGAAG
		CTTCCCGCACCCCCGGCACTTTTCCTTCTCCTCACAGCTG
c.48 + 5C > T	IVS1	GAGGAGAAGGAAAAGGTGCTGGGGGTGCGGGAAGGGCGGA
		TCCGCCCTTCCCGCACCCCCAGCACCTTTTCCTTCTCCTC
c.49-2del	IVS1	TGCCCAGTATTGTTGGTGTTTTCTTCTTCCGTTAAAGGA
		TCCTTTAACGGAAGAAGAAAAACACCAACAATACTGGGCA
c.49-1del	IVS1	TGCCCAGTATTGTTGGTGTTTTCTTCTTCCATTAAAGGA
		TCCTTTAATGGAAGAAGAAAAACACCAACAATACTGGGCA
c.49-1G > A	IVS1	TTCTTCCAATTAAAGGAGAAATTAGCATTCTTGAAAAGGG
		CCCTTTTCAAGAATGCTAATTTCTCCTTTAATTGGAAGAA
c.108 + 1_108 + 2insC	IVS2	CCTTCAGGCTAAGTGAATCGTATTCTCAAATTAAGGTGTT
		AACACCTTAATTTGAGAATACGATTCACTTAGCCTGAAGG
c.108 + 5G > A	IVS2	TAGCCCGCCTTCAGGTAAATGAATCGTATTCTCAAATTAA
		TTAATTTGAGAATACGATTCATTTACCTGAAGGCGGGCTA
c.109-2A > C	IVS2	TTTGTCTCCTCTCGCGTGCCCAAAGAGCTGAAAAGATTAA
		TTAATCTTTTCAGCTCTTTGGGCACGCGAGAGGAGACAAA
c.210A > G	Ex3	CCGCAGCTAAAACACTCGGGTAAATCTAGACCATTCACTT
		AAGTGAATGGTCTAGATTTACCCGAGTGTTTTAGCTGCGG
c.210A > C	Ex3	CGCAGCTAAAACACTCCGGTAAATCTAGACCATTCACTTA
		TAAGTGAATGGTCTAGATTTACCGGAGTGTTTTAGCTGCG
c.211 + 1G > T	IVS3	CCGCAGCTAAAACACTCAGTTAAATCTAGACCATTCACTT
		AAGTGAATGGTCTAGATTTAACTGAGTGTTTTAGCTGCGG
c.211 + 2T > C	IVS3	ACCGCAGCTAAAACACTCAGGCAAATCTAGACCATTCACT
		AGTGAATGGTCTAGATTTGCCTGAGTGTTTTAGCTGCGGT

2.4. Splicing Functional Assays

Approximately 2×10^5 MCF-7 and MDA-MB-231 cells were seeded in four-well plates (Nunc, Roskilde, Denmark) to grow up to 90% confluency in 0.5 mL of medium (MEME, 10% fetal bovine serum, 2 mM glutamine, 1% non-essential amino acids, and 1% penicillin/streptomycin). Then, using a standard protocol of transfection, MCF-7 cells were transfected with either the wild-type or the mutant minigenes. To inhibit nonsense-mediated decay (NMD), cells were incubated with cycloheximide 300 µg/mL (Sigma-Aldrich, St. Louis, MO) for 4 h. RNA was extracted after 48 h and purified with the Genematrix Universal RNA purification Kit (EURx, Gdansk, Poland) with on-column DNAse I digestion to degrade genomic DNA that could interfere in RT-PCR. Retrotranscription was carried out with specific primers of exons V1 and V2 of the pSAD® vector as previously described [26,28,38]. The expected size of the minigene mgPALB2_ex1–3 full-length (mgFL) transcript was 366 nt. To estimate the relative abundance of all transcripts, semi-quantitative fluorescent RT-PCRs (26 cycles) were performed with pSPL3_RT-FW and FAM-RTpSAD-RV. FAM-labeled products were run with LIZ-600 Size Standards at the Macrogen facility and analyzed with the Peak Scanner software V1.0 (Life Technologies, Carlsbad, CA, USA). Three independent experiments for each variant were carried out to calculate the average relative proportions of each transcript and the corresponding standard deviations.

2.5. Clinical Classification of PALB2 Variants

We performed a tentative clinical classification of 16 *PALB2* variants according to ACMG/AMP-based guidelines. We used a Bayesian-ACMG/AMP point system that shows higher plasticity in combining different ACMG/AMP criteria and strengths of evidence [39,40]. Point-based variant classification categories are defined as follows: pathogenic (P) $\geq$ +10; likely pathogenic (LP) +6 to +9; variant of uncertain significance (VUS) 0 to +5; likely benign (LB) −1 to −6; and benign (B) $\leq$ −7. The mgPALB2 read-outs were included in the classification system as observable PVS1_O or BP7_O evidence codes of variable strength depending on the splicing outcome (P, supporting ($\pm$1 point); M, moderate ($\pm$2); S, strong ($\pm$4); VS, very strong ($\pm$8)) [29,41]. This score is deduced from the presumed impact of all the transcripts generated by a particular variant. To interpret variants producing $\geq$2 transcripts, we applied the following rules: (i) decode/separate mgPALB2-readouts into individual components (transcripts); (ii) apply ACMG/AMP-based evidence levels to each individual transcript; and (iii) deduce a global PVS1_O (or BP7_O) code strength based on the relative contribution of individual transcripts to the overall expression. Thus, if pathogenic (or benign) supporting transcripts contribute $\geq$90% to the overall expression level, PVS1_O (or BP7_O) codes are applied. If different transcripts support different pathogenic evidence strengths, the lowest strength contributing >10% to the overall expression is selected as overall evidence strength. At present, $\geq$90% and $\geq$10% cut-offs of the overall mgPALB2 expression are merely operational. Recently, we already used a similar approach to deal with those *PALB2/ATM/RAD51C* minigene readouts that yielded several transcripts per variant [28,29,41].

We considered that functional splicing data (PVS1_O/BP7_O) override predictive splicing codes PVS1 (GT-AG splice site variants) and PP3/BP4 (non-GT-AG variants) so that the latter does not contribute to our variant classification. Otherwise, internal inconsistencies would arise in the ACMG/AMP classification system (e.g., IVS + 1 and IVS + 5 variants with identical splicing impact would score very differently). Furthermore, the ACMG/AMP system implicitly assumes that each piece of evidence contributing to the final classification is independent, which is an assumption barely met by predictive and functional splicing codes, as most splicing analyses (including our mgPALB2 ones) are performed for bioinformatically pre-selected variants. These issues have been extensively discussed elsewhere [28,29,41]. The rarity code PM2 was considered with allele frequency $\leq$ 0.001% at gnomADv2.1.1 (https://gnomad.broadinstitute.org; accessed on 21 June 2022) decreasing, so PM2 evidence strength to "supporting" as previously reported [29]. For *PALB2* variants absent on gnomADv2.1.1, the number of interrogated alleles (allele number) was determined using data of the closest available SNP ($\leq$5 nt apart from the variant of interest).

Since no specific *PALB2* recommendations exist for missense variants, we applied general recommendations recently published by ClinGen SVI [42]. Specifically, REVEL $\geq$0.8 supporting pathogenic (moderate strength), REVEL $\leq$ 0.4 supporting benign (moderate strength), and 0.4 < REVEL < 0.8 supporting neither pathogenic nor benign. To obtain REVEL scores, we ran the built-in Ensembl Variant Effect Predictor (www.ensembl.org/Tools/VEP; accessed on 1 June 2022).

3. Results and Discussion
3.1. Bioinformatics Analysis of ClinVar Variants

A total of 31 ClinVar variants comprising 66 submissions to the ClinVar database were chosen from the intron/exon boundaries of *PALB2* exons 1 to 3. All the 31 variants were bioinformatically analyzed with MaxEntScan, 16 of which met the criteria indicated in Materials and Methods, so they were selected for subsequent minigene RNA assays (Table 2). Twelve of these variants targeted splice donor sites, while the remaining four targeted acceptor sites. The 16 MES-selected variants were also analyzed by SpliceAI (Table 3). Changes c.48 + 5C > T and c.108 + 5G > A were not predicted to affect splicing.

3.2. Minigene Splicing Assays of Candidate Variants

The 16 variants were introduced into the wild-type minigene mgPALB2ex1–3 by site-directed mutagenesis and assayed in MCF-7 cells. Twelve variants impaired splicing, eleven of which showed a total impact, as the minigene full-length transcript was absent (Figure 1b, Table 4). These 11 variants affected the AG/GT (±1,2) dinucleotides of the 3′SS and 5′SS and showed the strongest impacts on MES scores (Table 2). In contrast, partial splicing anomalies were found in variants at other splice-site positions. Actually, we noticed weak or no splicing effects for those variants involving the antepenultimate nt of exon 1 (c.46A > G), +5 nt of introns 1 and 2 (c.48 + 5C > T and c.108 + 5G > A, respectively), and penultimate nt of exon 3 (c.210A > G and c.210A > C). Splicing disruptions of variants at positions other than ±1,2 are particularly difficult to predict, as we have pointed out in previous reports [28]. In this study, leaky variants (those that generate non-negligible levels of full-length transcripts) were associated with moderate reductions in the MES score (-19.3% to -29.8%, Table 2). To test the reproducibility of the minigene assay in different cell lines, four variants (c.46A > G, c.48 + 1G > T, c.49-2del, and c.210A > C) were also assayed in the triple-negative breast cancer cell line MDA-MB-231. All the variants mimicked the splicing patterns characterized in MCF-7 cells (Figure 2). Moreover, variant c.49-1G > A replicated the splicing outcomes formerly characterized in patient RNA [43], confirming the reproducibility of minigene assays (Table 3).

A total of eight different anomalous transcripts were characterized (Table 4, Figure 3). Three transcripts (Δ(E1q17), Δ(E3p11), Δ(E3)])are predicted to introduce a premature termination codon triggering the NMD surveillance mechanism (PTC-NMD) [28,44], while the remaining five isoforms, including two versions of ▼(E3q48) (a and b), maintained the reading frame. Minigene assays, together with fluorescent fragment analysis, displayed simplicity, robustness, high resolution, and sensitivity. This strategy allowed us to detect splicing alterations introducing small size changes (i.e., insertion of 9 nt or ▼(E1q9) or deletion of 6 nt, Δ(E2p6)) as well as some transcripts representing a minor contribution to the overall mgPALB2 expression (i.e., c.46A > G: Δ(E1q17), 7.5%; c.48 + 1G > C: ▼(E1q9), 9.2%; Table 4).

Table 2. Bioinformatics analysis of *PALB2* variants with Max Ent Scan.

PALB2 VARIANTS [1]	# ClinVar Records [2]	EXON/INTRON	MES wt	MES mut	MES Score Change [3]	Cryptic/De novo Splice Sites [4]
c.46A > G	1	Exon 1	5.74	4.05	−29.4%	
c.48 + 1del	1	IVS1	5.74	−12.45	316.9%	
c.48 + 1G > C	3	IVS1	5.74	−2.53	−144.1%	
c.48 + 1G > T	1	IVS1	5.74	−2.76	−148.1%	
c.48 + 2T > G	1	IVS1	5.74	−1.9	133.1%	
c.48 + 5C > T	3	IVS1	5.74	4.05	−29.4%	
c.48 + 6G > C	1	IVS1	5.74	5.96	+3.8%	
c.49-2del	1	IVS1	9.28	1.16	−87.5%	3'SS: 5,47 26 nt upstream; 3'SS: 8,65, 6 nt downstream
c.49-1del	1	IVS1	9.28	−7.59	181.8%	3'SS: 5,47 26 nt upstream; 3'SS: 8,76, 6 nt downstream
c.49-1G > A	1	IVS1	9.28	0.53	−94.3%	3'SS: 5,47 26 nt upstream; 3'SS: 7,53, 6 nt downstream
c.50T > G	2	Exon 2	9.28	9.02	−2.8%	3'SS: 5,47 26 nt upstream
c.50dup	1	Exon 2	9.28	9.25	−0.3%	3'SS: 5,47 26 nt upstream
c.106C > T	4	Exon 2	10.86	9.66	−11%	
c.108G > A	1	Exon 2	10.86	10.08	−7.2%	de novo 5'SS: 3,81 4 nt downstream
c.108 + 1_108 + 2insC	1	IVS2	10.86	−4.16	−138.3%	
c.108 + 4A > G	3	IVS2	10.86	10.28	−5.3%	
c.108 + 5C > A	1	IVS2	10.86	8.76	−19.3%	
c.108 + 6T > C	1	IVS2	10.86	9.88	−9%	
c.109-2A > C	3	IVS2	10.06	2.02	−79.9%	3'SS: 5,47, 11 nt downstream
c.109C > G	2	Exon 3	10.06	11.86	+11.8%	
c.109C > T	5	Exon 3	10.06	9.82	−2.4%	
c.109C > A	7	Exon3	10.06	10.18	+1.2%	
c.110G > T	2	Exon 3	10.06	9.69	−3.7%	
c.110G > A	9	Exon 3	10.06	9.64	−4.2%	
c.111T > C	3	Exon 3	10.06	10.3	+2.4%	
c.210A > G	2	Exon 3	8.76	6.15	29.8%	5'SS: 7,88, 48 nt downstream
c.210A > C	1	Exon 3	8.76	6.89	21.3%	5'SS: 7,88, 48 nt downstream
c.211 + 1G > T	1	IVS3	8.76	0.26	−97.0%	5'SS: 7,88, 48 nt downstream
c.211 + 2T > C	1	IVS3	8.76	1.01	88.5%	5'SS: 7,88, 48 nt downstream
c.211 + 4A > G	1	IVS3	8.76	7.25	−17.2%	5'SS: 7,88, 48 nt downstream
c.211 + 6T > A	1	IVS3	8.76	8.59	−1.9%	5'SS: 7,88, 48 nt downstream

[1] Selected variants are shown in red. [2] #, number of ClinVar Records; [3] MES score changes (Δ%): mutant (mut) vs. wild type (wt). [4] Positions of cryptic/de novo splice sites are relative to the corresponding canonical splice site.

Table 3. SpliceAI predictions, mgPALB2 read-outs, and experimental splicing data in carriers.

PALB2 Variants [1]	SpliceAI [2]				Predicted Splicing Outcome	mgPALB2 Read-out (>10%)	Experimental Data in RNA from Carriers
	AL (>20%)	DL (>20%)	AG (>20%)	DG (>20%)			
c.46A > G	-	-	-	0.27 (+11)	-	mgFL (92.5%); Δ(E1q17) (7.5%)	Normal [45]
c.48 + 1del	-	0.94 (−2)	-	0.25 (−171)	Δ(E1q169)	Δ(E1q17) (100%)	
c.48 + 1G > C	-	0.94 (−1)	-	0.45 (+8)	▼(E1q9)	Δ(E1q17) (90.8%) / ▼(E1q9) (9.2%)	
c.48 + 1G > T	-	0.94 (−1)	-	0.30 (+8)	▼(E1q9)	Δ(E1q17) (100%)	
c.48 + 2T > G	-	0.94 (−2)	-	-	-	Δ(E1q17) (100%)	
c.48 + 5C > T	-	-	-	-	-	FL (100%)	
c.49-2del	0.98 (+1)	-	0.74 (+7)	-	Δ(E2p6)	Δ(E2p6) (100%)	
c.49-1del	0.98 (+1)	-	0.79 (+6)	-	Δ(E2p6)	Δ(E2p6) (100%)	
c.49-1G > A	0.98 (+1)	-	0.65 (+7)	-	Δ(E2p6)	Δ(E2p6) (100%)	Δ(E2p6) [43]
c.108 + 1_108 + 2insC	0.96 (−61)	0.99 (−2)	-	-	Δ(E2)	Δ(E2) (100%)	
c.108 + 5G > A	-	-	-	-	-	FL (100%)	
c.109-2A > C	1 (+2)	0.33 (+104)	0.55 (+13)	-	Δ(E3p11)	Δ(E3p11) (85%) / Δ(E3) (15%)	
c.210A > G	-	-	-	0.25 (+49)	-	FL (100%)	
c.210A > C	-	-	-	0.28 (+49)	-	FL (100%)	
c.211 + 1G > T	0.42 (−103)	1 (−1)	-	0.47 (+47)	▼(E3q48)	Δ(E3) (73.3%) / ▼(E3q48a) (26.7%)	
c.211 + 2T > C	0.32 (−104)	0.99 (−2)	-	0.59 (+46)	▼(E3q48)	Δ(E3) (48.1%) / ▼(E3q48b) (51.9%)	

[1] Bold-highlighted variants for which SpliceAI predictions are, in our opinion, accurate, rightly predicting the exact experimental read-out. [2] SpliceAI parameters were as follows (genome version hg38; score type raw; max distance 10,000 nt; Illumina's pre-computed scores yes). Acceptor loss (AL), donor loss (DL), acceptor gain (AG), and donor gain (DG) scores (and positions) are shown. Color codes indicate scores in the 20–49 (high recall), 50–79 (recommended), and 80–100 (high precision) ranges, as per Illumina's specifications. Scores < 20% are not shown. SpliceAI positions are annotated as (−) if upstream of the variant or (+) if downstream. Yet, the SpliceAI annotation (relative to the forward strand) becomes confusing for genes located in the antisense strand, such as *PALB2*. For that reason, in the present table, upstream (+) and downstream (−) positions are not shown as per SpliceAI but relative to *PALB2* coding strand. A minimum of two scores above the threshold are required to predict a specific aberrant outcome (e.g., for a variant damaging a donor site, an acceptor loss scoring at the right position predicts exon skipping, while a donor gain will predict use of a cryptic/de novo site). Since SpliceAI predictions for c.46A >G, c.210A >G, and c.210A >C do not fulfill the two score approach, they were considered negative (no splicing alteration) and therefore accurate.

Table 4. Splicing outcomes of *PALB2* variants.

Variant (HGVS) [1]	Bioinformatics Summary (MES) [2]	Canonical Transcript	PTC-Transcripts [3]	In-Frame Transcripts [4]
Wild type mgPB2_ex1–3		100%		
c.46A > G	(↓) 5′SS (5.74 → 4.05)	92.5% ± 0.1%	Δ(E1q17) (7.5% ± 0.1%)	
c.48 + 1del	(−) 5′SS (5.74 → −12.45)	-	Δ(E1q17) (100%)	
c.48 + 1G > C	(−) 5′SS (5.74 → −2.53)	-	Δ(E1q17) (90.8% ± 0.6%)	▼(E1q9) (9.2% ± 0.6%)
c.48 + 1G > T	(−) 5′SS (5.74 → −2.76)	-	Δ(E1q17) (100%)	
c.48 + 2T > G	(−) 5′SS (5.74 → −1.9)	-	Δ(E1q17) (100%)	
c.48 + 5C > T	(↓) 5′SS (5.74 → 4.05)	100%		
c.49-2del	(−) 3′SS (9.28 → 1.16) (+) 3′SS (8.65) 6 nt downstream	-		Δ(E2p6) (100%)
c.49-1del	(−) 3′SS (9.28 → −7.59) (+) 3′SS (8.76) 6 nt downstream	-		Δ(E2p6) (100%)
c.49-1G > A	(−) 3′SS (9.28 → 0.53) (+) 3′SS (7.53) 6 nt downstream	-		Δ(E2p6) (100%)
c.108 + 1_108 + 2insC	(−) 5′SS (10.86 → −4.16)	-		Δ(E2) (100%)
c.108 + 5G > A	(↓) 5′SS (10.86 → 8.76)	100%		
c.109-2A > C	(−) 5′SS (10.06 → 2.02) (+) 3′SS (5.47) 11 nt downstream	-	Δ(E3p11) (85% ± 0.5%) Δ(E3) (15% ± 0.5%)	
c.210A > G	(↓) 5′SS (8.76 → 6.15)	100%		
c.210A > C	(↓) 5′SS (8.76 → 6.89)	100%		
c.211 + 1G > T	(↓) 3′SS (8.76 → 0.26)	-	Δ(E3) (73.3% ± 0.6%)	▼(E3q48a) (26.7% ± 0.6%)
c.211 + 2T > C	(−) 3′SS (8.76 → 1.01)	-	Δ(E3) (48.1% ± 7.4%)	▼(E3q48b) (51.9% ± 7.4%)

[1] Bold font: No traces or <5% of the full-length transcript. [2] (−) site disruption; (+) New site; (↓) Reduction of MES score; Cr, Cryptic. [3] PTC, Premature Termination Codon; [3,4] Δ, loss of exonic sequences; ▼, inclusion of intronic sequences; E (exon), p (acceptor shift), q (donor shift). When necessary, the exact number of nt inserted or deleted is indicated. For example, transcript ▼(E1q9) denotes the use of an alternative donor site that is located nine nucleotides downstream of exon 1, causing the addition of 9 nt to the mature mRNA.

As above mentioned, total splicing disruptions were exclusively due to changes in the canonical AG/GT dinucleotides (Table 4). There are only a few exceptions of non-spliceogenic ±1,2 variants, basically consisting of the change of the consensus AG or GT dinucleotides into atypical splice sites, such as the GC 5′ splice sites that account for about 1% of human 5′SS [46,47]. Thus, it has been assessed that about 15–18% of + 2T > C variants, which generate an atypical GC donor site, are able to produce the full-length transcript [48], as is the case of the *PALB2* c.108 + 2T > C variant [28]. However, in this study, we have shown that c.211 + 2T > C produced just aberrant transcripts similarly to variant c.48 + 2T > C [28]. SpliceAI analysis of c.211 + 2T > C (donor loss = 0.99) correctly predicted a total impact on splicing. Curiously, we found another atypical splice-site recognition in a previous study [29]. ATM variant c.1898 + 2T > G creates an intronic GG dinucleotide that might represent an extremely rare 5′SS (~0.01% of human exons) [47]. In fact, we found that this GG 5′SS was used in 13% of minigene transcripts producing the full-length isoform [29]. Therefore, the splicing outcomes of any variant should be carefully analyzed since the generation and use of active atypical sites may rescue the production of the full-length transcript, and thus, these data may modify the clinical classification of variants. Most importantly, up to now, the use of uncommon splice sites cannot be predicted, so they can only be detected by splicing assays. In this regard, minigenes provide a substantial advantage over RNA assays in carriers since variant read-out is not mistaken with wt allele expression. Then, any residual full-length transcript produced by the variant can be tracked by the highly sensitive fluorescent fragment electrophoresis. Conversely, partial splicing outcomes producing the full-length transcript are not simply identified in patient RNA assays unless a coding heterozygous SNP was also present so that the wild-type and variant alleles can be distinguished.

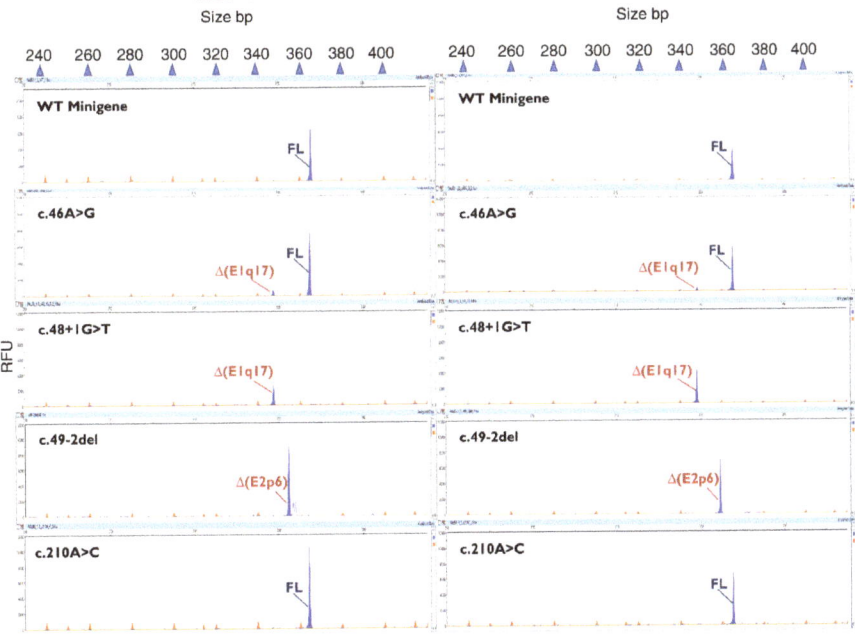

Figure 2. Reproducibility of PALB2 RNA assays in MDA-MB-231 (left) and MCF-7 (right) cells. The wild-type and mutant minigenes of c.46A > G, c.48 + 1G > T, c.49-2del, and c.210A > C were tested in MCF-7 and MDA-MB-231 cells. RT-PCR products were run by fluorescent fragment electrophoresis using LIZ-600 as size standard. The x-axis indicates size in bp (electropherograms on the top) and the y-axis represents relative fluorescence units (RFU).

Concerning the splicing output, SpliceAI produced reliable predictions for 12 out of the 16 assayed variants (Table 3). Interestingly, two false-positive variants selected on MES score (c.48 + 5C > T and c.108 + 5G > A) were ruled out by SpliceAI. MES accurately predicted splice-site disruptions or their weakening for the twelve spliceogenic variants although estimations failed in the case of four variants. By increasing the MES threshold to −30%, the specificity of the selection procedure would have considerably improved. We firmly believe that bioinformatics predictions are only useful to filter out variants and select those potentially spliceogenic, but at present, RNA assays are critical at validating a splicing effect.

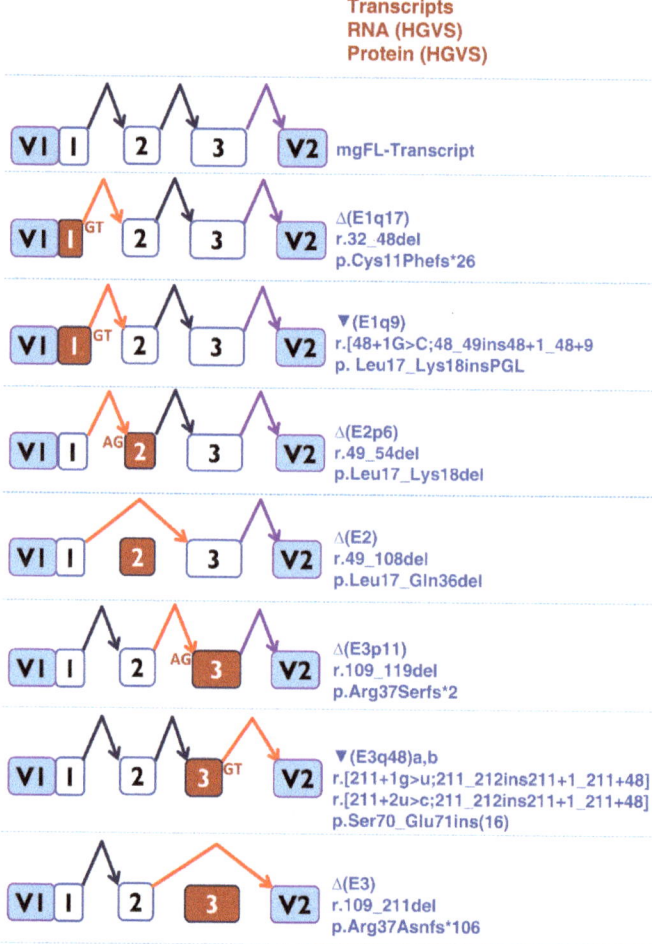

Figure 3. Transcripts produced by *PALB2* variants. Diagrams of the splicing reactions. Exons and the splicing reactions are indicated by boxes and elbow arrows, respectively. Anomalous events, exon skipping or alternative site usage (AG or GT sites) and exons are indicated in red. The impact of each transcript at the RNA and protein levels are described following the Human Genome Variation Society (HGVS) recommendations (right).

3.3. ACMG/AMP-Based Interpretation of Variants

PALB2 expert panel specifications of the ACMG/AMP guidelines are not yet available (https://clinicalgenome.org/, last accessed on 07 July 2022); so, as indicated in Materials and Methods, we classified 16 *PALB2* variants according to generic ACMG/AMP-based classification guidelines combined with some *PALB2* specifications previously developed by our group [28]. This approach integrates mgPALB2 readouts as observable PVS1_O/BP7_O evidence codes (Table 5). Thus, the three PTC-NMD transcripts (Δ(E1q17), Δ(E3p11), and Δ(E3)) are considered a very strong evidence of pathogenicity (P_VS). Likewise, the in-frame transcript Δ(E2) deletes a key PALB2 domain (CC domain), where residues Leu17, Leu21, Leu24, Tyr28, Thr31, and Leu35 mediate important interactions in the PALB2 homodimer and/or the PALB2/BRCA1 heterodimer [28,49]. Then, Δ(E2) was deemed a very strong evidence of pathogenicity (P_VS). In addition, the in-frame isoforms ▼(E1q9) and Δ(E2p6) are predicted to disrupt critical regions for PALB2, inserting three or deleting two amino acids at the CC domain, respectively. However, in both cases, a functional impact on protein function cannot be predicted. Therefore, as we had previously pointed out [28], we think that both transcripts provide a moderate evidence of pathogenicity (P_M).

On the other hand, the contribution of ▼(E3q48) a and b (insertion of 16 new amino acids: VKSRPFTYACFIIHFP and GKSRPFTYACFIIHFP, respectively) is unclear. As we previously reported, the 16-aminoacids insertion was classified as a supporting evidence of pathogenicity (P_P) based on bioinformatics predictions (PROVEAN score of −15.84, deleterious) [28]. Finally, the FL-transcript with the missense variant c.46A > G (p.Lys16Glu) was considered a supporting benign evidence BP4 (−1) since the REVEL score (0.075) suggests no impact on protein function.

All the 16 variants are absent in the gnomAD database, so they meet the PM2 rarity code (Table 5) that we have considered a supporting evidence of pathogenicity (PM2_P; +1 point) as previously mentioned [29]. As indicated above (see Section 2.5), once we incorporate minigene readouts into the classification scheme, predictive splicing codes PVS1 (GT-AG variants) or PP3/BP4 (non GT-AG variants) are no longer taken into consideration.

Finally, we considered that some pathogenic (PS2, PM1, PM6, PP2, PP4, PP5) and benign (BS2, BP1, BP3, BP5, BP6) codes are not applicable to the classification of any of the herein described *PALB2* variants. In addition, the PM3 evidence (in trans with a pathogenic variant in a recessive disorder) was not applied to any of the variants because they were not found in Fanconi Anemia patients (based on ClinVar database, Leiden Open Variation Database, https://databases.lovd.nl/shared/genes/PALB2, accessed 8 July 2022, and literature searches).

Taking these considerations altogether, six variants were classified as likely pathogenic (+9 points of the Bayesian scale), five as VUS (+2 or +3 points), and five as likely benign (−1 or −3 points) (Table 5). Remarkably, five ±1,2 variants (c.49-2del, c.49-1del, c.49-1G >A, c.211 + 1G >T, and c.211 + 2T >C) were catalogued as VUS because they produced the in-frame transcripts Δ(E2p6) (100% of the overall expression) or ▼(E3q48) (27%–52% of the overall expression), whose impact on PALB2 function is uncertain. Therefore, it is essential to elucidate if these transcripts retain the DNA repair activity to ascertain the pathogenicity of these five variants. Hence, the PVS1 splicing predictive evidence of ±1,2 variants may lead to their clinical misinterpretation [50].

Table 5. ACMG/AMP-based classification of 16 *PALB2* variants at exons 1 to 3.

Variants	ClinVar [1]	ACMG-AMP [2] Classification	Splicing Predictive PVS1/PP3 [3]	PVS1_O/BP7_O (mgPALB2 Readouts) [4]	PM2 [5]
c.46A > G (p.Lys16Glu)	B	LB (−1)	PP3	BP7_O_M (-2): 93% [BP7_O_M, FL] [6] + 7% [PVS1_O, Δ(E1q17)]	PM2_P (+1)
c.48 + 1del	LP	LP (+9)	PVS1	PVS1_O (+8): 100% [PVS1_O, Δ(E1q17)]	PM2_P (+1)
c.48 + 1G > C	Conflicting	LP (+9)	PVS1	PVS1_O (+8): 91% [PVS1_O, Δ(E1q17)]+ 9% [PVS1_O_M, ▼(E1q9)]	PM2_P (+1)
c.48 + 1G > T	P/LP	LP (+9)	PVS1	PVS1_O (+8): 100% [PVS1_O, Δ(E1q17)]	PM2_P (+1)
c.48 + 2T > G	LP	LP (+9)	PVS1	PVS1_O (+8): 100% [PVS1_O, Δ(E1q17)]	PM2_P (+1)
c.48 + 5C > T	Conflicting	LB (−3)	PP3	BP7_O_S (-4): 100% [BP7_O_S, FL] [7]	PM2_P (+1)
c.49-2del	VUS	VUS (+3)	PVS1	PVS1_O_M (+2): 100% [PVS1_O_M, Δ(E2p6)]	PM2_P (+1)
c.49-1del	P	VUS (+3)	PVS1	PVS1_O_M (+2): 100% [PVS1_O_M, Δ(E2p6)]	PM2_P (+1)
c.49-1G > A	LP	LP (+9)	PVS1	PVS1_O (+8): 100% [PVS1_O, Δ(E2)]	PM2_P (+1)
c.108 + 1_108 + 2insC	LP	LB (−3)	PP3	BP7_O_S (-4): 100% [BP7_O_S, FL] [7]	PM2_P (+1)
c.108 + 5G > A	VUS	LP (+9)	PVS1	PVS1_O (+8): 85% [PVS1_O, Δ(E3p11)] + 15% [PVS1_O, Δ(E3)]	PM2_P (+1)
c.109-2A > C	LP	LB (−3)	PP3	BP7_O_S (-4): 100% [BP7_O_S, FL] [8]	PM2_P (+1)
c.210A > G (p.Ser70=)	Conflicting	LB (−3)	PP3	BP7_O_S (-4): 100% [BP7_O_S, FL] [8]	PM2_P (+1)
c.210A > C (p.Ser70=)	LB	VUS (+2)	PVS1	PVS1_O_P (+1): 73% [PVS1_O_P, ▼(E3q48a)] + 27% [PVS1_O_P, ▼(E3q48a)]	PM2_P (+1)
c.211 + 1G > T	P/LP	VUS (+2)	PVS1	PVS1_O_P (+1): 48% [PVS1_O, Δ(E3)] + 52% [PVS1_O_P, ▼(E3q48b)]	PM2_P (+1)
c.211 + 2T > C	LP				

[1] Clinical interpretation at the ClinVar database (accessed on 9 September 2022) are defined as follows: pathogenic (P) ≥+10; likely pathogenic (LP) +6 to +9; variant of uncertain significance (VUS) 0 to +5; likely benign (LB) −1 to −6; and benign (B) ≤−7. [3] The predictive splicing codes were not taken into account in this study since they were considered redundant when splicing assay data are available. [4] Deconvolution of minigene readouts and assigned score according to the rules indicated in Materials and Methods. Note that transcripts representing <10% of the overall expression (e.g., Δ(E1q17) in c.46A > G) do not contribute to the final PVS1_O/BP7_O evidence strength assignment. If two transcripts representing >10% of the overall expression each support different evidence strengths, the most conservative strength is assigned (e.g., c.211 + 1G > T minigene readout ends up as PVS1_O_P even if the major signal supports PVS1_O). [5] Rarity code PM2 with allele frequency ≤0.01% at gnomADv2.1.1. [6] The FL transcript carries a missense variant r.46A>G (p.Lys16Glu) that qualifies for protein predictive evidence BP4 (multiple lines of computational evidence suggest no impact) with moderate strength (REVEL score = 0.075). Based on that, FL expression as observed in the assay qualifies for BP7_O_M. [7] The FL transcripts has a wt sequence that qualifies for BP7_S. [8] The FL transcripts carries a synonymous variant r.210A > G or r.210A > C that, once an impact on splicing has been excluded, qualifies for BP7_O.

4. Conclusions

We tested 16 variants at *PALB2* exons 1 to 3 by hybrid minigenes. Twelve variants impaired splicing, and eleven produced negligible levels of the mgFL-transcript. Integrating our previous results for *PALB2* [28], we analyzed a total 58 potential spliceogenic variants, 47 of which (81%) induced splicing anomalies, supporting the high sensitivity and specificity of our selection criteria as well as the efficacy of our minigene approach. By an ACMG/AMP-based strategy, a total of 29 variants were classified as pathogenic/likely pathogenic and, equally relevant, 13 variants as likely benign, whereas 16 variants were kept as VUS. Interestingly, another 56 ClinVar variants at exons 4 to 12 (accessed on 3 August 2021) would be potentially spliceogenic as per MES scores (data not shown), so in future projects, they could be assayed in our two previously reported *PALB2* minigenes: mgPALB2_ex4-6 and mgPALB2_ex5-12 [28]. Moreover, the ACMG/AMP-based guidelines provide a useful framework for the clinical interpretation of variants when splicing data are available. Finally, minigene assays allowed assessing more than 600 variants of the main breast cancer susceptibility genes up to now, demonstrating their high simplicity and robustness. Furthermore, this tool has been used to successfully assay variants at other disease genes, such as *UGT1A1* (Crigler–Najjar syndrome) [51], *CHD7* (Charge syndrome) [52], or *TRPM4* (colorectal cancer) [53], among others (http://www.ibgm.med.uva.es/servicios/servicio-de-splicing-minigenes/, accessed on 13 July 2022).

Author Contributions: Conceptualization, E.A.V.-S.; data curation, A.V.-P., formal analysis, A.V.-P., E.B.-M., L.S.-M., A.E.-S., M.d.l.H. and E.A.V.-S.; funding acquisition, M.d.l.H. and E.A.V.-S.; investigation, A.V.-P., E.B.-M., L.S.-M., A.E.-S., I.L.-B., P.P.-S., A.G.-Á., S.G.-B., M.d.l.H. and E.A.V.-S.; methodology, A.V.-P., L.S.-M., E.B.-M., I.L.-B., A.G.-Á., M.d.l.H. and E.A.V.-S.; supervision, E.A.V.-S.; writing—original draft, A.V.-P. and E.A.V.-S.; writing—review and editing, A.V.-P., S.G.-B., L.S.-M., M.d.l.H. and E.A.V.-S. All authors have read and agreed to the published version of the manuscript.

Funding: The EAV lab is supported by grants from the Spanish Ministry of Science and Innova-tion, Plan Nacional de I+D+I 2013–2016, ISCIII (PI20/00225), co-funded by FEDER (the European Regional Development Fund, European Union) and the Consejería de Educación, Junta de Castilla y León, ref. CSI242P18 (actuación cofinanciada P.O. FEDER 2014–2020 de Castilla y León) and Programa Estratégico Instituto de Biología y Genética Molecular (IBGM), Escalera de Excelencia, Junta de Castilla y León (Ref. CLU-2019-02). The MdlH lab is supported by a grant from the Spanish Ministry of Science and Innovation, Plan Nacional de I+D+I 2013–2016, ISCIII (PI20/00110), co-funded by FEDER. L.S.-M. is supported by a predoctoral fellowship from the AECC Scientific Foundation, Sede Provincial de Valladolid (2019–2023). E.B.-M. is a postdoctoral researcher funded by the University of Valladolid (POSTDOC-UVA05, 2022–2025). I.L.-B. is supported by a predoctoral fellowship from the Consejería de Educación, Junta de Castilla y León (2022–2025). A.E.-S. is supported through the Operational Program for Youth Employment and the Youth Employment Initiative (YEI), set up by the Community of Madrid in 2020 and co-financed by the European Social Fund.

Institutional Review Board Statement: Not applicable.

Informed Consent Statement: Not applicable.

Data Availability Statement: All sequencing and fragment analysis data will be available after publication at Digital. CSIC.

Conflicts of Interest: The authors declare no conflict of interest.

References

1. Nielsen, F.C.; van Overeem Hansen, T.; Sørensen, C.S. Hereditary breast and ovarian cancer: New genes in confined pathways. *Nat. Rev. Cancer* **2016**, *16*, 599–612. [CrossRef] [PubMed]
2. Gerhardus, A.; Schleberger, H.; Schlegelberger, B.; Gadzicki, D. Diagnostic accuracy of methods for the detection of BRCA1 and BRCA2 mutations: A systematic review. *Eur. J. Hum. Genet.* **2007**, *15*, 619–627.
3. Velasco, E.; Infante, M.; Durán, M.; Esteban-Cardeñosa, E.; Lastra, E.; García-Girón, C.; Miner, C.; Duran, M.; Esteban-Cardenosa, E.; Lastra, E.; et al. Rapid mutation detection in complex genes by heteroduplex analysis with capillary array electrophoresis. *Electrophoresis* **2005**, *26*, 2539–2552. [CrossRef] [PubMed]

4. Dorling, L.; Carvalho, S.; Allen, J.; González-Neira, A.; Luccarini, C.; Wahlström, C.; Pooley, K.A.; Parsons, M.T.; Fortuno, C.; Wang, Q.; et al. Breast Cancer Risk Genes — Association Analysis in More than 113,000 Women. *N. Engl. J. Med.* **2021**, *384*, 428–439.
5. Hu, C.; Hart, S.N.; Gnanaolivu, R.; Huang, H.; Lee, K.Y.; Na, J.; Gao, C.; Lilyquist, J.; Yadav, S.; Boddicker, N.J.; et al. A Population-Based Study of Genes Previously Implicated in Breast Cancer. *N. Engl. J. Med.* **2021**, *384*, 440–451. [CrossRef]
6. Narod, S.A. Which Genes for Hereditary Breast Cancer? *N. Engl. J. Med.* **2021**, *384*, 471–473.
7. Reid, S.; Schindler, D.; Hanenberg, H.; Barker, K.; Hanks, S.; Kalb, R.; Neveling, K.; Kelly, P.; Seal, S.; Freund, M.; et al. Biallelic mutations in PALB2 cause Fanconi anemia subtype FA-N and predispose to childhood cancer. *Nat. Genet.* **2007**, *39*, 162–164. [CrossRef]
8. Zhao, W.; Wiese, C.; Kwon, Y.; Hromas, R.; Sung, P. The BRCA tumor suppressor network in chromosome damage repair by homologous recombination. *Annu. Rev. Biochem.* **2019**, *88*, 221–245. [CrossRef]
9. Nepomuceno, T.C.; De Gregoriis, G.; de Oliveira, F.M.B.; Suarez-Kurtz, G.; Monteiro, A.N.; Carvalho, M.A. The role of PALB2 in the DNA damage response and cancer predisposition. *Int. J. Mol. Sci.* **2017**, *18*, 1886. [CrossRef]
10. Rahman, N.; Seal, S.; Thompson, D.; Kelly, P.; Renwick, A.; Elliott, A.; Reid, S.; Spanova, K.; Barfoot, R.; Chagtai, T.; et al. PALB2, which encodes a BRCA2-interacting protein, is a breast cancer susceptibility gene. *Nat. Genet.* **2007**, *39*, 165–167. [CrossRef]
11. Antoniou, A.C.; Foulkes, W.D.; Tischkowitz, M. Breast cancer risk in women with PALB2 mutations in different populations. *Lancet Oncol.* **2015**, *16*, e375. [CrossRef]
12. Yang, X.; Leslie, G.; Doroszuk, A.; Schneider, S.; Allen, J.; Decker, B.; Dunning, A.M.; Redman, J.; Scarth, J.; Plaskocinska, I.; et al. Cancer risks associated with germline PALB2 pathogenic variants: An international study of 524 families. *J. Clin. Oncol.* **2020**, *38*, 674–685. [CrossRef]
13. Eccles, D.M.; Mitchell, G.; Monteiro, A.N.A.; Schmutzler, R.; Couch, F.J.; Spurdle, A.B.; Gómez-García, E.B. ENIGMA Clinical Working Group BRCA1 and BRCA2 genetic testing—pitfalls and recommendations for managing variants of uncertain clinical significance. *Ann. Oncol.* **2015**, *26*, 2057–2065. [CrossRef]
14. Radice, P.; de Summa, S.; Caleca, L.; Tommasi, S. Unclassified variants in BRCA genes: Guidelines for interpretation. *Ann. Oncol.* **2011**, *22*, i18–i23. [CrossRef]
15. De Vooght, K.M.K.; Van Wijk, R.; Van Solinge, W.W. Management of gene promoter mutations in molecular diagnostics. *Clin. Chem.* **2009**, *55*, 698–708. [CrossRef]
16. Fraile-Bethencourt, E.; Valenzuela-Palomo, A.; Díez-Gómez, B.; Infante, M.; Durán, M.; Marcos, G.; Lastra, E.; Gómez-Barrero, S.; Velasco, E.A. Genetic dissection of the BRCA2 promoter and transcriptional impact of DNA variants. *Breast Cancer Res. Treat.* **2018**, *171*, 53–63. [CrossRef]
17. Buratti, E.; Baralle, M.; Baralle, F.E. Defective splicing, disease and therapy: Searching for master checkpoints in exon definition. *Nucleic Acids Res.* **2006**, *34*, 3494–3510. [CrossRef]
18. Manning, K.S.; Cooper, T.A. The roles of RNA processing in translating genotype to phenotype. *Nat. Rev. Mol. Cell Biol.* **2017**, *18*, 102–114. [CrossRef]
19. Wang, G.-S.S.; Cooper, T.A. Splicing in disease: Disruption of the splicing code and the decoding machinery. *Nat. Rev. Genet.* **2007**, *8*, 749–761. [CrossRef]
20. Baralle, D.; Lucassen, A.; Buratti, E. Missed threads. The impact of pre-mRNA splicing defects on clinical practice. *EMBO Rep.* **2009**, *10*, 810–816. [CrossRef]
21. Scotti, M.M.; Swanson, M.S. RNA mis-splicing in disease. *Nat. Rev. Genet.* **2016**, *17*, 19–32. [CrossRef]
22. Lopez-Bigas, N.; Audit, B.; Ouzounis, C.; Parra, G.; Guigo, R.; López-Bigas, N.; Audit, B.; Ouzounis, C.; Parra, G.; Guigó, R. Are splicing mutations the most frequent cause of hereditary disease? *FEBS Lett.* **2005**, *579*, 1900–1903. [CrossRef]
23. Rhine, C.L.; Cygan, K.J.; Soemedi, R.; Maguire, S.; Murray, M.F.; Monaghan, S.F.; Fairbrother, W.G. Hereditary cancer genes are highly susceptible to splicing mutations. *PLoS Genet.* **2018**, *14*, e1007231. [CrossRef]
24. Sanz, D.J.; Acedo, A.; Infante, M.; Durán, M.; Pérez-Cabornero, L.; Esteban-Cardeñosa, E.; Lastra, E.; Pagani, F.; Miner, C.; Velasco, E.A. A high proportion of DNA variants of BRCA1 and BRCA2 is associated with aberrant splicing in breast/ovarian cancer patients. *Clin. Cancer Res.* **2010**, *16*, 1957–1967. [CrossRef]
25. Fraile-Bethencourt, E.; Díez-Gómez, B.; Velásquez-Zapata, V.; Acedo, A.; Sanz, D.J.; Velasco, E.A. Functional classification of DNA variants by hybrid minigenes: Identification of 30 spliceogenic variants of BRCA2 exons 17 and 18. *PLoS Genet.* **2017**, *13*, e1006691. [CrossRef]
26. Sanoguera-Miralles, L.; Valenzuela-Palomo, A.; Bueno-Martínez, E.; Llovet, P.; Díez-Gómez, B.; Caloca, M.J.; Pérez-Segura, P.; Fraile-Bethencourt, E.; Colmena, M.; Carvalho, S.; et al. Comprehensive Functional Characterization and Clinical Interpretation of 20 Splice-Site Variants of the RAD51C Gene. *Cancers* **2020**, *12*, 3771. [CrossRef]
27. Bueno-Martínez, E.; Sanoguera-Miralles, L.; Valenzuela-Palomo, A.; Lorca, V.; Gómez-Sanz, A.; Carvalho, S.; Allen, J.; Infante, M.; Pérez-Segura, P.; Lázaro, C.; et al. Rad51d aberrant splicing in breast cancer: Identification of splicing regulatory elements and minigene-based evaluation of 53 dna variants. *Cancers* **2021**, *13*, 2845. [CrossRef]
28. Valenzuela-Palomo, A.; Bueno-Martínez, E.; Sanoguera-Miralles, L.; Lorca, V.; Fraile-Bethencourt, E.; Esteban-Sánchez, A.; Gómez-Barrero, S.; Carvalho, S.; Allen, J.; García-Álvarez, A.; et al. Splicing predictions, minigene analyses, and ACMG-AMP clinical classification of 42 germline PALB2 splice-site variants. *J. Pathol.* **2022**, *256*, 321–334. [CrossRef]

29. Bueno-Martínez, E.; Sanoguera-Miralles, L.; Valenzuela-Palomo, A.; Esteban-Sánchez, A.; Lorca, V.; Llinares-Burguet, I.; Allen, J.; García-Álvarez, A.; Pérez-Segura, P.; Durán, M.; et al. Minigene-based splicing analysis and ACMG/AMP-based tentative classification of 56 ATM variants. *J. Pathol.* **2022**, *258*, 83–101. [CrossRef]
30. Lopez-Perolio, I.; Leman, R.; Behar, R.; Lattimore, V.; Pearson, J.F.; Castéra, L.; Martins, A.; Vaur, D.; Goardon, N.; Davy, G.; et al. Alternative splicing and ACMG-AMP-2015-based classification of PALB2 genetic variants: An ENIGMA report. *J. Med. Genet.* **2019**, *56*, 453–460. [CrossRef]
31. Fraile-Bethencourt, E.; Valenzuela-Palomo, A.; Díez-Gómez, B.; Caloca, M.J.; Gómez-Barrero, S.; Velasco, E.A. Minigene Splicing Assays Identify 12 Spliceogenic Variants of BRCA2 Exons 14 and 15. *Front. Genet.* **2019**, *10*, 503. [CrossRef] [PubMed]
32. Yeo, G.; Burge, C.B. Maximum entropy modeling of short sequence motifs with applications to RNA splicing signals. *J. Comput. Biol.* **2004**, *11*, 377–394. [CrossRef] [PubMed]
33. Houdayer, C.; Caux-Moncoutier, V.; Krieger, S.; Barrois, M.; Bonnet, F.; Bourdon, V.; Bronner, M.; Buisson, M.; Coulet, F.; Gaildrat, P.; et al. Guidelines for splicing analysis in molecular diagnosis derived from a set of 327 combined in silico/in vitro studies on BRCA1 and BRCA2 variants. *Hum. Mutat.* **2012**, *33*, 1228–1238. [CrossRef] [PubMed]
34. Moles-Fernández, A.; Duran-Lozano, L.; Montalban, G.; Bonache, S.; López-Perolio, I.; Menéndez, M.; Santamariña, M.; Behar, R.; Blanco, A.; Carrasco, E.; et al. Computational Tools for Splicing Defect Prediction in Breast/Ovarian Cancer Genes: How Efficient Are They at Predicting RNA Alterations? *Front. Genet.* **2018**, *9*, 366. [CrossRef]
35. Jaganathan, K.; Kyriazopoulou Panagiotopoulou, S.; McRae, J.F.; Darbandi, S.F.; Knowles, D.; Li, Y.I.; Kosmicki, J.A.; Arbelaez, J.; Cui, W.; Schwartz, G.B.; et al. Predicting Splicing from Primary Sequence with Deep Learning. *Cell* **2019**, *176*, 535–548.e24. [CrossRef]
36. De Garibay, G.R.; Acedo, A.; García-Casado, Z.; Gutiérrez-Enríquez, S.; Tosar, A.; Romero, A.; Garre, P.; Llort, G.; Thomassen, M.; Díez, O.; et al. Capillary Electrophoresis Analysis of Conventional Splicing Assays: IARC Analytical and Clinical Classification of 31 BRCA2 Genetic Variants. *Hum. Mutat.* **2014**, *35*, 53–57. [CrossRef]
37. Acedo, A.; Hernández-Moro, C.; Curiel-García, Á.; Díez-Gómez, B.; Velasco, E.A. Functional classification of BRCA2 DNA variants by splicing assays in a large minigene with 9 exons. *Hum. Mutat.* **2015**, *36*, 210–221. [CrossRef]
38. Fraile-Bethencourt, E.; Valenzuela-Palomo, A.; Díez-Gómez, B.; Goina, E.; Acedo, A.; Buratti, E.; Velasco, E.A. Mis-splicing in breast cancer: Identification of pathogenic BRCA2 variants by systematic minigene assays. *J. Pathol.* **2019**, *248*, 409–420. [CrossRef]
39. Tavtigian, S.V.; Greenblatt, M.S.; Harrison, S.M.; Nussbaum, R.L.; Prabhu, S.A.; Boucher, K.M.; Biesecker, L.G. ClinGen Sequence Variant Interpretation Working Group (ClinGen SVI) Modeling the ACMG/AMP variant classification guidelines as a Bayesian classification framework. *Genet. Med.* **2018**, *20*, 1054–1060. [CrossRef]
40. Tavtigian, S.V.; Harrison, S.M.; Boucher, K.M.; Biesecker, L.G. Fitting a naturally scaled point system to the ACMG/AMP variant classification guidelines. *Hum. Mutat.* **2020**, *41*, 1734–1737. [CrossRef]
41. Sanoguera-Miralles, L.; Bueno-Martínez, E.; Valenzuela-Palomo, A.; Esteban-Sánchez, A.; Llinares-Burguet, I.; Pérez-Segura, P.; García-Álvarez, A.; de la Hoya, M.; Velasco-Sampedro, E.A. Minigene Splicing Assays Identify 20 Spliceogenic Variants of the Breast/Ovarian Cancer Susceptibility Gene RAD51C. *Cancers* **2022**, *14*, 2960. [CrossRef]
42. Wilcox, E.H.; Sarmady, M.; Wulf, B.; Wright, M.W.; Rehm, H.L.; Biesecker, L.G.; Abou Tayoun, A.N. Evaluating the impact of in silico predictors on clinical variant classification. *Genet. Med.* **2022**, *24*, 924–930. [CrossRef]
43. Tsaousis, G.N.; Papadopoulou, E.; Apessos, A.; Agiannitopoulos, K.; Pepe, G.; Kampouri, S.; Diamantopoulos, N.; Floros, T.; Iosifidou, R.; Katopodi, O.; et al. Analysis of hereditary cancer syndromes by using a panel of genes: Novel and multiple pathogenic mutations. *BMC Cancer* **2019**, *19*, 535. [CrossRef]
44. Lykke-Andersen, S.; Jensen, T.H. Nonsense-mediated mRNA decay: An intricate machinery that shapes transcriptomes. *Nat. Rev. Mol. Cell Biol.* **2015**, *16*, 665–677. [CrossRef]
45. Casadei, S.; Gulsuner, S.; Shirts, B.H.; Mandell, J.B.; Kortbawi, H.M.; Norquist, B.S.; Swisher, E.M.; Lee, M.K.; Goldberg, Y.; O'Connor, R.; et al. Characterization of splice-altering mutations in inherited predisposition to cancer. *Proc. Natl. Acad. Sci. USA* **2019**, *116*, 26798–26807. [CrossRef]
46. Thanaraj, T.A.; Clark, F. Human GC-AG alternative intron isoforms with weak donor sites show enhanced consensus at acceptor exon positions. *Nucleic Acids Res.* **2001**, *29*, 2581–2593. [CrossRef]
47. Parada, G.E.; Munita, R.; Cerda, C.A.; Gysling, K. A comprehensive survey of non-canonical splice sites in the human transcriptome. *Nucleic Acids Res.* **2014**, *42*, 10564–10578. [CrossRef]
48. Lin, J.H.; Tang, X.Y.; Boulling, A.; Zou, W.B.; Masson, E.; Fichou, Y.; Raud, L.; Le Tertre, M.; Deng, S.J.; Berlivet, I.; et al. First estimate of the scale of canonical 5′ splice site GT>GC variants capable of generating wild-type transcripts. *Hum. Mutat.* **2019**, *40*, 1856–1873. [CrossRef]
49. Song, F.; Li, M.; Liu, G.; Swapna, G.V.T.; Daigham, N.S.; Xia, B.; Montelione, G.T.; Bunting, S.F. Antiparallel Coiled-Coil Interactions Mediate the Homodimerization of the DNA Damage-Repair Protein PALB2. *Biochemistry* **2018**, *57*, 6581–6591. [CrossRef]
50. Richards, S.; Aziz, N.; Bale, S.; Bick, D.; Das, S.; Gastier-Foster, J.; Grody, W.W.; Hegde, M.; Lyon, E.; Spector, E.; et al. Standards and guidelines for the interpretation of sequence variants: A joint consensus recommendation of the American College of Medical Genetics and Genomics and the Association for Molecular Pathology. *Genet. Med.* **2015**, *17*, 405–424. [CrossRef]
51. Gailite, L.; Valenzuela-Palomo, A.; Sanoguera-Miralles, L.; Rots, D.; Kreile, M.; Velasco, E.A. UGT1A1 Variants c.864+5G>T and c.996+2_996+5del of a Crigler-Najjar Patient Induce Aberrant Splicing in Minigene Assays. *Front. Genet.* **2020**, *11*, 169. [CrossRef]

52. Villate, O.; Ibarluzea, N.; Fraile-Bethencourt, E.; Valenzuela, A.; Velasco, E.A.; Grozeva, D.; Raymond, F.L.; Botella, M.P.; Tejada, M.-I. Functional Analyses of a Novel Splice Variant in the CHD7 Gene, Found by Next Generation Sequencing, Confirm Its Pathogenicity in a Spanish Patient and Diagnose Him with CHARGE Syndrome. *Front. Genet.* **2018**, *9*, 26–31. [CrossRef]
53. Zhu, L.; Miao, B.; Dymerska, D.; Kuswik, M.; Bueno-Martínez, E.; Sanoguera-Miralles, L.; Velasco, E.A.; Paramasivam, N.; Schlesner, M.; Kumar, A.; et al. Germline Variants of CYBA and TRPM4 Predispose to Familial Colorectal Cancer. *Cancers* **2022**, *14*, 670. [CrossRef]

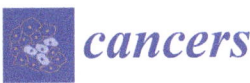

Article

Mitochondrial Protein Cox7b Is a Metabolic Sensor Driving Brain-Specific Metastasis of Human Breast Cancer Cells

Marine C. N. M. Blackman [1], Tania Capeloa [1], Justin D. Rondeau [1], Luca X. Zampieri [1], Zohra Benyahia [1], Justine A. Van de Velde [1], Maude Fransolet [2], Evangelos P. Daskalopoulos [3], Carine Michiels [2], Christophe Beauloye [3] and Pierre Sonveaux [1,4,*]

1. Pole of Pharmacology and Therapeutics, Institut de Recherche Expérimentale et Clinique (IREC), Walloon Excellence in Life Sciences and Biotechnology (WELBIO), Université Catholique de Louvain (UCLouvain), Avenue Hippocrate 57 Box B1.53.09, 1200 Brussels, Belgium
2. URBC-NARILIS, University of Namur, 5000 Namur, Belgium
3. Pole of Cardiology, Institut de Recherche Expérimentale et Clinique (IREC), Université Catholique de Louvain (UCLouvain), Avenue Hippocrate 55 Box B1.55.05, 1200 Brussels, Belgium
4. Walloon Excellence in Life Sciences and Biotechnology (WELBIO) Research Institute, 1300 Wavre, Belgium
* Correspondence: pierre.sonveaux@uclouvain.be

Simple Summary: What controls organotropism during cancer metastasis is still largely unknown. The "seed-and-soil hypothesis" of Stephen Paget (1889) proposes that metastatic onset strictly depends on a match between the needs of a given metastatic progenitor cell (the seed) and the resources provided by a given organ (the soil). Here, we decided to challenge this old theory in the context of cancer metabolism. Considering that metastasis can be prevented, we focused on triple-negative breast cancer brain metastasis. Comparing RNAseq data from wild-type human cancer cells and two independent brain-seeking variants, we identified cyclooxygenase 7b (Cox7b) in Complex IV of the mitochondrial electron transport chain as a driver of triple-negative breast cancer brain metastasis. Cox7b is not an easy therapeutic target and is most probably not unique in driving brain metastasis. Therefore, our general approach could be used to identify other metabolic proteins responsible for organotropism and amenable for metastasis-prevention therapy.

Abstract: Distant metastases are detrimental for cancer patients, but the increasingly early detection of tumors offers a chance for metastasis prevention. Importantly, cancers do not metastasize randomly: depending on the type of cancer, metastatic progenitor cells have a predilection for well-defined organs. This has been theorized by Stephen Paget, who proposed the "seed-and-soil hypothesis", according to which metastatic colonization occurs only when the needs of a given metastatic progenitor cell (the seed) match with the resources provided by a given organ (the soil). Here, we propose to explore the seed-and-soil hypothesis in the context of cancer metabolism, thus hypothesizing that metastatic progenitor cells must be capable of detecting the availability of metabolic resources in order to home in a secondary organ. If true, it would imply the existence of metabolic sensors. Using human triple-negative MDA-MB-231 breast cancer cells and two independent brain-seeking variants as models, we report that cyclooxygenase 7b (Cox7b), a structural component of Complex IV of the mitochondrial electron transport chain, belongs to a probably larger family of proteins responsible for breast cancer brain tropism in mice. For metastasis prevention therapy, this proof-of-principle study opens a quest for the identification of therapeutically targetable metabolic sensors that drive cancer organotropism.

Keywords: breast cancer; brain metastasis; tissue-specific metastasis; organotropism; cancer metabolism; oxidative phosphorylation (OXPHOS); mitochondria; cyclooxygenase 7b (Cox7b)

Citation: Blackman, M.C.N.M.; Capeloa, T.; Rondeau, J.D.; Zampieri, L.X.; Benyahia, Z.; Van de Velde, J.A.; Fransolet, M.; Daskalopoulos, E.P.; Michiels, C.; Beauloye, C.; et al. Mitochondrial Protein Cox7b Is a Metabolic Sensor Driving Brain-Specific Metastasis of Human Breast Cancer Cells. *Cancers* **2022**, *14*, 4371. https://doi.org/10.3390/cancers14184371

Received: 8 August 2022
Accepted: 5 September 2022
Published: 8 September 2022

Publisher's Note: MDPI stays neutral with regard to jurisdictional claims in published maps and institutional affiliations.

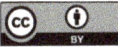

Copyright: © 2022 by the authors. Licensee MDPI, Basel, Switzerland. This article is an open access article distributed under the terms and conditions of the Creative Commons Attribution (CC BY) license (https://creativecommons.org/licenses/by/4.0/).

1. Introduction

Entry in the metastatic phase often represents a point of no return for cancer patients, as it is associated with a transition from curative to palliative care. This is mainly due to a limitation of therapeutic options, as local treatments are not always an option for (poly)metastatic patients, and secondary tumors are generally more resistant to treatments than primary tumors [1]. Treating brain metastasis offers the additional challenge of blood–brain barrier (BBB) protection in an initially immunopreserved environment [2]. Consequently, poorly symptomatic cancers that are often detected at an advanced, post-metastatic stage are associated with poor 5-year overall survival rates, while slowly evolutive cancers that are commonly detected at the premetastatic stage are, in contrast, associated with much longer patient survival rates. Between these two extremes, improvements of detection methodologies and their systematic use in individuals at risk allow an early detection of some aggressive types of cancers. This is typically the case of triple-negative breast cancer (TNBC), which is most often detected at the premetastatic stage [3]. However, these cancers usually evolve quite rapidly despite early treatment delivery, and distant metastases have a high prediction to occur. About 35% of TNBC patients develop metastases in the course of the disease, despite surgery, chemotherapy, and radiotherapy [4]. Furthermore, immunotherapy with checkpoint inhibitors has only shown modest efficacy in a subset of patients [5]. Overall, polymetastatic TNBC is currently still regarded as a largely incurable disease [6].

While the vast majority of solid tumors primarily colonize regional lymph nodes, distant metastases do not occur randomly: different cancer types present different metastatic patterns, with different frequencies. For example, malignant melanomas preferentially metastasize to the lungs (frequency of 85%, including micrometastases), the liver (54–77%), the gastrointestinal tract (~60%), the brain (36–54%), the bones (23–49%), and distant skin and subcutis (~18%) [7–9]. In the case of TNBC, metastases occur in the central nervous system (~46% of patients), lungs (~41%), liver (~29%), bones (~24%), and breast or chest wall (~22%) [10]. Brain metastasis is particularly detrimental, with a median patient survival time of 4 to 7 months [10,11]. These numbers further highlight that several organs can be colonized at the same time. Thus, in both cases, a large proportion of patients that were metastasis-free at diagnosis become polymetastatic over the course of the diseases.

Among circulating tumor cells (CTCs), only a minority, termed "metastatic progenitor cells" [12,13], possess all the characteristics that are mandatory to successfully establish a metastasis. The preference of these cells for a limited panel of secondary organs has been theorized by Stephen Paget [14] in 1889 and revisited several times since then (see reference [15] for a recent review). In the "seed and soil" hypothesis, Paget proposed that metastases do not occur randomly in secondary organs but, rather, colonize a given organ based on a match between the needs of a (sub)population of metastatic progenitor cells ("the seed") and the resources provided by the secondary organ ("the soil"). His proposition highlighted the importance of the tumor microenvironment at both primary and secondary tumor locations. Further interpretation also suggests the possible coexistence of several different populations of metastatic progenitor cells with different tropisms for secondary organs in the same patient.

So, what does the seed-and-soil hypothesis implicate? On the one hand, the capabilities of metastatic progenitor cells would depend on the genetic and epigenetic characteristics inherited from their tissue of origin as well as from genetic and epigenetic changes acquired over time, from the onset of malignancy until dissemination. Indeed, metastatic progenitor cells are, nowadays, consensually believed to originate from metabolically hostile cancer areas characterized by a combination of hypoxia, nutrient deprivation, and metabolic waste accumulation causing, e.g., microenvironmental acidification [16–23]. Each parameter, per se, contributes to the metastatic switch, defined as a discrete event converting non-metastatic cancer cells to their metastatic version [24]. However, it is the coexistence of these parameters and their fluctuation over time and space that constitutes an ideal situation for cancer cell adaptation and evolution, which both necessitate environmental changes to operate [25]. The outcome of these processes is the generation of subsets of cancer cells that simultaneously possess mesenchymal characteristics, resist anoïkis, migrate and invade directionally, resist redox and shear stresses in the systemic circulation, and possess stem cell characteristics [26]. On the other hand, resources available at the secondary site would depend not only on the basal composition and mode of function of the organ to be colonized but also on the organ's "education" by the primary tumor, a paradigm formulated as "premetastatic niche" formation [27]. In the process, cancer cells at the initial site produce and secrete soluble factors (including, e.g., VEGF-A, PLGF, G-CSF, CCL2, TGFβ, TNF, and enzymes such as lysyl oxidase that remodel the extracellular matrix) and exosomes that modify the composition and integrity of the secondary site (see reference [28] for a detailed review). As a result, vascular leakiness is increased; resident cells, such as fibroblasts, modify their behavior; non-resident cells, such as bone-marrow-derived cells and neutrophils, are recruited; a proinflammatory milieu offering immunoprotection is formed; and the structure of the extracellular matrix is remodeled to yield a provisional matrix promoting cell migration, invasion, and, hence, colonization [28].

The homing of metastatic progenitor cells at the secondary site is facilitated by the enhanced permeability of blood vessels lining premetastatic niches. In an active process, CTCs expressing E-selectin ligands (that may include CD44, PSGL-1, ESL-1, β2-integrins, and L-selectin [29]) roll on and adhere on endothelial cells expressing E-selectin at their luminal surface, extravasate (which may require proteolytic activities by CTCs, especially to cross the BBB during brain metastasis [30]), and invade the niche. There, they anchor to host cells and undergo a process of differentiation to generate a secondary tumor. Intravascular metastasis is a rare event.

In the general context of metastasis, we previously observed that mitochondria act as metabolic sensors of the primary tumor microenvironment, producing superoxide and activating the prometastatic transforming growth factor β (TGFβ) pathway in metabolically hostile tumor microenvironments [31]. Inactivating mitochondrial superoxide with specific drugs MitoTEMPO or MitoQ blocked the metastatic process as a whole [13,31,32]. Others showed that transferring superoxide-producing mitochondria from metastatic to nonmetastatic cancer cells was sufficient to turn recipient cells into metastatic progenitor cells [33]. In the context of the seed-and-soil hypothesis, we, therefore, hypothesized that a successful metastatic process would require a match between the metabolic needs of a given subset of metastatic progenitor cells and the availability of specific metabolites at a given secondary site. In other words, we propose that the metabolic preferences of a metastatic progenitor cell would participate in, and perhaps drive, organotropism. Thus, metabolic pairing between different "seeds" and different "soils" would be responsible for the existence of a restricted panel of secondary sites for a given tumor type.

This study on brain tropism is the first of a series addressing this general hypothesis. Using the human TNBC MDA-MB-231 cell line as a working model, we report a cause–effect relationship between the expression of cyclooxygenase 7b (Cox7b) in Complex IV of the electron transport chain (ETC) of metastatic progenitor cells and the brain tropism of these cells. In brain-seeking variants, Cox7b expression enhances oxidative phosphorylation (OXPHOS), while, compared to other organs, the brain is well-known to be enriched in OXPHOS substrates glucose, lipids, and lactate. Cox7b most probably belongs to a larger family of proteins driving brain metastasis, and other organs would offer other substrates to other subsets of metastatic progenitor cells, which could lead to the potential identification of several targets for the therapeutic prevention of tissue-specific metastasis.

2. Materials and Methods

2.1. Chemicals and Reagents

Unless stated otherwise, all chemicals and reagents were from Sigma-Aldrich (Overijse, Belgium).

2.2. Cells and Cell Culture

Parental MDA-MB-231 human triple-negative breast adenocarcinoma cancer cells were from Caliper (Mechelen, Belgium; catalogue #119369). MDA-MB-231-derived brain-seeking variants 231-BR [34] and 231-BR-2 [35,36] were kind gifts from Patricia Steeg (National Cancer Institute, Bethesda, MD, USA) and Harikrishna Nakshatri (Indiana University School of Medicine, Indianapolis, IN, USA), respectively. Cells were routinely cultured in DMEM containing glutaMAX and 4.5 g/L glucose (Thermo Fisher, Erembodegem, Belgium; catalogue #61965026) supplemented with 10% FBS and maintained at 37 °C in a 5% CO_2 humidified atmosphere. Cells were authenticated using short tandem repeat (STR) profiling (Eurofins Genomics, Ebersberg, Germany).

Human astrocytes (T0281, expressing hTERT), mouse astrocytes (T0289, expressing the SV40 large T antigen), human hepatocytes (T0063, expressing HPV E6/E7, hTERT and MycT58A), and human bronchial epithelial cells (T0753, expressing hTERT and Cdk4) used in migration assays were immortalized cells from Applied Biological Materials Inc. (ABM, Richmond, BC, Canada). Astrocytes were routinely cultured in DMEM with glutaMAX and 4.5 g/L glucose (Thermo Fisher; catalogue #61965026) supplemented with 10% FBS and 5% astrocyte growth supplement (Sanbio, Uden, The Netherlands; catalogue #1852; for human astrocytes only). Hepatocytes were maintained in PriGrow IX medium (ABM; catalogue #TM019) supplemented with 10% FBS and then were progressively transferred to the same medium as cancer cells. Bronchial cells were maintained in Prigrow X medium (ABM; catalogue #TM0753), and then were progressively transferred to bronchial epithelial cell growth medium (BEGM; Lonza, Verviers, Belgium; catalogue #CC-3170).

2.3. Genetic Manipulations

For constitutive luciferase and GFP expression, cells were infected with lentiviruses carrying the luciferase and GFP sequences along with puromycin resistance gene (Amsbio, Alkmaar, The Netherlands; catalogue #LPV020), as detailed in Appendix A.1.

COX7B gene silencing was performed using a CRISPR-Cas9 strategy following Zhang's lab protocol [37], and Cox7b overexpression using the pCMV3 expression vector (Bio-Connect, Te Huissen, The Netherlands; catalogue #HG20762-UT), as detailed in Appendix A.2. and Appendix A.3. pSpCas9(BB)-2A-Puro (PX459) V2.0 and pU6-(BbsI) CBh-Cas9-T2A-mCherry were kind gifts from Feng Zhang (Addgene, Watertown, MA, USA; plasmid #62988) and Ralf Kuehn (Addgene; plasmid #64324), respectively.

2.4. Metastatic Take in Mice

On day 0, 6-week-old female NMRI nude mice (Janvier, Le Genest-Saint-Isle, France) received image-guided intraventricular injections of 100,000 cancer cells, using a Vevo 2100 imaging system (FUJIFILM VisualSonics, Toronto, ON, Canada) equipped with a 30 MHz transducer. Briefly, mice were anesthetized (80 mg/Kg ketamine and 8 mg/Kg xylazine) and secured on the animal platform in supine position, and their thoraxes were shaved. Two-dimensional (2D) parasternal long-axis ultrasound images of the left ventricle were acquired, in order to ascertain the optimal point in the apex of the heart for the intraventricular injection. A microinjector system with a 26G hypodermic needle was used to perform a precise echocardiography-guided intraventricular injection of 100,000 cancer cells constitutively expressing luciferase and GFP. Following injection, the blood flow within the left ventricle was closely observed (and images were recorded), confirming that the cancer cells were successfully injected intraventricularly. All mice were followed-up for a few minutes with echography, to ascertain that the injection did not lead to any injury, and were closely monitored until recovery.

Metastasis development was monitored using a Xenogen IVIS 50 bioluminescence imaging system (PerkinElmer, Seer Green, UK) and quantified with Living Image software (PerkinElmer). Every week, mice were injected i.p with 0.15 mg/g bodyweight of luciferin (PerkinElmer) and were anesthetized using isoflurane after a 10-min incubation. Chemiluminescence was detected with a 1–12 s acquisition time. Mice were sacrificed after

4 weeks by cervical dislocation under terminal anesthesia, and organ chemiluminescence was acquired ex vivo before fixation in 4% paraformaldehyde (PFA).

2.5. Cell Migration and Invasion

Corning transwell inserts (Avantor, Leuven, Belgium; catalogue #62406-198) were used to measure cell migration and invasion capacities, as detailed in Appendix A.4. FBS 1% (general migration/invasion) or confluent nonmalignant cells (astrocytes, hepatocytes, bronchial cells) seeded in the lower chamber were used as chemoattractants.

2.6. Cell Numbers

Cell numbers were determined over time on a SpectraMax i3 spectrophotometer equipped with a MiniMax imaging cytometer (Molecular Devices, Munich, Germany), after seeding 5000 cells per well in a 96-well plate. Results were normalized to initial cell numbers.

2.7. Metabolic Assays

Oxygen consumption rates (OCRs) were measured on a Seahorse XF96 bioenergetics analyzer using the XF Cell Mito Stress Test Kit and the Fuel Flex test kit, in accordance with the instructions of the manufacturer (Agilent, Machelen, Belgium). Details are provided in Appendix A.5. Glucose and lactate concentrations were measured using an enzymatic CMA600 analyzer (Aurora Borealis, Schoonebeek, The Netherlands), in accordance with the instructions of the manufacturer, in the supernatant of 150,000 (for 24 h assays) and 250,000 (for 48 h assays) cells seeded in exactly 1 mL of culture medium. Wells containing medium only were used as controls for the calculation of glucose consumption and lactate production. The ATP content of 10,000 cells per well (96-well plate) was measured using the Cell titer Glo assay of Promega (Leiden, The Netherlands; catalogue #G7570). All metabolic measurements were normalized to total protein content determined after overnight incubation with 0.5 M NaOH using the Bio-Rad protein assay (Temse, Belgium; catalogue #5000006) on a SpectraMax i3 spectrophotometer equipped with a MiniMax imaging cytometer.

2.8. Electron Microscopy

Cells were collected and resuspended in 400 µL of a 2.5% glutaraldehyde solution containing 0.1 M of sodium cacodylate at pH 7.4 in a pyramidal BEEM capsule (Agar Scientific, Stansted, UK; catalogue #G360). Samples were then processed as previously described [38]. Images were acquired on a TECNAI G^2 20 LaB6 transmission microscope (Field Electron and Ion Company, Hillsboro, OR, USA).

2.9. Mitochondrial Abundance and Mitochondrial DNA Content

Mitochondrial DNA (mtDNA) content was measured using RT-qPCR as previously described [39]. Briefly, total DNA was isolated with a QIAmp DNA kit (Qiagen, Antwerp, Belgium). The 12S-rRNAA mitochondrial gene (forward primer: 5′-GTA CCC ACG TAA AGA CGT TAG G-3′; reverse primer: 3′-TAC TGC TAA ATC CAC CTT CG-5′; labeled probe: 5′-CCC ATG AGG TGG CAA GAA AT-3′ FAM), in parallel with nuclear gene RNAseP (RNAseP VIC-labeled probe; Thermo Fisher Scientific; catalogue #4401631), were then analyzed by RT-qPCR (50 ng of sample and 1 µL of each primer pair [10µM]), with TaqMan universal master mix II with UNG (Thermo Fisher). For presentation, mtDNA content was normalized to nuclear DNA (nDNA) content [40].

2.10. Microarray Database Analysis

According to Gene Expression Omnibus (GEO) and reference [36], database #GSE66495 reports on the whole genome expression, determined using Illumina Human HT-12 V4 expression beadchips, of MDA-MB-231 parental cells and tissue-specific metastatic variants derived thereof (including 231-BR), which were maintained in MEM with 10% FBS. For database reanalysis, we first extracted metabolic genes related to glycolysis, OXPHOS, and the TCA cycle. We next retained only genes that were differentially expressed ($p < 0.05$, using one-way ANOVA) in brain (231-BR), adrenal (ADMD-231), bone (BMD-231) and/or lung (LMD-231) metastatic variants, compared to parental MDA-MB-231 cells. They are displayed in Table 1. We then identified the genes that were differently expressed ($p < 0.05$, using one-way ANOVA) in 231-BR versus ADMD-231, BMD-231, and LMD-231 cells. Expression changes were independently confirmed by RT-qPCR using fresh lysates from brain-seeking variants 231-BR and 231-BR-2 and MDA-MB-231 parental cells.

Table 1. Metabolic genes differentially expressed in 231-BR versus other tissue-specific variants of parental MDA-MB-231 human breast cancer cells.

Gene ID	231-BR (Brain-Seeking)	ADMD-231 (Adrenal-Glands-Seeking)	BMD-231 (Bone-Seeking)	LMD-231 (Lung-Seeking)	p^4	p^5
HK2 [1]	1.62 [2,3]	1.83	1.66	1.70	>0.05	>0.05
ALDH1A3	1.18	1.53	1.43	1.48	<0.05	>0.05
ALDH9A1	**1.55**	1.04	1.07	1.09	>0.05	<0.05
ALDH3A1	1.18	1.03	1.21	1.16	>0.05	>0.05
PCK2	1.08	−1.43	**−1.21**	**−1.33**	<0.05	<0.05
IDH1	−1.18	**−1.31**	−1.13	−1.14	>0.05	>0.05
FH	**1.54**	1.08	1.04	1.11	>0.05	<0.05
MDH2	−1.10	**−1.19**	**−1.17**	−1.27	>0.05	>0.05
ATP5I	1.25	**1.36**	1.33	1.33	>0.05	>0.05
ATP5G2	−1.06	**−1.21**	−1.07	−1.11	>0.05	>0.05
ATP6V0E2	**1.62**	1.43	1.41	1.34	>0.05	>0.05
ATP6V1D	1.69	**2.45**	1.83	1.96	>0.05	>0.05
ATP6V0D1	−1.02	**−1.23**	−1.14	−1.11	>0.05	>0.05
ATP6V0D2	**1.21**	1.08	1.03	1.20	>0.05	>0.05
ATP6V1B1	**1.25**	−1.09	−1.07	1.03	<0.05	>0.05
COX17	−1.47	−1.46	**−1.50**	−1.52	>0.05	>0.05
COX7B	**2.02**	1.06	−1.06	−1.20	<0.05	<0.05
NDUFB7	1.45	**1.54**	1.27	1.21	>0.05	>0.05
NDUFB8	**−1.43**	**1.46**	**1.45**	**1.54**	<0.05	<0.05
NDUFV3	1.10	**1.51**	1.42	1.37	>0.05	>0.05
UQCRB	**1.31**	1.05	1.27	1.30	>0.05	>0.05
PGM5	−1.11	**6.42**	**4.32**	**4.51**	<0.05	<0.05

[1] From the GEO #GSE66495 microarray database ($n = 3$ per cell line), including only those genes involved in glycolysis, the TCA cycle, and oxidative phosphorylation. [2] Numbers report on fold changes, compared to parental MDA-MB-231 cells used as control. [3] Bold numbers are fold changes with $p < 0.05$ compared to parental MDA-MB-231 cells using one-way ANOVA. [4] p value for 231-BR compared to all other tissue-seeking variants using one-way ANOVA. [5] p value for 231-BR compared to all other tissue-seeking variants and parental cells using one-way ANOVA. Genes of interest ($p < 0.05$) are highlighted in gray.

2.11. Real-Time Quantitative PCR

Total RNA was collected using the NucleoSpin RNA kit (Filter Service, Eupen, Belgium; catalogue #740955.50), quantified with a NanoDrop 1000 Spectrophotometer (Thermo Fisher), and reverse-transcribed in cDNA with the RevertAid First Strand cDNA synthesis kit (Thermo Fisher; catalogue #K1621), using the same quantity (500–1000 ng) for all RNA samples and a 90-min incubation time. cDNAs were diluted 1:10 in DNase/RNase-free distilled water (Thermo Fisher), and 2 µL were used with 5 µL of 2X Takyon qPCR Master Mix and 0.2 µL of each primer (10 µM) and completed to 10 µL with water for RT-qPCR analysis (ViiA 7417 Real-Time instrument, Thermo Fisher). Primers were: *ALDH9A1* Forward 5′-AAG GAG CAG GGT GCT AAA GT-3′ and Reverse 5′-TCG TCT CTG CAA TTA GTT AAT ACA C-3′; *FH* Forward 5′-TGC CAA CCC CAG TTA TTA AAG C-3′ and Reverse 5′-CTT CAG CTA CCT CAT CTG CTG-3′; *NDUFB8* Forward 5′-CGG ATG ATG GCA TGG GGT A-3′ and Reverse 5′-GGT GCC AGT GCA TCG GTT-3′; *COX7B* Forward 5′-TAC CTG AAG CGA ATT GGC AC-3′ and Reverse 5′-GCT TCG AAC TTG GAG ACG

AT-3'; and *β-actin* Forward 5'-CCC GCG AGC ACA GAG C-3' and Reverse 5'-TCA TCA TCC ATG GTG AGC TGG- 3'. All gene expression data were normalized to *β-actin* gene expression.

2.12. Western Blotting

Western blotting was performed, as previously described [41], after protein collection in RIPA buffer containing phosphatase (PhosSTOP) and protease (proteases inhibitor cocktail) inhibitors. Membranes were incubated overnight with primary rabbit antibodies against ALDH9A1 (Proteintech; catalogue #26621), FH (BIOKE, Leiden, The Netherlands; catalogue #4567S), NDUFB8 (Proteintech, Manchester, UK; catalogue #14794), COX7b (Abcam, Cambridge, UK; catalogue #ab137094), and Vinculin (BIOKE; catalogue #4650S), or mouse antibodies against β-actin (Sigma-Aldrich; catalogue #A5441). Staining was revealed with an Amersham Imager 600 (Diegem, Belgium). All data are normalized to vinculin or β-actin expression.

2.13. Immunohistochemistry

Brains were collected, cut along the separation between right and left hemispheres, and embedded in paraffin. Sections (5 µm thick) were performed from the center of each hemisphere, to produce 10 slides for each sample. For each hemisphere, 3 slides from the beginning, the middle, and the end were used for immunostaining, and the process was repeated up to 3 times in order to analyze slices representative of the whole brain.

Brain sections were immunostained for GFP (Bio-Techne, Abingdon, UK; catalogue #600-308; BIOKE; catalogue #2956), with a secondary Envision anti-rabbit antibody coupled to HRP (Agilent; catalogue #K4003), and hematoxylin and eosin counterstained. Slides were scanned at 20x magnification with a SCN400 bright field Slide Scanner (Leica Biosystems, Diegem, Belgium). Metastasis number and surface area were determined using cytomine (Liège, Belgium; cytomine.org; accessed on 1 December 2021) and QuPath software version 0.1.2 (Belfast, UK) [42].

2.14. Clinical Database Analysis

Overall Survival (OS) curves were generated on Kaplan–Meier plotter (kmplot.com) with the auto select best cutoff for the 202110 Affy ID (*COX7B*) on the RNA-seq mRNA dataset (breast cancer and renal clear cell carcinoma in pan-cancer) and on gene chip mRNA datasets for lung cancers [43]. Sources for the databases include GEO, EGA, and TCGA.

2.15. Statistics

Data are shown as means ± SEM (error bars are sometimes smaller than symbols) or as individual values with the median. n indicates the total number of replicates per group/condition. Graphpad Prism version 9.2.0. (San Diego, CA, USA) was used for statistical analyses. Mann–Whitney U test, Student's t-test, one-way ANOVA, and two-ways ANOVA were used where indicated. $p < 0.05$ was considered to be statistically significant.

3. Results

3.1. Validation of Brain-Seeking Variant Models Derived from Human MDA-MB-231 Triple-Negative Breast Cancer Cells

The objective of our study was to identify metabolic protein(s) responsible for the brain tropism of human metastatic breast cancer. As models, we used MDA-MB-231 triple-negative breast cancer (TNBC) cells and two independently derived brain-seeking variant cell lines, 231-BR and 231-BR-2 [34–36], which were generated by serial cycles of in vivo selection in mice. The selection protocol involved intracardiac cancer cell injection in the left ventricle of female nude mice, surgical isolation, expansion of metastatic cancer cells retrieved from the brain, and intracardiac injection of these cells sequentially in additional animals for several rounds, until metastatic dissemination became restricted to the brain [34–36]. To identify metabolic drivers of brain-specific metastasis, we first ascertained the validity of the two model cell lines in vitro and in vivo. Short tandem repeat (STR) profiling confirmed that all variants were genomically similar to the parental MDA-MB-231 cells (Table S1). For in vivo assays, cells were infected with lentiviruses to constitutively express luciferase and green fluorescent protein (GFP). An intracardiac injection of 100,000 MDA-MB-231 parental cells (Figure 1a) did not generate brain metastases in female nude mice, whereas the use of either the 231-BR or 231-BR-2 variants yielded metastases in most animals (4/5 for 231-BR and 6/9 for 231-BR-2) 4 weeks after injection, which were detected by ex vivo bioluminescence imaging on isolated brains (Figure 1b).

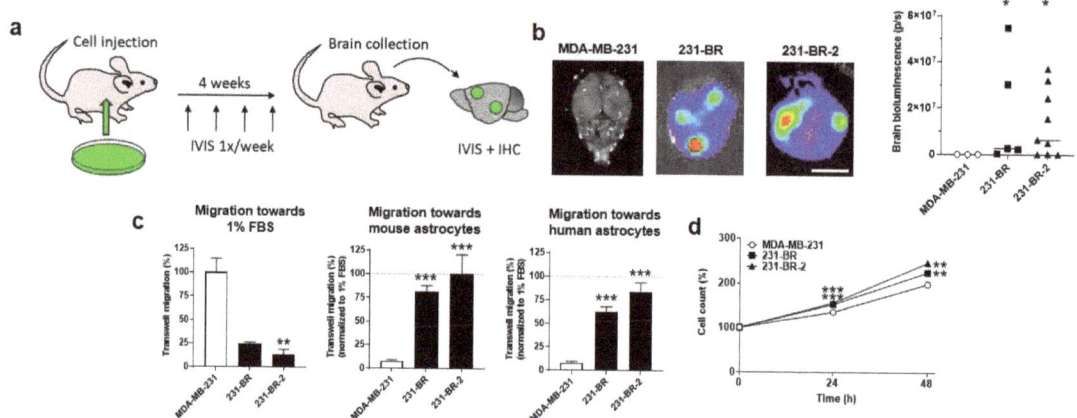

Figure 1. Validation of the brain tropism of MDA-MB-231-derived brain-seeking variants. (**a**) Schematic representation of in vivo experiments, where 6-week-old female mice were injected intracardially with 100,000 luciferase- and green fluorescent protein (GFP)-expressing cancer cells on Day 0, imaged once a week to track metastases, and sacrificed at Week 4 for organ collection, followed by ex vivo bioluminescence imaging and immunohistochemistry. (**b**) Ex vivo bioluminescence imaging of mouse brains at the end of the protocol illustrated in (**a**). Pictures on the left are representative of mouse brains in luciferin-containing medium captured using a Xenogen IVIS 50 bioluminescence imaging system. The right graph shows brain bioluminescence intensity in mice having received parental MDA-MB-231 cancer cells or 231-BR or 231-BR-2 brain-seeking variants (n = 3–9). Bar = 5 mm. (**c**) Migration of MDA-MB-231, 231-BR, and 231-BR-2 cells was assayed in transwells towards 1% FBS (n = 2–3), towards mouse astrocytes (n = 6) or towards human astrocytes (n = 6). (**d**) Cell count (%) over time on a SpectraMax i3 spectrophotometer equipped with a MiniMax imaging cytometer, after seeding 5000 cells per well in a 96-well plate (n = 18–19). Data are shown as individual values and medians (**b**) or as means ± SEM (**c**,**d**). * p < 0.05, ** p < 0.01, *** p < 0.005; compared to MDA-MB-231; using Mann–Whitney test (**b**), one-way ANOVA with Dunnett's post hoc test (**c**), or two-way ANOVA with Dunnett's post hoc test (**d**).

For in vitro model validation, we developed a transwell assay aimed to test the general and organotropic migration of the human breast cancer cells in the upper well towards 1% FBS or towards living immortalized nonmalignant astrocytes in the lower well, respectively. Since the selection of the brain-seeking variants was made in mice, we tested both mouse and human astrocytes as attractants. While parental MDA-MB-231 cells had a higher capacity to migrate towards 1% FBS compared to the two brain-seeking variants, conversely, 231-BR and 231-BR-2 cells migrated much more efficiently towards mouse or human astrocytes (Figure 1c), thus validating their preferential tropism for the brain. Of note, both brain-seeking variants were slightly, yet significantly, more proliferative than the parental cells, as determined by direct cell counting over time (Figure 1d).

3.2. Brain-Seeking Variants of MDA-MB-231 Cells Undergo an Oxidative Switch

Using Seahorse oximetry and the dedicated Fuel Flex test kit of Agilent, we next determine the oxidative metabolic preferences of the parental and brain-seeking variant cells. The assay involves sequential inhibition of glucose-fueled (using 2 μM of mitochondrial pyruvate carrier inhibitor UK5099), glutamine-fueled (using 3 μM of glutaminase 1 inhibitor BPTES), and lipid-fueled (using 4 μM of carnitine palmitoyl-transferase 1A inhibitor Etomoxir) OXPHOS. The results show that OXPHOS in MDA-MB-231 cells was supported almost equally by glutamine (52%) and fatty acids (48%), but not at all by glucose, whereas OPXHOS in the two brain-seeking variants was supported not only by glutamine and fatty acids but also by glucose (5.1 ± 0.6 % for 231-BR and 8.4 ± 1.4% for 231-BR-2 cells) (Figure 2a). Glucose uptake, lactate release, and, hence, the glycolytic ratio ([glucose]/[lactate]) were unchanged in full medium (DMEM containing glutaMAX, 4.5g/L glucose, and 10% FBS) (Figure 2b). Therefore, changes in the capacity to use OXPHOS fuels reflected an increased oxidative flexibility of brain-seeking variants compared to parental cells, rather than an increased dependency on glucose. Accordingly, both 231-BR and 231-BR-2 cell lines presented improved basal and maximal respiration activities as well as an improved oxidative ATP production, compared to parental cells (Figure 2c).

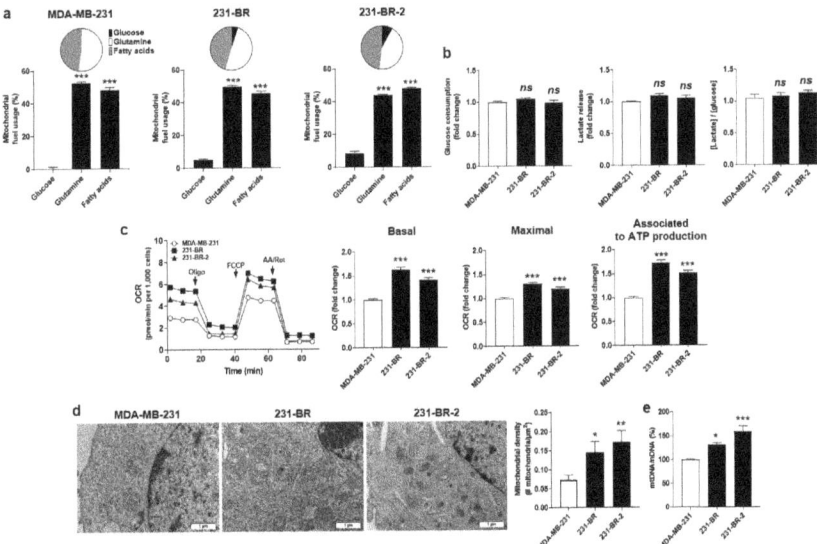

Figure 2. Brain-seeking variants are more oxidative than parental MDA-MB-231 human breast cancer cells. (**a**) Mitochondrial fuel usage of MDA-MB-231 (**left**, n = 14), 231-BR (**middle**, n = 14–16), and 231-BR-2 (**right**, n = 14–15) cancer cells was determined using the Fuel Flex test kit (Agilent) on a Seahorse XF96 bioenergetics analyzer. Data are presented as pie and column graphs, where total fuel usage = 100%. (**b**) Glucose consumption (**left**, n = 11–16), lactate production (middle, n = 16–17), and the lactate/glucose ratio (**right**, n = 13–16) were determined from measurements in deproteinized cell supernatants using an enzymatic CMA600 analyzer. (**c**) Basal (**left**, n = 29–32) and maximal (**middle**, n = 28–32) oxygen consumption rates (mtOCRs), as well as the OCR of the cells associated to mitochondrial ATP production (**right**, n = 29–32), were measured using a XF Cell Mito Stress Test kit (Agilent) on a Seahorse XF96 bioenergetics analyzer. Representative Seahorse traces are shown on far left. (**d**) Transmission electron microscopy pictures of the cells are shown on the left (bars = 1 μm), and the mitochondrial density is quantified on the right graph (n = 6–12). (**e**) Mitochondrial DNA/nuclear DNA (mtDNA/nDNA) cell content determined using RT-qPCR (n = 5). All data are shown as means ± SEM. * $p < 0.05$, ** $p < 0.01$, *** $p < 0.005$, ns: $p > 0.05$; compared to first column; using one-way ANOVA with Dunnett's post hoc test (**a**–**c**,**e**).

The oxidative switch evidenced in brain-seeking variants was linked to qualitative and quantitative changes affecting mitochondria. Qualitatively, electron microscopy revealed enlarged mitochondria in 231-BR compared to the parental cells, whereas they were smaller but more abundant in 231-BR-2 compared to MDA-MB-231 cells (Figure 2d). The mitochondrial to nuclear DNA ratio (mtDNA/nDNA) was determined using RT-qPCR, revealing a significantly increased mtDNA abundance in both 231-BR and 231-BR-2 compared to the parental cells (Figure 2e). Collectively, we concluded that the oxidative efficiency of mitochondria was increased in the brain-seeking variants of MDA-MB-231 cells.

3.3. Identification of Four Candidate Metabolic Genes That Could Account for the Brain Tropism of Human Breast Cancer Cells

Based on our working hypothesis of a metabolic preference of brain-seeking variants for metabolites present in the brain and on the above evidence of metabolic differences in the filiation, we next aimed to identify metabolic genes/proteins associated to the brain tropism of 231-BR and 231-BR-2 cells. We first analyzed the publicly available microarray database GEO #GSE66495, reporting on the whole genome expression of not only MDA-MB-231 and 231-BR cells but also MDA-MD-231-derived adrenal (ADMD-231), bone (BMD-231), and lung (LMD-231) metastatic variants [36]. We focused on genes involved in glycolysis, the TCA cycle, and OXPHOS.

Using the two-step methodology described in the materials and methods, we identified 22 metabolic genes differentially expressed in at least one metastatic variant compared to parental MDA-MB-231 cells, among which 6 were further differentially expressed in 231-BR cells compared to any other metastatic variant (Table 1). Significantly upregulated genes were *ALDH9A1* (Genbank ID 223, on chromosome 1) encoding aldehyde dehydrogenase 9 family member A1, *FH* (Genbank ID 2271, on chromosome 1) encoding fumarate hydratase, and *COX7B* (Genbank ID 1349, on chromosome X) encoding cytochrome c oxidase subunit 7B. Significantly downregulated genes were *ALDH1A3* (Genbank ID 220, on chromosome 15) encoding aldehyde dehydrogenase 1 family member A3, *NDUFB8* (Genbank ID 4714, on chromosome 10) encoding NADH:ubiquinone oxidoreductase subunit B8, and *PGM5* (Genbank ID 5239, on chromosome 9) encoding phosphoglucomutase 5.

Among the six genes, *ALDH1A3* and *PGM5* expression was not significantly different ($p > 0.05$) between 231-BR and parental MDA-MB-231 cells (Table 1). They were, therefore, excluded from further analysis.

3.4. Cytochrome c Oxidase Subunit 7b in Mitochondrial Complex IV Is a Candidate Protein Supporting the Brain Tropism of Human Breast Cancer Cells

We next aimed to validate our short list of four genes: *ALDH9A1*, *FH*, *NDUFB8*, and *COX7B*. To avoid idiosyncrasies that would have been associated to 231-BR cells, changes in gene expression were independently tested using RT-qPCR in both 231-BR and 231-BR-2 brain-seeking variants. We further verified that the changes in protein matched the changes in mRNA expression. Uncropped western blots are displayed in Figure S1.

ALDH9A1 encodes a cytosolic aldehyde dehydrogenase that catalyzes the oxidation of γ-aminobutyraldehyde and aminoaldehydes derived from polyamines. It is involved in carnitine biosynthesis [44], which facilitates the transport of fatty acids across the inner mitochondrial membrane for β-oxidation and, potentially, in a marginal pathway for the biosynthesis of neurotransmitter γ-aminobutyric acid (GABA) [45] (Figure 3a, left). Compared to parental MDA-MB-231 cells, *ALDH9A1* mRNA expression was significantly increased in 231-BR, but it was slightly decreased in 231-BR-2 cells (Figure 3a, middle). The corresponding protein was overexpressed in 231-BR but not in 231-BR-2 cells (Figure 3a, right), which disqualified it as a shared metabolic sensor for brain tropism in our model cell lines.

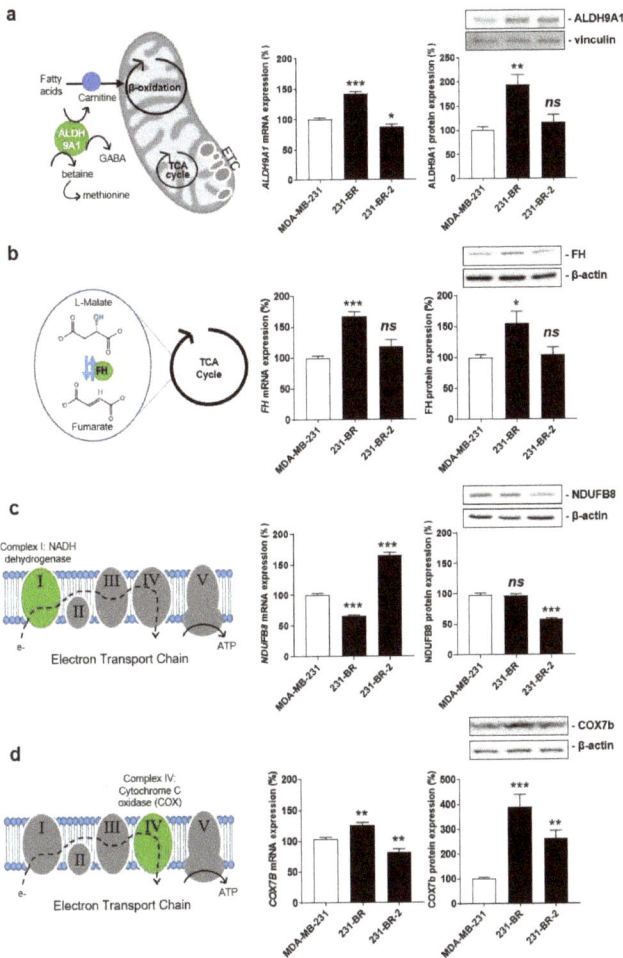

Figure 3. Identification of Cox7b as a candidate protein for the brain tropism of human breast cancer. (**a**) The left drawing depicts the three main functions of aldehyde hydrogenase 9A1 (ALDH9A1) that catalyzes the biosynthesis of γ-aminobutyric acid (GABA) in the cytosol, the biosynthesis of carnitine to facilitate the transport of fatty acids across the inner mitochondrial membrane, and the oxidation of γ-aminobutyraldehyde and aminoaldehydes derived from polyamines in the mitochondrial matrix. The middle graph shows *ALDH9A1* mRNA expression normalized to β-actin (n = 5–6), and the right graph shows ALDH9A1 protein expression normalized to vinculin (n = 6), in MDA-MB-231, 231-BR, and 231-BR-2 cancer cells. (**b**) The left drawing depicts fumarate hydratase (FH) activity, which catalyzes the reversible hydration of fumarate to malate in the TCA cycle. The middle graph shows *FH* mRNA expression normalized to β-actin (n = 5–6), and the right graph shows FH protein expression normalized to β-actin (n = 9). (**c**) The left drawing localizes NDUFB8 as a component of electron transport chain (ETC) Complex I (green). The middle graph shows *NDUFB8* mRNA expression normalized to β-actin (n = 6), and the right graph shows NDUFB8 protein expression normalized to β-actin (n = 3). (**d**) The left drawing depicts cyclooxygenase 7b (COX7b) as a component of ETC Complex IV (green). The middle graph shows *COX7B* mRNA expression normalized to β-actin (n = 5–6), and the right graph shows Cox7b protein expression normalized to β-actin (n = 9). All data are shown as means ± SEM. * $p < 0.05$, ** $p < 0.01$, *** $p < 0.005$, ns: $p > 0.05$; compared to MDA-MB-231 cells; using one-way ANOVA with Dunnett's post hoc test (**a**–**d**).

FH encodes fumarate hydratase, the seventh enzyme of the TCA cycle that catalyzes the hydration of fumarate to *L*-malate (Figure 3b, left). When mutated/inactivated, FH can cause various diseases, including hereditary and sporadic forms of cancer [46]. In the context of brain-specific breast cancer metastasis, FH mRNA and protein expression was increased in 231-BR but not in 231-BR-2 cells (Figure 3b, middle and right), thus disqualifying this enzyme as a shared metabolic sensor for brain tropism.

NDUFB8 encodes an accessory subunit of NADH ubiquinone oxidoreductase, a large protein complex known as ETC Complex I at the inner mitochondrial membrane (Figure 3c, left). The subunit is bound to NADH dehydrogenase 5 (ND5) in the proton-pumping module of Complex I [47]. Similar to microarray data analysis, RT-qPCR showed significantly reduced *NDUFB8* mRNA expression in 231-BR compared to MDA-MB-231 cells (Figure 3c, middle). However, it was significantly increased in 231-BR-2 cells, and the changes in protein expression did not match the changes in mRNA expression (Figure 3c, middle and right). Overall, this disqualified NDUFB8 as a metabolic sensor for brain-selective metastasis.

COX7B encodes subunit 7b of cytochrome c oxidase (Cox), a large protein complex known as ETC Complex IV that catalyzes the transfer of electrons from reduced cytochrome c to molecular oxygen at the inner mitochondrial membrane (Figure 3d, left) [48]. Cox7b is a short 80 amino acid protein that stabilizes the complex and modulates Cox activity [49]. *COX7B* mRNA expression was increased in 231-BR but decreased in 231-BR-2 cells (Figure 3d, middle). However, the expression of the corresponding protein was increased in both variants (Figure 3d, right). Considering that among the four candidate proteins only Cox7b expression showed a similar change in both brain-seeking variants, we retained Cox7b for further investigation.

3.5. Cox7b Expression Drives Human Breast Cancer Cell Migration towards Astrocytes

Transwell migration assays were used to establish a causal link between Cox7b expression and MDA-MB-231 brain chemoattraction, mimicked by cell migration towards immortalized human and mouse astrocytes. Chemoattraction at other important metastatic sites [34] was mimicked by immortalized human hepatocytes (T0063) and human bronchial epithelial cells (T0763). All four cell lines were nonmalignant.

As expected, *COX7b* silencing in brain-seeking variant cells, using a CRISPR-Cas9 strategy (Figure S2a), significantly decreased 231-BR cell migration towards human and mouse astrocytes but not towards human hepatocytes and human bronchial cells (Figure 4a). The general migratory phenotype towards serum (1% FBS, used as a control) was unaffected. Similarly, *COX7B* silencing significantly reduced 231-BR-2 migration towards human and mouse astrocytes but not towards human hepatocytes, human bronchial cells, or serum (Figure 4b). Conversely, experimental Cox7b protein overexpression in parental MDA-MB-231 cells (Figure S2b) increased their migration towards human and mouse astrocytes, while migration towards human hepatocytes, human bronchial cells, or serum was not changed (Figure 4c).

Together, these in vitro results supported a cause–effect relationship between Cox7b protein expression and the brain tropism of human metastatic breast cancer cells. In particular, Cox7b protein overexpression was sufficient to trigger a selective brain tropism of otherwise pan-metastatic, wild-type MDA-MB-231 cells. This finding does not exclude that other proteins could have a similar function in other cancer cell lines.

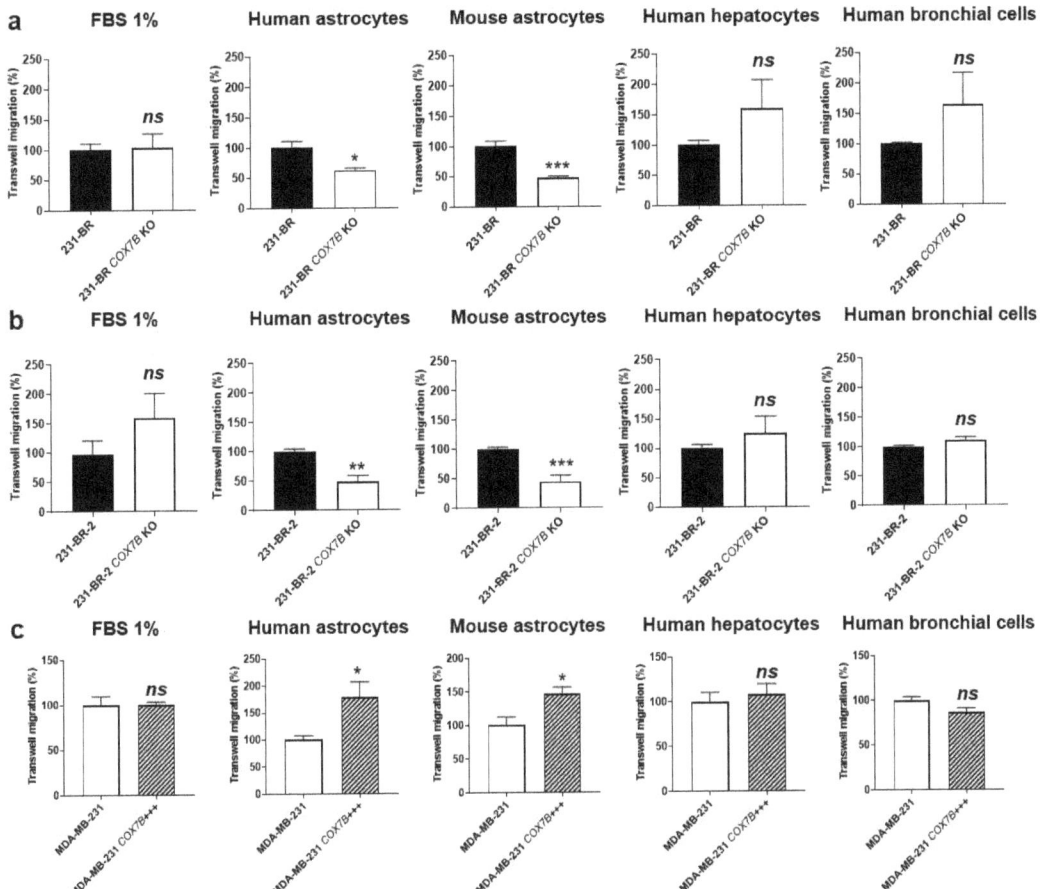

Figure 4. Cause–effect relationship between Cox7b expression and the selective migration of human breast cancer cells towards astrocytes. (**a**) Migration assayed in transwells of 231-BR brain-seeking variants, expressing or not expressing (KO using a CRISP-Cas9 strategy) Cox7b, towards 1% FBS ($n = 9$), human astrocytes ($n = 3$), mouse astrocytes ($n = 5$), human hepatocytes ($n = 6$), or human bronchial cells ($n = 6$). (**b**) Migration of 231-BR-2 brain-seeking variants, expressing or not expressing Cox7b, towards 1% FBS ($n = 9$), human astrocytes ($n = 5$–6), mouse astrocytes ($n = 7$), human hepatocytes ($n = 6$), or human bronchial cells ($n = 6$). (**c**) Migration of MDA-MB-231 parental cancer cells, overexpressing Cox7b or expressing basal levels of Cox7b, towards 1% FBS ($n = 7$), human astrocytes ($n = 9$), mouse astrocytes ($n = 6$), human hepatocytes ($n = 6$), or human bronchial cells ($n = 6$). All data are normalized to control (first columns) and are shown as means ± SEM. * $p < 0.05$, ** $p < 0.01$, *** $p < 0.005$, ns: $p > 0.05$; using Student's t-test (**a**–**c**).

3.6. Cox7b Expression Promotes the Oxidative Phenotype of Human Metastatic Breast Cancer Cells

The data displayed in Figure 2 showed that increased OXPHOS is a major metabolic characteristic of 231-BR and 231-BR-2 brain-seeking variants compared to parental cells. Since Cox7b resides in the ETC [49], we reasoned that its expression might modulate the OCR of the cells, which was measured using Seahorse oximetry.

COX7B silencing reduced 231-BR basal OCR and OCR associated to ATP production, but maximal OCR, reflecting the respiration spare capacity, was unchanged (Figure 5a). Comparatively, *COX7B* silencing reduced all basal OCR, maximal OCR, and OCR associated to ATP production in 231-BR-2 cells (Figure 5b), demonstrating that loss of *COX7B* represses

OXPHOS in brain-seeking variants of metastatic breast cancer. Of note, *COX7B* silencing did not decrease cell numbers (Figure S3), suggesting the existence of rescue metabolic pathways preventing cell death. Cox7b overexpression in wild-type MDA-MB-231 cells induced the opposite effect, i.e., an oxidative switch characterized by a rise in all basal OCR, maximal OCR, and OCR associated to ATP production (Figure 5c).

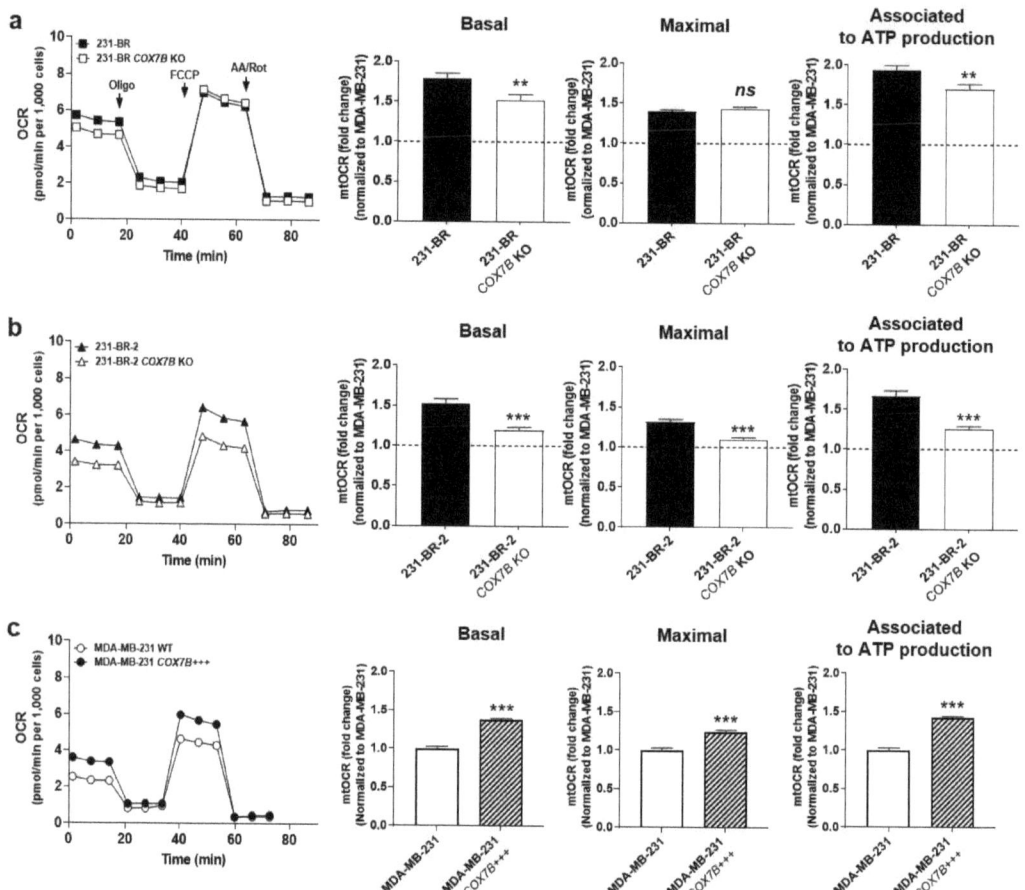

Figure 5. Cox7b expression drives the oxidative switch of brain-seeking variants. (**a**) 231-BR brain-seeking variants expressing or not expressing (KO using a CRISP-Cas9 strategy) Cox7b. Basal (**left**) and maximal (**middle**) oxygen consumption rates (mtOCRs), as well as the OCR of the cells associated to mitochondrial ATP production (**right**), were measured using a XF Cell Mito Stress Test Kit (Agilent) on a Seahorse XF96 bioenergetics analyzer (n = 20 all). Representative Seahorse traces are shown on far left. (**b**) As in (**a**), but using 231-BR-2 brain-seeking variants expressing or not expressing Cox7b (n = 15–20). (**c**) As in (**a**), but using MDA-MD-231 parental cancer cells overexpressing or expressing basal levels of Cox7b (n = 23–32). All data are normalized to control (dotted lines) and are shown as means ± SEM. ** $p < 0.01$, *** $p < 0.005$, ns: $p > 0.05$; using Student's t-test (**a–c**).

Together, these experiments demonstrated that Cox7b is an OXPHOS inducer. They further established a positive correlation between the oxidative activities of human metastatic breast cancer cells and their preferential migration towards astrocytes. Of note, Cox7b expression did not modulate the OXPHOS substrate preference of the brain-seeking variants (Figure S4).

3.7. Cox7b Expression Is Responsible for the Brain Tropism of Metastatic Human Breast Cancer Cells in Mice

To experimentally establish a cause–effect relationship between Cox7b expression and breast cancer brain metastasis, we ran a series of in vivo experiments in nude mice, as depicted in Figure 1a. Briefly, because our investigation interrogated metastatic tropism linked to metastatic take (a late metastatic event) but not metastatic cell dissemination from a primary tumor (an early metastatic event), breast cancer cells were injected in the left cardiac ventricle, which is known to generate systemic metastatic lesions to the bones, brain, ovary, and adrenal glands using MDA-MB-231 cells [34,35]. The constitutive and concurrent expression of luciferase and GFP by our model cell lines allowed for a confirmation of bioluminescence data with immunohistochemistry.

Following the protocol depicted in Figure 1a, *COX7B* silencing with a CRISPR-cas9 strategy in 231-BR and 231-BR-2 brain-seeking variants resulted in an almost total loss of brain tropism following intracardiac injection (Figure 6a). This was evidenced using ex vivo luciferase bioluminescence imaging on brains isolated at the time of mouse sacrifice. Conversely, parental MDA-MB-231 cells, which did not generate detectable brain metastasis for 4 weeks, gained a strong increase in the occurrence of brain metastases upon Cox7b overexpression (Figure 6a). For validation, brains were collected at the end of the experiments, sliced, stained with an antibody against GFP, and counterstained with hematoxylin and eosin. Figure 6b shows representative pictures of the brains, with insets representing typical metastasis-positive areas. Analyses revealed a strong decrease in the number of metastases per mouse and in the metastasis-positive tumor area per slice in mice injected with 231-BR and 231-BR-2 cells lacking *COX7B*, compared to wild-type 231-BR and 231-BR-2 cells (Figure 6b, left and middle graphs). The opposite effects were seen in mice that received parental MDA-MB-231 cells overexpressing Cox7b compared to wild-type MDA-MB-231 cells (Figure 6b, right graphs). Collectively, these in vivo data established a cause–effect relationship between Cox7b expression and the brain tropism of human TNBC in mice.

We concluded our study by analyzing publicly available gene chip and RNA-seq mRNA expression databases [43] reporting on clinical human breast and lung cancers, as wells as on renal clear cell carcinoma, all subtypes included. High Cox7B expression was identified as an independent poor prognosis factor for overall patient survival in all three cancer types (Figure 6c).

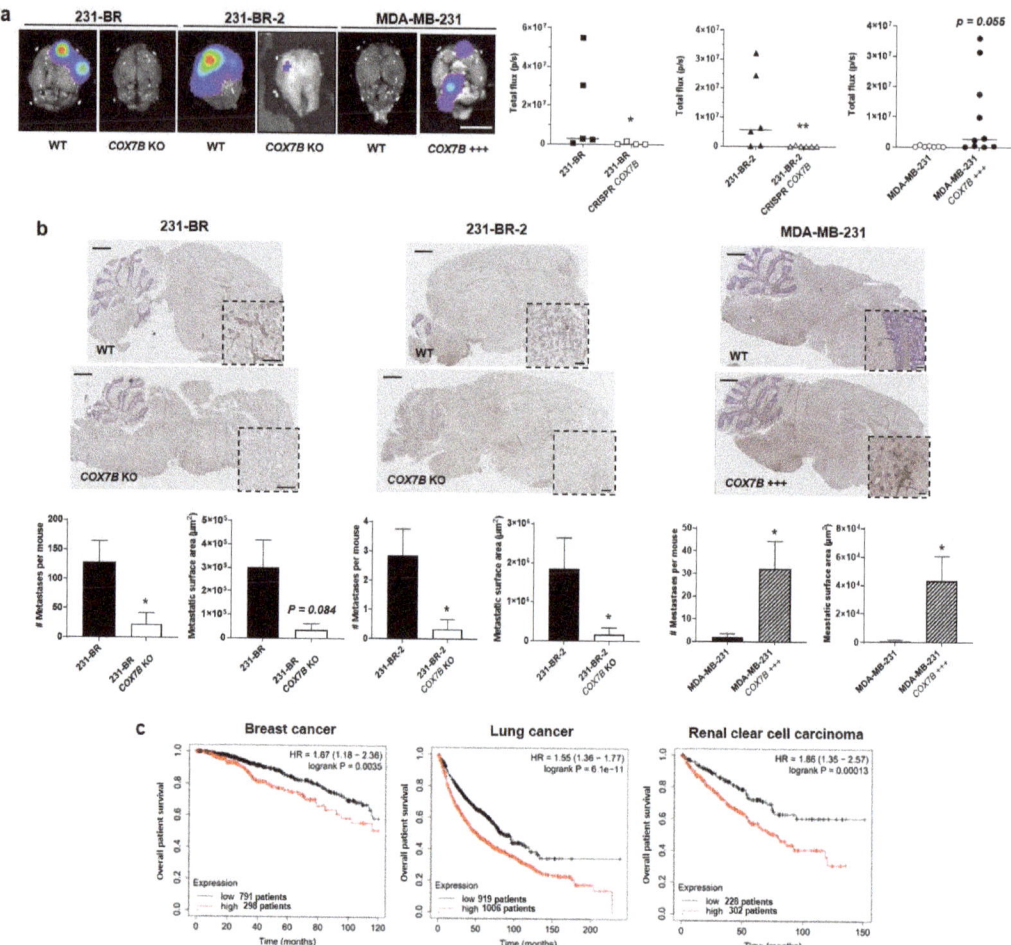

Figure 6. Cox7b drives the tropism of metastatic human breast cancer cells to the brain. (**a,b**) The brain tropism of 231-BR and 231-BR-2 brain-seeking variants, expressing or not Cox7b (KO using a CRISP-Cas9 strategy), and of parental MDA-MB-231 human breast cancer cells, overexpressing or not overexpressing Cox7b, was assessed using the protocol depicted in Figure 1a. The cells constitutively expressed luciferase and GFP. (**a**) Ex vivo bioluminescence imaging of mouse brains 4 weeks after the intracardiac injection of cancer cells. Pictures on the **left** are representative of mouse brains in luciferin-containing medium captured using a Xenogen IVIS 50 bioluminescence imaging system. Graphs on the right show brain bioluminescence intensity (n = 4–10). (**b**) Central sections of the brains were immunostained for GFP and counterstained for hematoxylin and eosin. Representative pictures are shown on top (bars = 1 mm). Insets represent typical GFP-positive metastatic lesions (bars = 100 μm). On the bottom, the left graphs represent the number of detected metastases (**left**) and the metastasis-positive surface area per mouse (n = 4–10). Representative images of the brains are shown. (**c**) Overall survival of patients with breast cancer (**left**, all types combined, 1090 patients), lung cancer (**middle**, all types combined, 1925 patients) and renal clear cell carcinoma (RCC, **right**, 530 patients). Data are shown as individual values and medians (**a**), means ± SEM (**b**), or individual values (**c**). * $p < 0.05$, ** $p < 0.01$, using Mann–Whitney test (**a**), Student's t-test (**b**), or log rank test (**c**).

4. Discussion

In the context of the seed-and-soil hypothesis proposing that secondary organs should fulfill the specific needs of metastatic progenitor cells [14], this study aimed to investigate the existence of a metabolic control of tissue-specific metastasis. We used breast cancer brain metastasis as an example, and we selected the human MDA-MB-231 TNBC cancer cell line as a working model for the generally high propensity of this breast cancer subtype to metastasize in humans [50] and because two brain-seeking variants derived from the same parental cell line were already available from two independent laboratories [34–36]. It allowed us to validate characteristics identified in one variant by those of the other. In this model, we report that Cox7b, a structural subunit of ETC Complex IV [51,52], drives metastatic breast cancer cell homing to the brain: repression of Cox7b expression selectively blocked the migration of brain-seeking variants towards astrocytes and their capacity to generate brain metastases in mice; conversely, pan-metastatic parental cells manipulated to gain Cox7b expression increased their selective migration towards astrocytes and their capability to generate brain metastases. This series of experiments established a cause–consequence relationship between Cox7b expression and metastatic brain tropism in the MDA-MB-231 model. Other proteins could exert a similar function in other cancer cell lines and models.

Mammalian Cox, also known as Complex IV, is a 13-subunit multiheteromeric enzyme that catalyzes the oxidation of cytochrome c and the reduction of molecular oxygen to water at the terminal step of OXPHOS in the mitochondrial ETC [48]. Complex IV is located at the inner mitochondrial membrane. In the complex, Cox7b is a short 80 amino acid nuclear-encoded transmembrane protein that associates with mitochondria-encoded subunits Cox1, Cox2, and Cox3, which contain the four catalytic redox centers of the enzyme [49]. Cox7b is ubiquitously expressed. It has no enzymatic activity but stabilizes the complex and positively modulates Cox activity. Its expression is increased in several degenerative pathologies characterized by high OXPHOS activities (see reference [53] for a recent review), and inactivating mutations have been associated with the development of microphthalmia with linear skin lesions (MLS) [54]. The fact that Cox7b stabilizes Complex IV is in line with our observation that high Cox7b expression triggers OXPHOS, whereas *COX7B* silencing has the opposite effect. To date, nothing is known about the regulation of Cox7b expression in mammalian cells.

Interestingly, high Cox7b expression was enhanced through rounds of in vivo selection using intracardiac delivery in mice, thus bypassing adaptation and selection in a primary tumor. This highlights a key characteristic of metastatic cancer cells: selective homing. Homing is an active process involving cancer cell interactions with vascular endothelial cells at given body locations; transvascular diapedesis; nesting in the premetastatic niche; the establishment of molecular relationships with host cells at the new location; and a phenotypic reversion from a stem to a proliferative phenotype for most post-metastatic cancer cells [26,55]. This succession of events would be incomplete without answering to the question: how do metastatic progenitor cells sense that they have arrived at the metastatic location, while they are still in the blood stream? If they exist, sensor systems should be sensitive enough to discriminate changes in the composition of the blood between different organs.

For homing, physical interactions between metastatic progenitor cells and host cells in the metastatic niche can be excluded as a triggering event, because they occur after extravasation. Theses interactions would rather primarily retain and re-educate/redifferentiate cancer cells at the metastatic site. Similarly, physical interactions between metastatic progenitor cells and endothelial cells lining blood vessels along premetastatic niches might not be the primary event for homing. Indeed, our in vitro experiments demonstrate that selective cancer cell migration towards host cells, seen as feeder cells, can be manipulated in the absence of vascular cells in vitro. In other words, metastatic progenitor cells would sense soluble molecules produced by host cells that act as chemoattractants. These molecules are expected to reach the blood stream in concentrations high enough to be sensed and with a concentration gradient steep enough to be followed by metastatic progenitors. Our data suggest that Cox7b could be such a sensor in human TNBC cells, but the exact nature of the metabolic signal(s) recognized by Cox7b is still unknown. Based on the observation that Cox7b expression increases OXPHOS activity, candidate chemoattractants should be primarily sought among TCA cycle substrates and intermediates. These chemoattractants would be produced by human and mouse astrocytes in culture and in vivo, but not by human bronchial cells nor by human hepatocytes. Lactate, which is produced and secreted by astrocytes to feed neurons [56], pyruvate, acetate, and glutamate are attractive candidates [57,58]. Of note, brain-seeking variants also gained metabolic flexibility to fuel OXPHOS, but this was not linked to Cox7b expression.

Our study was primarily aimed at proving the concept of a metabolic control of organotropism, and our data support that idea, even if additional experiments are still warranted to demonstrate our initial hypothesis. Cox7b was identified using the MDA-MB-231 model solely. This TNBC cell line was used because it represents a cancer type that is often detected in patients before entry in the metastatic phase, but that evolves to this phase despite treatments in a significant number of patients. Hence, in a cohort study where 25,362 TNBC patients were included, only 6% were at the metastatic stage and only 0.68% had brain metastases at the time of diagnosis; however, even for those with localized disease, approximately 25% of patients relapsed with distant metastasis [59,60]. Overall, brain metastasis affected up to 50% of TNBC patients in the course of the disease [10]. Our choice of the model was, thus, driven by the possibility to identify a suitable target for the prevention of brain metastasis. At the end of the study, one must recognize that Cox7b is not a suitable pharmacological target, as this structural protein has no enzymatic activity and is buried within Complex IV at the mitochondrial inner membrane. However, we believe that the use of the same selection approach for in vivo organotropism starting from different types of cancer cells (e.g., other breast cancer cells, prostate cancer, cervix cancer, melanoma) will reveal additional metabolic proteins controlling tissue-specific homing. Candidates have already been proposed [61] that must still be validated as being causal in organotropism. Among these, some could be amenable for therapy, with the ultimate intention of interfering with the metabolic sensing of different subtypes of metastatic progenitor cells at different secondary sites. Some of these targets could further be shared by different types of tumors (as illustrated here, with high Cox7b expression in primary tumors being a poor predictive factor of overall survival not only in breast cancer but also in lung cancer and in renal clear cell carcinoma), and others could be specific for a particular cancer type metastasizing to a particular secondary organ. Furthermore, a metabolic sensor could have additional effects unrelated to metastasis. This is the case of Cox7b, which sensitizes cancers to cisplatin chemotherapy, with high Cox7b expression in primary tumors being a favorable factor for overall patient survival upon cisplatin treatment [62].

5. Conclusions

This study is the first of a series investigating the existence of metabolic sensors for tissue-specific metastasis in the context of the seed-and-soil hypothesis and the premetastatic niche theory. Using parental human MDA-MB-231 TNBC cells and two independent brain-seeking variants selected in mice as models, we identified mitochondrial protein Cox7b in ETC Complex IV as a selective regulator of brain metastasis. Silencing and overexpression experiments established a causal link between Cox7b expression and metastatic brain tropism in vivo, where metabolically active astrocytes were sufficient to chemoattract brain-seeking metastatic variants expressing high levels of Cox7b. While Cox7b is not adapted as a direct target for the therapeutic prevention of brain metastasis, we believe that our general strategy, applied to other cancer types and/or different secondary sites, has the potential to unravel other, unprecedented target candidates.

6. Patent

M.C.N.M.B. and P.S. are inventors of patent application EP22191920, entitled "Stem Cells with Brain Tropism", which is related to the work reported in this manuscript.

Supplementary Materials: The following supporting information can be downloaded at: https://www.mdpi.com/article/10.3390/cancers14184371/s1. Figure S1: uncropped western blots; Figure S2: Validation of *COX7B* silencing and overexpression; Figure S3: *COX7B* silencing does not alter brain-seeking variant cell numbers in vitro; Figure S4: *COX7B* silencing does not alter the metabolic plasticity of brain-seeking variant cells; Table S1: Short tandem repeat profiles.

Author Contributions: Conceptualization, M.C.N.M.B., C.B. and P.S.; methodology, M.C.N.M.B., T.C. and P.S.; investigation, M.C.N.M.B., T.C., L.X.Z., J.D.R., Z.B., J.A.V.d.V., M.F. and E.P.D.; formal analysis, M.C.N.M.B., T.C. and P.S.; validation, C.M., C.B., and P.S.; resources, C.B. and P.S.; data curation, P.S.; writing—original draft preparation, M.C.N.M.B. and P.S.; writing—review and editing, M.C.N.M.B., T.C., J.D.R., L.X.Z., Z.B., J.A.V.d.V., M.F., E.P.D., C.M., C.B. and P.S.; visualization, M.C.N.M.B. and P.S.; supervision, P.S.; project administration, P.S.; funding acquisition, P.S. All authors have read and agreed to the published version of the manuscript.

Funding: This work was supported by the FRFS-WELBIO strategic axis of the Walloon Region of Belgium (WELBIO-CR-2022A-13), the Belgian Fonds National de la Recherche Scientifique (F.R.S.-FNRS, CDR J.0135.18, CDR J.0177.22), the Belgian Télévie (project n° 7.4529.17), the European Union's Horizon 2020 research innovation program under the Marie Skłodowska–Curie grant agreements No. 722605 TRANSMIT, and the Louvain Foundation. M.C.N.M.B. is a Ph.D. Fellow of the Télévie; L.X.Z. is a Ph.D. Fellow of Marie Skłodowska–Curie grant No 722605 TRANSMIT.; P.S. is a F.R.S.-FNRS Research Director and a WELBIO Investigator.

Institutional Review Board Statement: Mouse experiments were performed with the approval of UCLouvain Comité d'Ethique pour l'Expérimentation Animale (approval IDs: 2016/UCL/MD/018 and 2020/UCL/MD/033), according to national and European animal care regulations.

Informed Consent Statement: Not applicable.

Data Availability Statement: All data are contained within the article and the Supplementary Materials.

Acknowledgments: The authors thank François P. Duhoux (Department of Medical Oncology, Institut Roi Albert II, Cliniques Universitaires Saint-Luc, Brussels, Belgium) for sharing his medical expertise; Thibaut Vazeille, Loïc Hamelin, and Marie Bedin for excellent technical assistance; the Morph-Im technological platform and electron microscopy services of UNamur; and Davide Bruza, Caroline Bouzin, Michèle De Beukelaer, Aurélie Daumerie, and Marc De Burnonville at UCLouvain IREC's core facilities. The authors further thank Patricia Steeg (NIH) and Harikrishna Nakshatri (Indiana University School of Medicine) for the kind gift of MDA-MB-231-derived brain-seeking variants 231-BR and 231-BR-2, respectively. The plasmids used in this study were provided by the laboratories of Feng Zhang and Ralf Kuehn, via Addgene.

Conflicts of Interest: M.C.N.M.B. and P.S. are inventors of a patent application entitled "Stem Cells with Brain Tropism". The authors declare no other conflicts of interest related to the present study. The funders had no role in the design of the study; in the collection, analyses, or interpretation of data; in the writing of the manuscript; or in the decision to publish the results.

Appendix A

Appendix A.1 Cell Infection for Constitutive Luciferase and GFP Expression

For constitutive luciferase and GFP expression, cells were infected with lentiviruses carrying the luciferase and GFP sequences along with a puromycin resistance gene (Amsbio; catalogue #LPV020). Briefly, 70%–80% of the confluent cells in a 24-well plate were transduced with 2 μL per well of the lentivirus solution in 1mL medium with 10 μL/mL polybrene. Cells were selected by a 48–72 h incubation with 1 μg/mL puromycin (InvivoGen, Toulouse, France) and FACS-sorted for GFP expression on a Becton Dickinson FACSAriaIII system (Erembodegem, Belgium).

Appendix A.2 COX7B Gene Silencing

CRISPR plasmids were constructed following Zhang's laboratory protocol [37] with pX459 (Addgene; catalogue #62988, puromycin selection) or pU6-(BbsI)_CBh-Cas9-T2A-mCherry (Addgene; catalogue #64324, red fluorescence selection) plasmids [37,63,64]. These plasmids contain both Cas9 and guide RNA (gRNA) expression cassettes, with BbsI restriction sites for the insertion of gRNA sequences. Prevalidated gRNA sequences were chosen in the GenScript genome-wide database [65] for a non-overlapping duo of gRNAs: 5'-AGCGCACTAAATCGTCTCCA-3' and 5'-GAGTTACCCCAAAGGAATGG-3'. Sticky ends were created for insertion in the vector plasmids, with CACCG at the 5' of the gRNA sense sequence and AAAC at the 5' and C at the 3' of the gRNA antisense sequence.

gRNA oligonucleotides (Eurogentec, Seraing, Belgium) were annealed into double-stranded DNA, with 1 µL of stock solutions containing 100 µM of each sense and antisense oligonucleotides in 2 µL of 5X T4 ligase buffer (Thermo Fisher; catalogue #46300018), 0.5 µL of T4 PNK (BIOKE; catalogue #M0201) and 5.5 µL of DNase/RNase-free distilled water. Incubation times were 37 °C for 30 min, followed by 95 °C for 5 min, and then the temperature was decreased at a rate of 5 °C/min until reaching 25 °C.

The Golden Gate DNA Assembly protocol [66] was then used for inserting 1 µL of annealed gRNA at 1 µM into 100 ng of vector plasmid, in a solution containing 5 µL of 10x Fast Digest buffer (Thermo Fisher; catalogue #B64), 0.5 µL of ATP 0.1 M (Thermo Fisher; catalogue #R1441), 0.5 µL of BSA 10 mg/mL (Promega; catalogue #R396D), 1 µL of restriction enzyme BpiI (Thermo Fisher; catalogue #FD1014), and 2 µL of T4 ligase 5 U/µL (Thermo Fisher; catalogue #EL0014) in a total volume of 50 µL completed with water. The mixture was incubated for 20 cycles at 37 °C for 5 min and 20 °C for 5 min, followed by 80 °C for 20 min.

Five microliters of the resulting solution were used for TOP10 bacteria (Thermo Fisher; catalogue #C404003) transformation using prewarmed LB agar plates (Thermo Fisher; catalogue #22700-025) containing 100 µg/mL of ampicillin, in accordance with the instructions of the manufacturer. Single colonies were inoculated in LB broth (Thermo Fisher; catalogue #12780-052) with 50 µg/mL ampicillin and incubated at 37 °C overnight. Plasmid DNA was then collected with the PureYield Plasmid Miniprep System (Promega; catalogue #A1223), and its concentration was obtained using a NanoDrop device (Thermo Fisher). Sequences were verified by Sanger Sequencing (Genewiz, Leipzig, Germany).

Cancer cells at 70%–80% confluence were transfected with the Lipofectamine LTX/Plus transfection kit (Thermo Fisher; catalogue #15338100) or with the jetOPTIMUS kit (Westburg, Leusden, The Netherlands; catalogue #117-01). The first kit was used with 0.25 µg of each gRNA plasmid, for a total of 0.5 µg of DNA in 100 µL of OptiMEM, containing 0.5 µL of Plus and 2.25 µL of lipofectamine LTX, with incubation times of 15 and 30 min, respectively. The second kit was used with 0.5 µg of each gRNA plasmid, for a total of 1 µg of DNA, with 1 µL of reagent in 200 µL of buffer for each well in a 6-well plate. Cells were selected with puromycin (1 µg/mL)-containing medium for 48–72 h or FACS-sorted for mCherry fluorescence 48 h after transfection on a Becton Dickinson FACSAriaIII system.

Appendix A.3 Cox7b Overexpression

The human untagged *COX7B* cDNA ORF Clone in expression vector pCMV3 (BioConnect; catalogue #HG20762-UT) was used to overexpress Cox7b in MDA-MB-231 cancer cells. Cells at 70–80% confluence were transfected with 10 µg of the plasmid and Lipofectamine 3000 (Thermo Fisher; catalogue #L3000001) in a 10 cm dish, allowed to recover the next day in fresh DMEM containing glutaMAX and 4.5 g/L glucose (Thermo Fisher; catalogue #61965026) supplemented with 10% FBS, and selected with hygromycin (400 µg/mL)-containing medium for 10 days. Medium was renewed every 3–4 days. Colonies were individually picked, expanded, and tested by western blotting for the expression of Cox7b.

Appendix A.4 Cell Migration and Invasion

Invasion was assessed by coating the inserts with 250 μg/mL of Matrigel (Corning, Tewksbury, MA, USA; #356231) for 2 h at 37 °C, and migration without Matrigel coating. Fifty thousand cancer cells were seeded in the upper chamber of each transwell in 500 μL of serum-free culture medium, while the lower chamber contained FBS 1% (general migration/invasion) or confluent nonmalignant astrocytes, hepatocytes, or bronchial cells, which were used as attractants. Cancer cells were allowed to migrate/invade for 24 h at 37 °C in a 5% CO_2 humidified atmosphere. At the end of the assay, cells were fixed with 4% PFA in PBS for 10 min, rinsed three times with PBS, and immobile cells (upper compartment of the insert) were wiped away. Mobile cells were stained with DAPI for 30 min, rinsed three times with PBS, and imaged at 5x on an AxioVert microscope equipped with an AxioCam-MRc camera (Zeiss). Two images were taken per well, thus covering the upper and lower halves. Nuclei were counted using QuPath software version 0.1.2. with the Positive Cell Detection analysis tool.

Appendix A.5 Seahorse Oximetry

Basal, maximal, and ATP-linked oxygen consumption rates (OCRs) were quantified using the XF Cell Mito Stress Test Kit (Agilent) on a Seahorse XF96 bioenergetics analyzer (Agilent). Briefly, 10,000 cells were seeded in XF96 culture plates 16 h before the experiments in DMEM, containing glutaMAX and 4.5 g/L glucose (Thermo Fisher; catalogue #61965026) supplemented with 10% FBS. On the day of analysis, the culture medium was replaced by DMEM containing 10 mM glucose, 2 mM glutamine, 1.85 g/L NaCl, and 3 mg/L phenol red, pH 7.4. Cells were further incubated for 1 h in a CO_2-free incubator before analysis. Sequentially, basal OCR was acquired without treatment, ATP-linked OCR after the addition of 1 μM of ATP synthase inhibitor oligomycin, maximal OCR after mitochondrial potential disruption using 1 μM of ionophore carbonyl cyanide-4-(trifluoromethoxy)phenylhydrazone (FCCP), and non-mitochondrial OCR after the addition of 0.5 μM of Complex I inhibitor rotenone together with 0.5 μM of Complex III inhibitor antimycin A.

Mitochondrial fuel dependency was determined using the Fuel Flex test kit (Agilent) with either 2 μM of mitochondrial pyruvate carrier (MPC) inhibitor UK5099, 3 μM of glutaminase inhibitor BPTES, or 4 μM of carnitine palmitoyltransferase-1 (CPT-1) inhibitor etomoxir, to challenge oxidative glucose metabolism, glutaminolysis, and lipolysis, respectively.

Mitochondrial OCRs (mtOCRs) were calculated by subtracting non-mitochondrial OCRs from the corresponding basal, maximal, and ATP-linked OCRs. Respiration used for ATP production is the difference between basal OCR and OCR in the presence of ATP-synthase inhibitor oligomycin. All data were normalized by the total protein content.

References

1. Weiss, F.; Lauffenburger, D.; Friedl, P. Towards targeting of shared mechanisms of cancer metastasis and therapy resistance. *Nat. Rev. Cancer* **2022**, *22*, 157–173. [CrossRef] [PubMed]
2. Seoane, J.; De Mattos-Arruda, L. Brain metastasis: New opportunities to tackle therapeutic resistance. *Mol. Oncol.* **2014**, *8*, 1120–1131. [CrossRef] [PubMed]
3. Kuksis, M.; Gao, Y.; Tran, W.; Hoey, C.; Kiss, A.; Komorowski, A.S.; Dhaliwal, A.J.; Sahgal, A.; Das, S.; Chan, K.K.; et al. The incidence of brain metastases among patients with metastatic breast cancer: A systematic review and meta-analysis. *Neuro. Oncol.* **2021**, *23*, 894–904. [CrossRef] [PubMed]
4. Dent, R.; Trudeau, M.; Pritchard, K.I.; Hanna, W.M.; Kahn, H.K.; Sawka, C.A.; Lickley, L.A.; Rawlinson, E.; Sun, P.; Narod, S.A. Triple-negative breast cancer: Clinical features and patterns of recurrence. *Clin. Cancer. Res.* **2007**, *13*, 4429–4434. [CrossRef]
5. Hugo, H.S.; Cortes, J.; Cescon, D.W.; Im, S.; Md Yusof, M.; Gallardo, C.; Lipatov, O.; Barrios, C.H.; Perez-Garcia, J.; Iwata, H.; et al. KEYNOTE-355: Final results from a randomized, double-blind phase III study of first-line pembrolizumab + chemotherapy vs placebo + chemotherapy for metastatic TNBC. *Annals Oncol.* **2021**, *32* (Suppl. 5), S1283–S1346.
6. Gennari, A.; Stockler, M.; Puntoni, M.; Sormani, M.; Nanni, O.; Amadori, D.; Wilcken, N.; D'Amico, M.; DeCensi, A.; Bruzzi, P. Duration of chemotherapy for metastatic breast cancer: A systematic review and meta-analysis of randomized clinical trials. *J. Clin. Oncol.* **2011**, *29*, 2144–2149. [CrossRef]
7. Damsky, W.E.; Rosenbaum, L.E.; Bosenberg, M. Decoding melanoma metastasis. *Cancers* **2010**, *3*, 126–163. [CrossRef]

8. Blecker, D.; Abraham, S.; Furth, E.E.; Kochman, M.L. Melanoma in the gastrointestinal tract. *Am. J. Gastroenterol.* **1999**, *94*, 3427–3433. [CrossRef]
9. Tas, F. Metastatic behavior in melanoma: Timing, pattern, survival, and influencing factors. *J. Oncol.* **2012**, *2012*, 647684. [CrossRef]
10. Lin, N.U.; Claus, E.; Sohl, J.; Razzak, A.R.; Arnaout, A.; Winer, E.P. Sites of distant recurrence and clinical outcomes in patients with metastatic triple-negative breast cancer: High incidence of central nervous system metastases. *Cancer* **2008**, *113*, 2638–2645. [CrossRef]
11. Jin, J.; Gao, Y.; Zhang, J.; Wang, L.; Wang, B.; Cao, J.; Shao, Z.; Wang, Z. Incidence, pattern and prognosis of brain metastases in patients with metastatic triple negative breast cancer. *BMC Cancer* **2018**, *18*, 446. [CrossRef]
12. Patrawala, L.; Calhoun, T.; Schneider-Broussard, R.; Li, H.; Bhatia, B.; Tang, S.; Reilly, J.G.; Chandra, D.; Zhou, J.; Claypool, K.; et al. Highly purified CD44+ prostate cancer cells from xenograft human tumors are enriched in tumorigenic and metastatic progenitor cells. *Oncogene* **2006**, *25*, 1696–1708. [CrossRef] [PubMed]
13. Capeloa, T.; Krzystyniak, J.; d'Hose, D.; Canas Rodriguez, A.; Payen, V.L.; Zampieri, L.X.; Van de Velde, J.A.; Benyahia, Z.; Pranzini, E.; Vazeille, T.; et al. MitoQ inhibits human breast cancer cell migration, invasion and clonogenicity. *Cancers* **2022**, *14*, 1516. [CrossRef] [PubMed]
14. Paget, S. The distribution of secondary growths in cancer of the breast. *Cancer Metastasis Rev.* **1889**, *8*, 98–101. [CrossRef]
15. Ribelles, N.; Santonja, A.; Pajares, B.; Llacer, C.; Alba, E. The seed and soil hypothesis revisited: Current state of knowledge of inherited genes on prognosis in breast cancer. *Cancer Treat. Rev.* **2014**, *40*, 293–299. [CrossRef] [PubMed]
16. Jang, A.; Hill, R.P. An examination of the effects of hypoxia, acidosis, and glucose starvation on the expression of metastasis-associated genes in murine tumor cells. *Clin. Exp. Metastasis* **1997**, *15*, 469–483. [CrossRef]
17. Vaupel, P. The role of hypoxia-induced factors in tumor progression. *Oncologist* **2004**, *9* (Suppl. 5), 10–17. [CrossRef]
18. Lunt, S.J.; Chaudary, N.; Hill, R.P. The tumor microenvironment and metastatic disease. *Clin. Exp. Metastasis* **2009**, *26*, 19–34. [CrossRef]
19. Gilkes, D.M.; Semenza, G.L.; Wirtz, D. Hypoxia and the extracellular matrix: Drivers of tumour metastasis. *Nat. Rev. Cancer* **2014**, *14*, 430–439. [CrossRef]
20. Rankin, E.B.; Giaccia, A.J. Hypoxic control of metastasis. *Science* **2016**, *352*, 175–180. [CrossRef]
21. Payen, V.L.; Porporato, P.E.; Baselet, B.; Sonveaux, P. Metabolic changes associated with tumor metastasis, part 1: Tumor pH, glycolysis and the pentose phosphate pathway. *Cell. Mol. Life Sci.* **2016**, *73*, 1333–1348. [CrossRef] [PubMed]
22. Porporato, P.E.; Payen, V.L.; Baselet, B.; Sonveaux, P. Metabolic changes associated with tumor metastasis, part 2: Mitochondria, lipid and amino acid metabolism. *Cell. Mol. Life Sci.* **2016**, *73*, 1349–1363. [CrossRef] [PubMed]
23. DeClerck, K.; Elble, R.C. The role of hypoxia and acidosis in promoting metastasis and resistance to chemotherapy. *Front. Biosci.* **2010**, *15*, 213–225. [CrossRef] [PubMed]
24. Pietila, M.; Ivaska, J.; Mani, S.A. Whom to blame for metastasis, the epithelial-mesenchymal transition or the tumor microenvironment? *Cancer Lett.* **2016**, *380*, 359–368. [CrossRef]
25. Klein, C.A. Selection and adaptation during metastatic cancer progression. *Nature* **2013**, *501*, 365–372. [CrossRef]
26. Gupta, G.P.; Massague, J. Cancer metastasis: Building a framework. *Cell* **2006**, *127*, 679–695. [CrossRef]
27. Kaplan, R.N.; Riba, R.D.; Zacharoulis, S.; Bramley, A.H.; Vincent, L.; Costa, C.; MacDonald, D.D.; Jin, D.K.; Shido, K.; Kerns, S.A.; et al. VEGFR1-positive haematopoietic bone marrow progenitors initiate the pre-metastatic niche. *Nature* **2005**, *438*, 820–827. [CrossRef]
28. Peinado, H.; Zhang, H.; Matei, I.R.; Costa-Silva, B.; Hoshino, A.; Rodrigues, G.; Psaila, B.; Kaplan, R.N.; Bromberg, J.F.; Kang, Y.; et al. Pre-metastatic niches: Organ-specific homes for metastases. *Nat. Rev. Cancer* **2017**, *17*, 302–317. [CrossRef]
29. Laubli, H.; Borsig, L. Selectins promote tumor metastasis. *Semin. Cancer Biol.* **2010**, *20*, 169–177. [CrossRef]
30. Sevenich, L.; Bowman, R.L.; Mason, S.D.; Quail, D.F.; Rapaport, F.; Elie, B.T.; Brogi, E.; Brastianos, P.K.; Hahn, W.C.; Holsinger, L.J.; et al. Analysis of tumour- and stroma-supplied proteolytic networks reveals a brain-metastasis-promoting role for cathepsin S. *Nat. Cell Biol.* **2014**, *16*, 876–888. [CrossRef]
31. Porporato, P.E.; Payen, V.L.; Perez-Escuredo, J.; De Saedeleer, C.J.; Danhier, P.; Copetti, T.; Dhup, S.; Tardy, M.; Vazeille, T.; Bouzin, C.; et al. A mitochondrial switch promotes tumor metastasis. *Cell Rep.* **2014**, *8*, 754–766. [CrossRef]
32. Capeloa, T.; Krzystyniak, J.; Canas Rodriguez, A.; Payen, V.L.; Zampieri, L.X.; Pranzini, E.; Derouane, F.; Vazeille, T.; Bouzin, C.; Duhoux, F.P.; et al. MitoQ prevents human breast cancer recurrence and lung metastasis in mice. *Cancers* **2022**, *14*, 1488. [CrossRef] [PubMed]
33. Ishikawa, K.; Takenaga, K.; Akimoto, M.; Koshikawa, N.; Yamaguchi, A.; Imanishi, H.; Nakada, K.; Honma, Y.; Hayashi, J. ROS-generating mitochondrial DNA mutations can regulate tumor cell metastasis. *Science* **2008**, *320*, 661–664. [CrossRef] [PubMed]
34. Yoneda, T.; Williams, P.J.; Hiraga, T.; Niewolna, M.; Nishimura, R. A bone-seeking clone exhibits different biological properties from the MDA-MB-231 parental human breast cancer cells and a brain-seeking clone in vivo and in vitro. *J. Bone Miner. Res.* **2001**, *16*, 1486–1495. [CrossRef] [PubMed]
35. Patel, J.B.; Appaiah, H.N.; Burnett, R.M.; Bhat-Nakshatri, P.; Wang, G.; Mehta, R.; Badve, S.; Thomson, M.J.; Hammond, S.; Steeg, P.; et al. Control of EVI-1 oncogene expression in metastatic breast cancer cells through microRNA miR-22. *Oncogene* **2011**, *30*, 1290–1301. [CrossRef] [PubMed]

36. Burnett, R.M.; Craven, K.E.; Krishnamurthy, P.; Goswami, C.P.; Badve, S.; Crooks, P.; Mathews, W.P.; Bhat-Nakshatri, P.; Nakshatri, H. Organ-specific adaptive signaling pathway activation in metastatic breast cancer cells. *Oncotarget* **2015**, *6*, 12682–12696. [CrossRef]
37. Ran, F.A.; Hsu, P.D.; Wright, J.; Agarwala, V.; Scott, D.A.; Zhang, F. Genome engineering using the CRISPR-Cas9 system. *Nat. Protoc.* **2013**, *8*, 2281–2308. [CrossRef]
38. Piret, J.P.; Vankoningsloo, S.; Mejia, J.; Noel, F.; Boilan, E.; Lambinon, F.; Zouboulis, C.C.; Masereel, B.; Lucas, S.; Saout, C.; et al. Differential toxicity of copper (II) oxide nanoparticles of similar hydrodynamic diameter on human differentiated intestinal Caco-2 cell monolayers is correlated in part to copper release and shape. *Nanotoxicology* **2012**, *6*, 789–803. [CrossRef]
39. Grasso, D.; Medeiros, H.C.D.; Zampieri, L.X.; Bol, V.; Danhier, P.; van Gisbergen, M.W.; Bouzin, C.; Brusa, D.; Gregoire, V.; Smeets, H.; et al. Fitter mitochondria are associated with radioresistance in human head and neck SQD9 cancer cells. *Front. Pharmacol.* **2020**, *11*, 263. [CrossRef]
40. Li, H.; Durbin, R. Fast and accurate short read alignment with Burrows-Wheeler transform. *Bioinformatics* **2009**, *25*, 1754–1760. [CrossRef]
41. Van Hee, V.F.; Perez-Escuredo, J.; Cacace, A.; Copetti, T.; Sonveaux, P. Lactate does not activate NF-kappaB in oxidative tumor cells. *Front. Pharmacol.* **2015**, *6*, 228. [CrossRef]
42. Bankhead, P.; Loughrey, M.B.; Fernandez, J.A.; Dombrowski, Y.; McArt, D.G.; Dunne, P.D.; McQuaid, S.; Gray, R.T.; Murray, L.J.; Coleman, H.G.; et al. QuPath: Open source software for digital pathology image analysis. *Sci. Rep.* **2017**, *7*, 16878. [CrossRef] [PubMed]
43. Gyorffy, B. Survival analysis across the entire transcriptome identifies biomarkers with the highest prognostic power in breast cancer. *Comput. Struct. Biotechnol. J.* **2021**, *19*, 4101–4109. [CrossRef] [PubMed]
44. Vaz, F.M.; Fouchier, S.W.; Ofman, R.; Sommer, M.; Wanders, R.J. Molecular and biochemical characterization of rat gamma-trimethylaminobutyraldehyde dehydrogenase and evidence for the involvement of human aldehyde dehydrogenase 9 in carnitine biosynthesis. *J. Biol. Chem.* **2000**, *275*, 7390–7394. [CrossRef] [PubMed]
45. Zhao, D.; McCaffery, P.; Ivins, K.J.; Neve, R.L.; Hogan, P.; Chin, W.W.; Drager, U.C. Molecular identification of a major retinoic-acid-synthesizing enzyme, a retinaldehyde-specific dehydrogenase. *Eur. J. Biochem.* **1996**, *240*, 15–22. [CrossRef]
46. Schmidt, C.; Sciacovelli, M.; Frezza, C. Fumarate hydratase in cancer: A multifaceted tumour suppressor. *Semin. Cell. Dev. Biol.* **2020**, *98*, 15–25. [CrossRef]
47. Zhu, J.; Vinothkumar, K.R.; Hirst, J. Structure of mammalian respiratory complex I. *Nature* **2016**, *536*, 354–358. [CrossRef]
48. Kadenbach, B.; Huttemann, M. The subunit composition and function of mammalian cytochrome c oxidase. *Mitochondrion* **2015**, *24*, 64–76. [CrossRef]
49. Tsukihara, T.; Aoyama, H.; Yamashita, E.; Tomizaki, T.; Yamaguchi, H.; Shinzawa-Itoh, K.; Nakashima, R.; Yaono, R.; Yoshikawa, S. The whole structure of the 13-subunit oxidized cytochrome c oxidase at 2.8 A. *Science* **1996**, *272*, 1136–1144. [CrossRef]
50. Nakhjavani, M.; Samarasinghe, R.M.; Shigdar, S. Triple-negative breast cancer brain metastasis: An update on druggable targets, current clinical trials, and future treatment options. *Drug Discov. Today* **2022**, *27*, 1298–1314. [CrossRef]
51. Kadenbach, B.; Jarausch, J.; Hartmann, R.; Merle, P. Separation of mammalian cytochrome c oxidase into 13 polypeptides by a sodium dodecyl sulfate-gel electrophoretic procedure. *Anal. Biochem.* **1983**, *129*, 517–521. [CrossRef]
52. Kuhn-Nentwig, L.; Kadenbach, B. Immunological identification of four different polypeptides in 'subunit VII' of mammalian cytochrome c oxidase. *FEBS Lett.* **1984**, *172*, 189–192. [CrossRef]
53. Cunatova, K.; Reguera, D.P.; Houstek, J.; Mracek, T.; Pecina, P. Role of cytochrome c oxidase nuclear-encoded subunits in health and disease. *Physiol. Res.* **2020**, *69*, 947–965. [CrossRef] [PubMed]
54. Indrieri, A.; van Rahden, V.A.; Tiranti, V.; Morleo, M.; Iaconis, D.; Tammaro, R.; D'Amato, I.; Conte, I.; Maystadt, I.; Demuth, S.; et al. Mutations in COX7B cause microphthalmia with linear skin lesions, an unconventional mitochondrial disease. *Am. J. Hum. Genet.* **2012**, *91*, 942–949. [CrossRef] [PubMed]
55. Jolly, M.K.; Ware, K.E.; Gilja, S.; Somarelli, J.A.; Levine, H. EMT and MET: Necessary or permissive for metastasis? *Mol. Oncol.* **2017**, *11*, 755–769. [CrossRef] [PubMed]
56. Perez-Escuredo, J.; Van Hee, V.F.; Sboarina, M.; Falces, J.; Payen, V.L.; Pellerin, L.; Sonveaux, P. Monocarboxylate transporters in the brain and in cancer. *Biochim. Biophys. Acta* **2016**, *1863*, 2481–2497. [CrossRef]
57. Mashimo, T.; Pichumani, K.; Vemireddy, V.; Hatanpaa, K.J.; Singh, D.K.; Sirasanagandla, S.; Nannepaga, S.; Piccirillo, S.G.; Kovacs, Z.; Foong, C.; et al. Acetate is a bioenergetic substrate for human glioblastoma and brain metastases. *Cell* **2014**, *159*, 1603–1614. [CrossRef]
58. Bergers, G.; Fendt, S.M. The metabolism of cancer cells during metastasis. *Nat. Rev. Cancer* **2021**, *21*, 162–180. [CrossRef]
59. Martin, A.M.; Cagney, D.N.; Catalano, P.J.; Warren, L.E.; Bellon, J.R.; Punglia, R.S.; Claus, E.B.; Lee, E.Q.; Wen, P.Y.; Haas-Kogan, D.A.; et al. Brain metastases in newly diagnosed breast cancer: A population-based study. *JAMA Oncol.* **2017**, *3*, 1069–1077. [CrossRef]
60. O'Reilly, D.; Sendi, M.A.; Kelly, C.M. Overview of recent advances in metastatic triple negative breast cancer. *World J. Clin. Oncol.* **2021**, *12*, 164–182. [CrossRef]
61. Wang, C.; Luo, D. The metabolic adaptation mechanism of metastatic organotropism. *Exp. Hematol. Oncol.* **2021**, *10*, 30. [CrossRef] [PubMed]

62. Tanaka, N.; Katayama, S.; Reddy, A.; Nishimura, K.; Niwa, N.; Hongo, H.; Ogihara, K.; Kosaka, T.; Mizuno, R.; Kikuchi, E.; et al. Single-cell RNA-seq analysis reveals the platinum resistance gene COX7B and the surrogate marker CD63. *Cancer Med.* **2018**, *7*, 6193–6204. [CrossRef] [PubMed]
63. Cong, L.; Ran, F.A.; Cox, D.; Lin, S.; Barretto, R.; Habib, N.; Hsu, P.D.; Wu, X.; Jiang, W.; Marraffini, L.A.; et al. Multiplex genome engineering using CRISPR/Cas systems. *Science* **2013**, *339*, 819–823. [CrossRef] [PubMed]
64. Chu, V.T.; Weber, T.; Wefers, B.; Wurst, W.; Sander, S.; Rajewsky, K.; Kuhn, R. Increasing the efficiency of homology-directed repair for CRISPR-Cas9-induced precise gene editing in mammalian cells. *Nat. Biotechnol.* **2015**, *33*, 543–548. [CrossRef]
65. Sanjana, N.E.; Shalem, O.; Zhang, F. Improved vectors and genome-wide libraries for CRISPR screening. *Nat. Methods* **2014**, *11*, 783–784. [CrossRef]
66. Engler, C.; Kandzia, R.; Marillonnet, S. A one pot, one step, precision cloning method with high throughput capability. *PLoS ONE* **2008**, *3*, e3647. [CrossRef]

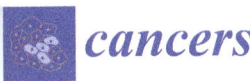

Article

Connected-SegNets: A Deep Learning Model for Breast Tumor Segmentation from X-ray Images

Mohammad Alkhaleefah [1,†], Tan-Hsu Tan [1,†], Chuan-Hsun Chang [2,*], Tzu-Chuan Wang [1], Shang-Chih Ma [1], Lena Chang [3] and Yang-Lang Chang [1,*]

1 Department of Electrical Engineering, National Taipei University of Technology, Taipei 10608, Taiwan
2 Division of General Surgery, Cheng Hsin General Hospital, Taipei 112, Taiwan
3 Department of Communications, Navigation and Control Engineering, National Taiwan Ocean University, Keelung 202301, Taiwan
* Correspondence: ch6358@chgh.org.tw (C.-H.C.); ylchang@ntut.edu.tw (Y.-L.C.)
† These authors contributed equally to this work.

Simple Summary: The segmentation of breast tumors is an important step in identifying and classifying benign and malignant tumors in X-ray images. Mammography screening has proven to be an effective tool for breast cancer diagnosis. However, the inspection of breast mammograms for early-stage cancer can be a challenging task due to the complicated structure of dense breasts. Several deep learning models have been proposed to overcome this particular issue; however, the false positive and false negative rates are still high. Hence, this study introduced a deep learning model, called Connected-SegNets, that combines two SegNet architectures with skip connections to provide a robust model to reduce false positive and false negative rates for breast tumor segmentation from mammograms.

Citation: Alkhaleefah, A.; Tan, T.-H.; Chang, C.-H.; Wang, T.-C.; Ma, S.-C.; Chang, L.; Chang, Y.-L. Connected-SegNets: A Deep Learning Model for Breast Tumor Segmentation from X-ray Images. *Cancers* 2022, 14, 4030. https://doi.org/10.3390/cancers14164030

Academic Editors: Enrico Cassano and Filippo Pesapane

Received: 18 July 2022
Accepted: 18 August 2022
Published: 20 August 2022
Corrected: 11 April 2023

Publisher's Note: MDPI stays neutral with regard to jurisdictional claims in published maps and institutional affiliations.

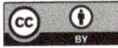

Copyright: © 2022 by the authors. Licensee MDPI, Basel, Switzerland. This article is an open access article distributed under the terms and conditions of the Creative Commons Attribution (CC BY) license (https://creativecommons.org/licenses/by/4.0/).

Abstract: Inspired by Connected-UNets, this study proposes a deep learning model, called Connected-SegNets, for breast tumor segmentation from X-ray images. In the proposed model, two SegNet architectures are connected with skip connections between their layers. Moreover, the cross-entropy loss function of the original SegNet has been replaced by the intersection over union (IoU) loss function in order to make the proposed model more robust against noise during the training process. As part of data preprocessing, a histogram equalization technique, called contrast limit adapt histogram equalization (CLAHE), is applied to all datasets to enhance the compressed regions and smooth the distribution of the pixels. Additionally, two image augmentation methods, namely rotation and flipping, are used to increase the amount of training data and to prevent overfitting. The proposed model has been evaluated on two publicly available datasets, specifically INbreast and the curated breast imaging subset of digital database for screening mammography (CBIS-DDSM). The proposed model has also been evaluated using a private dataset obtained from Cheng Hsin General Hospital in Taiwan. The experimental results show that the proposed Connected-SegNets model outperforms the state-of-the-art methods in terms of Dice score and IoU score. The proposed Connected-SegNets produces a maximum Dice score of 96.34% on the INbreast dataset, 92.86% on the CBIS-DDSM dataset, and 92.25% on the private dataset. Furthermore, the experimental results show that the proposed model achieves the highest IoU score of 91.21%, 87.34%, and 83.71% on INbreast, CBIS-DDSM, and the private dataset, respectively.

Keywords: breast tumor segmentation; convolutional neural network; deep learning; X-ray images

1. Introduction

The United States of America reported a total of 43,250 female deaths and 530 male deaths due to breast cancer in 2022 [1]. Researchers are motivated by these statistics to develop accurate tools for early breast cancer diagnosis, which will offer physicians more options for treatment. Mammograms are still being widely used to detect the presence of any abnormalities in breasts [2–4]. Mammogram images show different types of breast tissues as pixel clusters with different intensities [5]. These tissues include fiber-glandular, fatty, and pectoral muscle tissues [6]. On mammography, abnormal tissues such as lesions, tumors, lumps, masses, or calcifications may be indicators of breast cancer [7,8]. However, there is always the possibility of human error when analyzing and diagnosing breast cancer due to dense breasts and the high variability between patients [9–11]. Additionally, mammography screening sensitivity is affected by image quality and radiologist experience [12,13].

Automated techniques are being developed to analyze and diagnose breast mammograms with the goal of counteracting this variability and standardizing diagnostic procedures [14,15]. The rapid emergence of artificial intelligence (AI) and deep learning (DL) has significant implications for breast cancer diagnosis [16–18]. The advancements in image segmentation using convolutional neural networks (CNNs) have been applied to segment breast cancer from X-ray images [19–23]. The earlier works on mass segmentation faced some challenges, such as low signal to noise ratio, indiscernible mass boundaries, high false positives, and high false negative rates. To address these challenges, one study proposed a deeply supervised UNet model (DS U-Net) coupled with dense conditional random fields (CRFs) for lesion segmentation from whole mammograms [19]. The DS U-Net model has produced a Dice score of 79% on the INbreast dataset and 83% on the CBIS-DDSM dataset, whereas its IoU score is 83% and 86% on the INbreast and CBIS-DDSM datasets, respectively. Another study [20] proposed an attention-guided dense up-sampling network (AU-Net) for accurate breast mass segmentation from mammograms. An asymmetrical encoder–decoder structure is employed in this AU-Net and it uses an effective up-sampling block and attention-guided dense up-sampling block (AU block). The AU block is designed to have three merits. First, dense upsampling compensates for the information loss experienced during bilinear up-sampling. Second, it integrates high- and low-level features more effectively. Third, it highlights channels with rich information via the channel attention function. Compared to the state-of-the-art FCNs, AU-Net achieved the best performance, with a Dice score of 90% on the INbreast dataset and 89% on the CBIS-DDSM dataset.

However, such models do not capture the features of different scales of masses effectively, and therefore they suffer from low segmentation accuracy. Hence, a new model, called UNet, was presented to mitigate the limitations of the previous models [21]. UNet integrates the high-level features of the encoder with the low-level features of the decoder. Through skip connections, the UNet architecture was able to maintain this form of fusion for a variety of medical applications. The UNet architecture achieves better performance on different biomedical segmentation applications. Asma Baccouche et al. [22] introduced Connected-UNets to segment breast masses. This method integrated atrous spatial pyramid pooling (ASPP) in the two standard UNets. The architecture of Connected-UNets was built on the attention network (AUNet) and residual network (ResUNet). To augment and enhance the images, cycle-consistent generative adversarial networks (CycleGANs) were used between two unpaired datasets. Additionally, a regional deep learning approach called you-only-look-once (YOLO) has been used to detect breast lesions from mammograms. Finally, a full-resolution convolutional network (FrCN) has been implemented to segment breast lesions. The Connected-UNets model has produced a Dice score of 94% and 92% on the INbreast and CBIS-DDSM datasets, respectively. Moreover, it has achieved an IoU score of 90% and 86% on INbreast and CBIS-DDSM, respectively. Badrinarayanan et al. [23] proposed a practical deep fully convolutional neural network architecture for semantic pixel-wise segmentation, termed SegNet. Its segmentation architecture consists of an encoder network and a decoder network followed by a pixel-wise classification layer. Topologically, the architecture of the encoder network matches that of the 13 convolutional layers in the VGG16 network. The role of the decoder network is to map the low-resolution encoder feature maps to full-input-resolution feature maps for pixel-wise classification.

The SegNet model has achieved satisfactory segmentation performance. However, since the SegNet architecture does not consist of skip connections, incorporating fine multiscale information during the training process is challenging.

This study combines the characteristics of the Connected-UNets and SegNet models to form Connected-SegNets from two standard SegNets with skip connections for breast tumor segmentation from breast mammograms. The flow chart of the proposed system is illustrated in Figure 1. The major contributions of this study include the following.

1. This study proposes a deep learning model called Connected-SegNets for breast tumor segmentation from X-ray images.
2. The proposed model, Connected-SegNets, is designed using skip connections, which helps to recover the spatial information lost during the pooling operations.
3. The original SegNet cross-entropy loss function has been replaced by the IoU loss function to overcome any noisy features and enhance the detection of the false negative and false positive cases.
4. The histogram equalization method of the contrast limit adapt histogram equalization (CLAHE) is applied to all datasets to enhance the compressed areas and smooth the pixel distribution.
5. Image augmentation methods including rotation and flipping have been used to increase the number of training data and to reduce the impact of overfitting.

The rest of this paper is organized as follows. Section 2 describes the datasets and architectural details of the proposed method. Section 3 presents the experimental results. Section 4 discusses the merits of this study. Finally, the article is concluded with its primary findings in Section 5.

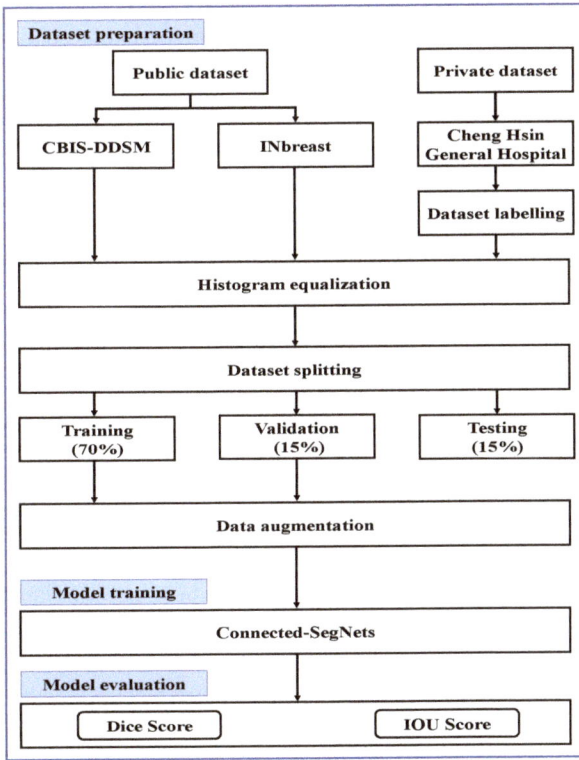

Figure 1. Flow chart of the proposed tumor segmentation system.

2. Materials and Methods

This research uses the two publicly available datasets of INbreast and CBIS-DDSM, and one private dataset obtained from Cheng Hsin General Hospital in Taiwan. Initially, a histogram equalization, CLAHE, is applied to all datasets to enhance the compressed areas and smooth the pixel distribution. Then, each X-ray dataset is randomly divided into 70%, 15%, and 15% for training, validation, and testing, respectively. Finally, the training and validation samples are augmented to increase the amount of data before feeding them to the proposed Connected-SegNets model.

2.1. Datasets

The proposed model, Connected-SegNets, has been evaluated on the following datasets.

2.1.1. INbreast Dataset

The INbreast dataset is a collection of mammograms from Centro de Mama Hospital de S. João, Breast Centres Network, Porto, Portugal. A total of 410 images with 115 cases were collected from August 2008 to July 2010 [24,25], and 95 of 115 cancer cases involved both breasts in women. Four different types of breast diseases are recorded in the database, including calcification, mass, distortions, and asymmetries. This database includes images from craniocaudal (CC) and mediolateral oblique (MLO) perspectives. Moreover, the breast density is divided into four categories according to the breast imaging reporting and data system (BI-RADS) assessment categories, which are: entirely fat (BI-RADS 1), scattered fibroglandular (BI-RADS 2), heterogeneously dense (BI-RADS 3), and extremely dense (BI-RADS 4). All the images were saved in two sizes: 3328×4084 or 2560×3328 pixels. Among the 410 mammograms, 107 images contain breast tumors. Hence, these 107 images were selected for this study. The 107 images were randomly split into 90 images for training and 17 images for testing, as shown in Table 1. The image augmentation methods, including rotation and flipping, were applied to the training data. The augmentation methods increased the number of breast tumor mammography images to 720 images. The 720 images were randomly split into 576 images for training data and 174 images for validation data, as shown in Table 2.

2.1.2. CBIS-DDSM Dataset

The DDSM is a public dataset provided by the University of South Florida Computer Science and Engineering Department, Sandia National Laboratories, and Massachusetts General Hospital [26]. The CBIS-DDSM is an updated and standardized version of the DDSM [27]. It contains a variety of pathologically verified cases, including malignant, benign, and normal cases. DDSM is an extremely useful database for the development and testing of computer-aided diagnosis (CAD) systems due to its scale and the ground truth validation it offers. The CBIS-DDSM collection includes a subset of the DDSM data organized by expert radiologists. It also comprises pathological diagnosis, bounding boxes, and region of interest (ROI) segmentation for training data. Among all mammography images with tumors in the CBIS-DDSM dataset, 838 images were selected for this study. The 838 images were randomly split into 728 images for training data and 110 images for testing data, as shown in Table 1. The image augmentation methods, including rotation and flipping, were applied to the training samples. Through image augmentation, the number of breast tumor mammography images was increased to 5824. The 5824 images were randomly split into 4659 images for training data and 1165 images for validation data, as shown in Table 2.

2.1.3. Private Dataset

The private dataset comprised mammography images from the Cheng Hsin General Hospital, Taipei City, Taiwan. Initially, VGG image annotator (VIA) software was used by an expert radiologist from the department of medical imaging to mark the tumor location based on the pathological data [28]. Then, all the labeled images were verified and confirmed by the department of hematology and oncology. Finally, the dataset was de-identified for patient privacy. A total of 196 mammography images were collected from January 2019 to December 2019. All the mammograms consist of tumors with a grade of breast imaging reporting and data system assessment category 4 (BIRADS 4) or higher. A total of 196 mammography images were randomly split into 148 images for training and 48 images for testing, as shown in Table 1. The image augmentation methods, including rotation and flipping, were applied to the training samples. Through image augmentation methods, the number of breast tumor mammography images was increased to 1184. The 1184 images were randomly split into 947 images for training and 237 images for validation, as shown in Table 2.

Table 1. Distribution of the mammography datasets.

Dataset	Raw ROIs	Training Samples	Testing Samples
INbreast dataset	107	90	17
CBIS-DDSM dataset	838	728	110
Private dataset	196	148	48
Total	1141	966	175

Table 2. The number of training and validation samples before and after data augmentation.

Dataset	Raw Images	Augmented Images	Training	Validation
INbreast Dataset	90	720	576	144
CBIS-DDSM dataset	728	5824	4659	1165
Private dataset	148	1184	947	237
Total	966	7728	6182	1546

2.2. Data Preprocessing

This research study only focused on the segmentation step. Initially, the ROI of the tumor was cropped manually. The ROI of the tumor was resized into 256×256. In order to eliminate additional noise and degradation caused by the scanning process of digital X-ray mammography, all images were preprocessed [29,30].

2.2.1. Histogram Equalization

Histogram equalization is a well-known technique widely used for contrast enhancement [31]. It is used in a variety of applications, including medical image processing and radar signal processing, due to its simple function and effectiveness [32–35]. Histogram equalization well distributes the pixels over the full dynamic intensity range. One drawback of histogram equalization is that the background noise can be increased when the image is too bright or too dark in the local area after the histogram equalization, which is mainly due to the flattening property of the histogram equalization. This study applied the local histogram equalization method called CLAHE to address the above challenges. CLAHE is an adaptive extension of histogram equalization. It helps in the dynamic preservation of the local contrast features of an image. CLAHE has been applied to all datasets of this study. The sample results on the datasets after applying the CLAHE are shown in Figure 2. From Figure 2, it is noted that the edges of the tumors became clearer after applying the CLAHE technique. A total of 107, 838, and 196 ROIs were obtained from the INbreast, CBIS-DDSM, and the private datasets, respectively. The complete details of the mammography datasets are listed in Table 1.

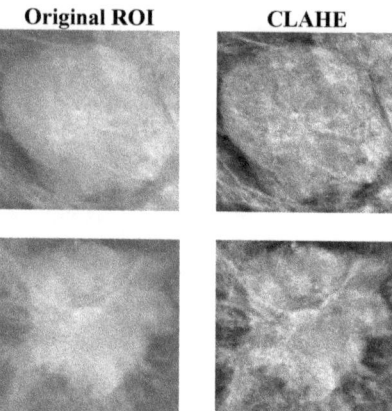

Figure 2. Sample results after applying the histogram equalization (CLAHE) to random ROI images from the datasets.

2.2.2. Image Augmentation

The most common problem that DL models might face is the overfitting problem due to the limited amount of training samples [36–38]. As a result of overfitting, a model might detect or classify features derived from the training samples, but the same model will not be able to detect or classify features derived from unseen samples. To address the issue of overfitting, this study has used two image augmentation methods, namely rotation and flipping. First, bi-linear interpolation has been used to rotate each image around its center point by a value of 90° degrees counter-clockwise up to 360°. By using the bi-linear interpolation method, the rotated image has the same aspect ratio as the original image, without losing any part of the image. Second, mirroring or flipping is the simplest augmentation approach. It results in a dataset with twice as many images. The flipping technique is basically the same as the rotation technique; however, it transforms rotation in the reverse direction. The sample results on the datasets after applying the augmentation methods are shown in Figure 3.

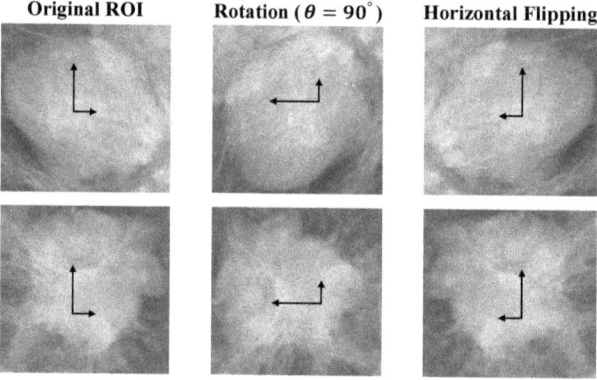

Figure 3. Random sample results after applying the rotation and flipping augmentation methods on the original ROIs. Arrows refer to the direction of the image.

The raw ROIs of the training data were augmented by rotating at an angle of 90° and horizontal flipping. Hence, a total of 720, 5824, and 1184 ROIs were generated from the INbreast, CBIS-DDSM, and private datasets, respectively. Then, the data were randomly split into training and validation. Detailed information of the mammography datasets in terms of the training data is provided in Table 2.

2.3. Proposed Model

SegNet can record pooling indices when applying Max pooling. These pooling indices are used to up-sample the images to the original size. Hence, the required graphics processing unit (GPU) memory for training the model can be lower. Inspired by the success of SegNet and Connected-UNets, this research proposed a model, called Connected-SegNets, which connects two standard SegNets using additional adapted skip connections. The overall architecture of the proposed Connected-SegNets model is shown in Figure 4.

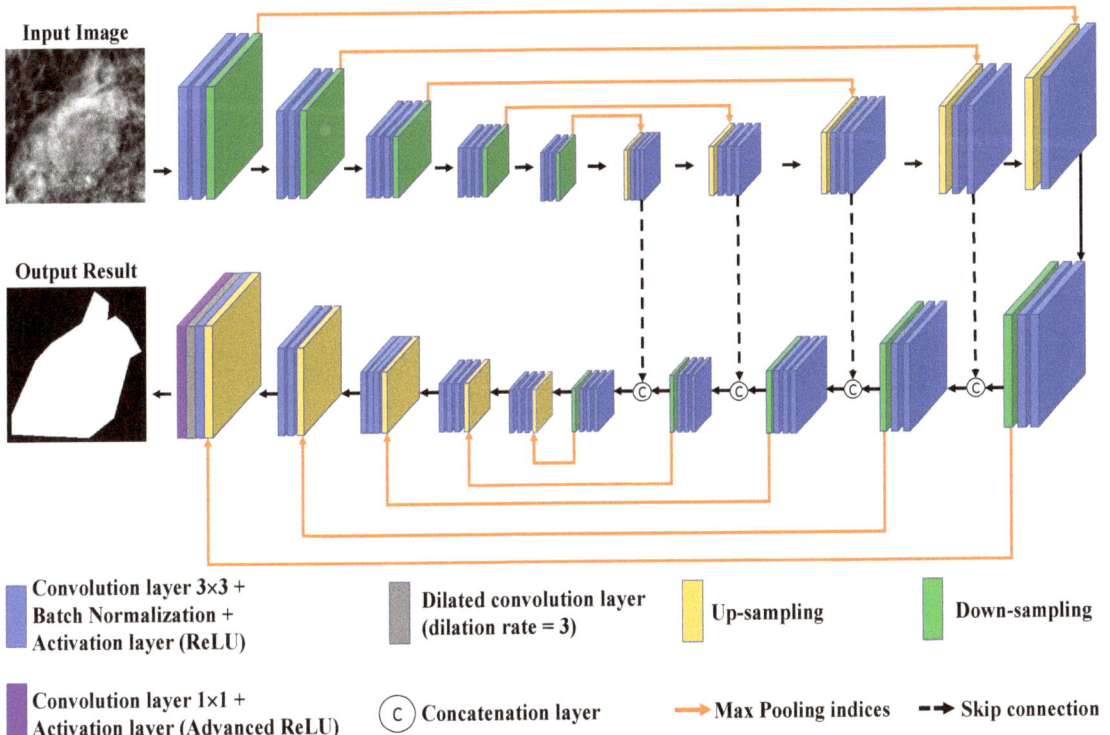

Figure 4. Architecture of the proposed Connected-SegNets model.

The proposed model consists of two encoder and two decoder networks. The first decoder network and the second encoder network are connected with additional skip connections after cascading a second SegNet. This helps to recover the fine-grained features that are lost in the encoding of the SegNet and apply them to encode the high-resolution features by connecting them to the previously decoded features. The proposed Connected-SegNets architecture is deepened by stacking two SegNets. The upper half of the proposed architecture is similar to SegNet, which uses the first 13 convolutional layers in the VGG16 network as the encoder network [39]. In the decoder network, the last convolutional layer is removed. Each encoder network comprises two convolutional kernels, which includes 3×3 convolutional layers followed by an activation rectified linear unit (ReLU) and a batch normalization (BN) layer. Then, a maximum pooling indices operation is applied to the output of each encoder network before passing the information to the next encoder. Each decoder network consists of a 2×2 transposed convolution unit that is concatenated with the previous encoder output, and then the result is fed into two convolution blocks, which consist of 3 × 3 convolutions followed by an activation ReLU and a BN layer. Additionally, a second SegNet is attached to the first SegNet through new skip connections that use information from the first up-sampling pathway. The result of the last decoder block is concatenated with the same result after being fed into a 3 × 3 convolution layer followed by an activation ReLU and a BN layer. This serves as the input of the first encoder network to the second SegNet. The output of the maximum pooling indices operations of each of the three encoder networks is fed into 3 × 3 convolution layers and then concatenated with the output of the last previous decoder network. The result is next down-sampled to the next encoder network. Finally, the last output is given to a dilation layer with a dilation rate of 3, followed by an advanced ReLU activation layer to generate the predicted mask. In order to obtain more features, a dilation layer with a dilation rate of 3 is used in the last layer. Moreover, an activation ReLU limits the maximum value to 1, which is called an advanced ReLU. The details of the Connected-SegNets layers are listed in Table 3.

Table 3. The detailed architecture of the proposed Connected-SegNet.

	SegNet1				
No.	Layer Name	Output	Filter Size	No. of Filters	No. of Layers
1	Input	256 × 256 × 1			1
2	Conv1	256 × 256 × 64	3 × 3	64	2
3	Maxpool [1]	128 × 128 × 64			1
4	Conv2	128 × 128 × 128	3 × 3	128	2
5	Maxpool [1]	64 × 64 × 128			1
6	Conv3	64 × 64 × 256	3 × 3	256	3
7	Maxpool [1]	32 × 32 × 256			1
8	Conv4	32 × 32 × 512	3 × 3	512	3
9	Maxpool [1]	16 × 16 × 512			1
10	Conv5	16 × 16 × 512	3 × 3	512	3
11	Maxpool [1]	8 × 8 × 512			1
12	Upsampling [2]	16 × 16 × 512			1
13	Conv6	16 × 16 × 512	3 × 3	512	3
14	Upsampling [2]	32 × 32 × 512			1
15	Conv7	32 × 32 × 512	3 × 3	512	2
16	Conv8	32 × 32 × 256	3 × 3	256	1
17	Upsampling [2]	64 × 64 × 256			1
18	Conv9	64 × 64 × 256	3 × 3	256	2
19	Conv10	64 × 64 × 128	3 × 3	128	1
20	Upsampling [2]	128 × 128 × 128			1
21	Conv11	128 × 128 × 128	3 × 3	128	2
22	Conv12	128 × 128 × 64	3 × 3	64	1
23	Upsampling [2]	256 × 256 × 64			1
24	Conv13	256 × 256 × 64	3 × 3	64	1
25	Conv13	256 × 256 × 64			
26	Conv14	256 × 256 × 64	3 × 3	64	2
27	Maxpool [1]	128 × 128 × 64			1
28	Concatenate	128 × 128 × 128			1
29	Conv15	128 × 128 × 128	3 × 3	128	2
30	Maxpool [1]	64 × 64 × 128			1
31	Concatenate	64 × 64 × 256			1
32	Conv16	64 × 64 × 256	3 × 3	256	3
33	Maxpool [1]	32 × 32 × 256			1
34	Concatenate	16 × 16 × 512			1
35	Conv17	32 × 32 × 512	3 × 3	512	3
36	Maxpool [1]	16 × 16 × 512			1
37	Concatenate	16 × 16 × 1024			1
38	Conv18	16 × 16 × 512	3 × 3	512	3
39	Maxpool [1]	8 × 8 × 512			1
40	Upsampling [2]	16 × 16 × 512			1

Table 3. Cont.

	SegNet2				
No.	Layer Name	Output	Filter Size	No. of Filters	No. of Layers
41	Conv19	16 × 16 × 512	3 × 3	512	3
42	Upsampling [2]	32 × 32 × 512			1
43	Conv20	32 × 32 × 512	3 × 3	512	2
44	Conv21	32 × 32 × 256	3 × 3	256	1
45	Upsampling [2]	64 × 64 × 256			1
46	Conv22	64 × 64 × 256	3 × 3	256	2
47	Conv23	64 × 64 × 128	3 × 3	128	1
48	Upsampling [2]	128 × 128 × 128			1
49	Conv24	128 × 128 × 128	3 × 3	128	2
50	Conv25	128 × 128 × 64	3 × 3	64	1
51	Upsampling [2]	256 × 256 × 64			1
52	Conv26	256 × 256 × 64	3 × 3	64	1
53	Conv27	256 × 256 × 64	3 × 3 (D [3] = 3)	64	1
54	Output	256 × 256 × 1	1 × 1	1	1

[1] Maxpooling: Maxpooling and recording of the indices. [2] Upsampling: Upsampling with the recorded indices. [3] D: Dilation rate.

2.4. Experimental Environment and Parameter Settings

All experiments were performed using a PC with an Intel i7-9700K CPU, 55 GB of DDR4 RAM, and an NVIDIA GeForce RTX 2080Ti GPU with 11 GB of memory. The software environment used a Windows 10 64-bit operating system, python 3.8.12, CUDA 10.1, cuDNN 7.6.5, and TensorFlow 2.8.0. The learning rate was set to 0.0001 using the Adam optimizer [40] and the batch size was 4. The loss function was the IoU loss function.

2.5. Evaluation Metrics

In this research, precision, recall, IoU score, and Dice score evaluation metrics have been used to evaluate the proposed model based on the confusion matrix. The confusion matrix is an evaluation metric often used to evaluate classification, detection, and segmentation algorithms. The confusion matrix shows information about the true classes and the predicted classes. The true class and the predicted class can be positive or negative. The true negative (TN) case is when both the true case and the predicted case are tumors. False negatives (FN) occur when the true case is not a tumor, but the predicted case is. The false positive (FP) case occurs when the true case is a tumor while the prediction is a non-tumor. True positives (TP) occur when the actual case is non-tumor and the predicted case is tumor. The Dice score is also known as the F1-score, which represents the harmonic mean of precision and recall, as expressed in Equation (3). Additionally, the IoU evaluation metric represents the percentage of overlap between the predicted classes and the true classes, as represented in Equation (4).

$$Precision = \frac{TP}{TP + FP} \quad (1)$$

$$Recall = \frac{TP}{TP + FN} \quad (2)$$

$$Dice\ score = 2 \times \frac{Precision \times Recall}{Precision + Recall} \quad (3)$$

$$IoU\ score = \frac{TP}{TP + FP + FN} \quad (4)$$

3. Results

3.1. Results on INbreast Dataset

The confusion matrix results of Connected-SegNets on the INbreast dataset are listed in Table 4. From the Table 4, it is observed that the proportion of actual tumors that was correctly identified as tumors (TP) by Connected-SegNets is 96%. This is the highest TP rate compared to the other datasets. In addition, the proportion of non-tumors that was correctly identified as non-tumors (TN) by Connected-SegNets is 88%.

Table 4. Confusion matrix results of the proposed Connected-SegNets on INbreast dataset.

		Connected-SegNets	
		Ground Truth	
		Tumor	Non-Tumor
Prediction	Tumor	96% (TP)	4% (FN)
	Non-Tumor	12% (FP)	88% (TN)

3.2. Results on CBIS-DDSM Dataset

The identification results of Connected-SegNets on the CBIS-DDSM dataset are listed in Table 5. From the Table 5, it can be seen that the proportion of true tumors that was correctly identified as tumors (TP) by Connected-SegNets is 93%. Moreover, the proportion of non-tumors that was correctly identified as non-tumors (TN) by Connected-SegNets is 87%.

Table 5. Confusion matrix results of the proposed Connected-SegNets on CBIS-DDSM dataset.

		Connected-SegNets	
		Ground Truth	
		Tumor	Non-Tumor
Prediction	Tumor	93% (TP)	7% (FN)
	Non-Tumor	13% (FP)	87% (TN)

3.3. Results on Private Dataset

The results of the Connected-SegNets model on the private dataset are listed in Table 6. It is observed that the proportion of actual tumors that was correctly identified as tumors (TP) by Connected-SegNets is 92%. On the other hand, the proportion of tumors that were not tumors and were correctly identified as non-tumors (TN) by Connected-SegNets is 89%. This TN rate is considered to be the highest compared to other datasets.

Table 6. Confusion matrix results of the proposed Connected-SegNets on the private dataset.

		Connected-SegNets	
		Ground Truth	
		Tumor	Non-Tumor
Prediction	Tumor	92% (TP)	8% (FN)
	Non-Tumor	11% (FP)	89% (TN)

The accuracy and loss curves of the training and validation for Connected-SegNets are shown in Figures 5 and 6, respectively. It can be noted from Figures 5 and 6 that the training and validation curves behave similarly, which is an indication that the proposed Connected-SegNets can be generalized and does not suffer from overfitting.

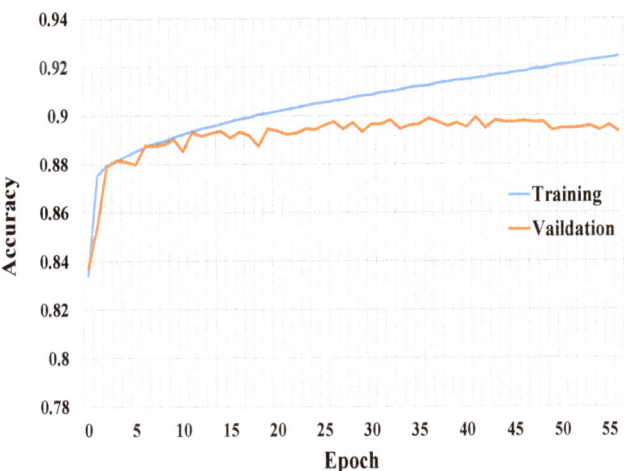

Figure 5. The training and validation accuracy curves of Connected-SegNets.

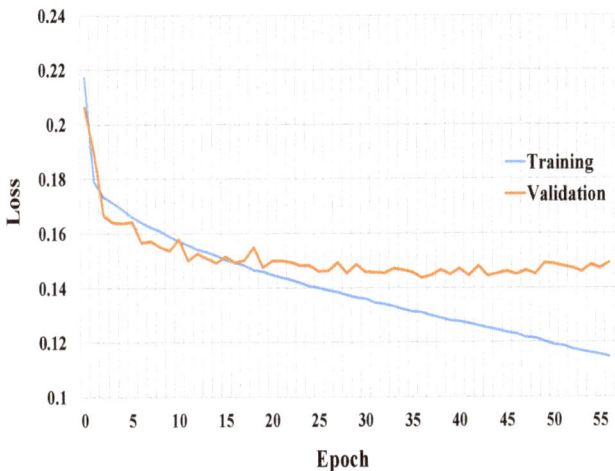

Figure 6. The training and validation loss curves of Connected-SegNets.

A large number of epochs might cause a deep learning model to overfit the data, whereas a small number of epochs can lead to smooth convergence. Therefore, the early stop technique has been utilized during the model training to avoid overfitting. The validation dataset is used to track the model training performance. The early stop method can help to set a suitable training epoch by tracking the best performance on the validation dataset. Therefore, when the validation performance stops improving, an early stop mode of the training process will be activated. Moreover, using the early stop algorithm not only can avoid the overfitting problem, but it also can help with choosing the optimal hyperparameter configurations for training the model. The early stop algorithm steps are shown in Algorithm 1. In this research, the validation tracking, ActStepSetting, was set to 20 iterations. Hence, if the validation performance did not improve after 20 iterations, the training was stopped automatically.

Algorithm 1 Validation Loss Tracking for Early Stop

Input: LatestValLoss, ActStepSetting
Output: BestValLossScore
1: $EarlyStop \leftarrow False$;
2: **if** $BestValidationRepeatNum <= ActStepSetting$ **then**
3:    **if** $LatestValLoss < BestValLossScore$ **then**
4:       $BestValidationRepeatNum \leftarrow 0$;
5:       $BestValLossScore \leftarrow LatestValLoss$;
6:    **else**
7:       $BestValidationRepeatNum \leftarrow BestValidationRepeatNum + 1$;
8:    **end if**
9: **else**
10:    $EarlyStop \leftarrow True$;
11: **end if**
12: **return** ($BestValLossScore$)

3.4. Comparison of Segmentation Results

As shown in Table 7, the segmentation results of each testing datum were evaluated by the two evaluation metrics, Dice score and IoU score, for the segmented maps per pixel, and compared with the original ground truth. It is noted that the proposed Connected-SegNets model produced the highest Dice score of 96.34%, 92.86%, and 92.25% on the INbreast, CBIS-DDSM, and private datasets, respectively. Moreover, the proposed model achieved the highest IoU Score of 91.21%, 87.34%, and 83.71% on the INbreast, CBIS-DDSM, and private datasets, respectively. Finally, the comparative results show that the proposed model, Connected-SegNets, outperformed the related models in terms of Dice score and IoU score on the three datasets.

Table 7. Comparison results between the proposed Connected-SegNets and the related segmentation models on the testing datasets of INbreast, CBIS-DDSM, and the private dataset, respectively.

Model	INbreast Dataset		CBIS-DDSM Dataset		Private Dataset	
	Dice Score (%)	IoU Score (%)	Dice Score (%)	IoU Score (%)	Dice Score (%)	IoU Score (%)
DS U-Net [19]	79.00	83.40	82.70	85.70	NA	NA
AUNet [20]	90.12	86.51	89.03	82.65	89.44	80.87
UNet [21]	92.14	88.23	90.47	84.79	89.11	80.21
Connected-UNets [22]	94.45	89.72	90.66	85.81	90.41	81.33
SegNet [23]	92.01	88.77	90.52	85.30	88.49	81.97
Connected-SegNets	**96.34**	**91.21**	**92.86**	**87.34**	**92.25**	**83.71**

Figure 7 shows some examples of the segmented ROI results generated by different models against their ground truth images. It is clearly observed that the quality of the segmentation maps of the Connected-SegNets model contain less error and produce more precise segmentation compared to other methods.

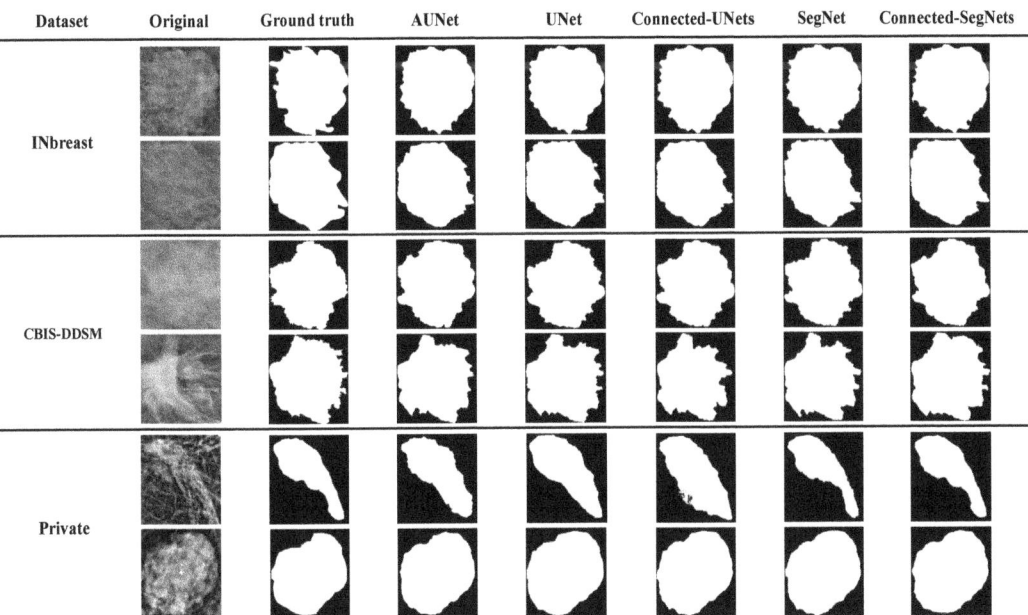

Figure 7. Example of the breast tumor segmentation results using AUNet, UNet, Connected-UNets, SegNet, and the proposed Connected-SegNets on the testing data of INbreast, CBIS-DDSM, and the private dataset.

4. Discussion

In recent years, several DL models have been developed and applied for breast tumor segmentation. These DL models have achieved remarkable success in segmenting breast tumors in mammograms. Nevertheless, many of these DL models produce high false positive and false negative rates [41]. The SegNet model is considered to be one of the deep learning models that is easy to modify and further optimize to provide better segmentation performance in different fields. Therefore, this study proposed a DL model, called Connected-SegNets, based on SegNet, for better breast tumor segmentation. The main goal of the proposed Connected-SegNets model is to improve the overall performance of breast tumor segmentation. Hence, several techniques have been implemented and incorporated into the proposed method in order to achieve this goal. These techniques include deepening the architecture with two SegNets, replacing the cross-entropy loss function of the standard SegNet with the IoU loss function, applying histogram equalization (CLAHE), and performing image augmentation. Figure 7 illustrates the segmentation results of AUNet, Standard UNet, Connected-UNets, Standard SegNet, and the proposed Connected-SegNets on the testing data of the INbreast, CBIS-DDSM, and private datasets. The segmentation results of the proposed Connected-SegNets are the closest to the ground truth compared to those of the AUNet, UNet, Connected-UNets, and SegNet models. The proposed model fully connects two single SegNets using additional skip connections. These are helpful to recover the spatial information that is lost during the pooling operations. Moreover, the IoU loss function leads to a more robust model. Furthermore, the histogram equalization (CLAHE) has been applied to smoothen the distribution of the image pixels for better pixel segmentation. Additionally, image augmentation methods, including rotation and flipping, have been applied to increase the number of training samples and reduce the impact of overfitting. This has led to more accurate segmentation performance compared to the other models. The significant improvement is shown in Tables 4–6, where the Connected-SegNets model has the TP value of 96%, 93%, and 92%, on the

INbreast, CBIS-DDSM, and private datasets, respectively. Similarly, the TN value is of 88%, 87%, and 89%, on INbreast, CBIS-DDSM, and the private dataset, respectively. The results of the proposed model, Connected-SegNets, showed a significant segmentation improvement compared to the other models, with a maximum Dice score of 96.34% on the INbreast dataset, 92.86% on the CBIS-DDSM dataset, and 92.25% on the private dataset. Similarly, the Connected-SegNets model has achieved the highest IoU score of 91.21% on the INbreast dataset, 87.34% on the CBIS-DDSM dataset, and 83.71% on the private dataset. Overall, the proposed Connected-SegNets model has outperformed DS U-Net, AUNet, UNet, Connected-UNets, and SegNet in terms of Dice score and IoU score. This shows the power of the proposed model to learn complex features through the connections added between the two SegNets in the proposed Connected-SegNets, which take advantage of the decoded features as another input in the encoder pathway.

5. Conclusions

This research proposed a deep learning model, namely Connected-SegNets, for breast tumor segmentation from X-ray images. Two SegNets were used in the proposed model, both of which were fully connected via additional skip connections. The cross-entropy loss function of the original SegNet was replaced by the IoU loss function to make the proposed model more robust against sparse data. Additionally, the contrast limit adapt histogram equalization (CLAHE) was applied to enhance the compressed areas and smooth the pixel distribution. Moreover, two augmentation methods including rotation and flipping were used to increase the number of training samples and prevent overfitting. The experimental results showed that Connected-SegNets outperformed the existing models, with the highest Dice scores of 96.34%, 92.86%, and 92.25%, and the highest IoU scores of 91.21%, 87.34%, and 83.71% on the INbreast, CBIS-DDSM, and private datasets, respectively. Future work will focus on implementing new deep learning algorithms for tumor detection and classification for automatic breast cancer diagnosis.

Author Contributions: Conceptualization, M.A., L.C. and Y.-L.C.; Data curation, C.-H.C. and T.-C.W.; Formal analysis, M.A., T.-H.T., C.-H.C., S.-C.M. and L.C.; Funding acquisition, C.-H.C., S.-C.M. and Y.-L.C.; Investigation, T.-H.T.; Methodology, M.A., T.-H.T. and T.-C.W.; Project administration, C.-H.C., S.-C.M. and Y.-L.C.; Resources, Y.-L.C.; Software, T.-C.W.; Supervision, C.-H.C.; Validation, T.-H.T., S.-C.M. and Y.-L.C.; Writing—original draft, T.-C.W. and L.C.; Writing–review and editing, M.A. All authors have read and agreed to the published version of the manuscript.

Funding: This work is supported by the Ministry of Science and Technology, Taiwan, Grant Nos. MOST 110-2119-M-027-001, MOST 110-2221-E-027-101, MOST 110-2622-E-027-025, MOST 111-2622-8-038-004-TD2, and National Taipei University of Technology and Cheng Hsin General Hospital, Grant No. NTUT-CHGH-110-01.

Institutional Review Board Statement: Not applicable.

Informed Consent Statement: Not applicable.

Data Availability Statement: The data presented in this study are available in this article.

Conflicts of Interest: The authors declare no conflict of interest.

References

1. Siegel, R.L.; Miller, K.D.; Fuchs, H.E.; Jemal, A. Cancer statistics, 2022. *CA Cancer J. Clin.* **2022**, *72*, 7–33. [CrossRef] [PubMed]
2. Zou, R.; Loke, S.Y.; Tan, V.K.M.; Quek, S.T.; Jagmohan, P.; Tang, Y.C.; Madhukumar, P.; Tan, B.K.T.; Yong, W.S.; Sim, Y.; et al. Development of a microRNA panel for classification of abnormal mammograms for breast cancer. *Cancers* **2021**, *13*, 2130. [CrossRef] [PubMed]
3. Li, J.; Guan, X.; Fan, Z.; Ching, L.M.; Li, Y.; Wang, X.; Cao, W.M.; Liu, D.X. Non-invasive biomarkers for early detection of breast cancer. *Cancers* **2020**, *12*, 2767. [CrossRef] [PubMed]
4. Almalki, Y.E.; Soomro, T.A.; Irfan, M.; Alduraibi, S.K.; Ali, A. Computerized Analysis of Mammogram Images for Early Detection of Breast Cancer. *Healthcare* **2022**, *10*, 801. [CrossRef] [PubMed]
5. Shi, P.; Zhong, J.; Rampun, A.; Wang, H. A hierarchical pipeline for breast boundary segmentation and calcification detection in mammograms. *Comput. Biol. Med.* **2018**, *96*, 178–188. [CrossRef]

6. Waks, A.G.; Winer, E.P. Breast cancer treatment: A review. *JAMA* **2019**, *321*, 288–300. [CrossRef] [PubMed]
7. Salgado, R.; Denkert, C.; Demaria, S.; Sirtaine, N.; Klauschen, F.; Pruneri, G.; Wienert, S.; Van den Eynden, G.; Baehner, F.L.; Pénault-Llorca, F.; et al. The evaluation of tumor-infiltrating lymphocytes (TILs) in breast cancer: Recommendations by an International TILs Working Group 2014. *Ann. Oncol.* **2015**, *26*, 259–271. [CrossRef]
8. Tariq, M.; Iqbal, S.; Ayesha, H.; Abbas, I.; Ahmad, K.T.; Niazi, M.F.K. Medical image based breast cancer diagnosis: State of the art and future directions. *Expert Syst. Appl.* **2021**, *167*, 114095. [CrossRef]
9. Petrillo, A.; Fusco, R.; Di Bernardo, E.; Petrosino, T.; Barretta, M.L.; Porto, A.; Granata, V.; Di Bonito, M.; Fanizzi, A.; Massafra, R.; et al. Prediction of Breast Cancer Histological Outcome by Radiomics and Artificial Intelligence Analysis in Contrast-Enhanced Mammography. *Cancers* **2022**, *14*, 2132. [CrossRef]
10. Ahmed, L.; Iqbal, M.M.; Aldabbas, H.; Khalid, S.; Saleem, Y.; Saeed, S. Images data practices for semantic segmentation of breast cancer using deep neural network. *J. Ambient. Intell. Humaniz. Comput.* **2020**, 1–17. [CrossRef]
11. Le, E.; Wang, Y.; Huang, Y.; Hickman, S.; Gilbert, F. Artificial intelligence in breast imaging. *Clin. Radiol.* **2019**, *74*, 357–366. [CrossRef] [PubMed]
12. Bi, W.L.; Hosny, A.; Schabath, M.B.; Giger, M.L.; Birkbak, N.J.; Mehrtash, A.; Allison, T.; Arnaout, O.; Abbosh, C.; Dunn, I.F.; et al. Artificial intelligence in cancer imaging: Clinical challenges and applications. *CA Cancer J. Clin.* **2019**, *69*, 127–157. [CrossRef] [PubMed]
13. Shah, S.M.; Khan, R.A.; Arif, S.; Sajid, U. Artificial intelligence for breast cancer analysis: Trends & directions. *Comput. Biol. Med.* **2022**, *142*, 105221. [PubMed]
14. Ketabi, H.; Ekhlasi, A.; Ahmadi, H. A computer-aided approach for automatic detection of breast masses in digital mammogram via spectral clustering and support vector machine. *Phys. Eng. Sci. Med.* **2021**, *44*, 277–290. [CrossRef]
15. Hosny, A.; Parmar, C.; Quackenbush, J.; Schwartz, L.H.; Aerts, H.J. Artificial intelligence in radiology. *Nat. Rev. Cancer* **2018**, *18*, 500–510. [CrossRef]
16. Vobugari, N.; Raja, V.; Sethi, U.; Gandhi, K.; Raja, K.; Surani, S.R. Advancements in Oncology with Artificial Intelligence—A Review Article. *Cancers* **2022**, *14*, 1349. [CrossRef]
17. Alkhaleefah, M.; Wu, C.C. A hybrid CNN and RBF-based SVM approach for breast cancer classification in mammograms. In Proceedings of the 2018 IEEE International Conference on Systems, Man, and Cybernetics (SMC), Miyazaki, Japan, 7–10 October 2018; pp. 894–899.
18. Kallenberg, M.; Petersen, K.; Nielsen, M.; Ng, A.Y.; Diao, P.; Igel, C.; Vachon, C.M.; Holland, K.; Winkel, R.R.; Karssemeijer, N.; et al. Unsupervised deep learning applied to breast density segmentation and mammographic risk scoring. *IEEE Trans. Med. Imaging* **2016**, *35*, 1322–1331. [CrossRef]
19. Ravitha Rajalakshmi, N.; Vidhyapriya, R.; Elango, N.; Ramesh, N. Deeply supervised u-net for mass segmentation in digital mammograms. *Int. J. Imaging Syst. Technol.* **2021**, *31*, 59–71.
20. Sun, H.; Li, C.; Liu, B.; Liu, Z.; Wang, M.; Zheng, H.; Feng, D.D.; Wang, S. AUNet: Attention-guided dense-upsampling networks for breast mass segmentation in whole mammograms. *Phys. Med. Biol.* **2020**, *65*, 055005. [CrossRef]
21. Ronneberger, O.; Fischer, P.; Brox, T. U-Net: Convolutional Networks for Biomedical Image Segmentation. In *Medical Image Computing and Computer-Assisted Intervention–MICCAI 2015*; Springer International Publishing: Cham, Switzerland, 2015; pp. 234–241.
22. Baccouche, A.; Garcia-Zapirain, B.; Castillo Olea, C.; Elmaghraby, A.S. Connected-UNets: A deep learning architecture for breast mass segmentation. *NPJ Breast Cancer* **2021**, *7*, 1–12. [CrossRef]
23. Badrinarayanan, V.; Kendall, A.; Cipolla, R. Segnet: A deep convolutional encoder-decoder architecture for image segmentation. *IEEE Trans. Pattern Anal. Mach. Intell.* **2017**, *39*, 2481–2495. [CrossRef] [PubMed]
24. Moreira, I.C.; Amaral, I.; Domingues, I.; Cardoso, A.; Cardoso, M.J.; Cardoso, J.S. Inbreast: Toward a full-field digital mammographic database. *Acad. Radiol.* **2012**, *19*, 236–248. [CrossRef] [PubMed]
25. Huang, M.L.; Lin, T.Y. Dataset of breast mammography images with masses. *Data Brief* **2020**, *31*, 105928. [CrossRef]
26. Heath, M.; Bowyer, K.; Kopans, D.; Kegelmeyer, P.; Moore, R.; Chang, K.; Munishkumaran, S. Current status of the digital database for screening mammography. In *Digital Mammography*; Springer: Cham, Switzerland, 1998; pp. 457–460.
27. Lee, R.S.; Gimenez, F.; Hoogi, A.; Miyake, K.K.; Gorovoy, M.; Rubin, D.L. A curated mammography data set for use in computer-aided detection and diagnosis research. *Sci. Data* **2017**, *4*, 1–9. [CrossRef] [PubMed]
28. Dutta, A.; Zisserman, A. The VIA Annotation Software for Images, Audio and Video. In Proceedings of the 27th ACM International Conference on Multimedia, Nice, France, 21–25 October 2019; ACM: New York, NY, USA, 2019; MM'19. [CrossRef]
29. Al-Masni, M.A.; Al-Antari, M.A.; Park, J.M.; Gi, G.; Kim, T.Y.; Rivera, P.; Valarezo, E.; Choi, M.T.; Han, S.M.; Kim, T.S. Simultaneous detection and classification of breast masses in digital mammograms via a deep learning YOLO-based CAD system. *Comput. Methods Programs Biomed.* **2018**, *157*, 85–94. [CrossRef]
30. Hai, J.; Qiao, K.; Chen, J.; Tan, H.; Xu, J.; Zeng, L.; Shi, D.; Yan, B. Fully convolutional densenet with multiscale context for automated breast tumor segmentation. *J. Healthc. Eng.* **2019**, *2019*, 8415485. [CrossRef] [PubMed]
31. Dhal, K.G.; Das, A.; Ray, S.; Gálvez, J.; Das, S. Histogram equalization variants as optimization problems: A review. *Arch. Comput. Methods Eng.* **2021**, *28*, 1471–1496. [CrossRef]
32. Huang, Z.; Zhang, Y.; Li, Q.; Zhang, T.; Sang, N. Spatially adaptive denoising for X-ray cardiovascular angiogram images. *Biomed. Signal Process. Control* **2018**, *40*, 131–139. [CrossRef]

33. Huang, Z.; Li, X.; Wang, N.; Ma, L.; Hong, H. Simultaneous denoising and enhancement for X-ray angiograms by employing spatial-frequency filter. *Optik* **2020**, *208*, 164287. [CrossRef]
34. Huang, Z.; Zhang, Y.; Li, Q.; Li, X.; Zhang, T.; Sang, N.; Hong, H. Joint analysis and weighted synthesis sparsity priors for simultaneous denoising and destriping optical remote sensing images. *IEEE Trans. Geosci. Remote Sens.* **2020**, *58*, 6958–6982. [CrossRef]
35. Rao, B.S. Dynamic histogram equalization for contrast enhancement for digital images. *Appl. Soft Comput.* **2020**, *89*, 106114. [CrossRef]
36. Alkhaleefah, M.; Ma, S.C.; Chang, Y.L.; Huang, B.; Chittem, P.K.; Achhannagari, V.P. Double-shot transfer learning for breast cancer classification from X-ray images. *Appl. Sci.* **2020**, *10*, 3999. [CrossRef]
37. Elasal, N.; Swart, D.M.; Miller, N. Frame augmentation for imbalanced object detection datasets. *J. Comput. Vis. Imaging Syst.* **2018**, *4*, 3.
38. Shorten, C.; Khoshgoftaar, T.M. A survey on image data augmentation for deep learning. *J. Big Data* **2019**, *6*, 1–48. [CrossRef]
39. Simonyan, K.; Zisserman, A. Very deep convolutional networks for large-scale image recognition. *arXiv* **2014**, arXiv:1409.1556.
40. Kingma, D.P.; Ba, J. Adam: A method for stochastic optimization. *arXiv* **2014**, arXiv:1412.6980.
41. Al-Antari, M.A.; Al-Masni, M.A.; Choi, M.T.; Han, S.M.; Kim, T.S. A fully integrated computer-aided diagnosis system for digital X-ray mammograms via deep learning detection, segmentation, and classification. *Int. J. Med. Infor.* **2018**, *117*, 44–54. [CrossRef]

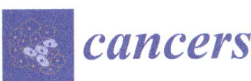

Article

Prediction of Breast Cancer Histological Outcome by Radiomics and Artificial Intelligence Analysis in Contrast-Enhanced Mammography

Antonella Petrillo [1,*], Roberta Fusco [2], Elio Di Bernardo [2], Teresa Petrosino [1], Maria Luisa Barretta [1], Annamaria Porto [1], Vincenza Granata [1], Maurizio Di Bonito [3], Annarita Fanizzi [4], Raffaella Massafra [5], Nicole Petruzzellis [5], Francesca Arezzo [6], Luca Boldrini [7] and Daniele La Forgia [8]

1 Radiology Division, Istituto Nazionale Tumori—IRCCS—Fondazione G. Pascale, 80131 Naples, Italy; t.petrosino@istitutotumori.na.it (T.P.); m.barretta@istitutotumori.na.it (M.L.B.); a.porto@istitutotumori.na.it (A.P.); v.granata@istitutotumori.na.it (V.G.)
2 Medical Oncology Division, Igea SpA, 80013 Naples, Italy; r.fusco@igeamedical.com (R.F.); e.dibernardo@igeamedical.com (E.D.B.)
3 Pathology Division, Istituto Nazionale Tumori—IRCCS—Fondazione G. Pascale, 80131 Naples, Italy; m.dibonito@istitutotumori.na.it
4 Direzione Scientifica—IRCCS Istituto Tumori Giovanni Paolo II, Via Orazio Flacco 65, 70124 Bari, Italy; a.fanizzi@oncologico.bari.it
5 SSD Fisica Sanitaria—IRCCS Istituto Tumori Giovanni Paolo II, Via Orazio Flacco 65, 70124 Bari, Italy; r.massafra@oncologico.bari.it (R.M.); n.petruzzellis@oncologico.bari.it (N.P.)
6 Obstetrics and Gynecology Unit, Department of Biomedical Sciences and Human Oncology, University of Bari Aldo Moro, Piazza Giulio Cesare 11, 70124 Bari, Italy; francescaarezzo@libero.it
7 Dipartimento di Diagnostica per Immagini, Radioterapia Oncologica ed Ematologia, Fondazione Policlinico Universitario A. Gemelli IRCCS, 00168 Roma, Italy; luca.boldrini@policlinicogemelli.it
8 Struttura Semplice Dipartimentale di Radiodiagnostica Senologica—IRCCS Istituto Tumori Giovanni Paolo II, Via Orazio Flacco 65, 70124 Bari, Italy; d.laforgia@oncologico.bari.it
* Correspondence: a.petrillo@istitutotumori.na.it

Simple Summary: The assessment of breast lesions through mammographic images is currently challenging, especially in dense breasts. Contrast-enhanced mammography has been shown to overcome the limitations of standard mammography but it greatly depends on the interpretative skills of the physician. The aim of this study was to evaluate the potentialities of statistical and artificial intelligence algorithms as a tool for helping the radiologists in the interpretation of images. The most remarkable results were achieved in discriminating benign from malignant lesions and in the identification of the presence of the hormone receptor. A tool to support the physician's decision-making process may be designed starting from simple logistic regression and tree-based algorithms. This type of tool may help the radiologist in assessing the investigated breast and in choosing the appropriate follow-up without resorting to histology.

Abstract: Purpose: To evaluate radiomics features in order to: differentiate malignant versus benign lesions; predict low versus moderate and high grading; identify positive or negative hormone receptors; and discriminate positive versus negative human epidermal growth factor receptor 2 related to breast cancer. Methods: A total of 182 patients with known breast lesions and that underwent Contrast-Enhanced Mammography were enrolled in this retrospective study. The reference standard was pathology (118 malignant lesions and 64 benign lesions). A total of 837 textural metrics were extracted by manually segmenting the region of interest from both craniocaudally (CC) and mediolateral oblique (MLO) views. Non-parametric Wilcoxon–Mann–Whitney test, receiver operating characteristic, logistic regression and tree-based machine learning algorithms were used. The Adaptive Synthetic Sampling balancing approach was used and a feature selection process was implemented. Results: In univariate analysis, the classification of malignant versus benign lesions achieved the best performance when considering the original_gldm_DependenceNonUniformity feature extracted on CC view (accuracy of 88.98%). An accuracy of 83.65% was reached in the classification of grading, whereas a slightly lower value of accuracy (81.65%) was found in the classification of the presence

Citation: Petrillo, A.; Fusco, R.; Di Bernardo, E.; Petrosino, T.; Barretta, M.L.; Porto, A.; Granata, V.; Di Bonito, M.; Fanizzi, A.; Massafra, R.; et al. Prediction of Breast Cancer Histological Outcome by Radiomics and Artificial Intelligence Analysis in Contrast-Enhanced Mammography. *Cancers* 2022, 14, 2132. https://doi.org/10.3390/cancers14092132

Academic Editors: Enrico Cassano, Filippo Pesapane and Oliver J. Ott

Received: 14 March 2022
Accepted: 21 April 2022
Published: 25 April 2022

Publisher's Note: MDPI stays neutral with regard to jurisdictional claims in published maps and institutional affiliations.

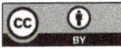

Copyright: © 2022 by the authors. Licensee MDPI, Basel, Switzerland. This article is an open access article distributed under the terms and conditions of the Creative Commons Attribution (CC BY) license (https://creativecommons.org/licenses/by/4.0/).

of the hormone receptor; the features extracted were the original_glrlm_RunEntropy and the original_gldm_DependenceNonUniformity, respectively. The results of multivariate analysis achieved the best performances when using two or more features as predictors for classifying malignant versus benign lesions from CC view images (max test accuracy of 95.83% with a non-regularized logistic regression). Considering the features extracted from MLO view images, the best test accuracy (91.67%) was obtained when predicting the grading using a classification-tree algorithm. Combinations of only two features, extracted from both CC and MLO views, always showed test accuracy values greater than or equal to 90.00%, with the only exception being the prediction of the human epidermal growth factor receptor 2, where the best performance (test accuracy of 89.29%) was obtained with the random forest algorithm. Conclusions: The results confirm that the identification of malignant breast lesions and the differentiation of histological outcomes and some molecular subtypes of tumors (mainly positive hormone receptor tumors) can be obtained with satisfactory accuracy through both univariate and multivariate analysis of textural features extracted from Contrast-Enhanced Mammography images.

Keywords: Contrast-Enhanced Mammography (CEM); Dynamic Contrast Magnetic Resonance Imaging (DCE-MRI); radiomics; artificial intelligence

1. Introduction

Mammography is one of the main techniques in the diagnosis of breast cancer, showing a key role in both screening and follow-up [1,2]. Mammographic screening has been shown to be highly accurate in detection of breast lesions; however, it suffers from some limitations, especially in the case of dense breasts. In fact, dense breasts show a hyper-intense signal over the mammary parenchyma, resulting in very little contrast between the latter and the lesions. For the mammographic screening of patients with dense breasts, other techniques, such as Magnetic Resonance Imaging (MRI), are commonly preferred [3,4]. In particular, one of the most recent novel approaches is Contrast-Enhanced Mammography (CEM). Combining the potential and benefits of Full-Field Digital Mammography (FFDM), CEM has been shown to be highly effective for the detection and the correct staging of cancer, particularly in dense breasts [4–10]. More specifically, CEM combines the enhancing properties of the intravenous administration of an iodinated contrast medium with the high precision of digital imaging from FFDM; therefore, the neo-vascularity associated with actively growing malignancy is remarkably emphasized. Due to this property, CEM is not only able to detect cancer with high accuracy, but it is also a powerful technique for the identification of cancers that are obscure at mammography; furthermore, it allows a more accurate evaluation of the disease extent and offers guidance in the planning of surgery and treatment [4–10]. However, as in all imaging techniques, the evaluation of CEM images depends on the experience and skills of the radiologist, making the identification of automated or semi-automated techniques, which can provide decision support, a considerable challenge.

Recent significant advancements in this sense rely on the application of artificial intelligence and radiomics for the processing of large quantities of data by different imaging modalities [11,12].

Radiomics is the process of extracting quantitative properties, named features, from medical images. This feature extraction generally includes pattern recognition algorithms and provides, as a result, a set of numbers, each representing a quantitative description of a specific either geometrical or physical property of the image portion under consideration. In the context of tumor characterization, the radiomics features typically considered are those that describe properties related to size, shape, intensity, and texture of the tumor [13–27].

Biological and molecular features related to breast cancer are commonly extracted by biopsy, which is invasive and not always able to detect tumor heterogeneity [28]. In recent years, there has been growing interest in non-invasive methods to directly derive insights from radiologic images. In this context, the radiomics analysis of tumor features extracted from CEM represents an important tool for breast tumor characterization. As several authors suggest, radiomics analysis combined with artificial intelligence techniques can be used to create a tool to support the physician's decision-making process in the classification of breast cancer [29–44]. In fact, through an appropriate tool, the physician would be able to discriminate the tumor nature and/or grading, identifying the adequate treatment for a single patient (e.g., neoadjuvant therapy) or even a more conservative approach (e.g., wait-and-see or conservative surgery). However, based on our knowledge, only some recent studies have used CEM in the prediction of histological grading and receptor status of breast cancer [45,46].

This work aimed to evaluate radiomics features to differentiate malignant versus benign lesions, to predict low versus moderate and high grading, to identify positive or negative hormone receptors, and to discriminate positive versus negative human epidermal growth factor receptor 2 related to breast cancer.

2. Methods

2.1. Patient Selection

From October 2017 to December 2021, according to regulations issued by the local Institutional Review Board, 182 patients (mean age ± standard deviation of 55.3 ± 10.9 years (range 31–80)) with known breast lesions were enrolled retrospectively. All women signed informed consent.

Inclusion criteria: patients with known breast lesions (from radiological or clinical screening, symptom of palpable lesions), histologically proven, and that underwent dual-energy CEM. CEM images of patients were acquired at Istituto Nazionale Tumori-IRCCS-Fondazione G. Pascale (Naples, Italy) and at Istituto Tumori "Giovanni Paolo II" of Bari (Bari, Italy).

Exclusion criteria: patient with breast implants, presence of non-removable drilling at the nipple, pacemakers, clips or other metal implants, pregnancy or possible pregnancy, inability to keep upright immobility during the examination, renal disease, or chemotherapy treatment at the time of imaging [41].

Overall, 118 malignant lesions and 64 benign lesions were analyzed.

2.2. Imaging Protocol

A total of 136 CEM examinations were performed using the Selenia® Dimensions® Unit dual-energy mammography system (Hologic, Bedford, MA, USA), whereas the remaining 46 CEM image were acquired with the Senographe Essential dual-energy mammography system (GE Healthcare, Princeton, NJ, USA).

The same acquisition protocol was implemented for all the images using both scanners. Specifically, two minutes after the intravenous injection of 1.5 mL/(kg bw) of iodinated contrast medium (Visipaque 320; GE Healthcare, Inc., Princeton, NJ, USA) at a rate of 2–3 mL/s, a set of images was acquired in quick succession, in both CC and MLO views. The CEM examination obtained two images: a low-energy (LE) acquisition at 26–30 kVp and a high-energy (HE) acquisition at 45–49 kVp, depending on breast density and thickness. CEM acquisition details were reported in previous studies [41,42,45].

2.3. Image Processing

Two expert radiologists, with 25 and 20 years of experience in breast imaging, manually segmented images by drawing slice-by-slice the contours of the lesions where contrast uptake was emphasized both in CC and MLO views.

MRI Post-Processing with PyRadiomics Tool

For each region of interest, 837 radiomics features were extracted as median values using the PyRadiomics Python package [47] including: First Order Statistics, Grey Level Co-occurrence Matrix, Grey Level Run Length Matrix, Grey Level Size Zone Matrix, Neighboring Grey Tone Difference Matrix, and Grey Level Dependence Matrix features before and after the wavelet filtering. The extracted features comply with feature definitions as described by the Imaging Biomarker Standardization Initiative (IBSI) [48] and as reported in (https://readthedocs.org/projects/pyradiomics/downloads/, accessed on 20 January 2017).

We used wavelet filtering, with all possible combinations of both high-pass (H) and low-pass (L) filters along the three axes (X, Y, and Z axes), to derive six different matrices:

- First Order (FIRST ORDER): Describes the individual values of voxels obtained as a result of ROI cropping. These are generally histogram-based properties (energy, entropy, kurtosis, skewness).
- Gray Level Co-occurrence Matrix (GLCM): Calculates how often the same and similar pixel values come together in an image and records statistical measurements according to this matrix. These resulting values numerically characterize the texture of the image.
- Gray Level Run Length Matrix (GLRLM): Defined as the number of homogeneous consecutive pixels with the same gray tone and quantifies the gray-level values.
- Gray Level Size Zone Matrix (GLSZM): Describes voxel counts according to the logic of measuring gray-level regions in an image.
- Neighboring Gray Tone Difference Matrix (NGTDM): Digitization of textures obtained from filtered images and their fractal properties.
- Gray Level Dependence Matrix (GLDM): Number of bound voxels at a fidex distance from the central voxel.

A graphical representation of the process for features extraction in a radiomics context is reported in Figure 1.

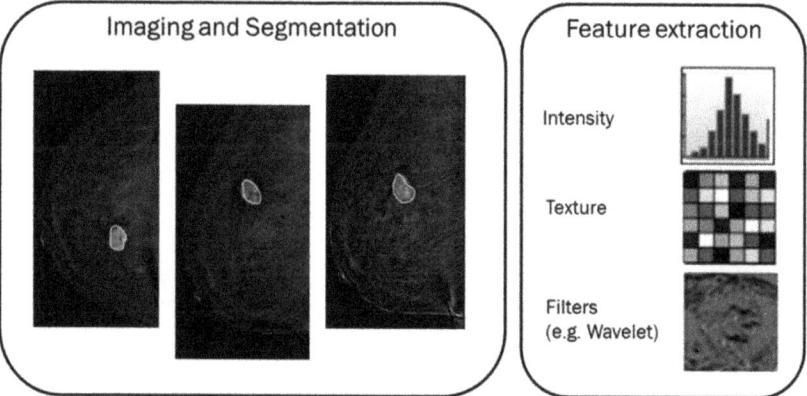

Figure 1. A graphical representation of the features extraction process in a radiomics context. The green lines represent the segmentation of lesion contours.

2.4. Histopathological Analysis

The reference standard (ground truth) was the histopathologic examination of tissue as reported in [41]. Breast lesions were categorized based on the American Joint Committee on Cancer staging. The histological grade and the expression of estrogen receptor (ER), progesterone receptor (PR), human epidermal growth factor receptor 2 (HER2), and Ki-67 antigen associated with cell proliferation were determined by immune-histochemical analysis.

The tumor grade G was defined on a three-grade scale according to the Elston–Ellis modification of the Scar–Bloom–Richardson grading system.

The hormone receptor (HR) was also considered; a breast cancer is classified as HR-positive if its cells have receptors for the hormones estrogen and progesterone.

2.5. Statistical Analysis

The statistical analysis was performed using the R programming language (version 4.0.2) with the RStudio software, version 1.3.959 (https://www.rstudio.com/, accessed on 20 January 2017) [49].

Considering the histologic results as ground truth, four different types of outcomes were used in both univariate and multivariate analysis: (1) nature of tumor (benign versus malignant); (2) grading (G1 versus G2 + G3); (3) presence of human epidermal growth factor receptor 2 (HER2+ versus HER2−); (4) presence of hormone receptor (HR+ versus HR−).

Before proceeding with statistical analysis, the dataset was balanced with respect of each outcome. The balancing was performed through the synthetization of samples for the less-represented classes using the Adaptive Synthetic Sampling (ADASYN) approach [50,51].

In the context of univariate analysis, the non-parametric Wilcoxon–Mann–Whitney test for continuous variables was used. Receiver operating characteristic (ROC) analysis and the Youden index were considered to obtain the optimal cut-off value for each feature; then, the area under ROC curve (AUC), sensitivity (SENS), specificity (SPEC), positive predictive value (PPV), negative predictive value (NPV), and accuracy (ACC) were computed. Bonferroni correction was used to adjust for multiple comparison.

In the context of multivariate analysis, logistic regression and tree-based algorithms were appropriately designed to predict each outcome individually; the main predictive features were also extracted. Before proceeding with the analysis, three pre-processing steps were performed.

Firstly, the dataset was randomly split into a training set and a test set, using the createDataPartition R function. Specifically, 90% of the entire dataset was used to train the algorithms, designing a cross-validated procedure; the remaining 10% of samples was used to estimate the accuracy of algorithms on 'new' samples, which are samples not used to train the algorithms themselves. Successively (and before running algorithms), a variable selection procedure was designed to remove redundant features from the training set. To achieve this aim, the cross-correlation between each predictor was calculated and all the features with a correlation higher than 0.7 (as an absolute value) with each single predictor were discarded. Finally, the input predictors were centered and scaled before running the logistic regression algorithm.

The machine learning approaches designed for the aim of this paper are described in the following. For each approach, the performance (accuracy) was assessed on both the training and test sets, also considering the values of sensitivity and specificity.

Logistic Regression. Considering the dichotomic nature of each outcome, a logistic regression was executed using all non-redundant features. The method was run using the glm R function.

Logistic Regression with least absolute shrinkage and selection operator (LASSO) method. In a different approach, the logistic regression model was fitted on training data, performing a further variable selection with the LASSO regularization method [52,53]. The LASSO was designed using the glmnet R function and the hyperparameter was tuned through a 10-fold cross validation procedure. The variables selected were saved to train the logistic regression algorithm.

Logistic Regression with two predictors. An additional variation of the logistic regression was considered predicting each outcome with all possible couples of features. All combinations that reached a test accuracy higher than 0.9 were saved and analyzed.

Tree-based algorithms. Among all tree-based algorithms, Classification and Regression Trees (CART) and Random Forest (RF) algorithms were chosen and designed. The CART algorithm was trained taking into account the possibility of obtaining a decision chart, whereas the RF method was used for a more robust evaluation of performances. Tuning of functions' hyperparameters was performed through a 10-fold cross validation procedure.

3. Results

Table 1 shows the distribution of characteristic of analyzed patients.

Table 1. Distribution of analyzed patients.

Characteristic	Distribution	
Age	Min value	25
	Max value	82
	Median value	52
Tumor nature	benign	64
	malignant	118
Tumor grading	G1	78
	G2 + G3	104
Human epidermal growth factor receptor 2	HER2+	135
	HER2−	47
Hormone receptor	HR+	93
	HR−	89
Histotype	0	16
	1	2
	2	80
	3	19
	4	14
	5	51

Table 2 reports the diagnostic accuracy of significant textural parameters for dual-energy CEM, in both CC and MLO views, obtained in the context of univariate analysis.

Table 2. Performance results of univariate analysis both on CC and MLO view.

Performance Results at Univariate Analysis	Benign Versus Malignant Lesions by CC-View	Benign Versus Malignant Lesions by MLO-View	G1 Versus G2 + G3 by CC-View	G1 Versus G2 + G3 by MLO-View	Identification of HER2+ by CC-View	Identification of HER2+ by MLO-View	Identification of HR+ by CC-View	Identification of HR+ by MLO-View
	original_gldm_ DependenceNonUniformity	wavelet_LLL_gldm_ DependenceNonUniformity	original_glrlm_ RunEntropy	wavelet_LLL_glrlm_ RunEntropy	wavelet_HLL_ glcm_Idn	wavelet_HLH_ glcm_Idm	original_gldm_ DependenceNonUniformity	wavelet_LLL_gldm_ DependenceNonUniformity
AUC	0.8587	0.8406	0.8237	0.7643	0.7150	0.7081	0.7500	0.7334
SENS	0.9237	0.8220	0.9038	0.7981	0.5481	0.5704	0.9699	0.8495
SPEC	0.8559	0.8814	0.7692	0.7692	0.8148	0.8148	0.6559	0.6882
PPV	0.8651	0.8739	0.7966	0.7757	0.7475	0.7549	0.7355	0.7315
NPV	0.9182	0.8320	0.8889	0.7921	0.6433	0.6548	0.9385	0.8205
ACC	0.8983	0.8517	0.8365	0.7837	0.6815	0.6926	0.8165	0.7688
Cut-off	2.3093	4.1147	0.8023	0.8732	0.8866	0.7384	2.5524	4.2121

As the table shows, in the classification of malignant versus benign lesions, the best performance was reached by the original_gldm_DependenceNonUniformity feature, extracted on CC view, with an accuracy of 89.83%, a sensitivity of 92.37%, and a specificity of 85.59%, and with a cut-off of 2.31.

In the classification of grading, the best performance was reached by the original_glrlm_RunEntropy feature, extracted on CC view, with an accuracy of 83.65%, a sensitivity of 90.38%, and a specificity of 76.92%, and with a cut-off of 0.80.

In the identification of HER2+, the best performance was reached by the wavelet_HLH_gldm_LargeDependenceHighGrayLevelEmphasis feature, extracted on MLO view, with an accuracy of 69.63%, a sensitivity of 62.22%, and a specificity of 77.04%, and with a cut-off of 0.74.

In the identification of HR+, the best performance was reached by the original_gldm_DependenceNonUniformity feature, extracted on CC view, with an accuracy of 81.65%, a sensitivity of 96.99%, and a specificity of 65.59%, and with a cut-off of 2.55.

Tables 3 and 4 show the results obtained with logistic regression-based and tree-based methods, respectively.

Table 3. Results for logistic regression with and without LASSO regularization.

Results for Single Outcome	Logistic Regression				Logistic Regression with LASSO			
	Trainset	Test Set			Trainset	Test Set		
	ACC	ACC	SENS	SPEC	ACC	ACC	SENS	SPEC
CC—Tumor nature	0.9583	0.9583	1.0000	0.9286	0.9167	0.9167	0.9000	0.9286
MLO—Tumor nature	0.7500	0.7500	0.8333	0.6667	0.8750	0.8750	1.0000	0.7500
CC—Grading	0.8333	0.8333	0.8571	0.8000	0.7917	0.7917	0.9286	0.6000
MLO—Grading	0.7083	0.7083	0.8462	0.5455	0.7917	0.7917	0.7692	0.8182
CC—HER2	0.7143	0.7143	0.7778	0.6000	0.7857	0.7857	1.0000	0.4000
MLO—HER2	0.6786	0.6786	0.5333	0.8462	0.8214	0.8214	0.8000	0.8462
CC—HR	0.8500	0.8500	0.8182	0.8889	0.8500	0.8500	0.7273	1.0000
MLO—HR	0.7500	0.7500	0.7500	0.7500	0.7000	0.7000	0.5000	1.0000

Table 4. Results for CART and RF methods.

Results for Single Outcome	CART				Random Forest			
	Trainset	Test Set			Trainset	Test Set		
	ACC	ACC	SENS	SPEC	ACC	ACC	SENS	SPEC
CC—Tumor nature	0.9122	0.9167	0.9000	0.9286	0.9259	0.9167	0.9000	0.9286
MLO—Tumor nature	0.8825	0.8333	1.0000	0.6667	0.8968	0.8750	1.0000	0.7500
CC—Grading	0.8073	0.9167	0.9286	0.9000	0.8265	0.8750	0.9286	0.8000
MLO—Grading	0.7660	0.8333	0.8462	0.8182	0.8021	0.8750	0.9231	0.8182
CC—HER2	0.6992	0.6071	0.4444	0.9000	0.7463	0.7143	0.6111	0.9000
MLO—HER2	0.7084	0.8214	0.8667	0.7692	0.8289	0.8929	0.8667	0.9231
CC—HR	0.8045	0.8000	0.6364	1.0000	0.8125	0.8500	0.7273	1.0000
MLO—HR	0.7331	0.7000	0.5000	1.0000	0.7756	0.8000	0.6667	1.0000

Considering the CC view, the best performances were obtained when predicting the tumor nature (malignant versus benign). Logistic regression proved to be the best performing model (test accuracy of 95.83%) when using an approach without LASSO regularization. The goodness of the logistic regression method was also observed with LASSO regularization (test accuracy of 91.67%). Almost comparable results were obtained when using the tree-based algorithms (Table 5), with a test accuracy of 91.67% in the prediction of tumor nature. The decisional chart obtained with the CART method is shown in Figure 2 and the goodness of training procedure on 500 trees with the RF method is shown in Figure 3.

Table 5. Examples of results for logistic regression methods run using all possible combinations of two predictors.

Results for Single Outcome	ACC	SENS	SPEC	Var 1	Var 2
CC—Tumor nature	0.9583	1.0000	0.9286	original_gldm_SmallDependenceEmphasis	original_firstorder_TotalEnergy
MLO—Tumor nature	0.9167	1.0000	0.8333	original_gldm_LargeDependenceHighGrayLevelEmphasis	wavelet_LHL_glcm_MaximumProbability
CC—Grading	0.9167	0.9286	0.9000	original_gldm_SmallDependenceEmphasis	wavelet_HLL_firstorder_Energy
MLO—Grading	0.9167	1.0000	0.8182	original_glrlm_RunPercentage	original_glszm_LargeAreaLowGrayLevelEmphasis
CC—HR	0.9000	0.8182	1.0000	original_glcm_InverseVariance	original_glcm_DifferenceVariance
MLO—HR	0.9500	0.9167	1.0000	original_firstorder_Maximum	wavelet_LHL_glrlm_RunPercentage

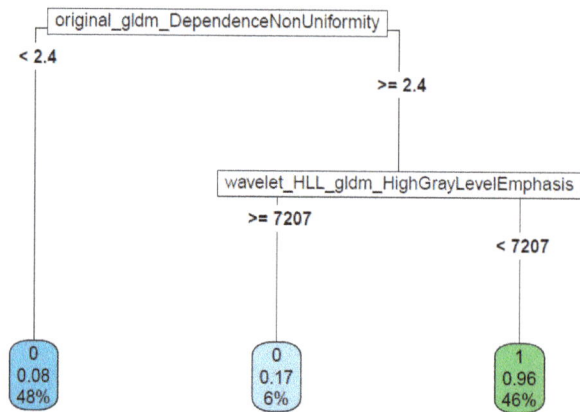

Figure 2. Decisional chart for the prediction of tumor nature from CC images.

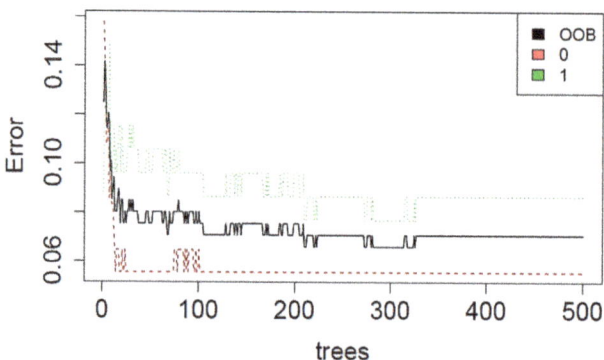

Figure 3. Error evolution during the training procedure of the RF method for the prediction of tumor nature from CC images.

Considering the features extracted from MLO view images, the best test accuracy (91.67%) was obtained when predicting the grading using a CART algorithm, while the use of all non-redundant features (44 predictors) in a logistic regression model significantly reduces the accuracy value (max test accuracy of 75.00%). The goodness of tree-based algorithms is confirmed by the error evolution plot of RF, reaching an accuracy value of 87.50% on the test set. The decision chart and error evolution are shown in Figure 4.

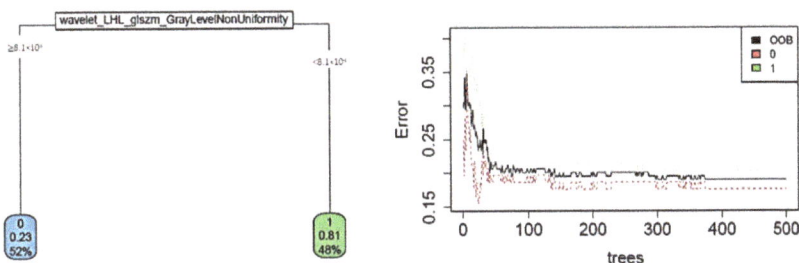

Figure 4. The decision chart and error evolution for the prediction of grading from MLO images.

Combinations of only two features, extracted from both CC and MLO views, always showed test accuracy values greater than or equal to 90.00% (Table 5), with the only exception being the HER2 outcome, where the best performance (test accuracy of 89.29%) was obtained with the RF algorithm.

4. Discussions

The radiomics analysis of tumor features extracted from CEM images represents an important tool for breast cancer characterization.

In this study, we aimed to perform radiomics analysis with texture features extracted by dual-energy CEM, evaluating its ability to classify malignant and benign breast lesions, and to predict grading and breast cancer receptors status (HER2+ and HR+).

In recent years, many studies have addressed the problem of breast lesion classification using several feature categories, such as morphological and textural features, in combination with different machine learning approaches, based on CEM and Dynamic Contrast-Enhanced MRI image analysis [29–40,54–58], whereas other studies used CEM to predict histological outcomes [45,46].

La Forgia et al. [45] assessed the discrimination power of the statistical features extracted from CEM images to predict histological outcomes and two particular subtypes of tumors, HER2-positive and triple-negative. In their work, they showed encouraging results for the differentiation between ER+/ER−, PR+/PR−, HER2+/HER2−, Ki67+/Ki67−, and High-Grade/Low-Grade. In particular, the highest performances were obtained for discriminating HER2+/HER2− (90.87%), ER+/ER− (83.79%), and Ki67+/Ki67− (84.80%).

In a retrospective study, Marino et al. [46] examined the potential of radiomics analysis using features from both CEM and MRI. In particular, they assessed the tumor invasiveness, the hormone receptor status, and the tumor grade in patients with primary breast cancer through common radiomics parameters. In their results, they showed remarkable accuracies when performing CEM radiomics analysis for discriminating HR+ versus HR− breast cancers (95.6%) and invasive versus non-invasive breast cancers (92.0%); slightly lower results were obtained, instead, in the classification of G1 + G2 versus G3 invasive cancers (77.8%).

The results of the univariate analysis of the present study show that the classification of malignant versus benign lesions achieved the best performance when considering the original_gldm_DependenceNonUniformity feature extracted on CC view (accuracy of 88.98%). The features extracted on CC view appeared to perform better, as the results in the classification of both grading and HR suggest. In fact, an accuracy of 83.65% was reached in the classification of grading, whereas a slightly lower value of accuracy (81.65%) was found in the classification of HR+; the features extracted were the original_glrlm_RunEntropy and the original_gldm_DependenceNonUniformity, respectively. In the identification of HER2+, the best performance, however low (accuracy of 69.63%), was reached when considering the wavelet_HLH_gldm_LargeDependenceHighGrayLevelEmphasis feature, extracted on MLO view images.

The results of multivariate analysis showed that better performances could be achieved when using two or more features as predictors for the classification of malignant and benign lesions and for the prediction of HR positive status. The best performance was achieved when predicting the tumor nature from the CC images through a logistic regression model, where the test accuracy reached a value of 95.83% without LASSO regulation. Nevertheless, the LASSO regularization selected 12 out of 27 predictors, significantly reducing the model complexity, at the price of an imperceptible reduction in performance (91.67%).

The same performance of logistic regression was not observed when predicting the same outcome (malignant versus benign classification) using MLO images, confirming the tendency of results in the univariate analysis context.

Features extracted from MLO images were shown to be useful in the prediction of grading with a CART algorithm. However, the results obtained with a logistic regression approach using only two predictors (minimum test accuracy of 90.00%, maximum test accuracy of 95.83%) suggest that simpler models are preferred, with the only exception of the HER2 outcome, where the best performance (test accuracy of 89.29%) was obtained with the RF algorithm.

Remarkable results were also obtained in the prediction of both the grading and the HR+, from both CC and MLO views; however, the performance of logistic regression (regularized or not) and of tree-based algorithms is surpassed by the accuracies obtained when using only two predictive features. Therefore, it can be stated that the prediction of all the outcomes is preferable with less complex models (that is, logistic regression with only two predictors or with a regularized approach). It is furthermore useful to note that the results of univariate analysis are less performant of those of the multivariate approach, suggesting that artificial intelligence can be powerfully used to extract insights from CEM images analysis.

The main limitation of this study is the need for manual segmentation of the images, which is time consuming and operator dependent. The problem of biased results due to this weakness was addressed by having two radiologists perform the segmentation. A foreseeable solution may be the use of automatic or semi-automatic segmentation; however, this may be difficult to implement, especially in the cases of multicentric lesions or background parenchymal enhancement. A further limit is that the interpretation of machine learning algorithm results is not always intuitive and may require specific expertise from the clinician.

5. Conclusions

The results of this study confirm that radiomics textural features extracted from CEM images can be highly informative about both the tumor nature and grading, and some molecular subtypes of tumors. Therefore, the results suggest that the combination of artificial intelligence algorithms with the concept of radiomics analysis can be successfully used to create a tool for supporting the physician's decision-making process in the classification of breast cancer. In particular, the identification of malignant breast lesions and HR positive status can be performed with a high predictive power, even using simpler models.

Author Contributions: Conceptualization, L.B.; Data curation, A.P. (Antonella Petrillo), R.F.; F.A. and D.L.F.; Formal analysis, R.F., E.D.B. and T.P.; Investigation, A.P. (Antonella Petrillo), M.L.B., A.P. (Annamaria Porto), V.G., M.D.B., A.F., R.M., N.P. and D.L.F.; Methodology, R.F., E.D.B., T.P., M.L.B., V.G., M.D.B., A.F., R.M., N.P., F.A. and D.L.F.; Project administration, A.P.(Annamaria Porto); Writing—original draft, A.P. (Antonella Petrillo); R.F.; E.D.B.; Writing—review and editing, A.P. (Antonella Petrillo), A.F., R.F., E.D.B.; R.M. and D.L.F. All authors have read and agreed to the published version of the manuscript.

Funding: This research was funded by the Italian Ministry of Health through the Project RCR-2021-23671213 of the "Alleanza Contro il Cancro (ACC)" network.

Institutional Review Board Statement: The study was conducted according to the guidelines of the Declaration of Helsinki, and approved by the Ethics Committee National Cancer Institute of Naples Pascale Foundation. The authorization number is: Executive Resolution No. 868 of 03/09/2020 of National Cancer Institute of Naples Pascale Foundation.

Informed Consent Statement: All patients enrolled signed the informed consent.

Data Availability Statement: Data are available at https://zenodo.org/record/6476156#.YmGi2tpBy3A, accessed on 13 March 2022.

Acknowledgments: The authors acknowledge the support from the Radiomics Group of "Alleanza Contro il Cancro" and the Italian Ministry of Health.

Conflicts of Interest: The authors declare that they have no known competing financial interests or personal relationships that could have appeared to influence the work reported in this paper.

References

1. Patel, B.K.; Lobbes, M.; Lewin, J. Contrast Enhanced Spectral Mammography: A Review. *Semin. Ultrasound CT MRI* **2018**, *39*, 70–79. [CrossRef] [PubMed]
2. Heywang-Köbrunner, S.; Viehweg, P.; Heinig, A.; Küchler, C. Contrast-enhanced MRI of the breast: Accuracy, value, controversies, solutions. *Eur. J. Radiol.* **1997**, *24*, 94–108. [CrossRef]
3. Satake, H.; Ishigaki, S.; Ito, R.; Naganawa, S. Radiomics in breast MRI: Current progress toward clinical application in the era of artificial intelligence. *Radiol. Med.* **2022**, *127*, 39–56. [CrossRef]
4. Dromain, C.; Balleyguier, C.; Muller, S.; Mathieu, M.C.; Rochard, F.; Opolon, P.; Sigal, R. Evaluation of tumor angiogenesis of breast carcinoma using contrast-enhanced digital mammography. *AJR Am. J. Roentgenol.* **2006**, *187*, 528–537. [CrossRef] [PubMed]
5. Dromain, C.; Balleyguier, C.; Adler, G.; Garbay, J.R.; Delalogeet, S. Contrast-enhanced digital mammography. *Eur. J. Radiol.* **2009**, *69*, 34–42. [CrossRef]
6. Li, L.; Roth, R.; Germaine, P.; Ren, S.; Lee, M.; Hunter, K.; Tinney, E.; Liao, L. Contrast-enhanced spectral mammography (CESM) versus breast magnetic resonance imaging (MRI): A retrospective comparison in 66 breast lesions. *Diagn. Interv. Imaging* **2017**, *98*, 113–123. [CrossRef] [PubMed]
7. Fallenberg, E.M.; Dromain, C.; Diekmann, F.; Engelken, F.; Krohn, M.; Singh, J.M.; Ingold-Heppner, B.; Winzer, K.J.; Bick, U.; Renz, D.M. Contrast-enhanced spectral mammography versus MRI: Initial results in the detection of breast cancer and assessment of tumour size. *Eur. Radiol.* **2014**, *24*, 256–264. [CrossRef]
8. Lewin, J.M.; Isaacs, P.K.; Vance, V.; Larke, F.J. Dual-energy contrast-enhanced digital subtraction mammography: Feasibility. *Radiology* **2003**, *229*, 261–268. [CrossRef]
9. Jochelson, M.S.; Dershaw, D.D.; Sung, J.S.; Heerdt, A.S.; Thornton, C.; Moskowitz, C.S.; Ferrara, J.; Morris, E.A. Bilateral contrast-enhanced dual-energy digital mammography: Feasibility and comparison with conventional digital mammography and MR imaging in women with known breast carcinoma. *Radiology* **2013**, *266*, 743–751. [CrossRef]
10. Tagliafico, A.S.; Bignotti, B.; Rossi, F.; Signori, A.; Sormani, M.P.; Valdora, F.; Calabrese, M.; Houssami, N. Diagnostic performance of contrast-enhanced spectral mammography: Systematic review and meta-analysis. *Breast* **2016**, *28*, 13–19. [CrossRef]
11. Liney, G.P.; Sreenivas, M.; Gibbs, P.; Garcia-Alvarez, R.; Turnbull, L.W. Breast lesion analysis of shape technique: Semiautomated vs. manual morphological description. *J. Magn. Reason. Imaging* **2006**, *23*, 493–498. [CrossRef] [PubMed]
12. Fusco, R.; Sansone, M.; Filice, S.; Carone, G.; Amato, D.M.; Sansone, C.; Petrillo, A. Pattern Recognition Approaches for Breast Cancer DCE-MRI Classification: A Systematic Review. *J. Med. Biol. Eng.* **2016**, *36*, 449–459. [CrossRef] [PubMed]
13. Nie, K.; Chen, J.H.; Yu, H.J.; Chu, Y.; Nalcioglu, O.; Su, M.Y. Quantitative analysis of lesion morphology and texture features for diagnostic prediction in breast MRI. *Acad. Radiol.* **2008**, *15*, 1513–1525. [CrossRef] [PubMed]
14. Hu, H.T.; Shan, Q.Y.; Chen, S.L.; Li, B.; Feng, S.T.; Xu, E.J.; Li, X.; Long, J.Y.; Xie, X.Y.; Lu, M.D.; et al. CT-based radiomics for preoperative prediction of early recurrent hepatocellular carcinoma: Technical reproducibility of acquisition and scanners. *Radiol. Med.* **2020**, *125*, 697–705. [CrossRef]
15. Rossi, F.; Bignotti, B.; Bianchi, L.; Picasso, R.; Martinoli, C.; Tagliafico, A.S. Radiomics of peripheral nerves MRI in mild carpal and cubital tunnel syndrome. *Radiol. Med.* **2020**, *125*, 197–203. [CrossRef]
16. Santone, A.; Brunese, M.C.; Donnarumma, F.; Guerriero, P.; Mercaldo, F.; Reginelli, A.; Miele, V.; Giovagnoni, A.; Brunese, L. Radiomic features for prostate cancer grade detection through formal verification. *Radiol. Med.* **2021**, *126*, 688–697. [CrossRef]
17. Fusco, R.; Sansone, M.; Filice, S.; Granata, V.; Catalano, O.; Amato, D.M.; Di Bonito, M.; D'Aiuto, M.; Capasso, I.; Rinaldo, M.; et al. Integration of DCE-MRI and DW-MRI Quantitative Parameters for Breast Lesion Classification. *BioMed. Res. Int.* **2015**, *2015*, 237863. [CrossRef]
18. Zhang, Y.; Zhu, Y.; Zhang, K.; Liu, Y.; Cui, J.; Tao, J.; Wang, Y.; Wang, S. Invasive ductal breast cancer: Preoperative predict Ki-67 index based on radiomics of ADC maps. *Radiol. Med.* **2020**, *125*, 109–116. [CrossRef]

19. Chianca, V.; Albano, D.; Messina, C.; Vincenzo, G.; Rizzo, S.; Del Grande, F.; Sconfienza, L.M. An update in musculoskeletal tumors: From quantitative imaging to radiomics. *Radiol. Med.* **2021**, *126*, 1095–1105. [CrossRef]
20. Kirienko, M.; Ninatti, G.; Cozzi, L.; Voulaz, E.; Gennaro, N.; Barajon, I.; Ricci, F.; Carlo-Stella, C.; Zucali, P.; Sollini, M.; et al. Computed tomography (CT)-derived radiomic features differentiate prevascular mediastinum masses as thymic neoplasms versus lymphomas. *Radiol. Med.* **2020**, *125*, 951–960. [CrossRef]
21. Karmazanovsky, G.; Gruzdev, I.; Tikhonova, V.; Kondratyev, E.; Revishvili, A. Computed tomography-based radiomics approach in pancreatic tumors characterization. *Radiol. Med.* **2021**, *126*, 1388–1395. [CrossRef] [PubMed]
22. Cellina, M.; Pirovano, M.; Ciocca, M.; Gibelli, D.; Floridi, C.; Oliva, G. Radiomic analysis of the optic nerve at the first episode of acute optic neuritis: An indicator of optic nerve pathology and a predictor of visual recovery? *Radiol. Med.* **2021**, *126*, 698–706. [CrossRef] [PubMed]
23. Benedetti, G.; Mori, M.; Panzeri, M.M.; Barbera, M.; Palumbo, D.; Sini, C.; Muffatti, F.; Andreasi, V.; Steidler, S.; Doglioni, C.; et al. CT-derived radiomic features to discriminate histologic characteristics of pancreatic neuroendocrine tumors. *Radiol. Med.* **2021**, *126*, 745–760. [CrossRef]
24. Nazari, M.; Shiri, I.; Hajianfar, G.; Oveisi, N.; Abdollahi, H.; Deevband, M.R.; Oveisi, M.; Zaidi, H. Noninvasive Fuhrman grading of clear cell renal cell carcinoma using computed tomography radiomic features and machine learning. *Radiol. Med.* **2020**, *125*, 754–762. [CrossRef] [PubMed]
25. Crivelli, P.; Ledda, R.E.; Parascandolo, N.; Fara, A.; Soro, D.; Conti, M. A New Challenge for Radiologists: Radiomics in Breast Cancer. *Biomed. Res. Int.* **2018**, *2018*, 6120703. [CrossRef]
26. Maglogiannis, I.; Zafiropoulos, E.; Anagnostopoulos, I. An intelligent system for automated breast cancer diagnosis and prognosis using SVM based classifiers. *Appl. Intell.* **2007**, *30*, 24–36. [CrossRef]
27. Zheng, Y.; Englander, S.; Baloch, S.; Zacharaki, E.I.; Fan, Y.; Schnall, M.D.; Shen, D. STEP: Spatiotemporal enhancement pattern for MR-based breast tumor diagnosis. *Med. Phys.* **2009**, *36*, 3192–3204. [CrossRef]
28. Turashvili, G.; Brogi, E. Tumor Heterogeneity in Breast Cancer. *Front. Med.* **2017**, *8*, 227. [CrossRef]
29. Lambin, P.; Rios-Velazquez, E.; Leijenaar, R.; Carvalho, S.; van Stiphout, R.G.; Granton, P.; Zegers, C.M.; Gillies, R.; Boellard, R.; Dekker, A.; et al. Radiomics: Extracting more information from medical images using advanced feature analysis. *Eur. J. Cancer* **2012**, *48*, 441–446. [CrossRef]
30. Sinha, S.; Lucas-Quesada, F.A.; DeBruhl, N.D.; Sayre, J.; Farria, D.; Gorczyca, D.P.; Bassett, L.W. Multifeature analysis of Gd-enhanced MR images of breast lesions. *J. Magn. Reson. Imaging* **1997**, *7*, 1016–1026. [CrossRef]
31. Vomweg, T.W.; Buscema, P.M.; Kauczor, H.U.; Teifke, A.; Intraligi, M.; Terzi, S.; Heussel, C.P.; Achenbach, T.; Rieker, O.; Mayer, D.; et al. Improved artificial neural networks in prediction of malignancy of lesions in contrast-enhanced MR-mammography. *Med. Phys.* **2003**, *30*, 2350–2359. [CrossRef] [PubMed]
32. Sathya, D.J.; Geetha, K. Mass classification in breast DCE-MR images using an artificial neural network trained via a bee colony optimization algorithm. *Science* **2013**, *39*, 294. [CrossRef]
33. Sathya, J.; Geetha, K. Experimental Investigation of Classification Algorithms for Predicting Lesion Type on Breast DCE-MR Images. *Int. J. Comput. Appl.* **2013**, *82*, 1–8. [CrossRef]
34. Fusco, R.; Sansone, M.; Petrillo, A.; Sansone, C. A Multiple Classifier System for Classification of Breast Lesions Using Dynamic and Morphological Features in DCE-MRI. *Comput. Vis.* **2012**, *7626*, 684–692. [CrossRef]
35. Degenhard, A.; Tanner, C.; Hayes, C.; Hawkes, D.J.O.; Leach, M. The UK MRI Breast Screening Study Comparison between radiological and artificial neural network diagnosis in clinical screening. *Physiol. Meas.* **2002**, *23*, 727–739. [CrossRef] [PubMed]
36. Haralick, R.M.; Shanmugam, K.; Dinstein, I. Textural Features for Image Classification. *IEEE Trans. Syst. Man. Cybern.* **1973**, *SMC-3*, 610–621. [CrossRef]
37. Fusco, R.; Sansone, M.; Sansone, C.; Petrillo, A. Segmentation and classification of breast lesions using dynamic and textural features in dynamic contrast enhanced-magnetic resonance imaging. In Proceedings of the 25th IEEE International Symposium on Computer-Based Medical Systems (CBMS), Rome, Italy, 20–22 June 2012; pp. 1–4.
38. Abdolmaleki, P.; Buadu, L.D.; Naderimansh, H. Feature extraction and classification of breast cancer on dynamic magnetic resonance imaging using artificial neural network. *Cancer Lett.* **2001**, *171*, 183–191. [CrossRef]
39. Agner, S.C.; Soman, S.; Libfeld, E.; McDonald, M.; Thomas, K.; Englander, S.; Rosen, M.A.; Chin, D.; Nosher, J.; Madabhushi, A. Textural Kinetics: A Novel Dynamic Contrast-Enhanced (DCE)-MRI Feature for Breast Lesion Classification. *J. Digit. Imaging* **2010**, *24*, 446–463. [CrossRef]
40. Levman, J.; Leung, T.; Causer, P.; Plewes, D.; Martel, A.L. Classification of dynamic contrast-enhanced magnetic resonance breast lesions by support vector machines. *IEEE Trans. Med. Imaging* **2008**, *27*, 688–696. [CrossRef]
41. Fusco, R.; Piccirillo, A.; Sansone, M.; Granata, V.; Rubulotta, M.R.; Petrosino, T.; Barretta, M.L.; Vallone, P.; Di Giacomo, R.; Esposito, E.; et al. Radiomics and Artificial Intelligence Analysis with Textural Metrics Extracted by Contrast-Enhanced Mammography in the Breast Lesions Classification. *Diagnostics* **2021**, *30*, 815. [CrossRef]
42. Fusco, R.; Piccirillo, A.; Sansone, M.; Granata, V.; Vallone, P.; Barretta, M.L.; Petrosino, T.; Siani, C.; Di Giacomo, R.; Petrillo, A.; et al. Radiomic and Artificial Intelligence Analysis with Textural Metrics, Morphological and Dynamic Perfusion Features Extracted by Dynamic Contrast-Enhanced Magnetic Resonance Imaging in the Classification of Breast Lesions. *Appl. Sci.* **2021**, *11*, 1880. [CrossRef]

43. Fanizzi, A.; Losurdo, L.; Basile, T.M.A.; Bellotti, R.; Bottigli, U.; Delogu, P.; Diacono, D.; Didonna, V.; Fausto, A.; Lombardi, A.; et al. Fully Automated Support System for Diagnosis of Breast Cancer in Contrast-Enhanced Spectral Mammography Images. *J. Clin. Med.* **2019**, *8*, 891. [CrossRef] [PubMed]
44. Massafra, R.; Bove, S.; Lorusso, V.; Biafora, A.; Comes, M.C.; Didonna, V.; Diotaiuti, S.; Fanizzi, A.; Nardone, A.; Nolasco, A.; et al. Radiomic Feature Reduction Approach to Predict Breast Cancer by Contrast-Enhanced Spectral Mammography Images. *Diagnostics* **2021**, *11*, 684. [CrossRef] [PubMed]
45. La Forgia, D.; Fanizzi, A.; Campobasso, F.; Bellotti, R.; Didonna, V.; Lorusso, V.; Moschetta, M.; Massafra, R.; Tamborra, P.; Tangaro, S.; et al. Radiomic Analysis in Contrast-Enhanced Spectral Mammography for Predicting Breast Cancer Histological Outcome. *Diagnostics* **2020**, *10*, 708. [CrossRef] [PubMed]
46. Marino, M.A.; Leithner, D.; Sung, J.; Avendano, D.; Morris, E.A.; Pinker, K.; Jochelson, M.S. Radiomics for Tumor Characterization in Breast Cancer Patients: A Feasibility Study Comparing Contrast-Enhanced Mammography and Magnetic Resonance Imaging. *Diagnostics* **2020**, *10*, 492. [CrossRef]
47. Radiomic Features. Available online: https://pyradiomics.readthedocs.io/en/latest/features.html (accessed on 20 January 2017).
48. Zwanenburg, A.; Vallières, M.; Abdalah, M.A.; Aerts, H.J.W.L.; Andrearczyk, V.; Apte, A.; Ashrafinia, S.; Bakas, S.; Beukinga, R.J.; Boellaard, R.; et al. The Image Biomarker Standardization Initiative: Standardized Quantitative Radiomics for High-Throughput Image-based Phenotyping. *Radiology* **2020**, *295*, 328–338. [CrossRef]
49. R-Tools Technology Inc. Available online: https://www.r-tt.com/ (accessed on 15 October 2020).
50. He, H.; Bai, Y.; Garcia, E.A.; Li, S. ADASYN: Adaptive synthetic sampling approach for imbalanced learning. In Proceedings of the 2008 IEEE International Joint Conference on Neural Networks (IEEE World Congress on Computational Intelligence), Hong Kong, China, 1–6 June 2008; pp. 1322–1328.
51. Gu, X.; Angelov, P.P.; Soares, E.A. A self-adaptive synthetic over-sampling technique for imbalanced classification. *Int. J. Intell. Syst.* **2020**, *35*, 923–943. [CrossRef]
52. Tibshirani, R. The lasso Method for Variable Selection in the Cox Model. *Statist. Med.* **1997**, *16*, 385–395. [CrossRef]
53. Tibshirani, R. Regression Shrinkage and Selection Via the Lasso. *J. R. Stat. Soc. Ser. B Statist. Methodol.* **1996**, *58*, 267–288. [CrossRef]
54. Bernardi, D.; Belli, P.; Benelli, E.; Brancato, B.; Bucchi, L.; Calabrese, M.; Carbonaro, L.A.; Caumo, F.; Cavallo-Marincola, B.; Clauser, P.; et al. Digital breast tomosynthesis (DBT): Recommendations from the Italian College of Breast Radiologists (ICBR) by the Italian Society of Medical Radiology (SIRM) and the Italian Group for Mammography Screening (GISMa). *Radiol. Med.* **2017**, *122*, 723–730. [CrossRef]
55. Bucchi, L.; Belli, P.; Benelli, E.; Bernardi, D.; Brancato, B.; Calabrese, M.; Carbonaro, L.A.; Caumo, F.; Cavallo-Marincola, B.; Clauser, P.; et al. Recommendations for breast imaging follow-up of women with a previous history of breast cancer: Position paper from the Italian Group for Mammography Screening (GISMa) and the Italian College of Breast Radiologists (ICBR) by SIRM. *Radiol. Med.* **2016**, *121*, 891–896. [CrossRef] [PubMed]
56. Losurdo, L.; Fanizzi, A.; Basile, T.M.A.; Bellotti, R.; Bottigli, U.; Dentamaro, R.; Didonna, V.; Lorusso, V.; Massafra, R.; Tamborra, P.; et al. Radiomics Analysis on Contrast-Enhanced Spectral Mammography Images for Breast Cancer Diagnosis: A Pilot Study. *Entropy* **2019**, *21*, 1110. [CrossRef]
57. Ahmed, S.A.; Samy, M.; Ali, A.M.; Hassan, R.A. Architectural distortion outcome: Digital breast tomosynthesis-detected versus digital mammography-detected. *Radiol. Med.* **2022**, *127*, 30–38. [CrossRef] [PubMed]
58. D'Angelo, A.; Orlandi, A.; Bufi, E.; Mercogliano, S.; Belli, P.; Manfredi, R. Automated breast volume scanner (ABVS) compared to handheld ultrasound (HHUS) and contrast-enhanced magnetic resonance imaging (CE-MRI) in the early assessment of breast cancer during neoadjuvant chemotherapy: An emerging role to monitoring tumor response? *Radiol Med.* **2021**, *126*, 517–526. [CrossRef] [PubMed]

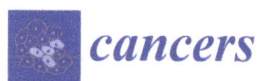

Article

A Model to Predict Upstaging to Invasive Carcinoma in Patients Preoperatively Diagnosed with Low-Grade Ductal Carcinoma In Situ of the Breast

Luca Nicosia [1,*], Anna Carla Bozzini [1], Silvia Penco [1], Chiara Trentin [1], Maria Pizzamiglio [1], Matteo Lazzeroni [2], Germana Lissidini [3], Paolo Veronesi [3,4], Gabriel Farante [3], Samuele Frassoni [5], Vincenzo Bagnardi [5], Cristiana Fodor [6], Nicola Fusco [4,7], Elham Sajjadi [4,7], Enrico Cassano [1,†] and Filippo Pesapane [1,†]

[1] Breast Imaging Division, Radiology Department, IEO, European Institute of Oncology, IRCCS, 20141 Milan, Italy; anna.bozzini@ieo.it (A.C.B.); silvia.penco@ieo.it (S.P.); chiara.trentin@ieo.it (C.T.); maria.pizzamiglio@ieo.it (M.P.); enrico.cassano@ieo.it (E.C.); filippo.pesapane@ieo.it (F.P.)
[2] Division of Cancer Prevention and Genetics, IEO, European Institute of Oncology, IRCCS, 20141 Milan, Italy; matteo.lazzeroni@ieo.it
[3] Division of Breast Surgery, IEO, European Institute of Oncology, IRCCS, 20141 Milan, Italy; germana.lissidini@ieo.it (G.L.); paolo.veronesi@ieo.it (P.V.); gabriel.farante@ieo.it (G.F.)
[4] Department of Oncology and Hemato-Oncology, University of Milan, 20133 Milan, Italy; nicola.fusco@ieo.it (N.F.); elham.sajjadi@ieo.it (E.S.)
[5] Department of Statistics and Quantitative Methods, University of Milan-Bicocca, 20126 Milan, Italy; samuele.frassoni@unimib.it (S.F.); vincenzo.bagnardi@unimib.it (V.B.)
[6] Division of Radiation Oncology, IEO, European Institute of Oncology, IRCCS, 20141 Milan, Italy; cristiana.fodor@ieo.it
[7] Division of Pathology, IEO, European Institute of Oncology, IRCSS, 20141 Milan, Italy
* Correspondence: luca.nicosia@ieo.it
† These authors contributed equally to this work.

Simple Summary: Surgical management is currently the main standard of care procedure used in order to treat ductal carcinoma in situ (DCIS) of the breast. Nevertheless, the survival benefit of surgical resection in patients with such lesions appears to be low, especially for low-grade DCIS. Low-grade DCIS typically exhibit a slow growth pattern and, in many cases, never fully develop into a clinically significant disease: discerning harmless lesions from potentially invasive ones could lead to avoid overtreatment in many patients. Nonetheless, up to 26% of patients with biopsy-proven DCIS can reveal a synchronous invasive carcinoma in surgical specimens. Here, we aimed to create a model of radiological and pathological criteria able to reduce the underestimation of vacuum assisted breast biopsy in DCIS, identifying patients at very low risk (e.g., <2%) of diagnostic underestimation.

Abstract: Background: We aimed to create a model of radiological and pathological criteria able to predict the upgrade rate of low-grade ductal carcinoma in situ (DCIS) to invasive carcinoma, in patients undergoing vacuum-assisted breast biopsy (VABB) and subsequent surgical excision. Methods: A total of 3100 VABBs were retrospectively reviewed, among which we reported 295 low-grade DCIS who subsequently underwent surgery. The association between patients' features and the upgrade rate to invasive breast cancer (IBC) was evaluated by univariate and multivariate analysis. Finally, we developed a nomogram for predicting the upstage at surgery, according to the multivariate logistic regression model. Results: The overall upgrade rate to invasive carcinoma was 10.8%. At univariate analysis, the risk of upgrade was significantly lower in patients with greater age ($p = 0.018$), without post-biopsy residual lesion ($p < 0.001$), with a smaller post-biopsy residual lesion size ($p < 0.001$), and in the presence of low-grade DCIS only in specimens with microcalcifications ($p = 0.002$). According to the final multivariable model, the predicted probability of upstage at surgery was lower than 2% in 58 patients; among these 58 patients, only one (1.7%) upstage was observed, showing a good calibration of the model. Conclusions: An easy-to-use nomogram for predicting the upstage at surgery based on radiological and pathological criteria is able to identify patients with low-grade carcinoma in situ with low risk of upstaging to infiltrating carcinomas.

Citation: Nicosia, L.; Bozzini, A.C.; Penco, S.; Trentin, C.; Pizzamiglio, M.; Lazzeroni, M.; Lissidini, G.; Veronesi, P.; Farante, G.; Frassoni, S.; et al. A Model to Predict Upstaging to Invasive Carcinoma in Patients Preoperatively Diagnosed with Low-Grade Ductal Carcinoma In Situ of the Breast. *Cancers* 2022, 14, 370. https://doi.org/10.3390/cancers14020370

Academic Editor: David Wong

Received: 21 December 2021
Accepted: 10 January 2022
Published: 12 January 2022

Publisher's Note: MDPI stays neutral with regard to jurisdictional claims in published maps and institutional affiliations.

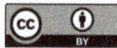

Copyright: © 2022 by the authors. Licensee MDPI, Basel, Switzerland. This article is an open access article distributed under the terms and conditions of the Creative Commons Attribution (CC BY) license (https://creativecommons.org/licenses/by/4.0/).

Keywords: ductal carcinoma in situ (DCIS); invasive breast carcinoma; breast; biopsy; overtreatment; active surveillance

1. Introduction

Breast cancer is one of the most prevalent malignancies among women worldwide, still leading to a considerable incidence of death; in 2020, almost 685,000 women were deceased owing to this malignancy [1]. Ductal carcinoma in situ (DCIS) represents almost 20–25% of all breast neoplastic lesions being diagnosed [2,3]. In DCIS, the cancer cells' growth is confined to the breast ducts or lobules with a minimal potential to spread [4]. As DCIS is mainly clinically occult (around 9% are symptomatic), more than 90% of cases are detected only through imaging studies. Prior to 1980, this condition could be rarely identified. Owing to the improvement of diagnostic and screening imaging tools, specifically mammography, DCIS incidence has rapidly increased [5].

According to the Current National Comprehensive Cancer Network (NCCN), the best therapeutic options are recommended as mastectomy, lumpectomy with radiation, or lumpectomy alone with the potential addition of tamoxifen for hormone receptor–positive carcinoma in situ [6]. There are few data available that compare the benefit obtained from the currently recommended treatments with those who did not receive treatment (active surveillance) [7].

Carcinoma in situ of the breast does not present a risk of invasion and metastasis and the mortality rate is as low as 4% [7]. Therefore, the main purpose of the treatment is to prevent the development of invasive carcinoma. However, a meta-analysis of underestimation and predictors of invasive breast cancer showed that up to 26% of patients with biopsy-proven DCIS can reveal a synchronous invasive carcinoma in surgical specimens [8]. As this percentage is unacceptable, it is necessary to reduce the diagnostic underestimation of the VABB before proposing active surveillance to patients.

How many low-grade breast carcinomas in situ are actually infiltrating carcinomas or high-grade carcinomas in situ? How can we identify patients at low risk of being underestimated with the VABB?

In our study, we examined surgical specimens of patients diagnosed with low-grade DCIS to identify potential indicators for upgrading [9].

By selecting a population with a low risk of upgrading, we may identify patients with low-grade breast cancer in which surgery may be safely spared.

Four prospective international study protocols (LORIS, COMET, LORD, and LORETTA) are currently in place to evaluate non-invasive treatment strategies for DCIS; however, a selection of patient population based on clinical and radiological features (which may reduce the diagnostic underestimation of the biopsy) appears to be neglected in these protocols [10]. We firmly believe that a better initial selection of patients, based on radiological, pathological, and clinical features, can make these protocols more effective, reducing the diagnostic underestimation of the biopsy. We can, therefore, hypothesize models that identify a population in which active surveillance could be safer.

The Loretta protocol is the only one that takes into account the initial size of the lesion. However, other radiological and pathological features, which would be easy to use to reduce the diagnostic underestimation of the biopsy, are not considered in the initial selection of patients in the four prospective international study protocols.

Details are shown in Table 1.

The purpose of our study is to identify a predictive model that identifies the features, mainly based on imaging, that can predict the diagnostic underestimation of low-grade DCIS to invasive carcinoma or worst grade DCIS.

Table 1. Main features of the four prospective international study protocols (LORIS, COMET, LORD and LORETTA).

Study	LORIS [11]	COMET [12]	LORD [13]	LORETTA [14]
Country	UK	USA	EU	JAPAN
Year of activation	2014	2017	2017	2017
Accrual target (number of patients)	932	1200	1240	340
Size of the lesion	Any	Any	Any	<2.5 cm
Type of guide for biopsy	Stereotactic (vacuum assisted)	Stereotactic (vacuum assisted)	Stereotactic (vacuum assisted)	Stereotactic and ultrasound (vacuum assisted)
Hormone receptor status	Any	Hr*-positive only	Any	Hr*-positive only
Endocrine therapy	Optional	Optional	Not allowed	Mandatory
Minimum age at diagnosis	48	40	45	40
Comedonecrosis	Excluded	Allowed	Excluded	Excluded

Hr*: Hestrogen receptor.

2. Materials and Methods

This retrospective study was notified to the Ethics Committee (Identification Number UID 2897, 24 September 2021) and was approved by the Institutional Review Board.

2.1. Study Design and Population

We retrospectively studied all patients who underwent a screening mammogram or an ultrasound for prevention, i.e., dense breasts in a single referral canter for breast cancer care (European Institute of Oncology, Milan, Italy). Among which those with doubtful lesions, between January 1999 and January 2019, were included in our study cohort. All the lesions were classified according to the Breast Imaging Reporting and Data System (BI-RADS), using the score BIRADS ≥ 3 as a threshold to define suspicious lesions. Ultrasound- or stereotactic-guided VABB was performed in patients with BIRADS ≥ 4; only in exceptional cases (3/295), with very high familiarity for breast cancer, patients with BIRADS 3 were biopsied too [15–17].

All the lesions undergoing stereotactic VABB presented as microcalcifications. Before each stereotactic VABB, two projection mammograms were performed in order to assess the precise extension of the lesion (Figure 1).

After the VABB procedure, all patients underwent two additional mammogram projections to confirm the complete macroscopic removal or the presence of residual lesion.

Before each ultrasound VABB, both transverse and longitudinal static images were acquired by US performed prior to the biopsy. After the procedure both transverse and longitudinal US images were taken to detect the complete macroscopic removal or the presence of residual of the lesion in all patients.

We collected and retrospectively analysed some of the features reported in the radiologist's and pathologist's report, in particular: the number of cores obtained for each biopsy, the complete macroscopical removal of the lesion, the diameter of the biopsy needle, and—for stereotactic VABB—if the disease was present only in the cores with microcalcifications (or even in the cores without microcalcifications, if any).

We investigated a potential correlation between patient's age, lesion size, diameter of the needle (with an equal number of biopsy samples, more tissue is collected with a larger needle), number of cores, complete macroscopic removal of the lesion, cases showing low-grade DCIS only in cores with microcalcifications, and the chance of upgrade to a worst grade DCIS or invasive ductal carcinoma (IDC). Since the BIRADS is often very subjective [18], we have excluded it from the analysis. Figure 2 represents a low-grade DCIS.

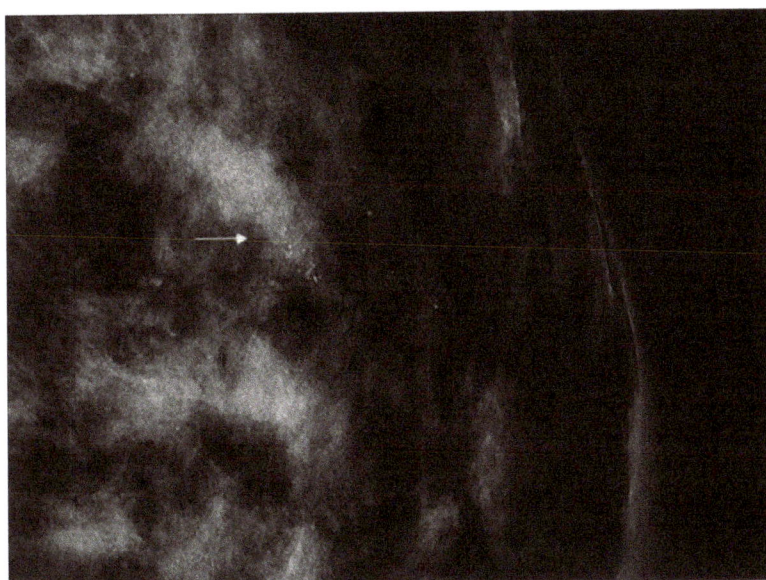

Figure 1. Full-field digital mammography showing a small cluster of pleomorphic microcalcifications (arrow) with a biopsy-proven histopathological result of low-grade ductal carcinoma in situ.

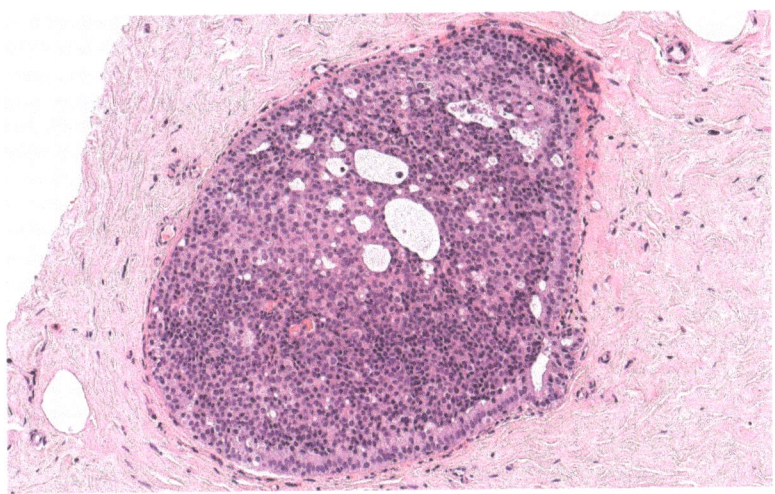

Figure 2. Histological features of low-grade DCIS from a breast biopsy showing bland homogeneous cells contained within the duct, forming rigid cell 'bridges' across the duct space in a cribriform architecture. In this case, the abnormal duct is surrounded by fibrotic stroma (hematoxylin and eosin, original magnification 100×).

In accordance with some recent studies that have shown a benefit in the change of therapy with patients presenting an intermediate grade DCIS with Ki-67 > 14%, we considered this threshold to be significant in our underestimation analyses of worst grade carcinoma in situ at the biopsy [19]. In our predictive model, we also considered underestimation of carcinoma in situ of the worst degree in case of finding of intermediate grade DCIS with Ki-67 > 14%.

2.2. Statistical Analysis

Continuous data are reported as median and range and categorical data are reported as counts and percentages.

Univariate and multivariate logistic regressions were performed to assess the association of age, biopsy needle, residual disease, residual lesion size, number of cores and disease only in cores with micro, with the risk of upgrade of low-grade DCIS to invasive carcinoma. Age, residual lesion size and number of cores were considered as continuous predictors in the models. Residual lesion size was log-transformed due to its skewed distribution.

According to the multivariate logistic regression model, a nomogram for predicting the upstage at surgery was reported.

To evaluate the predictive accuracy of the final multivariate model, in terms of discrimination, Area Under the ROC curve (AUC) was also reported. Moreover, to compare the actual vs. predicted by the model upstaging probabilities, a calibration plot was created. Patients were categorized in five classes, based on predicted probabilities ($\leq$2%, 2–5%, 5–10%, 10–25% and >25%). For each class, the average of the predicted probabilities and the observed relative frequency of patients with upstaging were calculated and reported in the plot.

All analyses were performed with SAS 9.4 (SAS Institute, Cary, NC, USA) and R version 4.0.3.

3. Results

Among the 3100 VABBs analysed, 295 were diagnosed as low-grade DCIS and all the patients underwent subsequent surgical excision.

The clinicopathological features of the patients are summarized in Table 2.

Table 2. Distribution of patients, diagnostic and tumor characteristics (N = 295 DCIS low grade).

Variable	Level	Overall (N = 295)
Year of Mammotome biopsy, N (%)	1999–2004	66 (22.4)
	2005–2009	65 (22.0)
	2010–2014	97 (32.9)
	2015–2018	67 (22.7)
Days between mammography and Mammotome biopsy, median (min–max)		33 (0–313)
Missing		16
Age at Mammotome biopsy, median (min–max)		51 (34–79)
Biopsy needle, N (%)	8G + 7G	45 (15.5)
	11G + 10G	245 (84.5)
	Missing	5
Post biopsy residual disease, N (%)	No	128 (43.4)
	Yes	167 (56.6)
Post biopsy residual lesion size (mm), median (min–max) BIRADS, N (%)		15 (4–100)
	3	3 (1.0)
	4a	124 (42.0)
	4b	95 (32.2)
	4c	61 (20.7)
	5	12 (4.1)
Number of cores, median (min–max)		13 (0–30)
Disease only in cores with microcalcifications, N (%)	No	132 (48.9)
	Yes	138 (51.1)
	Missing	25
Days between Mammotome biopsy and surgery, median (min–max)		51 (5–247)
Missing		3
Outcomes of the study		
Upstage (invasive at surgery), N (%)	No	263 (89.2)
	Yes	32 (10.8)
Upstage at surgery (implying change of therapy), N (%)	No	242 (82.0)
	Yes	53 (18.0)
Absence of disease at the surgery, N (%)	No	234 (79.3)
	Yes	61 (20.7)

Of these 295 patients, 272 were diagnosed by stereotactic VABB and identified by mammography (showing only microcalcifications), while 23 cases were diagnosed by ultrasound-guided VABB (showing as nodule).

Such disproportion is due to the usual radiological manifestation of DCIS as microcalcifications, instead of nodules [20].

At the biopsy, the median age of patients was 51 (34–79) years, the median size of the lesion was 15 mm (4–100); radiological diagnoses were: 3 BIRADS 3 (1%); 124 BIRADS 4a (42%); 95 BIRADS 4b (32.2%); 61 BIRADS 4c (20.7%); 12 BIRADS 5 (4.1%).

In 128 (43.4%) of cases, the lesion was macroscopically removed by VABB. In 138 cases (51.1%) we identified the disease only in the cores with macrocalcifications.

The histological exam of the surgical specimens of the 295 patients indicated that 32 cases (10.8%) were upgraded to IDC, and 53 cases (18.0%) were upgraded to worst grade DCIS, intermediate grade DCIS with Ki-67 > 14% and, high-grade ductal carcinoma in situ.

Interestingly, in 61 cases (20.7%) only benign findings were observed in subsequent surgical specimens; in some cases, the VABB seems to be able to completely remove the lesion.

At univariate analysis, the upgrade rate to IDC was statistically lower in patients with greater age ($p = 0.018$), without post-biopsy residual lesion ($p < 0.001$), with a smaller post-biopsy residual lesion size ($p < 0.001$), and in presence of low-grade DCIS only in specimens with microcalcifications ($p = 0.002$). At multivariate analysis, only post-biopsy residual lesion (OR (95% CI) for patients with vs. without residual disease was 7.14 (1.58–32.2)) and disease only in cores with microcalcifications (OR (95% CI) for patients with vs. without disease with microcalcifications was 0.33 (0.13–0.83)) were significantly associated with the upstage at surgery (Table 3).

Table 3. Association between variables and upstage (invasive at surgery). Results from univariate and multivariate logistic regression analyses.

Variable	Level	Upstage/Tot (%)	Univariate Analysis			Multivariate Analysis [1]		
			OR	95% CI	p-Value	OR	95% CI	p-Value
Overall	-	32/295 (10.8)	-	-	-	-	-	-
Age at Mammotome biopsy	+1 year		0.94	0.90–0.99	0.018	0.95	0.90–1.00	0.068
Biopsy needle	8G + 7G	7/45 (15.6)	Ref.	-	-	Ref.	-	-
	11G + 10G	25/245 (10.2)	0.62	0.25–1.53	0.30	0.77	0.29–2.06	0.60
	Missing	0/5						
Post biopsy residual disease	No	3/128 (2.3)	Ref.	-	-	Ref.	-	-
	Yes	29/167 (17.4)	8.76	2.60–29.4	<0.001	7.14	1.58–32.2	0.011
Post biopsy residual lesion size	+1 × $\log_2$ (mm)		1.76	1.26–2.46	<0.001	0.96	0.58–1.58	0.87
Number of cores	+1		0.98	0.91–1.05	0.53	0.98	0.90–1.05	0.53
Disease only in cores with microcalcifications	No	24/132 (18.2)	Ref.	-	-	Ref.	-	-
	Yes	7/138 (5.1)	0.24	0.10–0.58	0.002	0.33	0.13–0.83	0.018
	Missing	1/25						

[1] Twenty-nine patients with at least one missing value among independent variables were excluded from the model. Goodness of fit statistics: McFadden's R-Square = 0.16; AIC = 174.6; −2 Log Likelihood = 160.6.

A nomogram for predicting the upstage at surgery, based on the multivariate logistic regression model, was reported in Figure 3.

For example, a patient with: age at Mammotome biopsy = "67", biopsy needle = "11G or 10G", post biopsy residual disease = "No", $\log_2$ (Post biopsy residual lesion size) = "3.32", number of cores = "0", disease only in cores with microcalcifications = "Yes", has a probability of upstage (invasive at surgery) of 0.01. While a patient with: age at Mammotome biopsy = "62", biopsy needle = "8G or 7G", post biopsy residual disease = "Yes", $\log_2$ (Post biopsy residual lesion size) = "5.91", number of cores = "8", disease only in cores with microcalcifications = "No", has a probability of upstage (invasive at surgery) of 0.20.

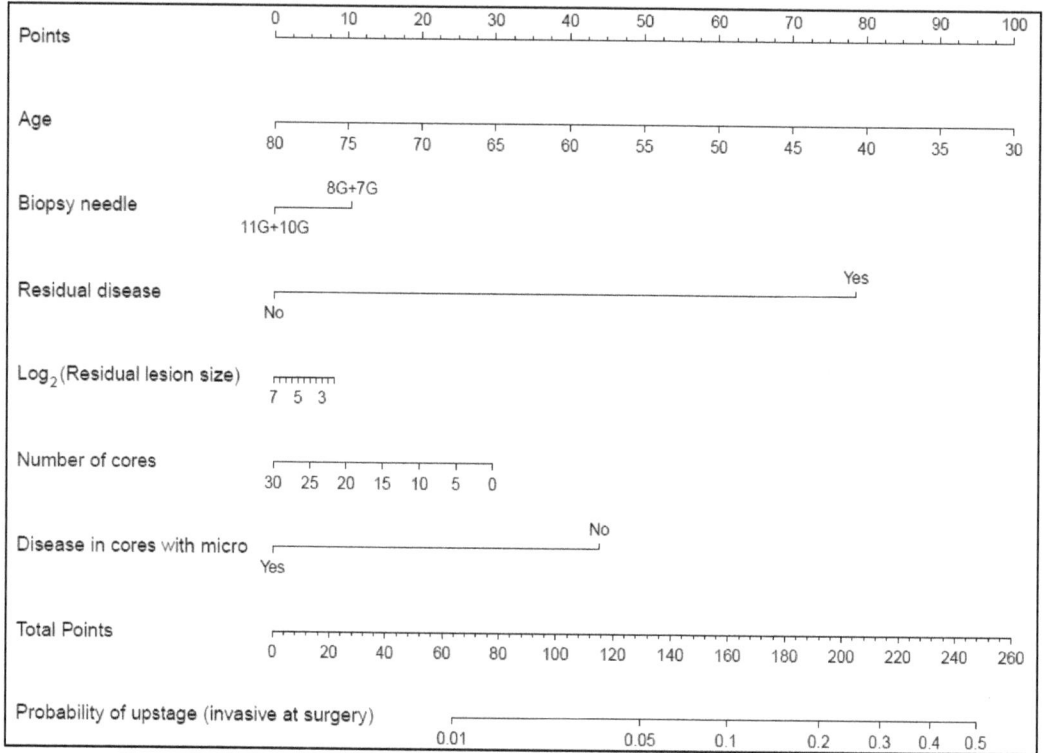

Figure 3. Nomogram for predicting the upstage (invasive at surgery) according to the multivariate logistic regression model. Instructions: to estimate the probability of upstage (invasive at surgery), locate the patient's age at Mammotome biopsy on the "Age" axis. Draw a line straight upward to the point axis to determine how many points they receives for their age. Repeat the process for each additional variable. Sum the points for each of the predictors. Locate the final sum on the "Total point" axis. Draw a line straight down to find the patient's probability of upstage (invasive at surgery). An online Shiny application was developed for users to easily access the model (https://bagnardi.shinyapps.io/DCIS_upstage/, accessed on 7 January 2022).

An online Shiny application was developed for users to easily access the model (https://bagnardi.shinyapps.io/DCIS_upstage/, accessed on 7 January 2022).

The AUC of the final multivariate model was 0.795 (Figure 4, Panel A). Panel B of Figure 4 showed the calibration plot: as an example, the predicted probability of upstage at surgery was lower than 2% in 58 patients (average predicted risk in this category: 1.3%) and, among these 58 patients, only one (1.7%) upstage was observed; the predicted risk was greater than 25% in 46 patients (average predicted risk in this category: 31%) and, among these 46 patients, 17 (37%) upstages were observed.

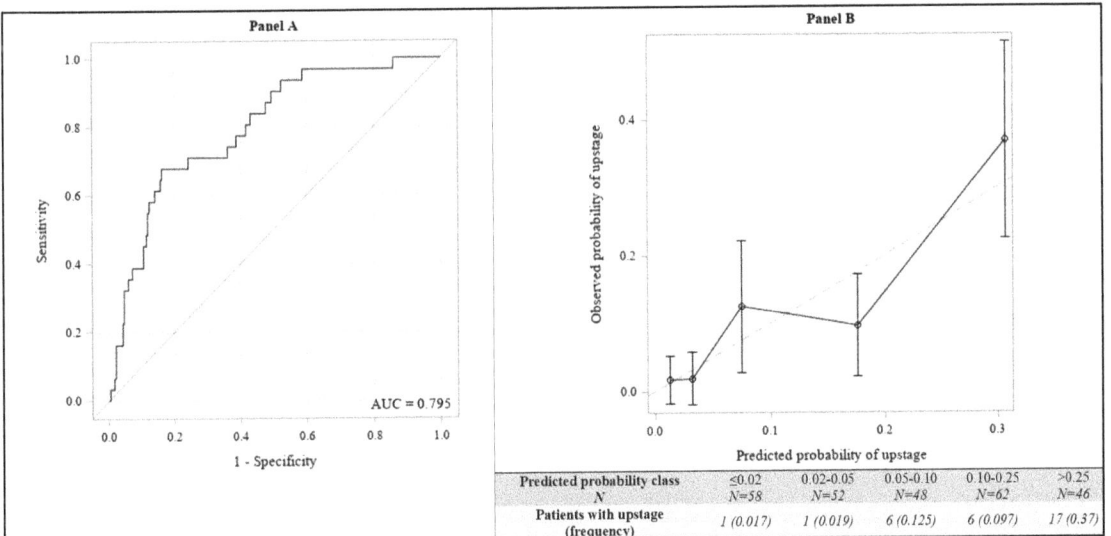

Figure 4. Predictive accuracy of the multivariate logistic regression model; ROC curve (**Panel A**) and Calibration plot (**Panel B**).

The results of the univariate and multivariate analyses considering upstage to worst grade ductal carcinoma in situ at surgery (intermediate grade DCIS with ki-67 > 14% and high-grade DCIS) as dependent variable, are shown in Table S1.

4. Discussion

DCIS is a non-life threatening condition and includes about 25% of all breast cancer cases. Most cases of DCIS will never progress to invasive breast cancer during a patient's lifetime and the 20-year breast cancer-specific mortality rate in patients with DCIS is low [21–23].

Sagara and colleagues [7], in a recent publication, analysed surveillance, epidemiology, and end-results (SEER) data from nine US states involving 57,222 women with a median 72 months' follow-up from diagnosis: the vast majority of patients diagnosed with all grades of DCIS (who did not receive surgery) did not decease from breast cancer. Considering this low long-term mortality, the surgical therapy and the radiotherapy of DCIS may be considered a sort of overtreatment and an unjustified cost to public health, especially for low-grade carcinomas in situ [24].

Four prospective international study protocols (LORIS, COMET, LORD, and LORETTA) are currently in place to evaluate non-invasive treatment strategies for DCIS the results of which will still be evaluated. However, the role of diagnostic underestimation of the breast biopsy is often overlooked. In a meta-analysis, Brennan et al. showed that 25.9% (18.6–37.2%) of presurgical cases diagnosed as DCIS were upgraded to IDC upon excision [8]. Considering only those undergoing VABB, this percentage dropped to around the 15% (regardless of the degree of DCIS) and to the 10% for the low-grade DCIS [25,26]. This percentage is still too high to propose active surveillance to a patient, as follow-up over surgery should be justified by an upgrade rate lower than 2%, as established for Breast Imaging Reporting and Data System, in which a possible diagnostic delay does not affect the outcome [15].

In our study, we propose a predictive model in order to minimize the risk of diagnostic underestimation in a smaller group of patients. Nomograms are predictive tools that allow, considering the multiples features, an assessment of the risk of underestimation [27]. With our nomogram, you are able to evaluate if a patient has a predicted probability of diagnostic underestimation below 2%. Notably, in almost 20% of those who underwent surgery, no residual disease was found in the surgical sample, suggesting a possible complete lesion removal by the VABB.

We believe that our predictive model, once validated in an external cohort, could help in the careful selection of patients to candidate to active surveillance rather than surgical excision. Our study may pose the basis for further future prospective studies where active surveillance can be suggested considering specific radiological and pathological criteria.

The major limitation of our study is represented by its monocentric and retrospective nature, by the low number of cases considered, and by the lack of an external validation cohort. Our study has an exploratory nature: a step towards a long path that can avoid overtreatment in this category of patients.

To be concretely used in clinical practice, our model needs a rigorous validation in an external cohort and to be applied in a large number of patients.

However, we are convinced that these preliminary results are promising, easy to apply in all breast units and deserve to be further investigated in other studies.

We believe that the near future will increasingly focus on enhancing studies that allow us to identify patients in whom the risk of upstaging is lower. In this regard, studies aimed at verifying a specific gene expression of high-risk patients and aimed at verifying specific image features of the lesion with radiomics and contrast enhanced spectral mammography (CESM) will certainly have a fundamental role in this issue [28–30].

5. Conclusions

An easy-to-use predictive model that considers the size of the lesion, its complete removal with VABB, patient's age, biopsy needle, number of cores and the presence of disease only in cores with microcalcifications is able to identify a population of patients with DCIS with low risk of upstaging to IDC.

These criteria, after validation in an external cohort, should be considered when selecting patients for active surveillance rather than surgical intervention.

Supplementary Materials: The following supporting information can be downloaded at: https://www.mdpi.com/article/10.3390/cancers14020370/s1, Table S1: Association between variables and upstage (implying change of therapy).

Author Contributions: Conceptualization, L.N. and F.P.; methodology, A.C.B., S.P., C.T. and M.P.; software, V.B. and S.F.; validation, A.C.B., P.V., G.L., G.F. and E.C.; formal analysis, S.F. and V.B.; investigation, L.N. and F.P.; resources, M.L.; data curation, C.F., S.F. and V.B.; writing—original draft preparation, L.N., F.P. and E.C.; writing—review and editing, N.F., E.S. and M.L.; visualization, M.L., N.F. and E.S.; supervision, L.N. and F.P.; project administration, M.L and E.C. All authors have read and agreed to the published version of the manuscript.

Funding: This research received no external funding.

Institutional Review Board Statement: The study was conducted according to the guidelines of the Declaration of Helsinki, and approved by the Ethics Committees of European Institute of Oncology (IEO, protocol code UID 2897, 24 September 2021).

Informed Consent Statement: Informed consent was obtained from all subjects involved in the study.

Data Availability Statement: The data presented in this study are available on request from the corresponding author. The data are not publicly available due to privacy concerns, in accordance with GDPR.

Conflicts of Interest: The authors declare no conflict of interest.

References

1. Sung, H.; Ferlay, J.; Siegel, R.L.; Laversanne, M.; Soerjomataram, I.; Jemal, A.; Bray, F. Global Cancer Statistics 2020: GLOBOCAN Estimates of Incidence and Mortality Worldwide for 36 Cancers in 185 Countries. *CA Cancer J. Clin.* **2021**, *71*, 209–249. [CrossRef] [PubMed]
2. Kerlikowske, K. Epidemiology of ductal carcinoma in situ. *J. Natl. Cancer Inst. Monogr.* **2010**, *2010*, 139–141. [CrossRef] [PubMed]

3. Salvatorelli, L.; Puzzo, L.; Vecchio, G.M.; Caltabiano, R.; Virzì, V.; Magro, G. Ductal Carcinoma In Situ of the Breast: An Update with Emphasis on Radiological and Morphological Features as Predictive Prognostic Factors. *Cancers* **2020**, *12*, 609. [CrossRef] [PubMed]
4. Parikh, U.; Chhor, C.M.; Mercado, C.L. Ductal Carcinoma In Situ: The Whole Truth. *Am. J. Roentgenol.* **2018**, *210*, 246–255. [CrossRef]
5. D'Orsi, C.J. Imaging for the diagnosis and management of ductal carcinoma in situ. *J. Natl. Cancer Inst. Monogr.* **2010**, *2010*, 214–217. [CrossRef]
6. Wehner, P.; Lagios, M.D.; Silverstein, M.J. DCIS treated with excision alone using the National Comprehensive Cancer Network (NCCN) guidelines. *Ann. Surg. Oncol.* **2013**, *20*, 3175–3179. [CrossRef]
7. Sagara, Y.; Mallory, M.A.; Wong, S.; Aydogan, F.; DeSantis, S.; Barry, W.T.; Golshan, M. Survival Benefit of Breast Surgery for Low-Grade Ductal Carcinoma In Situ: A Population-Based Cohort Study. *JAMA Surg.* **2015**, *150*, 739–745. [CrossRef]
8. Brennan, M.E.; Turner, R.M.; Ciatto, S.; Marinovich, M.L.; French, J.R.; Macaskill, P.; Houssami, N. Ductal carcinoma in situ at core-needle biopsy: Meta-analysis of underestimation and predictors of invasive breast cancer. *Radiology* **2011**, *260*, 119–128. [CrossRef]
9. Veronesi, U.; Viale, G.; Rotmensz, N.; Goldhirsch, A. Rethinking TNM: Breast cancer TNM classification for treatment decision-making and research. *Breast* **2006**, *15*, 3–8. [CrossRef]
10. Kanbayashi, C.; Thompson, A.M.; Hwang, E.S.; Partridge, A.H.; Rea, D.W.; Wesseling, J.; Shien, T.; Mizutani, T.; Shibata, T.; Iwata, H. The international collaboration of active surveillance trials for low-risk DCIS (LORIS, LORD, COMET, LORETTA). *J. Clin. Oncol.* **2019**, *37* (Suppl. 15), TPS603. [CrossRef]
11. Francis, A.; Thomas, J.; Fallowfield, L.; Wallis, M.; Bartlett, J.M.; Brookes, C.; Roberts, T.; Pirrie, S.; Gaunt, C.; Young, J.; et al. Addressing overtreatment of screen detected DCIS; the LORIS trial. *Eur. J. Cancer* **2015**, *51*, 2296–2303. [CrossRef]
12. Hwang, E.S.; Hyslop, T.; Lynch, T.; Frank, E.; Pinto, D.; Basila, D.; Collyar, D.; Bennett, A.; Kaplan, C.; Rosenberg, S.; et al. The COMET (Comparison of Operative versus Monitoring and Endocrine Therapy) trial: A phase III randomised controlled clinical trial for low-risk ductal carcinoma in situ (DCIS). *BMJ Open* **2019**, *9*, e026797. [CrossRef]
13. Elshof, L.E.; Tryfonidis, K.; Slaets, L.; van Leeuwen-Stok, A.E.; Skinner, V.P.; Dif, N.; Pijnappel, R.M.; Bijker, N.; Rutgers, E.J.; Wesseling, J. Feasibility of a prospective, randomised, open-label, international multicentre, phase III, non-inferiority trial to assess the safety of active surveillance for low risk ductal carcinoma in situ—The LORD study. *Eur. J. Cancer* **2015**, *51*, 1497–1510. [CrossRef]
14. Kanbayashi, C.; Iwata, H. Current approach and future perspective for ductal carcinoma in situ of the breast. *Jpn. J. Clin. Oncol.* **2017**, *47*, 671–677. [CrossRef]
15. American College of Radiology. *ACR BI-RADS Atlas: Breast Imaging Reporting and Data System*, 5th ed.; American College of Radiology: Reston, VA, USA, 2013.
16. American College of Radiology. ACR BI-RADS 5th Edition Changes. Available online: http://www.acr.org/$\sim$/media/acr/documents/pdf/qualitysafety/resources/birads/birads_v5_changes (accessed on 21 December 2021).
17. Spak, D.A.; Plaxco, J.S.; Santiago, L.; Dryden, M.J.; Dogan, B.E. BI-RADS® fifth edition: A summary of changes. *Diagn. Interv. Imaging* **2017**, *98*, 179–190. [CrossRef]
18. Spayne, M.C.; Gard, C.C.; Skelly, J.; Miglioretti, D.L.; Vacek, P.M.; Geller, B.M. Reproducibility of BI-RADS breast density measures among community radiologists: A prospective cohort study. *Breast J.* **2012**, *18*, 326–333. [CrossRef]
19. Lazzeroni, M.; Guerrieri-Gonzaga, A.; Botteri, E.; Leonardi, M.C.; Rotmensz, N.; Serrano, D.; Varricchio, C.; Disalvatore, D.; Del Castillo, A.; Bassi, F.; et al. Tailoring treatment for ductal intraepithelial neoplasia of the breast according to Ki-67 and molecular phenotype. *Br. J. Cancer* **2013**, *108*, 1593–1601. [CrossRef]
20. Wang, H.; Lin, J.; Lai, J.; Tan, C.; Yang, Y.; Gu, R.; Jiang, X.; Liu, F.; Hu, Y.; Su, F. Imaging features that distinguish pure ductal carcinoma in situ (DCIS) from DCIS with microinvasion. *Mol. Clin. Oncol.* **2019**, *11*, 313–319. [CrossRef]
21. Molinié, F.; Vanier, A.; Woronoff, A.S.; Guizard, A.V.; Delafosse, P.; Velten, M.; Daubisse-Marliac, L.; Arveux, P.; Tretarre, B. Trends in breast cancer incidence and mortality in France 1990–2008. *Breast Cancer Res. Treat.* **2014**, *147*, 167–175. [CrossRef]
22. Narod, S.A.; Iqbal, J.; Giannakeas, V.; Sopik, V.; Sun, P. Breast Cancer Mortality after a Diagnosis of Ductal Carcinoma In Situ. *JAMA Oncol.* **2015**, *1*, 888–896. [CrossRef]
23. Lazzeroni, M.; DeCensi, A. De-Escalating Treatment of Low-Risk Breast Ductal Carcinoma In Situ. *J. Clin. Oncol.* **2020**, *38*, 1252–1254. [CrossRef]
24. Fallowfield, L.; Francis, A. Overtreatment of Low-Grade Ductal Carcinoma In Situ. *JAMA Oncol.* **2016**, *2*, 382–383. [CrossRef]
25. Nicosia, L.; di Giulio, G.; Bozzini, A.C.; Fanizza, M.; Ballati, F.; Rotili, A.; Lazzeroni, M.; Latronico, A.; Abbate, F.; Renne, G.; et al. Complete Removal of the Lesion as a Guidance in the Management of Patients with Breast Ductal Carcinoma In Situ. *Cancers* **2021**, *13*, 868. [CrossRef]
26. Cheung, Y.C.; Chen, S.C.; Ueng, S.H.; Yu, C.C. Ductal Carcinoma In Situ Underestimation of Microcalcifications Only by Stereotactic Vacuum-Assisted Breast Biopsy: A New Predictor of Specimens without Microcalcifications. *J. Clin. Med.* **2020**, *9*, 2999. [CrossRef]
27. Nicosia, L.; Latronico, A.; Addante, F.; De Santis, R.; Bozzini, A.C.; Montesano, M.; Frassoni, S.; Bagnardi, V.; Mazzarol, G.; Pala, O.; et al. Atypical Ductal Hyperplasia after Vacuum-Assisted Breast Biopsy: Can We Reduce the Upgrade to Breast Cancer to an Acceptable Rate? *Diagnostics* **2021**, *11*, 1120. [CrossRef]

28. Solin, L.J.; Gray, R.; Baehner, F.L.; Butler, S.M.; Hughes, L.L.; Yoshizawa, C.; Cherbavaz, D.B.; Shak, S.; Page, D.L.; Sledge, G.W., Jr.; et al. A multigene expression assay to predict local recurrence risk for ductal carcinoma in situ of the breast. *J. Natl. Cancer Inst.* **2013**, *105*, 701–710. [CrossRef]
29. Li, J.; Song, Y.; Xu, S.; Wang, J.; Huang, H.; Ma, W.; Jiang, X.; Wu, Y.; Cai, H.; Li, L. Predicting underestimation of ductal carcinoma in situ: A comparison between radiomics and conventional approaches. *Int. J. Comput. Assist. Radiol. Surg.* **2019**, *14*, 709–721. [CrossRef]
30. Cheung, Y.C.; Chen, K.; Yu, C.C.; Ueng, S.H.; Li, C.W.; Chen, S.C. Contrast-Enhanced Mammographic Features of In Situ and Invasive Ductal Carcinoma Manifesting Microcalcifications Only: Help to Predict Underestimation? *Cancers* **2021**, *13*, 4371. [CrossRef]

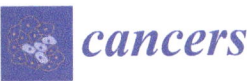

Review

Impact of the Cancer Cell Secretome in Driving Breast Cancer Progression

Syazalina Zahari, Saiful Effendi Syafruddin and M. Aiman Mohtar *

UKM Medical Molecular Biology Institute (UMBI), Universiti Kebangsaan Malaysia,
Kuala Lumpur 56000, Malaysia; p111431@siswa.ukm.edu.my (S.Z.); effendisy@ppukm.ukm.edu.my (S.E.S.)
* Correspondence: m.aimanmohtar@ppukm.ukm.edu.my

Simple Summary: Breast cancer is a complex disease that remains a significant public health challenge. The breast cancer cells secrete various substances collectively known as the secretome, which include proteins, lipids, and nucleic acids that contribute to the growth and spread of breast cancer. The secretome plays a crucial role in the development and progression of breast cancer by modifying signaling pathways and creating an environment supporting cancer growth while evading the immune system. Additionally, the secretome is responsible for the development of resistance to cancer drugs, making it a significant challenge for effective treatment. Therefore, understanding the role of the secretome in breast cancer is essential for developing innovative therapies. This review provides insights into the impact of the secretome on breast cancer progression and its interactions with the tumor microenvironment, and explores potential therapeutic opportunities targeting the secretome components. By identifying specific molecules and signaling pathways involved in the secretome, new targets for therapeutic intervention can be identified, which can ultimately improve outcomes for breast cancer patients.

Abstract: Breast cancer is a complex and heterogeneous disease resulting from the accumulation of genetic and epigenetic alterations in breast epithelial cells. Despite remarkable progress in diagnosis and treatment, breast cancer continues to be the most prevalent cancer affecting women worldwide. Recent research has uncovered a compelling link between breast cancer onset and the extracellular environment enveloping tumor cells. The complex network of proteins secreted by cancer cells and other cellular components within the tumor microenvironment has emerged as a critical player in driving the disease's metastatic properties. Specifically, the proteins released by the tumor cells termed the secretome, can significantly influence the progression and metastasis of breast cancer. The breast cancer cell secretome promotes tumorigenesis through its ability to modulate growth-associated signaling pathways, reshaping the tumor microenvironment, supporting pre-metastatic niche formation, and facilitating immunosurveillance evasion. Additionally, the secretome has been shown to play a crucial role in drug resistance development, making it an attractive target for cancer therapy. Understanding the intricate role of the cancer cell secretome in breast cancer progression will provide new insights into the underlying mechanisms of this disease and aid in the development of more innovative therapeutic interventions. Hence, this review provides a nuanced analysis of the impact of the cancer cell secretome on breast cancer progression, elucidates the complex reciprocal interaction with the components of the tumor microenvironment and highlights emerging therapeutic opportunities for targeting the constituents of the secretome.

Keywords: metastasis; secretome; immune modulation; tumor microenvironment; drug resistance; therapeutic targets; precision oncology

Citation: Zahari, S.; Syafruddin, S.E.; Mohtar, M.A. Impact of the Cancer Cell Secretome in Driving Breast Cancer Progression. *Cancers* 2023, 15, 2653. https://doi.org/10.3390/cancers15092653

Academic Editors: Enrico Cassano and Filippo Pesapane

Received: 14 April 2023
Revised: 4 May 2023
Accepted: 4 May 2023
Published: 8 May 2023

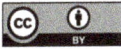

Copyright: © 2023 by the authors. Licensee MDPI, Basel, Switzerland. This article is an open access article distributed under the terms and conditions of the Creative Commons Attribution (CC BY) license (https://creativecommons.org/licenses/by/4.0/).

1. Introduction

Breast cancer is a disease that exhibits genetic and clinical heterogeneities with multiple cellular origins, encompassing various subtypes [1]. Breast cancer is the most diagnosed and life-threatening malignancy in women and the leading cause of cancer death in women worldwide [2]. According to GLOBOCAN 2020, the estimated prevalence of breast cancer in both sexes and for all ages is 7.79 million in 5 years, ranking number one in incidence at 2.26 million worldwide and fourth in the mortality rate [2]. In the United States, breast cancer is the second most significant cause of death by cancer among women overall, but ranks highest among Black and Hispanic women [3,4]. A localized breast cancer incidence has a good prognosis, with a five-year survival rate of more than 80% [5]. Usually, metastatic breast cancer is rare at initial diagnosis (around 6–7%). However, approximately 30% of patients diagnosed with early stages will eventually acquire recurrent or metastatic breast cancer [5–7]. Cases of patients with recurrent breast cancer are often fatal; survival is typically within five years of diagnosis [5].

Breast cancer has undergone several classifications over time, but the most used and widely accepted classification system of breast cancer involves the assessment of the expression of estrogen (ER), progesterone (PR), and human epidermal growth factor 2 (HER2) hormone receptors via immunohistochemical analysis. This renders breast cancer into four main subtypes: luminal A, luminal B, HER2-enriched, and basal-like [8,9]. Luminal-like breast cancer subtypes, characterized by ER and/or PR on the surface of breast cancer cells, are the most common breast cancer [10,11]. Luminal breast cancers are generally considered less aggressive than other breast cancer subtypes, such as the basal-like that do not express hormone receptors. Between the two Luminal subtypes, Luminal A breast cancers are less aggressive and have a better prognosis [12]. HER2-positive subtype overexpresses HER2, which accounts for about 20–25% of all breast cancer. Basal-like or triple-negative breast cancer (TNBC) lacks the above three key receptors. HER2 and TNBC tend to be more aggressive than other breast cancer subtypes, and are associated with a higher risk of recurrence and poorer prognosis if left untreated. Standard treatments for all subtypes would be surgical resection, radiotherapy, and chemotherapy, whereas targeted and immunotherapy would be the options to treat the specific subtypes [13–15]. This classification is, therefore, crucial to tailor specified treatment for the breast cancer patient. Recent therapeutic approaches have emerged, such as targeting metabolic pathways, immunotherapy, conjugated antibodies, and vaccines [16]. Therefore, it is crucial to comprehend the onset and course of breast cancer pathogenesis to create interventions that can improve cancer patients' health and well-being.

While there have been significant advances and breakthroughs in breast cancer research, there is still much to learn about this disease. This is partly due to the complexity and heterogeneity of the disease. In recent years, breast cancer's onset and metastatic properties have been linked to the extracellular moieties surrounding the tumor cells [17–19]. This includes the proteins secreted by cancer cells and other cellular constituents within the tumor microenvironment (TME). These secreted molecules released by tumor cells (termed the secretome) could influence the therapeutic response and clinical outcome, such as gaining resistance to cancer drugs and therapies, making its pathological evaluation indispensable in cancer management. Therefore, this review aims to evaluate the functional impacts of cancer cell secretome in the pathogenesis of breast cancer. While there have been several reviews linking the secretome and breast cancer progression previously, this review emphasized the recent findings, particularly on the protein molecules secreted in the tumor microenvironment and the secretome's interaction with major components of the TME that contribute to the hallmarks of breast cancer. Last, the relevance of targeting the components of breast cancer secretome is discussed.

2. The Topography of Breast Cancer Secretome

The secretome can be defined as both soluble and insoluble factors that are released or secreted into the extracellular environment. These include chemokines, cytokines, growth factors, coagulation factors, hormones, enzymes, glycoproteins, and nucleic acids. These factors can be secreted as naked components or cargo in vesicular compartments, such as extracellular vesicles (EVs). The latest human secretome atlas project highlighted that 2641 genes encode proteins predicted to be secreted in humans [20]. This number observably varies on cellular perturbation and disease development. Studies have shown that cancer cells, for example, have abnormal secretomes compared to their non-cancerous counterparts and therefore have functional impacts on cancer development [21–23]. The secretome is typically identified by high-throughput omics platforms, particularly protein identification by mass-spectrometry-based analysis.

The most basic and extensively researched secretome type is the cancer cell-derived conditioned medium (CM) of cancer cells grown in 2D or 3D culture [24]. Typically, serum proteins and scaffold-free (formation of spheroids without hydrogels, laminin, collagen, or ECM gel) are removed from the medium, and then culturing the cancer cells in serum-starved media in a short period (24 or 48 h). The medium is collected and centrifuged to remove apoptotic bodies, concentrated, and further subjected to secretome identification. This method's benefits include obtaining relatively large sample sizes and comparing data quantitatively following cancer cell modification [25,26]. In an in vivo setting, on the other hand, the cancer cell secretome, including breast cancer, can be isolated from the bodily fluids of the cancer patient. Often time, for most cancer types, serum or plasma is the primary source of secretomic studies.

In breast cancer patients, there are additional essential avenues to breast cancer research in that several localities of the breast ductal/lobular system are enriched with the secretome population. For example, the proteins can be secreted or shed by the tumor or stromal cells into the tumor interstitial fluid (TIF). This fluid, which surrounds the stromal and tumor cells, is thought to contain signaling constituents crucial for intercellular communication and the growth of the tumor. To obtain this TIF, small fragments of fresh tumor tissue are cultured in a buffered solution [27]. After centrifugation, the secretome will be released into the supernatant [28]. In addition, the secretome fractions from nipple aspirate fluid (NAF), pleural effusion (PE), stool, and ascites are other types of fluids that can be analyzed and have been previously shown to contain cancer-specific proteins as compared to the baseline patient. NAF extraction has been accomplished with varying success rates by using either a breast pump, massage, warming of the breast or combinations of these methods [29,30]. The release of NAF into the ducts could be enhanced by administering nasal oxytocin, increasing the yield of NAF in breast cancer patients [31]. It is known that breast cancer spreads into the pleural space via lymph vessels [32]. Hence, the PE sample is withdrawn from this pleural space localized between the inside of the chest wall and the outside of the lung via thoracentesis. Studies have shown that the gut microbiota induces multiple pathways linked to breast tumor growth [33,34] through endogenous estrogen regulation and systemic inflammation activation [33,35–37]. Therefore, stool samples are subjected to secretome studies that are usually extracted using a fecal swab test kit. Malignant ascites, a severe occurrence in cancer patients, are typically signs of late-stage cancer, particularly in those with stage IV breast cancer. Paracentesis is used to drain ascites from the abdominal cavity [38,39]. Overall, the breast components have the potential to add another essential avenue to the efforts to advance breast cancer research.

3. The Crosstalk between Cancer Cell Secretome and the Tumor Microenvironment

The tissue secretome is markedly changed during cancer development compared to normal tissue. The aberrant gene mutations in cancer cells cause high protein synthesis and secretion demand. The increased secretion levels resulted in the alteration of critical processes that augment tumor growth. The release of the secretome also could modulate the cancer extracellular space, particularly the TME behavior. The TME is an ecosystem that includes a heterogenous group of invading and resident host cells within a body surrounding the tumor [40]. TME composition is complex and varies according to tumor type.

Nevertheless, its hallmark features consist of cancer stem cells (CSC), immune cells, extracellular matrix (ECM), blood vessels, and cancer-associated fibroblast (CAFs) [41,42]. In the early onset of cancer, reciprocal heterotypic paracrine signaling between tumor cells and other TME components triggers a cascade of biochemical and biomechanical changes, leading to a dynamic interaction between TME components. The prerequisite of malignancy for many solid cancers is the alteration of ECM. This involves the secretion of ECM remodeling enzymes by newly transformed tumor cells to degrade the basement membrane, which provides a conducive environment for tumor invasion.

During malignancy, the stroma will undergo alterations to incite growth, invasion, and metastasis of cancer cells. These changes include CAF formation, which comprises a significant portion of the reactive tissue stroma and is critical in regulating tumor progression. The rearrangement of TME components via dynamic and mutual crosstalk is thought to drive tumor fitness and metastatic potentials [40,43,44]. The relationship between the components of TME also imposes a varying degree of response to therapy and drug resistance [45,46]. Most cancer types demonstrated fibrotic or rigid TME architecture [47,48]. Other TMEs have a more vascular microenvironment compacted with blood vessels [49,50]. The different architecture and variety of components of TMEs may also obscure the delivery of drugs to reach cancer cells [51]. Here, the interplay of breast cancer secretome with different members of TME is discussed.

3.1. Breast Cancer Cell Secretome and Stromal Components

Stromal cells are connective tissue cells found throughout the body in various organs and tissues that provide structural support and regulate cell growth, differentiation, and migration [52]. They are a diverse group of cells with different functions depending on their location, which includes fibroblasts, adipocytes, and pericytes. Stromal cells are essential in both normal tissue function and disease processes, with abnormalities in their function implicated in various diseases such as cancer, fibrosis, and autoimmune disorders [53,54]. The breast cancer stroma is a heterogeneous mixture of non-malignant cells comprising endothelial cells, lymphatic vessels, infiltrating immune cells, adipocytes, fibroblasts, and mesenchymal stem cells (MSCs) [55]. Breast cancer interacts bi-directionally with stromal cells by secreting cytokines, growth factors, and other signaling molecules. The interaction can either induce or inhibit stromal cells. Affected stromal cells then trigger the secretion of paracrine factors that promote the growth and progression of breast tumors, promoting epithelial-mesenchymal transition (EMT) and inducing invasive capabilities [56,57]. The most abundant breast cancer stroma cell is CAFs. CAFs facilitate several molecular interactions between the stroma and the breast cancer cells. For example, cancer cells secrete TGF-β and exert a paracrine effect to induce the differentiation of fibroblasts into CAFs [58]. As a result, CAFs secrete factors to promote angiogenesis and growth [59,60]. CAFs have a more proliferative capability and are aggressive compared to normal fibroblasts. CAFs are not always formed from the transformation of normal fibroblasts in the TME. Still, they may come from tissues or progenitor cells, such as stellate cells, bone marrow-derived fibrocytes, MSCs, adipocytes, pericytes, endothelial cells, and smooth muscle cells [61]. CAFs can induce the degradation of nearby ECM by secreting matrix metalloproteinases (MMPs) and urokinase-type plasminogen activators. At the same time, CAFs secrete large amounts of type I, III, IV, and V collagen, fibrinolytic protein, hyaluronic acid, and laminin to induce ECM remodeling. CAFs also secrete high amounts of growth factors such as transforming growth factor beta (TGF-β), hepatocyte growth factor (HGF), vascular endothelial growth factor (VEGF), and fibroblast growth factor (FGF) to induce EMT activation, angiogenic shift, metastasis, and metabolic reprogramming [62–65]. CAFs promote aggressive phenotypes in breast cancer by inducing the EMT by TGF-β1 through paracrine signaling [66]. The secretion of IL-1β, IL-6, IL-8, SDF-1, and NFκB by CAFs contributes to immune cell recruitment that may contribute to tumor progression, cancer survival and drug resistance by creating a protective niche in the TME [67,68].

Another cellular element that makes up breast cancer TME is adipocytes. Recent findings suggest that they promote the advancement of the tumor through a reciprocal and constantly evolving interaction with the cancerous cells and TME [69,70]. For example, breast cancer cells secrete pro-inflammatory cytokines such as IL-6 and tumor necrosis factor (TNF-α) that can promote adipose tissue inflammation and disrupt normal adipose tissue function [71]. In addition, adipokines such as leptin, adiponectin, autotaxin, and resistin are hormones produced by adipocytes that regulate metabolism and energy homeostasis [72]. In the TME, breast cancer cells can secrete adipokines such as adiponectin and leptin, promoting tumor growth and invasion [73].

3.2. Breast Cancer Cell Secretome and Immune Modulation

Breast cancer cells can secrete various factors such as cytokines, chemokines, growth factors, and EVs, which can modulate the immune response and promote tumor growth. Studies have shown dynamic interaction between tumor cells and tumor-infiltrating inflammatory cells such as lymphocytes (TILs), plasma cells, dendritic cells, macrophages, and neutrophils [74,75]. One of the mechanisms by which breast cancer cells modulate the immune response is by secreting cytokines such as interleukin 6 (IL-6), which can activate immune cells such as T cells, B cells, and macrophages [76,77]. IL-6 can also induce the production of other cytokines, such as IL-10 and transforming growth factor-beta (TGF-β), which can suppress the immune response and promote tumor growth [78,79]. Furthermore, breast cancer can recruit tumor-infiltrating lymphocytes (TILs) that are particularly abundant in ER and PR-negative or HER2-enriched cancers [80–83]. TILs in breast cancer are primarily T cells, with very few B cells [84,85]. Different types of T cells have varying effects on the TME. For example, CD8+ cytotoxic T cells kill tumor cells by secreting granzyme and perforin, which is mediated by interferon γ (IFN-γ). Type 1 helper T cells are induced by IFN-γ and IL-12 signals and activate antigen-presenting cells (APC) for effective CD8+ differentiation and progression [86,87]. Type 2 and type 17 helper T cells play more diverse roles in advancing breast cancer [88,89]. Follicular helper T cells perform critical functions in antigen-specific B cell maturation, increasing local memory cell differentiation and supporting the establishment of tertiary lymphoid organs, enhancing local anti-tumor immune response [90,91]. Regulatory T cells are essential for homeostasis and tolerance of the immune system. Their involvement in TME enhances immunosuppression via immunosuppressive cytokines (IL-10, TGF-β) and direct cell–cell contact suppression [92]. In general, the existence of type 1 helper T cell response is associated with a better prognosis, while regulatory T cells can aid in the progression of breast cancer [93,94]. B cells and T cells can be seen in close proximity within the TME, notably at tertiary lymphoid structures, and their presence is thought to have predictive value [85,95].

Dendritic cells are the most prominent APC that deliver antigens to T cells, including tumor-derived antigens [96]. High dendritic cell infiltration in breast cancer is associated with poor prognosis as it was shown to prevail metastasis via CXCR4/SDF-1 chemokine axis [97]. However, a high subset of dendritic cells in TNBC is also associated with better disease-free and disease-specific survival [98]. Tumor-associated macrophages (TAMs) are tumors' most common innate immune cells. An in vivo study on breast cancer bone metastasis revealed that bone metastases were markedly inhibited by macrophage ablation [99]. Furthermore, it was discovered that IL4R-dependent monocyte-derived macrophages drive bone metastases in breast cancer. Neutrophils are increasingly becoming identified as immune cells that infiltrate tumors. IFN-γ and IFN-β exposure generates N1 pro-inflammatory and anti-tumor of TAN, while TGF-β exposure induces N2 anti-inflammatory response and pro-tumor TAN [100,101]. In breast cancer mouse models, TAN can inhibit CD8+ proliferation and promote the recruitment of immunosuppressive cells in TME, but its effects in human patients are yet to be explored [102].

Breast cancer cells can also secrete EVs such as exosomes, which are small membrane-bound vesicles involved in cell-to-cell communication. Exosomes encapsulate various factors that can modulate the immune response and promote tumor growth. In breast cancer, exosomes carry miRNAs as one of their cargos that can target genes involved in immune regulation, suppressing the immune response and promoting tumor growth [103]. Exosomes can also carry proteins such as programmed death-ligand 1 (PD-L1), a checkpoint inhibitor involved in immune evasion by tumor cells. PD-L1 can bind to PD-1 receptors on T cells and suppress the immune response by inhibiting T cell activation and promoting

T cell apoptosis [83,104]. This allows the cancer cells to evade the immune system and proliferate uncontrollably.

3.3. Breast Cancer Cell Secretome and Metastasis

Tumor metastasis is a multi-step process comprising local invasion, intravasation, migration through the lymphatics or arteries, extravasation, and colonization, giving rise to metastases in distant organs [105]. Organ-specific colonization mainly depends on the dynamic and mutual interrelationship between tumor cells and the distant/secondary cells/organs secretome, as well as the components of TME [106]. Studies indicate that the genetic alterations found in breast cancer cells that have spread to the bone marrow are often different from those in primary tumors, and metastatic locations may be influenced by multiple microenvironments and cellular and molecular processes [107]. Different cancer types typically spread to multiple but preferred organ sites. Breast cancer, for example, has its preferential metastatic sites, including bones, lungs, liver and brain (Figure 1) [108]. All breast cancer subtypes can result in bone metastases, with the luminal A subtype posing a higher risk for bone recurrence, and luminal B patients are more likely to experience bone metastasis as the first site of relapse [109].

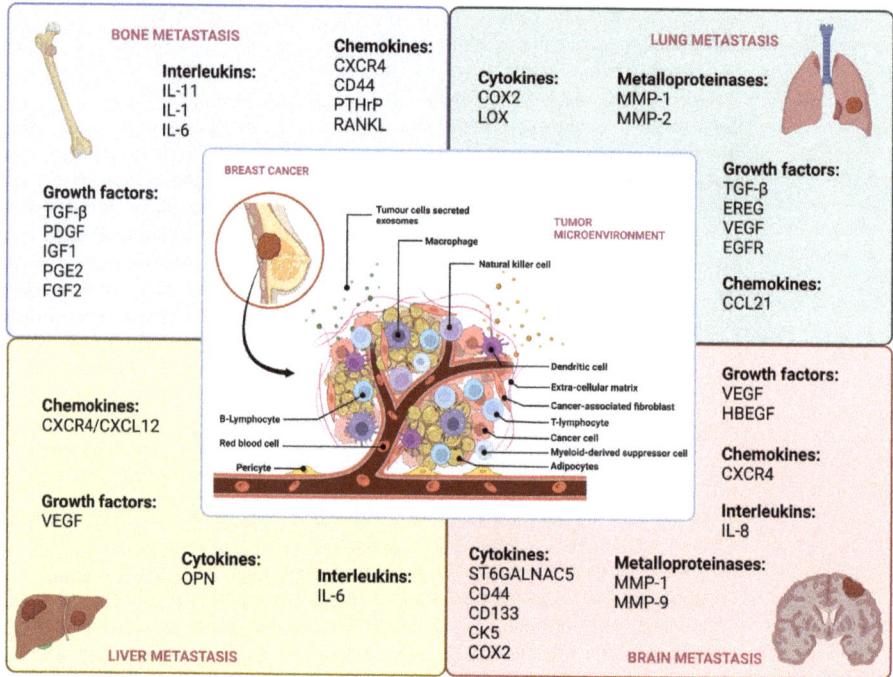

Figure 1. The summary of the signaling proteins that contribute to the site-specific metastasis in breast cancer.

In contrast, the incidence of bone metastasis is higher in luminal subtype tumors compared to other subtypes. Additionally, lung-specific metastasis is more common in luminal B and basal-like subtypes, while liver metastasis is more frequently observed in patients with HER2-enriched subtypes [109,110]. The basal-like subtype is more prone to spread to distant lymph nodes, the brain, and the lungs than to the liver and bones [111]. Through a complex system involving interaction between the stromal components of the primary tumors and organs, a pre-metastatic niche or a suitable microenvironment can be created in secondary tissues or organs before the occurrence of metastases [112]. It was reported that mobilized tumor bone marrow-derived cells (BMDCs) influence creating a favorable milieu for metastatic lung colonization [113]. The proteins secreted by the primary tumor, VEGF, and placental growth factor (PIGF) affect the bone marrow mesenchymal stem cells, causing the BMDCs to go to the preferred site for metastasis before the disseminated tumor cells do. During the process of EMT, ZEB1/2, SNAIL, GOOSECOID, and FOXC2 are upregulated, resulting in the loss of epithelial cell polarity and gap junction activities [62]. Breast cancer cells can alter the composition and organization of the ECM by secreting enzymes such as matrix metalloproteinases, cathepsins, and plasminogen activators, which break down ECM proteins and create space for tumor growth [114–116].

In contrast, during the mesenchymal-to-epithelial transition (MET), tumor cells regain their epithelial properties and interact through juxtacrine signaling (Notch and Wnt factors), colonizing the metastatic site. EMT significantly alters the dynamic environment of TME, drawing stromal and immune cells from different tissues to the TME through cytokines (such as TGF-β) and chemokines (such as CXCL2, CCL22, MMP, IL-6, and IL-8) released by breast cancer cells. It is worth noting that different breast cancer subtypes are involved in various pathways that mediate EMT and are regulated by diverse cell signaling mechanisms [117].

Endothelial cells create a continuous barrier in most organs, including the brain, which prevents cancer cells from freely entering. By establishing interactions with tumor cells via L-or-P-selectin secreted by endothelial cells, platelets and white blood cells can assist tumor cells in moving through the vasculature [118,119]. As a result, higher expression of selectin ligands by tumor cells is strongly associated with metastatic progression and poor prognosis. Moreover, TGF-β or small mother against decapentaplegic (SMAD) signaling pathway, has been found to increase cancer cells' retention in the lungs and give breast cancer cells the ability to damage the capillary wall of the lung and develop lung metastases [120]. In addition, target tissues where cancer cells can metastasize or migrate can secrete chemokines that cause directed cell migration, trigger signaling cascades and keep track of cytoskeletal rearrangement and adhesion [121].

3.4. Breast Cancer Cell Secretome-Mediated Chemoresistance and Recurrence

Breast cancer secretome-mediated chemoresistance is a complex process in which the secretome can create a supportive microenvironment for cancer cell growth and survival, leading to the development of drug resistance and, eventually, cancer recurrence. Post-therapy, various cells present in the TME, including CSCs, immune cells, fibroblasts, and endothelial cells, can be manipulated to promote tumor cell survival and relapse [122]. The secretome can also promote the survival of residual cancer cells that survive initial therapy. A common routine treatment for breast cancer patients with TNBC or high HER2 expression would be the administration of chemotherapy drugs as a neoadjuvant or adjuvant to surgery [123]. However, patients that relapsed with distant metastasis often develop chemoresistance with poor prognosis [122,124]. The development of chemoresistance can occur through two mechanisms, intrinsic or acquired resistance. Intrinsic resistance is caused by either inherent genetic mutations and/or by the heterogeneity and the protein interplay of the TME. In contrast, acquired resistance is by genetic modification, such as DNA damage repair or rewiring of intracellular signaling pathways during or after chemotherapy [51,125].

One of the key mechanisms of cancer cell secretome-mediated chemoresistance is the activation of the signaling pathway for survival and drug resistance in cancer cells. For example, cancer cells secrete IL-6 and TGF-β, which may encourage the expression of genes through autocrine or paracrine signaling. This includes genes that help to detoxify drugs (e.g., glutathione S-transferase P1 (GSTP1)), promote the activity of efflux pumps (e.g., multidrug resistance protein 1 (MDR1)), and regulate the effectiveness of chemotherapy to activate (e.g., STAT3 and SMAD) [76,77]. Alteration of the TME can also promote drug resistance. Secretion of ECM proteins such as collagen and fibronectin can create a dense matrix that limits drug penetration, creating a barrier that prevents chemotherapy drugs from reaching cancer cells. They can also induce the formation of abnormal blood vessels to further limit drug delivery [126]. Additionally, the breast cancer secretome components can induce the NF-κB pathway, which promotes cell survival by transcribing anti-apoptotic genes such as members of the B cell lymphoma 2 (Bcl-2) family and inhibitors of apoptosis (IAPs), as well as inhibits caspase cleavage [127].

Furthermore, the communication that occurs through EVs is becoming increasingly recognized as a significant factor in the development of chemoresistance in breast cancer. EVs have been found to carry anti-apoptotic proteins, Hsp 70, c-IAPs, and survivin [128]. Drug efflux pumps can be transported from chemoresistance cancer cells through EVs, either by directly packaging the functional protein or indirectly through encapsulation of mRNA [129]. When captured by chemosensitive cancer cells, this can result in effective drug efflux and subsequent chemoresistance. Findings indicate that EVs may also capture chemotherapeutic drugs, which could help to reduce drug toxicity. For example, EVs released by breast cancer cells are resistant to chemotherapy and can trap adriamycin [130].

4. Targeting the Breast Cancer Cell Secretome

Extensive studies of the breast cancer secretome have identified several potential targets for new cancer therapies, including antibodies or small molecules that can block the activity of specific proteins in the secretome [131,132]. In addition, analysis of the breast cancer secretome may also be useful for developing new biomarkers that can help for early detection and predict the likelihood of cancer recurrence or response to therapy. Therefore, it is imperative to develop novel therapeutic approaches to target secreted factors that are released into TME in order to prevent chemoresistance and relapse or enhance anti-tumor immunity. Several approaches have been used to target unique secretomes or constituents responsible for the secretion in breast cancer cells. For example, targeting the HER2 receptor using the FDA-approved monoclonal antibody trastuzumab to block its signaling pathway has been deemed efficacious for early and advanced breast cancer treatment [133]. Another FDA-approved alternative with the HER2 inhibitor lapatinib led to changes in the breast cancer cell secretome, promoting immune cell infiltration and activation [134,135]. The study found that lapatinib treatment led to an increase in the secretion of chemokines, such as CCL5 and CXCL10, that recruit immune cells, as well as an increase in the secretion of cytokines that activate immune cells, such as IFN-γ and TNF-α.

Another approach in targeting secretome is using drugs that block specific molecules' secretion rate, such as IL-6, to reduce breast cancer proliferation. In breast cancer, the IL-6 signaling axis is a promising therapeutic target since it promotes growth and invasion, mediates the spread of metastatic capabilities, and is associated with poor prognosis [76,77]. Anti-IL-6 monoclonal antibodies such as sirukumab, olokizumab, MEDI5117, and clazakizumab have been used as inhibitors of the IL-6/JAK/STAT3 signaling pathway in various cancers. Still, the FDA has yet to approve these drugs for breast cancer treatment [77]. Reports also show that the secretome can be induced by targeted therapy with kinase inhibitors, resulting in significant alterations in the expressed secretome and enhanced drug resistance [136]. However, the study was performed in melanoma and lung cancer models, but the observation could be transferable to breast cancer.

Targeting the epidermal growth factor receptor (EGFR) inhibitor in breast cancer with gefitinib was found to reduce the secretion of several proteins that promote tumor angiogenesis and invasion, including vascular endothelial growth factor (VEGF) and interleukin-8 (IL-8) [137]. The study also found that treatment with gefitinib increased the tumor suppressor protein thrombospondin-1 (TSP-1) secretion, which can inhibit tumor angiogenesis and promote apoptosis. Reports of other approved drugs targeting the secretome or TME components are listed in Table 1:

Table 1. Reports of drugs targeting the components of TME.

Drug	Target	Molecular Target	Ref.
Bevacizumab	Angiogenic factor	VEGF	[138]
Lapatinib	Kinase inhibitor	EGFR	[139]
Ramucirumab	Angiogenic factor	VEGFR2	[140]
Pembrolizumab	Immune checkpoint inhibitor	PD-1	[141]
Anakinra	Interleukin	IL-1α, IL-1β	[142]
Canakinumab	Interleukin	IL-1β	[143]
Cetuximab	Kinase inhibitor	EGFR	[144]
Nivolumab	Immune checkpoint inhibitor	PD-1	[145]
Atezolizumab	Immune checkpoint inhibitor	PD-L1	[146]

Breast cancer is a complex disease with a high recurrent rate. Drug combination therapy and precision medicine have emerged as promising strategies for improving treatment outcomes and reducing the risk of relapse [147–149]. The high relapse rate in breast cancer is caused by acquired resistance, which suggests the need for combination therapy [150]. Targeting one specialized microenvironment may lead to changes in other TME-related pathways because TME comprises numerous cells that frequently overlap and communicate. Therefore, a combination therapy targeting a specific microenvironment or niche may improve cancer treatment. Drug combination therapy involves using two or more drugs with different mechanisms of action to target multiple pathways involved in tumor survival and growth. This approach can improve treatment outcomes by enhancing the effectiveness of individual drugs, reducing the risk of drug resistance, and minimizing toxicity. Common practice would be the combination of chemotherapy and targeted therapy which has been shown to improve survival outcomes of patients compared to chemotherapy alone. For example, curcuminoid, a phenolic compound that has been utilized as a therapeutic agent in combination with chemotherapy, demonstrated enhanced efficacy in terms of reduced adverse effects and improved life quality in patients with solid tumors such as colorectal, gastric, and breast cancer in a phase II double-blind, randomized study [151–154].

The precision medicine approach would be tailoring treatment to the individual based on specific cancer characteristics, such as specific genetic mutations such as BRCA1/BRCA2 or the expression of specific biomarkers [155]. For example, the use of poly (ADP-ribose) polymerase (PARP) inhibitors has shown promising results in patients with BRCA mutations, which are associated with defects in DNA repair [156]. PARP inhibitors can block an alternative DNA repair pathway in these patients, leading to breast cancer cell death. In addition, emerging research suggests that combining precision medicine approaches with drug combination therapy may improve treatment outcomes and reduce the risk of relapse [157]. For example, combining a PARP inhibitor with a checkpoint inhibitor, pembrolizumab, enhances the immune system's ability to target improved treatment outcomes in patients with BRCA-mutated breast cancer [156].

Understanding the landscape of breast cancer cell secretomes is essential for developing new cancer therapies. By targeting specific proteins involved in cancer cell signaling, researchers may be able to create more effective treatments that can slow or halt tumor growth. In addition, understanding the breast cancer cell secretome may also lead to the development of new diagnostic tools that can detect cancer earlier.

5. Conclusions

The field of breast cancer secretome research is currently undergoing a dynamic phase of investigation as scientists are exploring novel methodologies and tools to unravel the intricate mechanisms underlying breast cancer progression and metastasis. Recent advancements in high-sensitivity and high-throughput technologies, such as mass spectrometry-based proteomics/metabolomics, have revolutionized our ability to accurately identify and quantify the complex array of proteins, lipids, and metabolites that comprise the breast cancer secretome. Leveraging these cutting-edge analytical tools, researchers can now conduct a comprehensive and detailed analysis of the breast cancer secretome, enabling a deeper understanding of the pathophysiological processes involved in cancer development and progression. This could ultimately lead to the discovery of new therapeutic targets and the development of more effective treatments for breast cancer.

Microenvironmental alterations contribute to tumor progression and are attractive therapeutic targets, especially with metastatic breast cancer where outcomes are poor, necessitating novel treatment approaches. One of the therapeutic approaches is to enhance stromal-targeted therapy, but this requires careful clinical trial design, including neoadjuvant therapy. Nevertheless, targeting the microenvironment is a promising approach that could improve outcomes in breast cancer patients. It is evident that the role of secretome contributes to the hallmarks of cancer and intersects with major cancer-related pathways, as summarized in Figure 2. In addition, a recent study highlighted that genomic alterations induce changes in the TME components by changing the landscape of cancer cell fitness [158]. These TME components had distinct enrichment blueprints among breast cancer subtypes, with ER status exerting utmost influence, and some were associated with genomic profiles indicative of immune escape. In addition, the TME components also assert a prognostic impact on the clinical outcome of breast cancer patients.

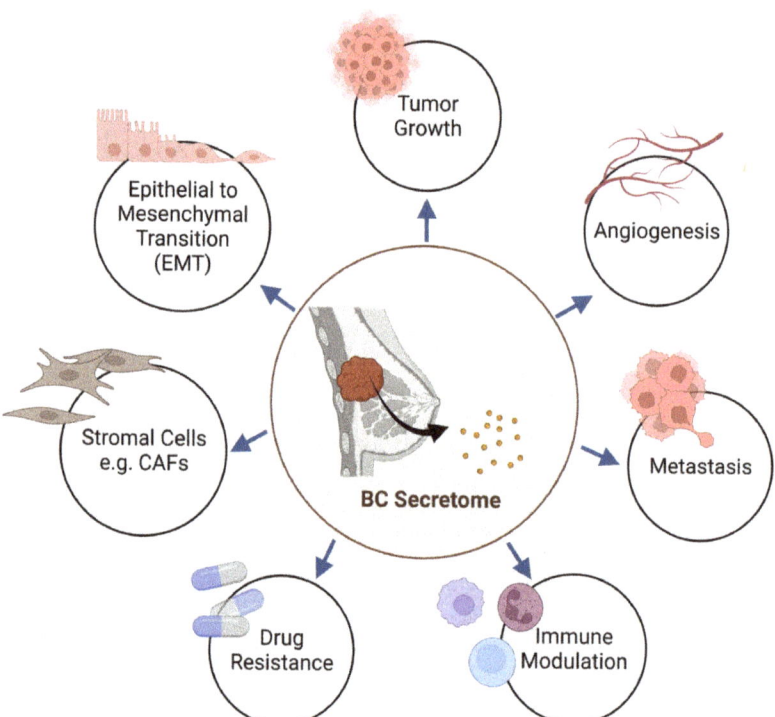

Figure 2. The breast cancer secretome contributes to the hallmarks of cancer.

While targeting specific proteins in the breast cancer secretome can be effective, it is essential to note that breast cancer is a complex disease requiring a multifaceted treatment approach. Henceforth, should precision medicine approaches in the treatment of breast cancer occur, the unique characteristics of each patient's genomic alteration and cancer cell secretome need to be considered. Therefore, continuous research into the breast cancer cell secretome and the role of TME is required to understand breast cancer progression further and develop new diagnostic and therapeutic strategies.

Author Contributions: Conceptualization, M.A.M.; writing—original draft preparation, S.Z.; writing—review and editing, M.A.M. and S.E.S.; funding acquisition, M.A.M. All authors have read and agreed to the published version of the manuscript.

Funding: This research was funded by Universiti Kebangsaan Malaysia, Dana Impak Perdana (DIP-2020-002).

Acknowledgments: We appreciate the work of the researchers cited in this review. We hope for the understanding of all authors whose influential work is in the field. Figures 1 and 2 were created using BioRender.com.

Conflicts of Interest: The authors declare no conflict of interest. The funders had no role in the writing of the manuscript; or in the decision to publish the results.

References

1. Sørlie, T. Molecular Portraits of Breast Cancer: Tumour Subtypes as Distinct Disease Entities. *Eur. J. Cancer* **2004**, *40*, 2667–2675. [CrossRef] [PubMed]
2. Cancer Today. Available online: http://gco.iarc.fr/today/home (accessed on 28 September 2022).
3. Giaquinto, A.N.; Miller, K.D.; Tossas, K.Y.; Winn, R.A.; Jemal, A.; Siegel, R.L. Cancer Statistics for African American/Black People 2022. CA. *Cancer J. Clin.* **2022**, *72*, 202–229. [CrossRef] [PubMed]
4. Giaquinto, A.N.; Sung, H.; Miller, K.D.; Kramer, J.L.; Newman, L.A.; Minihan, A.; Jemal, A.; Siegel, R.L. Breast Cancer Statistics, 2022. CA. *Cancer J. Clin.* **2022**, *72*, 524–541. [CrossRef] [PubMed]
5. Allemani, C.; Sant, M.; Weir, H.K.; Richardson, L.C.; Baili, P.; Storm, H.; Siesling, S.; Torrella-Ramos, A.; Voogd, A.C.; Aareleid, T.; et al. Breast Cancer Survival in the US and Europe: A CONCORD High-Resolution Study. *Int. J. Cancer* **2013**, *132*, 1170–1181. [CrossRef]
6. Redig, A.J.; McAllister, S.S. Breast Cancer as a Systemic Disease: A View of Metastasis. *J. Intern. Med.* **2013**, *274*, 113–126. [CrossRef]
7. Berman, A.T.; Thukral, A.D.; Hwang, W.-T.; Solin, L.J.; Vapiwala, N. Incidence and Patterns of Distant Metastases for Patients with Early-Stage Breast Cancer after Breast Conservation Treatment. *Clin. Breast Cancer* **2013**, *13*, 88–94. [CrossRef] [PubMed]
8. Perou, C.M.; Sørlie, T.; Eisen, M.B.; van de Rijn, M.; Jeffrey, S.S.; Rees, C.A.; Pollack, J.R.; Ross, D.T.; Johnsen, H.; Akslen, L.A.; et al. Molecular Portraits of Human Breast Tumours. *Nature* **2000**, *406*, 747–752. [CrossRef] [PubMed]
9. van 't Veer, L.J.; Dai, H.; van de Vijver, M.J.; He, Y.D.; Hart, A.A.M.; Mao, M.; Peterse, H.L.; van der Kooy, K.; Marton, M.J.; Witteveen, A.T.; et al. Gene Expression Profiling Predicts Clinical Outcome of Breast Cancer. *Nature* **2002**, *415*, 530–536. [CrossRef]
10. Miah, S.; Bagu, E.; Goel, R.; Ogunbolude, Y.; Dai, C.; Ward, A.; Vizeacoumar, F.S.; Davies, G.; Vizeacoumar, F.J.; Anderson, D.; et al. Estrogen Receptor Signaling Regulates the Expression of the Breast Tumor Kinase in Breast Cancer Cells. *BMC Cancer* **2019**, *19*, 78. [CrossRef]
11. Zhang, M.H.; Man, H.T.; Zhao, X.D.; Dong, N.; Ma, S.L. Estrogen Receptor-Positive Breast Cancer Molecular Signatures and Therapeutic Potentials (Review). *Biomed. Rep.* **2014**, *2*, 41–52. [CrossRef]
12. Inic, Z.; Zegarac, M.; Inic, M.; Markovic, I.; Kozomara, Z.; Djurisic, I.; Inic, I.; Pupic, G.; Jancic, S. Difference between Luminal A and Luminal B Subtypes According to Ki-67, Tumor Size, and Progesterone Receptor Negativity Providing Prognostic Information. *Clin. Med. Insights Oncol.* **2014**, *8*, CMO-S18006. [CrossRef]
13. Gibson, G.R.; Qian, D.; Ku, J.K.; Lai, L.L. Metaplastic Breast Cancer: Clinical Features and Outcomes. *Am. Surg.* **2005**, *71*, 725–730. [CrossRef]
14. Lehmann, B.D.; Pietenpol, J.A. Identification and Use of Biomarkers in Treatment Strategies for Triple-Negative Breast Cancer Subtypes. *J. Pathol.* **2014**, *232*, 142–150. [CrossRef]
15. Lehmann, B.D.; Bauer, J.A.; Chen, X.; Sanders, M.E.; Chakravarthy, A.B.; Shyr, Y.; Pietenpol, J.A. Identification of Human Triple-Negative Breast Cancer Subtypes and Preclinical Models for Selection of Targeted Therapies. *J. Clin. Investig.* **2011**, *121*, 2750–2767. [CrossRef]
16. Takahashi, R.; Toh, U.; Iwakuma, N.; Takenaka, M.; Otsuka, H.; Furukawa, M.; Fujii, T.; Seki, N.; Kawahara, A.; Kage, M.; et al. Feasibility Study of Personalized Peptide Vaccination for Metastatic Recurrent Triple-Negative Breast Cancer Patients. *Breast Cancer Res.* **2014**, *16*, R70. [CrossRef]
17. McHenry, P.R.; Prosperi, J.R. Proteins Found in the Triple-Negative Breast Cancer Secretome and Their Therapeutic Potential. *Int. J. Mol. Sci.* **2023**, *24*, 2100. [CrossRef]
18. Sirven, P.; Faucheux, L.; Grandclaudon, M.; Michea, P.; Vincent-Salomon, A.; Mechta-Grigoriou, F.; Scholer-Dahirel, A.; Guillot-Delost, M.; Soumelis, V. Definition of a Novel Breast Tumor-Specific Classifier Based on Secretome Analysis. *Breast Cancer Res.* **2022**, *24*, 94. [CrossRef]
19. Ritchie, S.; Reed, D.A.; Pereira, B.A.; Timpson, P. The Cancer Cell Secretome Drives Cooperative Manipulation of the Tumour Microenvironment to Accelerate Tumourigenesis. *Fac. Rev.* **2021**, *10*, 4. [CrossRef]
20. Uhlén, M.; Karlsson, M.J.; Hober, A.; Svensson, A.-S.; Scheffel, J.; Kotol, D.; Zhong, W.; Tebani, A.; Strandberg, L.; Edfors, F.; et al. The Human Secretome. *Sci. Signal.* **2019**, *12*, eaaz0274. [CrossRef]

21. Blanco, M.A.; LeRoy, G.; Khan, Z.; Alečković, M.; Zee, B.M.; Garcia, B.A.; Kang, Y. Global Secretome Analysis Identifies Novel Mediators of Bone Metastasis. *Cell Res.* **2012**, *22*, 1339–1355. [CrossRef]
22. Mustafa, S.; Pan, L.; Marzoq, A.; Fawaz, M.; Sander, L.; Rückert, F.; Schrenk, A.; Hartl, C.; Uhler, R.; Yildirim, A.; et al. Comparison of the Tumor Cell Secretome and Patient Sera for an Accurate Serum-Based Diagnosis of Pancreatic Ductal Adenocarcinoma. *Oncotarget* **2017**, *8*, 11963–11976. [CrossRef]
23. Pappa, K.I.; Kontostathi, G.; Makridakis, M.; Lygirou, V.; Zoidakis, J.; Daskalakis, G.; Anagnou, N.P. High Resolution Proteomic Analysis of the Cervical Cancer Cell Lines Secretome Documents Deregulation of Multiple Proteases. *Cancer Genom. Proteom.* **2017**, *14*, 507–521. [CrossRef]
24. Dowling, P.; Clynes, M. Conditioned Media from Cell Lines: A Complementary Model to Clinical Specimens for the Discovery of Disease-Specific Biomarkers. *Proteomics* **2011**, *11*, 794–804. [CrossRef]
25. Carter, K.; Lee, H.J.; Na, K.-S.; Fernandes-Cunha, G.M.; Blanco, I.J.; Djalilian, A.; Myung, D. Characterizing the Impact of 2D and 3D Culture Conditions on the Therapeutic Effects of Human Mesenchymal Stem Cell Secretome on Corneal Wound Healing in Vitro and Ex Vivo. *Acta Biomater.* **2019**, *99*, 247–257. [CrossRef]
26. Cases-Perera, O.; Blanco-Elices, C.; Chato-Astrain, J.; Miranda-Fernández, C.; Campos, F.; Crespo, P.V.; Sánchez-Montesinos, I.; Alaminos, M.; Martín-Piedra, M.A.; Garzón, I. Development of Secretome-Based Strategies to Improve Cell Culture Protocols in Tissue Engineering. *Sci. Rep.* **2022**, *12*, 10003. [CrossRef]
27. Celis, J.E.; Gromov, P.; Cabezón, T.; Moreira, J.M.A.; Ambartsumian, N.; Sandelin, K.; Rank, F.; Gromova, I. Proteomic Characterization of the Interstitial Fluid Perfusing the Breast Tumor Microenvironment: A Novel Resource for Biomarker and Therapeutic Target Discovery. *Mol. Cell. Proteom.* **2004**, *3*, 327–344. [CrossRef]
28. Fijneman, R.J.A.; de Wit, M.; Pourghiasian, M.; Piersma, S.R.; Pham, T.V.; Warmoes, M.O.; Lavaei, M.; Piso, C.; Smit, F.; Delis-van Diemen, P.M.; et al. Proximal Fluid Proteome Profiling of Mouse Colon Tumors Reveals Biomarkers for Early Diagnosis of Human Colorectal Cancer. *Clin. Cancer Res.* **2012**, *18*, 2613–2624. [CrossRef]
29. Sauter, E.R.; Ross, E.; Daly, M.; Klein-Szanto, A.; Engstrom, P.F.; Sorling, A.; Malick, J.; Ehya, H. Nipple Aspirate Fluid: A Promising Non-Invasive Method to Identify Cellular Markers of Breast Cancer Risk. *Br. J. Cancer* **1997**, *76*, 494–501. [CrossRef]
30. Shaheed, S.; Tait, C.; Kyriacou, K.; Linforth, R.; Salhab, M.; Sutton, C. Evaluation of Nipple Aspirate Fluid as a Diagnostic Tool for Early Detection of Breast Cancer. *Clin. Proteom.* **2018**, *15*, 3. [CrossRef]
31. Zhang, L.; Shao, Z.-M.; Beatty, P.; Sartippour, M.; Wang, H.-J.; Elashoff, R.; Chang, H.; Brooks, M.N. The Use of Oxytocin in Nipple Fluid Aspiration. *Breast J.* **2003**, *9*, 266–268. [CrossRef]
32. Skok, K.; Hladnik, G.; Grm, A.; Crnjac, A. Malignant Pleural Effusion and Its Current Management: A Review. *Medicina* **2019**, *55*, 490. [CrossRef]
33. Kwa, M.; Plottel, C.S.; Blaser, M.J.; Adams, S. The Intestinal Microbiome and Estrogen Receptor-Positive Female Breast Cancer. *J. Natl. Cancer Inst.* **2016**, *108*, djw029. [CrossRef]
34. Garcia-Estevez, L.; Moreno-Bueno, G. Updating the Role of Obesity and Cholesterol in Breast Cancer. *Breast Cancer Res. BCR* **2019**, *21*, 35. [CrossRef]
35. Flores, R.; Shi, J.; Fuhrman, B.; Xu, X.; Veenstra, T.D.; Gail, M.H.; Gajer, P.; Ravel, J.; Goedert, J.J. Fecal Microbial Determinants of Fecal and Systemic Estrogens and Estrogen Metabolites: A Cross-Sectional Study. *J. Transl. Med.* **2012**, *10*, 253. [CrossRef]
36. Maynard, C.L.; Elson, C.O.; Hatton, R.D.; Weaver, C.T. Reciprocal Interactions of the Intestinal Microbiota and Immune System. *Nature* **2012**, *489*, 11551. [CrossRef]
37. Belkaid, Y.; Hand, T. Role of the Microbiota in Immunity and Inflammation. *Cell* **2014**, *157*, 121–141. [CrossRef]
38. Ayantunde, A.A.; Parsons, S.L. Pattern and Prognostic Factors in Patients with Malignant Ascites: A Retrospective Study. *Ann. Oncol.* **2007**, *18*, 945–949. [CrossRef]
39. Elsherbiny, N.M.; Younis, N.N.; Shaheen, M.A.; Elseweidy, M.M. The Synergistic Effect between Vanillin and Doxorubicin in Ehrlich Ascites Carcinoma Solid Tumor and MCF-7 Human Breast Cancer Cell Line. *Pathol. Res. Pract.* **2016**, *212*, 767–777. [CrossRef]
40. Ni, C.; Huang, J. Dynamic Regulation of Cancer Stem Cells and Clinical Challenges. *Clin. Transl. Oncol.* **2013**, *15*, 253–258. [CrossRef]
41. Jahanban-Esfahlan, R.; Seidi, K.; Zarghami, N. Tumor Vascular Infarction: Prospects and Challenges. *Int. J. Hematol.* **2017**, *105*, 244–256. [CrossRef]
42. Jahanban-Esfahlan, R.; Seidi, K.; Banimohamad-Shotorbani, B.; Jahanban-Esfahlan, A.; Yousefi, B. Combination of Nanotechnology with Vascular Targeting Agents for Effective Cancer Therapy. *J. Cell. Physiol.* **2018**, *233*, 2982–2992. [CrossRef]
43. Jahanban-Esfahlan, R.; Seidi, K.; Monhemi, H.; Adli, A.D.F.; Minofar, B.; Zare, P.; Farajzadeh, D.; Farajnia, S.; Behzadi, R.; Abbasi, M.M.; et al. RGD Delivery of Truncated Coagulase to Tumor Vasculature Affords Local Thrombotic Activity to Induce Infarction of Tumors in Mice. *Sci. Rep.* **2017**, *7*, 8126. [CrossRef]
44. Truffi, M.; Sorrentino, L.; Corsi, F. Fibroblasts in the Tumor Microenvironment. In *Tumor Microenvironment: Non-Hematopoietic Cells*; Birbrair, A., Ed.; Advances in Experimental Medicine and Biology; Springer International Publishing: Cham, Switzerland, 2020; pp. 15–29. ISBN 978-3-030-37184-5.
45. Nassar, D.; Blanpain, C. Cancer Stem Cells: Basic Concepts and Therapeutic Implications. *Annu. Rev. Pathol. Mech. Dis.* **2016**, *11*, 47–76. [CrossRef]

46. Chen, K.; Huang, Y.; Chen, J. Understanding and Targeting Cancer Stem Cells: Therapeutic Implications and Challenges. *Acta Pharmacol. Sin.* **2013**, *34*, 732–740. [CrossRef]
47. Almagro, J.; Messal, H.A.; Elosegui-Artola, A.; van Rheenen, J.; Behrens, A. Tissue Architecture in Tumor Initiation and Progression. *Trends Cancer* **2022**, *8*, 494–505. [CrossRef]
48. Baghban, R.; Roshangar, L.; Jahanban-Esfahlan, R.; Seidi, K.; Ebrahimi-Kalan, A.; Jaymand, M.; Kolahian, S.; Javaheri, T.; Zare, P. Tumor Microenvironment Complexity and Therapeutic Implications at a Glance. *Cell Commun. Signal.* **2020**, *18*, 59. [CrossRef]
49. Fukumura, D.; Duda, D.G.; Munn, L.L.; Jain, R.K. Tumor Microvasculature and Microenvironment: Novel Insights Through Intravital Imaging in Pre-Clinical Models. *Microcirculation* **2010**, *17*, 206–225. [CrossRef]
50. Lamplugh, Z.; Fan, Y. Vascular Microenvironment, Tumor Immunity and Immunotherapy. *Front. Immunol.* **2021**, *12*, 811485. [CrossRef]
51. Cosentino, G.; Plantamura, I.; Tagliabue, E.; Iorio, M.V.; Cataldo, A. Breast Cancer Drug Resistance: Overcoming the Challenge by Capitalizing on MicroRNA and Tumor Microenvironment Interplay. *Cancers* **2021**, *13*, 3691. [CrossRef]
52. Valarmathi, M.T.; Bruna, F.A. *Stromal Cells—Structure, Function, and Therapeutic Implications*; IntechOpen: Rijeka, Croatia, 2019; ISBN 978-1-78984-985-1.
53. Chandler, C.; Liu, T.; Buckanovich, R.; Coffman, L.G. The Double Edge Sword of Fibrosis in Cancer. *Transl. Res.* **2019**, *209*, 55–67. [CrossRef]
54. Honan, A.M.; Chen, Z. Stromal Cells Underlining the Paths from Autoimmunity, Inflammation to Cancer With Roles Beyond Structural and Nutritional Support. *Front. Cell Dev. Biol.* **2021**, *9*, 658984. [CrossRef]
55. Balkwill, F.R.; Capasso, M.; Hagemann, T. The Tumor Microenvironment at a Glance. *J. Cell Sci.* **2012**, *125*, 5591–5596. [CrossRef]
56. Guido, C.; Whitaker-Menezes, D.; Capparelli, C.; Balliet, R.; Lin, Z.; Pestell, R.G.; Howell, A.; Aquila, S.; Andò, S.; Martinez-Outschoorn, U.; et al. Metabolic Reprogramming of Cancer-Associated Fibroblasts by TGF-β Drives Tumor Growth: Connecting TGF-β Signaling with "Warburg-like" Cancer Metabolism and L-Lactate Production. *Cell Cycle* **2012**, *11*, 3019–3035. [CrossRef]
57. Elenbaas, B.; Weinberg, R.A. Heterotypic Signaling between Epithelial Tumor Cells and Fibroblasts in Carcinoma Formation. *Exp. Cell Res.* **2001**, *264*, 169–184. [CrossRef]
58. Costanza, B.; Umelo, I.A.; Bellier, J.; Castronovo, V.; Turtoi, A. Stromal Modulators of TGF-β in Cancer. *J. Clin. Med.* **2017**, *6*, 7. [CrossRef]
59. Krishnamurty, A.T.; Turley, S.J. Lymph Node Stromal Cells: Cartographers of the Immune System. *Nat. Immunol.* **2020**, *21*, 369–380. [CrossRef]
60. Jalkanen, S.; Salmi, M. Lymphatic Endothelial Cells of the Lymph Node. *Nat. Rev. Immunol.* **2020**, *20*, 566–578. [CrossRef]
61. Giorello, M.B.; Borzone, F.R.; Labovsky, V.; Piccioni, F.V.; Chasseing, N.A. Cancer-Associated Fibroblasts in the Breast Tumor Microenvironment. *J. Mammary Gland Biol. Neoplasia* **2021**, *26*, 135–155. [CrossRef]
62. Felipe Lima, J.; Nofech-Mozes, S.; Bayani, J.; Bartlett, J.M.S. EMT in Breast Carcinoma—A Review. *J. Clin. Med.* **2016**, *5*, 65. [CrossRef]
63. Erdogan, B.; Webb, D.J. Cancer-Associated Fibroblasts Modulate Growth Factor Signaling and Extracellular Matrix Remodeling to Regulate Tumor Metastasis. *Biochem. Soc. Trans.* **2017**, *45*, 229–236. [CrossRef]
64. Hawsawi, N.M.; Ghebeh, H.; Hendrayani, S.-F.; Tulbah, A.; Al-Eid, M.; Al-Tweigeri, T.; Ajarim, D.; Alaiya, A.; Dermime, S.; Aboussekhra, A. Breast Carcinoma–Associated Fibroblasts and Their Counterparts Display Neoplastic-Specific Changes. *Cancer Res.* **2008**, *68*, 2717–2725. [CrossRef] [PubMed]
65. Aboussekhra, A. Role of Cancer-Associated Fibroblasts in Breast Cancer Development and Prognosis. *Int. J. Dev. Biol.* **2011**, *55*, 841–849. [CrossRef]
66. Yu, Y.; Xiao, C.-H.; Tan, L.-D.; Wang, Q.-S.; Li, X.-Q.; Feng, Y.-M. Cancer-Associated Fibroblasts Induce Epithelial–Mesenchymal Transition of Breast Cancer Cells through Paracrine TGF-β Signalling. *Br. J. Cancer* **2014**, *110*, 724–732. [CrossRef] [PubMed]
67. Straussman, R.; Morikawa, T.; Shee, K.; Barzily-Rokni, M.; Qian, Z.R.; Du, J.; Davis, A.; Mongare, M.M.; Gould, J.; Frederick, D.T.; et al. Tumor Microenvironment Induces Innate RAF-Inhibitor Resistance through HGF Secretion. *Nature* **2012**, *487*, 500–504. [CrossRef]
68. Houthuijzen, J.M.; Jonkers, J. Cancer-Associated Fibroblasts as Key Regulators of the Breast Cancer Tumor Microenvironment. *Cancer Metastasis Rev.* **2018**, *37*, 577–597. [CrossRef]
69. de Miranda, M.C.; Ferreira, A.d.F.; de Melo, M.I.A.; Kunrath-Lima, M.; de Goes, A.M.; Rodrigues, M.A.; Gomes, D.A.; Faria, J.A.Q.A. Adipose-Derived Stem/Stromal Cell Secretome Modulates Breast Cancer Cell Proliferation and Differentiation State towards Aggressiveness. *Biochimie* **2021**, *191*, 69–77. [CrossRef] [PubMed]
70. Ritter, A.; Kreis, N.-N.; Hoock, S.C.; Solbach, C.; Louwen, F.; Yuan, J. Adipose Tissue-Derived Mesenchymal Stromal/Stem Cells, Obesity and the Tumor Microenvironment of Breast Cancer. *Cancers* **2022**, *14*, 3908. [CrossRef]
71. Wu, Q.; Li, B.; Li, Z.; Li, J.; Sun, S.; Sun, S. Cancer-Associated Adipocytes: Key Players in Breast Cancer Progression. *J. Hematol. Oncol. J. Hematol. Oncol.* **2019**, *12*, 95. [CrossRef]
72. Schäffler, A.; Schölmerich, J.; Buechler, C. Mechanisms of Disease: Adipokines and Breast Cancer—Endocrine and Paracrine Mechanisms That Connect Adiposity and Breast Cancer. *Nat. Clin. Pract. Endocrinol. Metab.* **2007**, *3*, 345–354. [CrossRef]
73. Chu, D.-T.; Nguyen Thi Phuong, T.; Tien, N.L.B.; Tran, D.-K.; Nguyen, T.-T.; Thanh, V.V.; Luu Quang, T.; Minh, L.B.; Pham, V.H.; Ngoc, V.T.N.; et al. The Effects of Adipocytes on the Regulation of Breast Cancer in the Tumor Microenvironment: An Update. *Cells* **2019**, *8*, 857. [CrossRef]

74. Wu, L.; Saxena, S.; Awaji, M.; Singh, R.K. Tumor-Associated Neutrophils in Cancer: Going Pro. *Cancers* **2019**, *11*, 564. [CrossRef]
75. Salgado, R.; Denkert, C.; Demaria, S.; Sirtaine, N.; Klauschen, F.; Pruneri, G.; Wienert, S.; Van den Eynden, G.; Baehner, F.L.; Penault-Llorca, F.; et al. The Evaluation of Tumor-Infiltrating Lymphocytes (TILs) in Breast Cancer: Recommendations by an International TILs Working Group 2014. *Ann. Oncol.* **2015**, *26*, 259–271. [CrossRef]
76. Felcher, C.M.; Bogni, E.S.; Kordon, E.C. IL-6 Cytokine Family: A Putative Target for Breast Cancer Prevention and Treatment. *Int. J. Mol. Sci.* **2022**, *23*, 1809. [CrossRef]
77. Manore, S.G.; Doheny, D.L.; Wong, G.L.; Lo, H.-W. IL-6/JAK/STAT3 Signaling in Breast Cancer Metastasis: Biology and Treatment. *Front. Oncol.* **2022**, *12*, 866014. [CrossRef]
78. Sanguinetti, A.; Santini, D.; Bonafè, M.; Taffurelli, M.; Avenia, N. Interleukin-6 and pro Inflammatory Status in the Breast Tumor Microenvironment. *World J. Surg. Oncol.* **2015**, *13*, 129. [CrossRef]
79. Shi, J.; Feng, J.; Xie, J.; Mei, Z.; Shi, T.; Wang, S.; Du, Y.; Yang, G.; Wu, Y.; Cheng, X.; et al. Targeted Blockade of TGF-β and IL-6/JAK2/STAT3 Pathways Inhibits Lung Cancer Growth Promoted by Bone Marrow-Derived Myofibroblasts. *Sci. Rep.* **2017**, *7*, 8660. [CrossRef]
80. Beguinot, M.; Dauplat, M.-M.; Kwiatkowski, F.; Lebouedec, G.; Tixier, L.; Pomel, C.; Penault-Llorca, F.; Radosevic-Robin, N. Analysis of Tumour-Infiltrating Lymphocytes Reveals Two New Biologically Different Subgroups of Breast Ductal Carcinoma in Situ. *BMC Cancer* **2018**, *18*, 129. [CrossRef]
81. Denkert, C.; von Minckwitz, G.; Darb-Esfahani, S.; Lederer, B.; Heppner, B.I.; Weber, K.E.; Budczies, J.; Huober, J.; Klauschen, F.; Furlanetto, J.; et al. Tumour-Infiltrating Lymphocytes and Prognosis in Different Subtypes of Breast Cancer: A Pooled Analysis of 3771 Patients Treated with Neoadjuvant Therapy. *Lancet Oncol.* **2018**, *19*, 40–50. [CrossRef]
82. Kim, A.; Heo, S.-H.; Kim, Y.-A.; Gong, G.; Jin Lee, H. An Examination of the Local Cellular Immune Response to Examples of Both Ductal Carcinoma In Situ (DCIS) of the Breast and DCIS With Microinvasion, With Emphasis on Tertiary Lymphoid Structures and Tumor Infiltrating Lymphoctyes. *Am. J. Clin. Pathol.* **2016**, *146*, 137–144. [CrossRef]
83. Tsang, J.Y.S.; Au, W.-L.; Lo, K.-Y.; Ni, Y.-B.; Hlaing, T.; Hu, J.; Chan, S.-K.; Chan, K.-F.; Cheung, S.-Y.; Tse, G.M. PD-L1 Expression and Tumor Infiltrating PD-1+ Lymphocytes Associated with Outcome in HER2+ Breast Cancer Patients. *Breast Cancer Res. Treat.* **2017**, *162*, 19–30. [CrossRef]
84. Ruffell, B.; Au, A.; Rugo, H.S.; Esserman, L.J.; Hwang, E.S.; Coussens, L.M. Leukocyte Composition of Human Breast Cancer. *Proc. Natl. Acad. Sci. USA* **2012**, *109*, 2796–2801. [CrossRef]
85. Garaud, S.; Buisseret, L.; Solinas, C.; Gu-Trantien, C.; de Wind, A.; Van den Eynden, G.; Naveaux, C.; Lodewyckx, J.-N.; Boisson, A.; Duvillier, H.; et al. Tumor-Infiltrating B Cells Signal Functional Humoral Immune Responses in Breast Cancer. *JCI Insight* **2019**, *4*, e129641. [CrossRef]
86. Borst, J.; Ahrends, T.; Bąbała, N.; Melief, C.J.M.; Kastenmüller, W. CD4+ T Cell Help in Cancer Immunology and Immunotherapy. *Nat. Rev. Immunol.* **2018**, *18*, 635–647. [CrossRef]
87. Karasar, P.; Esendagli, G. T Helper Responses Are Maintained by Basal-like Breast Cancer Cells and Confer to Immune Modulation via Upregulation of PD-1 Ligands. *Breast Cancer Res. Treat.* **2014**, *145*, 605–614. [CrossRef]
88. Aspord, C.; Pedroza-Gonzalez, A.; Gallegos, M.; Tindle, S.; Burton, E.C.; Su, D.; Marches, F.; Banchereau, J.; Palucka, A.K. Breast Cancer Instructs Dendritic Cells to Prime Interleukin 13–Secreting CD4+ T Cells That Facilitate Tumor Development. *J. Exp. Med.* **2007**, *204*, 1037–1047. [CrossRef]
89. Tan, T.-T.; Coussens, L.M. Humoral Immunity, Inflammation and Cancer. *Curr. Opin. Immunol.* **2007**, *19*, 209–216. [CrossRef]
90. Cao, Y.; Dong, L.; He, Y.; Hu, X.; Hou, Y.; Dong, Y.; Yang, Q.; Bi, Y.; Liu, G. The Direct and Indirect Regulation of Follicular T Helper Cell Differentiation in Inflammation and Cancer. *J. Cell. Physiol.* **2021**, *236*, 5466–5481. [CrossRef]
91. Gu-Trantien, C.; Loi, S.; Garaud, S.; Equeter, C.; Libin, M.; de Wind, A.; Ravoet, M.; Buanec, H.L.; Sibille, C.; Manfouo-Foutsop, G.; et al. CD4+ Follicular Helper T Cell Infiltration Predicts Breast Cancer Survival. *J. Clin. Investig.* **2013**, *123*, 2873–2892. [CrossRef]
92. Wachstein, J.; Tischer, S.; Figueiredo, C.; Limbourg, A.; Falk, C.; Immenschuh, S.; Blasczyk, R.; Eiz-Vesper, B. HSP70 Enhances Immunosuppressive Function of CD4+CD25+FoxP3+ T Regulatory Cells and Cytotoxicity in CD4+CD25− T Cells. *PLoS ONE* **2012**, *7*, e51747. [CrossRef]
93. Datta, J.; Rosenblit, C.; Berk, E.; Showalter, L.; Namjoshi, P.; Mick, R.; Lee, K.P.; Brod, A.M.; Yang, R.L.; Kelz, R.R.; et al. Progressive Loss of Anti-HER2 CD4+ T-Helper Type 1 Response in Breast Tumorigenesis and the Potential for Immune Restoration. *OncoImmunology* **2015**, *4*, e1022301. [CrossRef]
94. Clark, N.M.; Martinez, L.M.; Murdock, S.; deLigio, J.T.; Olex, A.L.; Effi, C.; Dozmorov, M.G.; Bos, P.D. Regulatory T Cells Support Breast Cancer Progression by Opposing IFN-γ-Dependent Functional Reprogramming of Myeloid Cells. *Cell Rep.* **2020**, *33*, 108482. [CrossRef] [PubMed]
95. Nelson, B.H. CD20+ B Cells: The Other Tumor-Infiltrating Lymphocytes. *J. Immunol.* **2010**, *185*, 4977–4982. [CrossRef] [PubMed]
96. Harimoto, H.; Shimizu, M.; Nakagawa, Y.; Nakatsuka, K.; Wakabayashi, A.; Sakamoto, C.; Takahashi, H. Inactivation of Tumor-Specific CD8+ CTLs by Tumor-Infiltrating Tolerogenic Dendritic Cells. *Immunol. Cell Biol.* **2013**, *91*, 545–555. [CrossRef]
97. Gadalla, R.; Hassan, H.; Ibrahim, S.A.; Abdullah, M.S.; Gaballah, A.; Greve, B.; El-Deeb, S.; El-Shinawi, M.; Mohamed, M.M. Tumor Microenvironmental Plasmacytoid Dendritic Cells Contribute to Breast Cancer Lymph Node Metastasis via CXCR4/SDF-1 Axis. *Breast Cancer Res. Treat.* **2019**, *174*, 679–691. [CrossRef]

98. Oshi, M.; Newman, S.; Tokumaru, Y.; Yan, L.; Matsuyama, R.; Kalinski, P.; Endo, I.; Takabe, K. Plasmacytoid Dendritic Cell (PDC) Infiltration Correlate with Tumor Infiltrating Lymphocytes, Cancer Immunity, and Better Survival in Triple Negative Breast Cancer (TNBC) More Strongly than Conventional Dendritic Cell (CDC). *Cancers* **2020**, *12*, 3342. [CrossRef] [PubMed]
99. Ma, R.-Y.; Zhang, H.; Li, X.-F.; Zhang, C.-B.; Selli, C.; Tagliavini, G.; Lam, A.D.; Prost, S.; Sims, A.H.; Hu, H.-Y.; et al. Monocyte-Derived Macrophages Promote Breast Cancer Bone Metastasis Outgrowth. *J. Exp. Med.* **2020**, *217*, e20191820. [CrossRef] [PubMed]
100. Fridlender, Z.G.; Sun, J.; Kim, S.; Kapoor, V.; Cheng, G.; Ling, L.; Worthen, G.S.; Albelda, S.M. Polarization of Tumor-Associated Neutrophil Phenotype by TGF-β: "N1" versus "N2" TAN. *Cancer Cell* **2009**, *16*, 183–194. [CrossRef]
101. Ohms, M.; Möller, S.; Laskay, T. An Attempt to Polarize Human Neutrophils Toward N1 and N2 Phenotypes in Vitro. *Front. Immunol.* **2020**, *11*, 532. [CrossRef]
102. Burugu, S.; Asleh-Aburaya, K.; Nielsen, T.O. Immune Infiltrates in the Breast Cancer Microenvironment: Detection, Characterization and Clinical Implication. *Breast Cancer* **2017**, *24*, 3–15. [CrossRef]
103. Tai, Y.; Chen, K.; Hsieh, J.; Shen, T. Exosomes in Cancer Development and Clinical Applications. *Cancer Sci.* **2018**, *109*, 2364–2374. [CrossRef]
104. Wang, J.; Zeng, H.; Zhang, H.; Han, Y. The Role of Exosomal PD-L1 in Tumor Immunotherapy. *Transl. Oncol.* **2021**, *14*, 101047. [CrossRef] [PubMed]
105. Pelon, F.; Bourachot, B.; Kieffer, Y.; Magagna, I.; Mermet-Meillon, F.; Bonnet, I.; Costa, A.; Givel, A.-M.; Attieh, Y.; Barbazan, J.; et al. Cancer-Associated Fibroblast Heterogeneity in Axillary Lymph Nodes Drives Metastases in Breast Cancer through Complementary Mechanisms. *Nat. Commun.* **2020**, *11*, 404. [CrossRef] [PubMed]
106. Ungefroren, H.; Sebens, S.; Seidl, D.; Lehnert, H.; Hass, R. Interaction of Tumor Cells with the Microenvironment. *Cell Commun. Signal.* **2011**, *9*, 18. [CrossRef]
107. Izraely, S.; Witz, I.P. Site-Specific Metastasis: A Cooperation between Cancer Cells and the Metastatic Microenvironment. *Int. J. Cancer* **2021**, *148*, 1308–1322. [CrossRef]
108. Yousefi, M.; Nosrati, R.; Salmaninejad, A.; Dehghani, S.; Shahryari, A.; Saberi, A. Organ-Specific Metastasis of Breast Cancer: Molecular and Cellular Mechanisms Underlying Lung Metastasis. *Cell. Oncol.* **2018**, *41*, 123–140. [CrossRef]
109. Chen, W.; Hoffmann, A.D.; Liu, H.; Liu, X. Organotropism: New Insights into Molecular Mechanisms of Breast Cancer Metastasis. *NPJ Precis. Oncol.* **2018**, *2*, 4. [CrossRef]
110. Lu, X.; Kang, Y. Organotropism of Breast Cancer Metastasis. *J. Mammary Gland Biol. Neoplasia* **2007**, *12*, 153. [CrossRef]
111. Wu, Q.; Li, J.; Zhu, S.; Wu, J.; Chen, C.; Liu, Q.; Wei, W.; Zhang, Y.; Sun, S. Breast Cancer Subtypes Predict the Preferential Site of Distant Metastases: A SEER Based Study. *Oncotarget* **2017**, *8*, 27990–27996. [CrossRef]
112. Liu, Y.; Cao, X. Characteristics and Significance of the Pre-Metastatic Niche. *Cancer Cell* **2016**, *30*, 668–681. [CrossRef]
113. Kaplan, R.N.; Psaila, B.; Lyden, D. Bone Marrow Cells in the 'Pre-Metastatic Niche': Within Bone and Beyond. *Cancer Metastasis Rev.* **2006**, *25*, 521–529. [CrossRef]
114. Radisky, E.S.; Radisky, D.C. Matrix Metalloproteinases as Breast Cancer Drivers and Therapeutic Targets. *Front. Biosci. Landmark Ed.* **2015**, *20*, 1144–1163. [CrossRef]
115. Garcia, M.; Platet, N.; Liaudet, E.; Laurent, V.; Derocq, D.; Brouillet, J.P.; Rochefort, H. Biological and Clinical Significance of Cathepsin D in Breast Cancer Metastasis. *Stem. Cells Dayt. Ohio.* **1996**, *14*, 642–650. [CrossRef]
116. Tang, L.; Han, X. The Urokinase Plasminogen Activator System in Breast Cancer Invasion and Metastasis. *Biomed. Pharmacother. Biomed. Pharmacother.* **2013**, *67*, 179–182. [CrossRef] [PubMed]
117. Singh, S.; Chakrabarti, R. Consequences of EMT-Driven Changes in the Immune Microenvironment of Breast Cancer and Therapeutic Response of Cancer Cells. *J. Clin. Med.* **2019**, *8*, 642. [CrossRef] [PubMed]
118. Coupland, L.A.; Parish, C.R. Platelets, Selectins, and the Control of Tumor Metastasis. *Semin. Oncol.* **2014**, *41*, 422–434. [CrossRef]
119. Yadav, A.; Kumar, B.; Yu, J.-G.; Old, M.; Teknos, T.N.; Kumar, P. Tumor-Associated Endothelial Cells Promote Tumor Metastasis by Chaperoning Circulating Tumor Cells and Protecting Them from Anoikis. *PLoS ONE* **2015**, *10*, e0141602. [CrossRef]
120. Padua, D.; Zhang, X.H.-F.; Wang, Q.; Nadal, C.; Gerald, W.L.; Gomis, R.R.; Massagué, J. TGFβ Primes Breast Tumors for Lung Metastasis Seeding through Angiopoietin-like 4. *Cell* **2008**, *133*, 66–77. [CrossRef]
121. Yu, P.F.; Huang, Y.; Xu, C.L.; Lin, L.Y.; Han, Y.Y.; Sun, W.H.; Hu, G.H.; Rabson, A.B.; Wang, Y.; Shi, Y.F. Downregulation of CXCL12 in Mesenchymal Stromal Cells by TGFβ Promotes Breast Cancer Metastasis. *Oncogene* **2017**, *36*, 840–849. [CrossRef]
122. Madden, E.C.; Gorman, A.M.; Logue, S.E.; Samali, A. Tumour Cell Secretome in Chemoresistance and Tumour Recurrence. *Trends Cancer* **2020**, *6*, 489–505. [CrossRef]
123. Korde, L.A.; Somerfield, M.R.; Carey, L.A.; Crews, J.R.; Denduluri, N.; Hwang, E.S.; Khan, S.A.; Loibl, S.; Morris, E.A.; Perez, A.; et al. Neoadjuvant Chemotherapy, Endocrine Therapy, and Targeted Therapy for Breast Cancer: ASCO Guideline. *J. Clin. Oncol.* **2021**, *39*, 1485–1505. [CrossRef]
124. Dillekås, H.; Rogers, M.S.; Straume, O. Are 90% of Deaths from Cancer Caused by Metastases? *Cancer Med.* **2019**, *8*, 5574–5576. [CrossRef] [PubMed]
125. Holohan, C.; Van Schaeybroeck, S.; Longley, D.B.; Johnston, P.G. Cancer Drug Resistance: An Evolving Paradigm. *Nat. Rev. Cancer* **2013**, *13*, 714–726. [CrossRef] [PubMed]
126. Subrahmanyam, N.; Ghandehari, H. Harnessing Extracellular Matrix Biology for Tumor Drug Delivery. *J. Pers. Med.* **2021**, *11*, 88. [CrossRef] [PubMed]

127. Wang, W.; Nag, S.A.; Zhang, R. Targeting the NFκB Signaling Pathways for Breast Cancer Prevention and Therapy. *Curr. Med. Chem.* **2015**, *22*, 264–289. [CrossRef] [PubMed]
128. Kowal, J.; Arras, G.; Colombo, M.; Jouve, M.; Morath, J.P.; Primdal-Bengtson, B.; Dingli, F.; Loew, D.; Tkach, M.; Théry, C. Proteomic Comparison Defines Novel Markers to Characterize Heterogeneous Populations of Extracellular Vesicle Subtypes. *Proc. Natl. Acad. Sci. USA* **2016**, *113*, E968–E977. [CrossRef]
129. Hayatudin, R.; Fong, Z.; Ming, L.C.; Goh, B.-H.; Lee, W.-L.; Kifli, N. Overcoming Chemoresistance via Extracellular Vesicle Inhibition. *Front. Mol. Biosci.* **2021**, *8*, 629874. [CrossRef]
130. Ma, X.; Chen, Z.; Hua, D.; He, D.; Wang, L.; Zhang, P.; Wang, J.; Cai, Y.; Gao, C.; Zhang, X.; et al. Essential Role for TrpC5-Containing Extracellular Vesicles in Breast Cancer with Chemotherapeutic Resistance. *Proc. Natl. Acad. Sci. USA* **2014**, *111*, 6389–6394. [CrossRef]
131. Masoud, V.; Pagès, G. Targeted Therapies in Breast Cancer: New Challenges to Fight against Resistance. *World J. Clin. Oncol.* **2017**, *8*, 120–134. [CrossRef]
132. Swain, S.M.; Shastry, M.; Hamilton, E. Targeting HER2-Positive Breast Cancer: Advances and Future Directions. *Nat. Rev. Drug Discov.* **2023**, *22*, 101–126. [CrossRef]
133. Gajria, D.; Chandarlapaty, S. HER2-Amplified Breast Cancer: Mechanisms of Trastuzumab Resistance and Novel Targeted Therapies. *Expert Rev. Anticancer Ther.* **2011**, *11*, 263–275. [CrossRef]
134. Opdam, F.L.; Guchelaar, H.-J.; Beijnen, J.H.; Schellens, J.H.M. Lapatinib for Advanced or Metastatic Breast Cancer. *Oncologist* **2012**, *17*, 536–542. [CrossRef] [PubMed]
135. Yang, F.; Huang, X.; Sun, C.; Li, J.; Wang, B.; Yan, M.; Jin, F.; Wang, H.; Zhang, J.; Fu, P.; et al. Lapatinib in Combination with Capecitabine versus Continued Use of Trastuzumab in Breast Cancer Patients with Trastuzumab-Resistance: A Retrospective Study of a Chinese Population. *BMC Cancer* **2020**, *20*, 255. [CrossRef] [PubMed]
136. Obenauf, A.C.; Zou, Y.; Ji, A.L.; Vanharanta, S.; Shu, W.; Shi, H.; Kong, X.; Bosenberg, M.C.; Wiesner, T.; Rosen, N.; et al. Therapy-Induced Tumour Secretomes Promote Resistance and Tumour Progression. *Nature* **2015**, *520*, 368–372. [CrossRef]
137. Ye, J.; Tian, T.; Chen, X. The Efficacy of Gefitinib Supplementation for Breast Cancer. *Medicine* **2020**, *99*, e22613. [CrossRef]
138. Miyashita, M.; Hattori, M.; Takano, T.; Toyama, T.; Iwata, H. Risks and Benefits of Bevacizumab Combined with Chemotherapy for Advanced or Metastatic Breast Cancer: A Meta-Analysis of Randomized Controlled Trials. *Breast Cancer* **2020**, *27*, 347–354. [CrossRef]
139. Khan, M.; Zhao, Z.; Arooj, S.; Zheng, T.; Liao, G. Lapatinib Plus Local Radiation Therapy for Brain Metastases From HER-2 Positive Breast Cancer Patients and Role of Trastuzumab: A Systematic Review and Meta-Analysis. *Front. Oncol.* **2020**, *10*, 576926. [CrossRef]
140. Masuda, N.; Iwata, H.; Aogi, K.; Xu, Y.; Ibrahim, A.; Gao, L.; Dalal, R.; Yoshikawa, R.; Sasaki, Y. Safety and Pharmacokinetics of Ramucirumab in Combination with Docetaxel in Japanese Patients with Locally Advanced or Metastatic Breast Cancer: A Phase Ib Study. *Jpn. J. Clin. Oncol.* **2016**, *46*, 1088–1094. [CrossRef] [PubMed]
141. Schmid, P.; Cortes, J.; Dent, R.; Pusztai, L.; McArthur, H.; Kümmel, S.; Bergh, J.; Denkert, C.; Park, Y.H.; Hui, R.; et al. Event-Free Survival with Pembrolizumab in Early Triple-Negative Breast Cancer. *N. Engl. J. Med.* **2022**, *386*, 556–567. [CrossRef]
142. Tulotta, C.; Lefley, D.V.; Moore, C.K.; Amariutei, A.E.; Spicer-Hadlington, A.R.; Quayle, L.A.; Hughes, R.O.; Ahmed, K.; Cookson, V.; Evans, C.A.; et al. IL-1B Drives Opposing Responses in Primary Tumours and Bone Metastases; Harnessing Combination Therapies to Improve Outcome in Breast Cancer. *NPJ Breast Cancer* **2021**, *7*, 95. [CrossRef]
143. Zhou, J.; Tulotta, C.; Ottewell, P.D. IL-1β in Breast Cancer Bone Metastasis. *Expert Rev. Mol. Med.* **2022**, *24*, e11. [CrossRef]
144. Zhang, X.; Li, Y.; Wei, M.; Liu, C.; Yu, T.; Yang, J. Cetuximab-Modified Silica Nanoparticle Loaded with ICG for Tumor-Targeted Combinational Therapy of Breast Cancer. *Drug Deliv.* **2019**, *26*, 129–136. [CrossRef] [PubMed]
145. Barroso-Sousa, R.; Keenan, T.E.; Li, T.; Tayob, N.; Trippa, L.; Pastorello, R.G.; Richardson III, E.T.; Dillon, D.; Amoozgar, Z.; Overmoyer, B.; et al. Nivolumab in Combination with Cabozantinib for Metastatic Triple-Negative Breast Cancer: A Phase II and Biomarker Study. *NPJ Breast Cancer* **2021**, *7*, 110. [CrossRef] [PubMed]
146. Kang, C.; Syed, Y.Y. Atezolizumab (in Combination with Nab-Paclitaxel): A Review in Advanced Triple-Negative Breast Cancer. *Drugs* **2020**, *80*, 601–607. [CrossRef]
147. Correia, A.S.; Gärtner, F.; Vale, N. Drug Combination and Repurposing for Cancer Therapy: The Example of Breast Cancer. *Heliyon* **2021**, *7*, e05948. [CrossRef]
148. Fares, J.; Kanojia, D.; Rashidi, A.; Ulasov, I.; Lesniak, M.S. Landscape of Combination Therapy Trials in Breast Cancer Brain Metastasis. *Int. J. Cancer* **2020**, *147*, 1939–1952. [CrossRef]
149. Fisusi, F.A.; Akala, E.O. Drug Combinations in Breast Cancer Therapy. *Pharm. Nanotechnol.* **2019**, *7*, 3–23. [CrossRef] [PubMed]
150. Aumeeruddy, M.Z.; Mahomoodally, M.F. Combating Breast Cancer Using Combination Therapy with 3 Phytochemicals: Piperine, Sulforaphane, and Thymoquinone. *Cancer* **2019**, *125*, 1600–1611. [CrossRef]
151. Panahi, Y.; Saadat, A.; Beiraghdar, F.; Nouzari, S.M.H.; Jalalian, H.R.; Sahebkar, A. Antioxidant Effects of Bioavailability-Enhanced Curcuminoids in Patients with Solid Tumors: A Randomized Double-Blind Placebo-Controlled Trial. *J. Funct. Foods* **2014**, *6*, 615–622. [CrossRef]
152. Fuchs-Tarlovsky, V. Role of Antioxidants in Cancer Therapy. *Nutrition* **2013**, *29*, 15–21. [CrossRef]

153. Block, K.I.; Koch, A.C.; Mead, M.N.; Tothy, P.K.; Newman, R.A.; Gyllenhaal, C. Impact of Antioxidant Supplementation on Chemotherapeutic Efficacy: A Systematic Review of the Evidence from Randomized Controlled Trials. *Cancer Treat. Rev.* **2007**, *33*, 407–418. [CrossRef]
154. Mokhtari, R.B.; Homayouni, T.S.; Baluch, N.; Morgatskaya, E.; Kumar, S.; Das, B.; Yeger, H. Combination Therapy in Combating Cancer. *Oncotarget* **2017**, *8*, 38022–38043. [CrossRef] [PubMed]
155. Bettaieb, A.; Paul, C.; Plenchette, S.; Shan, J.; Chouchane, L.; Ghiringhelli, F. Precision Medicine in Breast Cancer: Reality or Utopia? *J. Transl. Med.* **2017**, *15*, 139. [CrossRef] [PubMed]
156. Tung, N.; Garber, J.E. PARP Inhibition in Breast Cancer: Progress Made and Future Hopes. *NPJ Breast Cancer* **2022**, *8*, 47. [CrossRef] [PubMed]
157. Barchiesi, G.; Roberto, M.; Verrico, M.; Vici, P.; Tomao, S.; Tomao, F. Emerging Role of PARP Inhibitors in Metastatic Triple Negative Breast Cancer. Current Scenario and Future Perspectives. *Front. Oncol.* **2021**, *11*, 769280. [CrossRef]
158. Danenberg, E.; Bardwell, H.; Zanotelli, V.R.T.; Provenzano, E.; Chin, S.-F.; Rueda, O.M.; Green, A.; Rakha, E.; Aparicio, S.; Ellis, I.O.; et al. Breast Tumor Microenvironment Structures Are Associated with Genomic Features and Clinical Outcome. *Nat. Genet.* **2022**, *54*, 660–669. [CrossRef]

Disclaimer/Publisher's Note: The statements, opinions and data contained in all publications are solely those of the individual author(s) and contributor(s) and not of MDPI and/or the editor(s). MDPI and/or the editor(s) disclaim responsibility for any injury to people or property resulting from any ideas, methods, instructions or products referred to in the content.

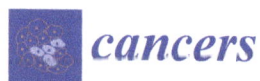

Review

Clinical Utility of Genomic Tests Evaluating Homologous Recombination Repair Deficiency (HRD) for Treatment Decisions in Early and Metastatic Breast Cancer

Loïck Galland [1,2,3,†], Nicolas Roussot [1,2,3,†], Isabelle Desmoulins [1], Didier Mayeur [1], Courèche Kaderbhai [1], Silvia Ilie [1], Audrey Hennequin [1], Manon Reda [1], Juliette Albuisson [4,5], Laurent Arnould [4,6], Romain Boidot [4,6], Caroline Truntzer [2,5,7], François Ghiringhelli [1,2,3,5] and Sylvain Ladoire [1,2,3,5,8,*]

1. Department of Medical Oncology, Georges-François Leclerc Center, 21000 Dijon, France
2. Platform of Transfer in Biological Oncology, Georges-François Leclerc Cancer Center, 21000 Dijon, France
3. University of Burgundy-Franche Comté, 21000 Dijon, France
4. Department of Pathology and Tumor Biology, Georges-François Leclerc Center, 21000 Dijon, France
5. Research Center INSERM LNC-UMR1231, 21000 Dijon, France
6. ICMUB UMR CNRS 6302, 21000 Dijon, France
7. Bioinformatic Core Facility Georges-François Leclerc Cancer Center, 21000 Dijon, France
8. Genomic and Immunotherapy Medical Institute, Dijon University Hospital, 21000 Dijon, France
* Correspondence: sladoire@cgfl.fr
† These authors contributed equally to this work.

Simple Summary: Breast cancer is the most frequently occurring cancer worldwide. With the help of next-generation sequencing, the development of biomedical technologies and the use of bioinformatics, it is now possible to identify specific molecular alterations in tumor cells, such as homologous recombination deficiencies, enabling us to consider using DNA-damaging agents such as platinum salts or PARP inhibitors. In this review, we summarize current knowledge on the clinical utility of genomic tests evaluating homologous recombination repair deficiency for treatment decisions in early and metastatic breast cancer.

Abstract: Breast cancer is the most frequently occurring cancer worldwide. With its increasing incidence, it is a major public health problem, with many therapeutic challenges such as precision medicine for personalized treatment. Thanks to next-generation sequencing (NGS), progress in biomedical technologies, and the use of bioinformatics, it is now possible to identify specific molecular alterations in tumor cells—such as homologous recombination deficiencies (HRD)—enabling us to consider using DNA-damaging agents such as platinum salts or PARP inhibitors. Different approaches currently exist to analyze impairment of the homologous recombination pathway, e.g., the search for specific mutations in homologous recombination repair (HRR) genes, such as *BRCA1/2*; the use of genomic scars or mutational signatures; or the development of functional tests. Nevertheless, the role and value of these different tests in breast cancer treatment decisions remains to be clarified. In this review, we summarize current knowledge on the clinical utility of genomic tests, evaluating HRR deficiency for treatment decisions in early and metastatic breast cancer.

Keywords: breast cancer; early breast cancer; metastatic breast cancer; *BRCA*; NGS; HRD score; homologous recombination deficiency; mutational signature; PARPi; platinum salts

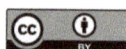

1. Background

Breast cancer is the most frequently occurring cancer in the world, with increasing incidence, and it is becoming a major public health problem [1]. It is therefore increasingly important to identify tools that can guide physicians in their therapeutic choices, both at the localized and metastatic stages. Among these tools, the evaluation of the homologous recombination (HR) process could prove to be of interest. Its clinical utility and its current place in the breast cancer landscape are the subject of this review.

1.1. Repair of DNA Double-Strand Breaks and Homologous Recombination (HR) Deficiency

DNA double-strand breaks (DSBs) may be linked to physiological (e.g., during meiosis or telomere erosions) and/or pathological mechanisms [2,3]. These pathological mechanisms may be the consequence of replication accidents or may result from the action of exogenous agents (such as radiotherapy or chemotherapy). If DSBs accumulate, the cell becomes non-viable and dies. Various pathways are involved in DNA repair, when DSBs arise [4].

First, non-homologous end joining (NHEJ) or micro-homologous end joining (AltEJ) pathways are active throughout the cell cycle and enable rapid but error-prone repair [5]. The second important pathway, called "homologous recombination repair (HRR) pathway", is the only one able to repair double-stranded DNA lesions *ad integrum*. This pathway involves several key proteins such as BRCA1 and BRCA2 but also many other actors such as RAD50, RAD51, or PALB2. During this process of HR, DSBs are recognized by the MRN complex (Mre11-Rad50-Nbs1), which transforms the double-stranded ends into single strands [6]. These single strands are initially passively coated with an RPA protein, and BRCA2 will replace RPA with the RAD51 protein [7]. The main steps and proteins involved in this HR process are summarized in Figure 1.

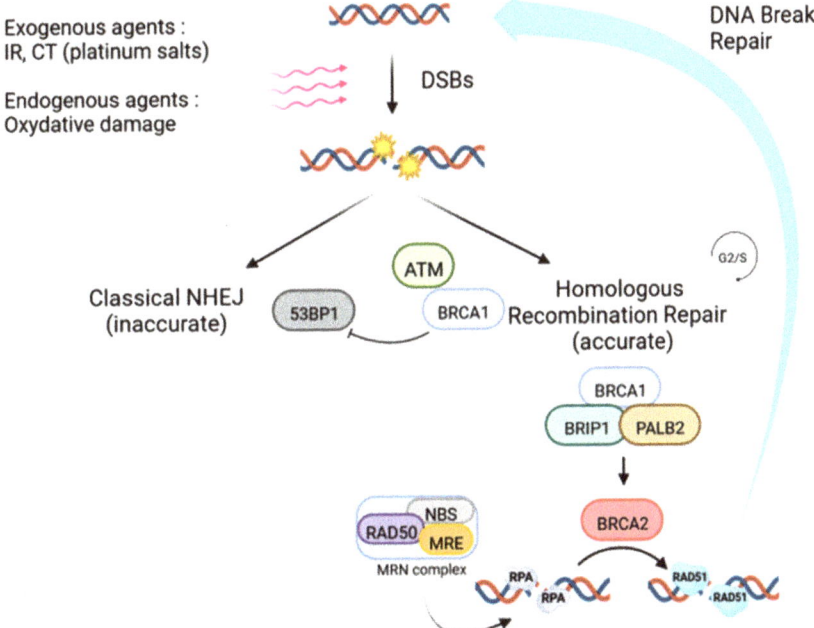

Figure 1. Homologous recombination repair pathway (made with Biorender). Repair begins at DSB sites by recruitment of ATM, which phosphorylates proteins such as BRCA1 in the case of HRR, or 53BP1 for NHEJ. Focusing on the HRR pathway, activation of BRCA1, via BRCA2 and PALB2, enables the transformation of DSBs into single-stranded DNA, to which the RPA proteins hybridize. This step also involves the MRN complex. RAD51 will then replace the RPA proteins bound to the single-stranded DNA, enabling the search for homology sequences, and involvement in strand invasion. The last step consists of DNA synthesis, ligation, and resolution of the Holliday junctions. IR: ionizing radiation, CT: chemotherapy, DSBs: DNA double-strand breaks, NHEJ: non-homologous end joining, DNA: deoxyribonucleic acid.

This pathway can be inactivated by numerous somatic events (mutations, deletions, and methylation of the promoters of the genes involved), with or without associated germline mutations in many solid tumors (breast, ovary, pancreas, prostate, and stomach or lung tumors) [8]. Deficiency of the HR pathway represents a mechanism of oncogenesis, increasing genetic instability, and promoting the activation of oncogenes and the inactivation of tumor suppressor genes. This is known as homologous recombination deficiency (HRD). As explained above, *BRCA1* and *2* genes are considered to be tumor suppressor genes, and their inactivation is responsible for a predisposition to breast or ovarian cancer [9]. This HR deficit is frequently found in high grade ovarian cancers and in breast cancers (BC). It is estimated that 70–80% of breast cancer patients with a *BRCA1* or *2* mutation have a TNBC subtype, and that about 20% of TNBC have a *BRCA1* or *2* mutation [10]. Approximately 10–36% of BCs that occur in *BRCA1/2* mutation carriers are estrogen-receptor (ER)-positive (ER+) [11]. Sometimes, the mutations found in this pathway do not affect *BRCA 1/2* but rather other genes involved, also leading to genomic instability and to a "*BRCA*ness or HRness phenotype" (such as *RAD51C* epimutations, inactivation of *PALB2, BRIP1,* or *BARD1*) [12]. Mutations caused by malfunction of the HR process occur in a specific pattern, or "signature". This mutation profile in cancer DNA thus appears to be a good way to identify breast cancers with a defect in HR DNA repair, regardless of the underlying cause [13].

1.2. Homologous Recombination Deficiency: Therapeutic Interest

The deficiency of the homologous recombination pathway also represents an "Achilles heel" of the tumor, with the development of molecules that take advantage of this inactivation (PARP inhibitors and chemotherapy with platinum salts in particular) [14–16]. Indeed, these molecules are able to create numerous DSBs in the DNA, which can no longer be repaired in cancer cells that are highly deficient in HR. The assessment of HRD status and the therapeutic value of treatments affecting this pathway initially originated in ovarian cancer.

Platinum salts are cytotoxic chemotherapies that induce binding of alkyl groups on the purine bases of DNA, enabling the creation of mono- or bi-functional adducts and intra- and/or inter-strand bridges [17,18]. The result is to halt the cell's transcription and replication processes. The HR pathway is required to repair platinum-induced double-strand breaks, which explains the greater sensitivity of HRD tumors to this therapeutic class. Thus, sensitivity to platinum salts could be considered indirectly as a possible clinical marker of tumor HRD.

In cells with inactivating mutations of the *BRCA1/2* genes, the HR pathway is deficient, and survival of these tumors relies on one or more accessory repair pathways. Poly-(ADP-ribose) polymerases (PARP) are enzymes that induce synthesis of a poly-ADP ribose chain, acting as a signal to initiate repair in the base excision repair (BER) pathway. PARP inhibitors (PARPi) are compounds that trap PARP on sites of DNA damage, leading to replication fork stalling and to the generation of DSBs, resulting from unresolved SSBs [19]. Thus, this accumulation of DSBs that cannot be repaired in HR-deficient cells leads to cell cycle arrest in G2/M and to apoptosis of the tumor cells. This phenomenon is now well known as "synthetic lethality" [14,16,20,21]. Olaparib, a selective PARP-1 inhibitor, was initially developed in advanced, high-grade, relapsing, platinum-sensitive ovarian cancer [22]. In addition, while the first trials and registrations only concerned *BRCA1* or *2* mutations, other trials have explored the extension of indications to tumors that are *BRCA1/2* wild-type (WT), but that are considered to harbor HRD.

1.3. Tools to Assess Homologous Recombination Deficiency in Tumors

Given the therapeutic challenges of identifying platinum salt or PARPi-sensitive tumors, a number of biological tools have been developed, primarily to detect *BRCA*-mutated tumors, but also to identify HRD tumors outside the context of *BRCA* mutations [23,24].

The first approach being developed to this end is the search for mutations in HR pathway genes [25]. Beyond germline *BRCA* mutations, there seems to be evidence of the value of identifying somatic exclusive mutations, notably in prostate [26] and ovarian [27] cancer. In breast cancer, the results of the TBCRC 048 study seem to confirm the potential interest of identifying exclusive *BRCA* somatic mutations to predict response to PARPi [28]. The clinical and therapeutic relevance of the detection of mutations other than *BRCA 1* or *2* seems to depend on the histological type of the cancer. For example, in the previously mentioned TBCRC 048 study, germline mutations in *PALB2* were also associated with response to PARP inhibitors. The results seemed interesting for some, but not all of these genes, raising the question of the panel of genes other than *BRCA* to study in each cancer.

An alternative method consists in the use of a genomic profile (or genomic signature) that reflects HRD in tumor cells, regardless of its molecular origin [24,29]. Indeed, DNA-based measures of genomic instability capturing large genomic aberrations ("genomic scars") resulting from HRD have been developed in recent years, and represent an alternative approach for identifying HR-deficient tumors. Three independent scores have been developed: The Curie Institute developed a profile based on the number of chromosomal status changes (or breaks), and more specifically, on breaks in large chromosomal regions >10 Mb (Large-scale state transition, LST). This profile was initially identified in TNBC, since Popova et al. showed that the number of LSTs was significantly associated with *BRCA1* inactivations in this tumor subtype [30]. Another team showed that an allelic imbalance in subtelomeric regions (Telomeric Allelic Imbalance, TAI) was significantly associated with platinum sensitivity in TNBC as well as in *BRCA* WT ovarian tumors [31]. *BRCA1* or *2* mutated tumors were also more likely to develop loss of heterozygosity (LOH). An overall measurement of allelic balance, with detection of large regions of LOH, which seems to correlate well with the deficit of HR has been developed under the name of "FoundationFocus CDx" [32]. This HRD-LOH profile is based on the detection of large regions (>15 Mb) of heterozygosity loss, and enables the detection of *BRCA* mutations in ovarian cancer.

Timms and colleagues subsequently demonstrated that the combined presence of LST, TAI, and LOH across the genome seems to be of even greater value in predicting HRD status, leading to the commercialization of a combined score called "myChoice HRD" (Myriad genetics) [33]. The assay yields a "HRD score", considered to be positive if the score is ≥ 42 (cutoff value validated in ovarian cancer). This score is currently the most widely used in the world. Moreover, as in ovarian cancer, this combined score could help to predict sensitivity to molecules that take advantage of the HR defect, such as platinum salts and PARPi [34]. However, it is important to note that these genomic profiles measure are established early in tumorigenesis. This profile will therefore persist during tumor progression, leading to the term "genomic scars". Thus, the profile provides valuable information about the initial HR status of the tumor, but not necessarily about the current status, especially at advanced stages of disease. HRD status (from a functional point a view) can evolve over time, with partial or complete restoration of HR pathway functionality, most often under the therapeutic pressure of HRD-targeting agents, and secondary mutations restoring HR function appear to be a mechanism of resistance [35,36].

Other tools are also available to assess the HR status of a tumor. Following the analysis of different mutations found in thousands of exomes from different tumors in the TCGA (The Cancer Genome Atlas) or the ICGC (International Cancer Genome Consortium), "mutational signatures" have been defined and referenced in the Catalogue of Somatic Mutations In Cancer (COSMIC) [37]. These different mutational profiles are characteristic patterns created on the cancer cell genome by each mutational process. Next-generation sequencing was used to obtain the mutational spectrum of these tumors, leading to the categorization into specific signatures [38]. In particular, signature 3 has been found to be predominantly expressed in breast or ovarian cancers and linked to a defect in HR [38–40] and response to platinum salts. However, all *BRCA* 1 or *BRCA* 2 pathogenic mutations do not result in a single mutational signature: other signatures [41] also seem to be associated with a deficit of HR, such as signature 8 for example [38,42,43]. Based on emerging knowledge of these mutational signatures, different algorithms have been developed to help define the HRD status of a given tumor, such as SignatureAnalyzer [44] or Signature Multivariate Analysis (SigMA) [45].

Recent advances in sequencing technologies, with reduced overall costs, have prompted the development of tools based on whole genome sequencing (WGS), such as the HRDetect tool, which has been developed and presented as a predictive score of HRD. This score combines different mutational signatures (incorporating COSMIC signatures 3, 5, and 8), as well as other elements mentioned above such as microhomology-mediated deletions, TAI, LOH, and LST. With this score, Davies et al. were able to detect *BRCA* deficiency (germline and/or somatic) with a sensitivity of 99% in a cohort of 560 TNBC, and identified 47 tumors with a functional *BRCA* deficiency without any mutation found [42]. Accordingly, the number of tumors with HRD increased from 1–5% to 22%, leading to increasing numbers of patients who could potentially benefit from platinum salts or PARPi.

As HRD tumors may evolve towards restoration of HRR and acquire resistance to DNA-damaging agents, such tumors may be misclassified by genomic scar/signature-based assays. Thus so-called "functional" tests have also been developed. These tests dynamically evaluate the ability of tumor cells to perform the HR mechanism. For example, it is possible to measure the nuclear accumulation of RAD 51 [46] and tumors classified as RAD 51-low (by immunofluorescence [47] or immunohistochemistry [48]) would have a functional HRD. The interest of this functional test has been evaluated in various cancers, including breast [49–51] and ovarian cancer [47,52,53], and may be a biomarker for PARPi and/or platinum response. The most well-known test, the REcombination CAPacity (RECAP test) [47,49], classified tumors in three HR groups (deficient, intermediate, or proficient), depending on their RAD 51 score [54]. Despite some technical limitations [46,48,55], these tests have the advantage of providing an assessment of the current HR status of the tumor, to detect resistance acquired under therapeutic pressure, and to detect restoration of homologous recombination in initially HRD tumors [56]. The RAD 51 test has been retrospectively validated on cohorts from prospective clinical trials in ovarian [57], prostate [58], and triple-negative breast [59] cancers but require further clinical validation and standardization for routine use.

Clearly, it is important, especially in the field of breast cancer, to critically evaluate the validity and clinical utility of these HRD tests (DNA-based and/or functional). The main objective is to help to predict the sensitivity of tumors to DNA-damaging agents such as PARPi inhibitors or platinum salts, both in localized and metastatic situations. Figure 2 summarizes the different assay strategies discussed in this last section.

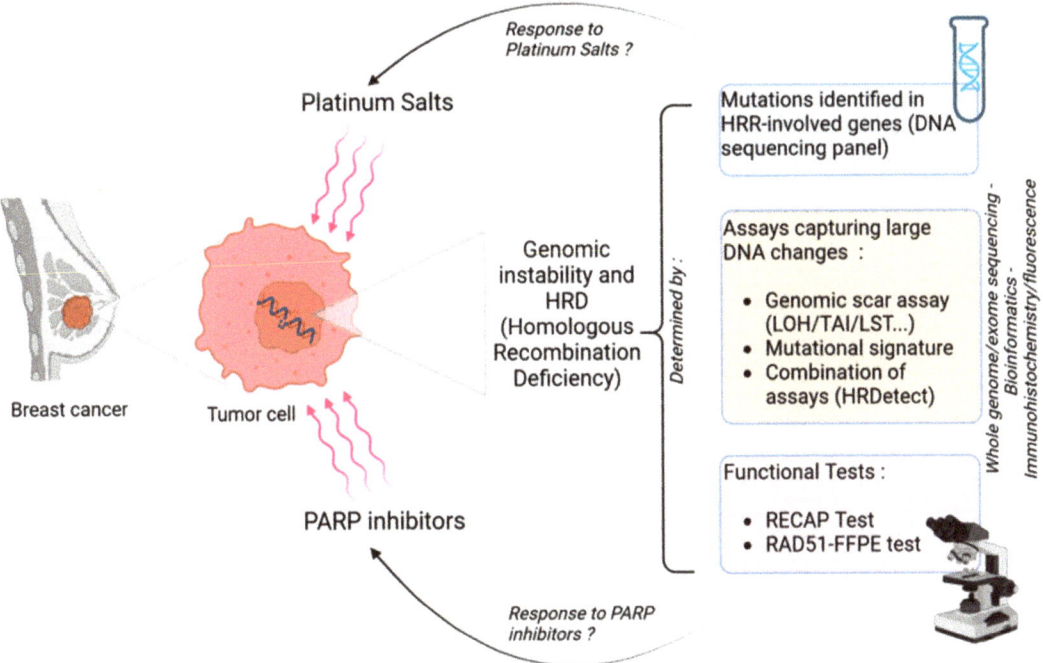

Figure 2. Homologous recombination deficiency (HRD) evaluation in breast cancer to predict platinum salts or PARP inhibitors response (made with Biorender). HRR: Homologous recombination repair, HRD: homologous recombination deficiency, DNA: deoxyribonucleic acid, LOH: loss of heterozygosity, TAI: telomeric allelic imbalance, LST: large-scale state transitions, PARP: poly(ADP-ribose) polymerase.

2. Early Breast Cancer (eBC)

Breast cancer represents nearly 30% of female cancers and patients harboring early stage disease are treated with a view to cure [1]. Nowadays, preoperative treatment is standard of care for a large proportion of early breast cancers enabling a down-staging and the assessment of treatment responsiveness, which is critical to adapting the adjuvant regimen. Evidence shows that pathologic complete response (pCR)—defined as the absence of infiltrative tumor cells in the breast and axilla (ypT0/is ypN0)—is associated with better outcomes, especially among the aforementioned aggressive subtypes [60]. Hence, achieving pCR with a preoperative regimen in this setting has become one of the main objectives of treatment in TNBC. Approximately 30–40% of TNBCs were shown to achieve pCR with a neoadjuvant cytotoxic regimen containing anthracyclines and taxanes [60,61]. Moreover, as previously mentioned, a majority of patients with *BRCA 1/2* mutations harbor this intrinsic subtype, and nearly a fifth of TNBC all-comers bear these mutations [10]. Given the relationship between TNBC and *BRCA 1/2* mutation, the use of additional therapies that target HRD—such as platinum salts or PARPi—is an attractive approach to improve the pathological response rate, and to achieve curative goals.

Here, we recap how evidence-based medicine has evolved in this setting, with the emergence of genomic tests evaluating HRD, to assist clinicians in treatment decision-making, and we review the clinical utility of these assays.

2.1. Platinum Salts and PARPi for BRCA-Mutated eBC

Firstly, the GEICAM/2006-03 trial [62] was the first randomized study to add platinum salts to standard neoadjuvant chemotherapy (NAC) in TNBC, regardless of *BRCA* status.

Of the 94 patients included, 49 received carboplatin in addition to an anthracycline-taxane based regimen, but the results failed to demonstrate any benefit in terms of pathologic response rate. A few years later, the CALG-B 40603 [63] phase II trial enrolled early TNBC to assess the addition of carboplatin. In that study, Sikov et al. demonstrated that adding carboplatin to standard chemotherapy increased the pCR rate, which was achieved in more than half of patients (54% vs. 41%, $p = 0.0029$). However, additional carboplatin did not result in any benefit in terms of event-free or overall survival benefit [63]. Considering these data, there was a keen interest in refining the selection of patients who might benefit from the addition of platinum salt in the neoadjuvant setting. Because of the centrality of *BRCA* in the homologous recombination process, the role of platinum salts in *BRCA*-mutated patients was studied first.

Byrski et al. assessed a single NAC regimen with cisplatin in a small cohort patients only with *gBRCA1* alteration, of whom 76.6% had the triple-negative subtype, achieving a promising pCR rate of 61% [64]. Of note, although there was a small proportion of estrogen receptor-positive (ER+) disease, 56% of them achieved ypT0/is ypN0 after single-platinum chemotherapy. Based on these data, the same regimen was compared to the standard doxorubicin-cyclophosphamide chemotherapy in the randomized phase II INFORM trial (TBCRC 031) [65]. Here again, only *gBRCA* mutation carriers were enrolled. Unexpectedly, only a few patients achieved complete response, 18% in the cisplatin arm and 26% in the comparative arm (HR = 0.70, 90% CI [0.39; 1.2]). Results were similar in the TNBC and ER+ populations, although the number of ER+ patients was small. One hypothesis that may explain these findings is that patients included in the INFORM trial had more advanced stage disease than in the study by Byrski et al. Nevertheless, the results were subsequently corroborated in large, phase III trials evaluating different NAC regimens in TNBC, such as the GeparSixto [66] and BrighTNess [67] trials. These trials demonstrated higher pCR rates for patients receiving carboplatin in addition to a standard anthracycline/taxane NAC backbone for TNBC in the whole population. In BrighTNess [67], 634 patients with TNBC were enrolled, and the authors showed an increased pCR rate with the combination of platinum and PARPi (veliparib) compared to standard chemotherapy (53% vs. 31%, $p < 0.0001$), but not when compared to patients receiving only additional carboplatin, in whom a promising 58% pCR was achieved ($p = 0.36$). A post-hoc analysis confirmed that the benefit obtained with carboplatin alone was significant ($p < 0.001$). While reinforcing NAC with platinum offered a significantly improved pCR rate, it seems that veliparib addition did not yield any benefit. Thus, since these results, the combination of carboplatin and paclitaxel has become standard of care in NAC for TNBC all-comers. Interestingly, the odds of pCR were not higher in patients with *BRCA* mutations receiving carboplatin, or carboplatin + veliparib, when compared with matched non *BRCA*-mutated patients [68]. Later, the assumption that patients harboring *gBRCA* mutation do not benefit from platinum addition, contrary to *BRCA* WT patients, was confirmed in a meta-analysis encompassing more than 300 *BRCA*-mutated patients [69]. These intriguing findings could be explained by the excellent results obtained with standard chemotherapy (which already contains some DNA-damaging agents such as alkylants or anthracyclines) in *BRCA*-mutated cases [66,67,70].

It therefore seemed essential to evaluate other potentially valuable drugs in these *BRCA*-mutated patients with eBC. In particular, cumulating lines of evidence pointed to PARPi activity in advanced ovarian, prostate, pancreatic, and breast cancers harboring *BRCA1/2* mutation [71–73]. Moreover, in the original phase II I-SPY-2 trial, Rugo et al. estimated that a carboplatin-PARPi regimen on top of the standard anthracycline-taxane based chemotherapy, had an estimated probability of pCR of 51% in TNBC [74]. Nevertheless, with such a combination in the experimental arm, deciphering the effectiveness of each drug alone remains problematic. Therefore, two neoadjuvant trials aimed to assess the efficacy of a single PARPi regimen in the setting of *gBRCA 1/2* mutation, and confirmed substantial activity, with pCR rates reaching 49% and 40% with talazoparib [75] and niraparib [76] respectively. However, it should be mentioned that a significant proportion did not respond to PARPi monotherapy in these two studies, which means that this strategy cannot currently constitute a standard treatment compared to NAC.

Later, Tutt et al. designed the OlympiA trial, to assess the efficacy of PARPi therapy (olaparib for 1 year) in the adjuvant setting. This phase III study enrolled eBC with gBRCA1/2 mutation carrying high-risk clinicopathological factors after definitive local treatment and neoadjuvant or adjuvant chemotherapy [77]. Results were in favor of olaparib in terms of invasive-free survival (HR = 0.58, 99.5% CI [0.41; 0.82]) which later translated into a significant overall survival benefit (HR = 0.68, $p = 0.009$) [78]. Although adjuvant capecitabine was not permitted in this trial (as in the CREATE-X trial [79]), therefore precluding direct comparison, data in the metastatic setting may suggest that olaparib is a better choice for gBRCA carriers harboring TNBC [80,81]. It is important to note that this study also included ER+ tumors, which may also benefit from this treatment. Accordingly, OlympiA is a practice-changing study that has demonstrated the clinical utility of gBRCA testing in this high-risk population of eBC.

2.2. Targeting BRCAness in eBC beyond BRCA1/2 Mutations

Whole genome sequencing analyses from a Swedish database revealed that among TNBC carriers harboring a high HRDetect mutational signature, 67% was explained by germline/somatic BRCA1/2, as well as by other genomic/epigenic abnormalities (BRCA1 promoter hypermethylation, RAD 51C hypermethylation, or biallelic loss of PALB 2), illustrating the existence of many alternative alterations that may lead to HRD tumor status [42]. Patients with HRDetect-high tumors were also found to have a better invasive-disease-free survival after adjuvant chemotherapy than those with HRDetect low tumors.

A number of authors have assessed the HRD score in the setting of early TNBC [29,33]. Three neoadjuvant trials reported that genomic instability, reflected by an HRD-score ≥ 42 or BRCA1/2 mutation significantly predicts pCR with NAC including platinum salts [29]. When restricted to the BRCA WT population, high-HRD score remains a predictor of response to platinum salts, demonstrating that an assay evaluating genomic instability may be able to identify a wider range of patients who might benefit from such a regimen, thus offering critical information for treatment decision-making.

More recently, translational analyses from the phase II randomized TBCRC 030 study comparing neoadjuvant cisplatin to paclitaxel chemotherapy, examined the role of HRD biomarkers and their associations with response to NAC in this TNBC population [82]. The threshold of positivity of the HRD score to define tumors deficient for HR was found to be 33 (and not 42). The results did not support an association between the presence of HRD and better response to platinum. Results remained unchanged in exploratory analysis using the more common threshold of ≥ 42 as a cut-off for HRD positivity.

Moreover, further exploratory analyses conducted in the BrighTNess trial, assessing the prognostic and predictive value of HRD-score, showed that patients with HRD-high tumors (with a cutoff value of either ≥ 42 or ≥ 33) had higher pCR rates, whatever the neoadjuvant treatment received. Patients treated with additional carboplatin had higher pCR, both in the HRD-high and HRD-low subgroups, and the odds of pCR were not better in patients with HRD-high tumors receiving carboplatin, or carboplatin + veliparib, compared to patients with HRD-low tumor [83]. Similar results were observed in the TNBC population from the GeparSixto study; these authors found HRD-high scores in 70.5% of TNBC, of whom 60.3% had high-HRD score without BRCA mutation [84]. Here again, HR deficiency was an independent predictor of pCR, but did not predict carboplatin benefit. Taken together, these results suggest that HR deficiency evaluated by HRD score may be a predictor of response to NAC, but not of the benefit of carboplatin on top of standard NAC. Therefore, this evidence does not support routine clinical use of this genomic assay in such decision making.

Later, assessment of genomic instability focusing on RAD 51 foci was undertaken in the same GeparSixto trial [59]. RAD 51-low score, reflecting a functional HRD phenotype, was closely concordant with genomic HRD-score, with 87% accuracy. As a HRD genomic test, RAD 51 score is able to identify tumors without *BRCA* mutation harboring epigenetic or other HR gene alterations that are supposed to sensitize them to DNA-damage therapy. RAD 51-low tumors treated with carboplatin were more prone to achieve pCR, contrary to RAD 51-high tumors. Furthermore, contrary to the HRD-score, the RAD 51 assay independently predicts platinum benefit. These results support further development of this assay to guide decisions about whether to add a carboplatin to standard NAC or not.

Rather than combining platinum salts with PARPi (as in the BrighTNess trial), the GeparOLA study aimed to replace platinum with a PARPi in a HR-deficient population (defined by high HRD score and/or germline or somatic *BRCA1/2* mutation) [85]. Although negative for its primary endpoint, this study reported better tolerance and a very promising pCR rate with paclitaxel + olaparib (55%). Interestingly, subgroup analyses failed to show any difference in pCR rates between olaparib and platinum in *BRCA*-mutated patients or in *BRCA* WT HRD-high subgroups of patients [85].

PARP inhibitors have also been tested as monotherapy before chemotherapy in TNBC in window of opportunity (WOO) trials. For example, the RIO study tested rucaparib exposure for 2 weeks before surgery or NAC, with a drop in Ki67 on the end-of-treatment biopsy as primary activity endpoint. HRD tumors were identified thanks to the HRDetect tool, and there was no association between Ki67 decrease and *BRCA* mutation status, nor was there any association with HRD-high status [86]. In the phase II PETREMAC study, patients with TNBC received olaparib for 10 weeks before NAC, and 56% of patients obtained an objective response. Interestingly, contrary to non-responders, most of the responders harbored various genomic alterations potentially leading to HRD-high status, other than *gBRCA1/2* mutations (somatic or germline mutations of other genes involved in HR and *BRCA* promoter methylation). Moreover, functional HR deficiency assessed by low RAD 51 foci was also related to response to olaparib, contrary to *BRCA*ness signature obtained by multiplex ligation-dependent probe amplification (MLPA) [87]. This study is in favor of the activity of PARPi in TNBC beyond *gBRCA* mutations alone.

In summary, neoadjuvant and adjuvant trials and studies that have assessed response to DNA-damage therapy, according to the presence or absence of genomic instability in the setting of early breast cancer are listed in Table 1.

All in all, while the identification of *gBRCA1/2* mutation is no longer debated to guide the prescription of adjuvant PARPi treatment (olaparib) for patients with clinico-pathological factors of high recurrent risk, it currently remains difficult to integrate other biomarkers of HRD into treatment decisions in routine clinical practice, especially when deciding whether or not to prescribe platinum-based chemotherapy. Moreover, apart from the fact that a deficiency in the HR pathway can help to predict the response to standard NAC, many uncertainties remain in TNBC, and even more so in other subtypes—such as ER+—which have not been widely studied [29,88,89]. Nevertheless, more and more data are emerging regarding *BRCA*-mutated tumors and *BRCA*ness, and perhaps in the future, it will be possible to use these HRD biomarkers more easily to predict tumor sensitivity to neoadjuvant or adjuvant DNA-damaging agents (PARPi and platinum salts). Moreover, several ongoing phase III trials such as PEARLY (NCT02441933) and PARTNER (NCT03150576) could be practice-changing, and may thus broaden the utilization of genomic tests. This perspective raises an exciting challenge for medical oncologists and oncogeneticists.

Table 1. Synthesis of trials and studies evaluating genomic instability and response to DNA-damaging treatments (platinum salts and PARPi) in early conditions.

Clinical Trials

Trial Name	Phase	Stage and Subtype	Treatment	HRD Status or Condition	Main Results
Neoadjuvant Platinum Regimen					
GeparSixto [66]	II	Stage II-III TNBC, HER2+/ER−, HER2+/ER+ (n = 595)	Paclitaxel + nonpeg. lipos. doxorubicin vs. carboplatin + PM - TNBC: + bevacizumab - ER−/HER2+: + trastuzumab + lapatinib	Among TNBC all comers: - 70.5% HRD (HRD score ≥42 or tBRCA1/2 mutation) - 29% tBRCA1/2 mutation - 20% gBRCA1/2 mutation	- Higher pCR rate with additional carboplatin - Longer DFS with Cb ($p = 0.02$) irrespective of BRCA status, trend towards better OS (n.s.) - Regarding pCR: no carboplatin benefit among gBRCA, carboplatin benefit among BRCA WT - HRD predicts pathological response but does not predict carboplatin benefit - Supports clinical utility of RAD51 assay (FFPE functional HRD assay): concordant with HRD genomic score, identifies non-tBRCA with functional HRD phenotype, predicts pCR and carboplatin benefit - Not a standard NAC regimen (nonpegylated liposomal anthracycline)
Byrski et al. [64]	II	Stage I-III, gBRCA1 mutation HER2− (77% TNBC, 16% ER+) (n = 107)	Cisplatin	- 100% gBRCA1 mutation	- 61% pCR rate: 61% in TNBC, 56% in ER+ - Evidence of a single platinum agent activity in gBRCA1 mutation - Not a standard NAC regimen (anthracycline-free), no randomized control
TBCRC 008 [90]	II	Stage II-III, HER2− (39% TNBC, 61% ER+) (n = 62)	Carboplatin + nab-paclitaxel vs. carboplatin + nab-paclitaxel + vorinostat	Among non tBRCA1/2 mutation: - 46% HRD (HRD score ≥ 42)	- 27% pCR (similar with or without vorinostat) - Small effective, not a standard NAC regimen (anthracycline-free regimen)
Kaklamani et al. [91]	II	Stage I-III, TNBC (n = 30)	Carboplatin + eribulin	Among TNBC all comers: - 46% HRD (HRD score ≥ 42 or gBRCA1/2 mutation) - 10% gBRCA1/2 mutation	- 43% pCR: 67% in gBRCA1/2 mutation, 75% in HRD, HRD score and HR deficiency associated with pCR (also in BRCA WT population) - Small effective, not a standard NAC regimen (anthracycline-free), no randomized control
INFORM [65]	II	Stage I (≥1.5 cm)-III, gBRCA1/2 mutation HER2− (70% TNBC, 30% ER+) (n = 118)	Cisplatin vs. AC	- 68% gBRCA1 mutation - 30% gBRCA2 mutation - 2% gBCRA1 + 2 mutation	- No higher pCR rate with cisplatin in both TNBC and ER+ - Does not support the use of a single platinum agent regimen in gBRCA1/2 mutation

Table 1. Cont.

Clinical Trials					
Trial Name	Phase	Stage and Subtype	Treatment	HRD Status or Condition	Main Results
TBCRC 030 [82]	II	Stage I (≥1.5 cm)-III, TNBC BRCA WT (n = 147)	Cisplatin or paclitaxel	Among BRCA WT : - 71% HRD positive (cut-off ≥ 33)	- HRD-score does not predict pathological response with single CT (RCB-0/1), does not support the use of HRD-score in the setting of a single platinum or taxane NAC regimen - Poor responder rate, does not support such a single NAC regimen in TNBC BRCA WT
Neoadjuvant platinum-PARPi regimen					
PreCOG 0105 [92]	II	Stage I-III, TNBC (97%) or gBRCA1/2 mutation (3% ER+) (n = 93)	Carboplatin + gemcitabine + iniparib → surgery → AC	Among 97% TNBC and 3% HR+/HER2- : - 24% gBRCA1/2 mutation	- 36% pCR : 33% in BRCA WT, 47% in gBRCA1/2 mutation, HRD-LOH scores associated with pCR - Small effective, not a standard NAC regimen (anthracycline-free), no randomized control
I-SPY-2 [74]	II	Stage II-III, TNBC, ER+/HER2 – (n = 116)	Paclitaxel → AC vs. paclitaxel + veliparib + carboplatin → AC	Among TNBC all comers : - 17% gBRCA	- 51% estimated probability of pCR rate with carboplatin-veliparib, need for results of the phase III NCT02032277
BrighTNess [67]	III	Stage II-III, TNBC all comers (n = 634)	Paclitaxel → AC vs. paclitaxel + carboplatin → AC vs. paclitaxel + carboplatin + veliparib → AC	Among TNBC all comers : - 67% HRD (HRD score ≥ 42 or tBRCA1/2 mutation) - 15% gBRCA1/2 mutation	- Higher pCR rate with additional Cb, no benefit from veliparib addition - Longer EFS with Cb (p = 0.02) irrespective of BRCA status, no difference in OS - Regarding pCR : no carboplatin benefit among gBRCA, carboplatin benefit among BRCA WT - HRD predicts pathological response but does not predict carboplatin benefit
GeparOLA [85]	II	Stage I-III, HRD-population HER2- (73% TNBC, 23% ER+) (n = 106)	Paclitaxel-olaparib EC → EC or paclitaxel-carboplatin → EC	Among HRD population : - 54% tBRCA1/2 mutation - 56% gBRCA1/2 mutation	- 55% pCR with PO but a potential lower rate not statistically excluded : not strong enough to change practice - Evidence of paclitaxel-PARPi combination efficacy in HRD-population with better safety
Neoadjuvant PARPi regimen					
NeoTALA [75]	II	Stage I (≥1 cm)-III, gBRCA1/2 mutation HER2- (75% TNBC, 25% ER+) (n = 20)	Talazoparib	- 80% gBRCA1 mutation - 20% gBRCA2 mutation	- 49% pCR - Evidence of a single PARPi agent activity in gBRCA1/2 mutation - Small effective, no randomized control

Table 1. Cont.

Clinical Trials					
Trial Name	Phase	Stage and Subtype	Treatment	HRD Status or Condition	Main Results
RIO [86]	II	TNBC ($n = 43$)	Rucaparib before surgery or NAC	- 69% HRD (HRDetect assay) - 19% gBRCA1/2 mutation	- Decrease Ki67 in 12% of BRCA WT tumors - No association between Ki67 drop and BRCA mutation status, nor with HRD - Association between Ki67 drop and early ctDNA decrease - Small effective, no randomized control
PETREMAC [87]	II	Stage II-III, TNBC ($n = 32$)	Olaparib before NAC	Among TNBC all comers: - 34% HRD (gBRCA1/2 and PALB2 or somatic HR mutations) - 14% gBRCA1/2 and PALB2 mutation	- 56% OR - Higher clinical response in HRD patients and/or BRCA1/2 hypermethylation and also in functional HRD harboring low RAD51 foci - Evidence of a single PARPi agent activity beyond gBRCA mutations - Small effective, no randomized control
Spring et al. [76]	I	Stage I (≥ 1 cm)-III, gBRCA1/2 mutation HER2- (71% TNBC, 29% ER+) ($n = 21$)	Niraparib	- 67% gBRCA1 mutation - 28% gBRCA2 mutation - 5% gBRCA1 + 2 mutation	- 40% pCR - Evidence of a single PARPi agent activity in gBRCA1/2 mutation - Small effective
Adjuvant PARPi regimen					
OlympiA [77]	III	gBRCA1/2 mutation with high risk HER2- (82% TNBC, 18% ER+) ($n = 1836$)	Olaparib	- 72% gBRCA1 mutation - 27% gBRCA2 mutation - <1% gBCRA1 + 2 mutation	- Longer iDFS and OS with olaparib - Strong evidence supporting HR gene analysis of BRCA in this setting

Adjuvant/neoadjuvant trials including platinum salts including PARP inhibitors alone are shown in blue, those with PARP inhibitors alone in green, and those with platinum salts and PARP inhibitors in orange. n = number of patients included. HR: homologous recombination; HRD: homologous recombination deficiency; TNBC: triple negative breast cancer; gBRCA1/2 mutation: germline BRCA1/2 mutation; tBRCA1/2 mutation: tumor BRCA1/2 mutation; BRCA WT: BRCA wild type; ER−: estrogen receptor negative cancer; ER+: estrogen receptor positive cancer; HER2−: HER2-negative cancer; HER2+: HER2-positive cancer; pCR: pathological complete response; RCB: residual cancer burden; CT: chemotherapy; DFS: disease free survival; iDFS: invasive disease free survival; Cb: carboplatin; FFPE: formalin fixed paraffin embedded; CT: chemotherapy; PARPi: poly ADP ribose polymerase inhibitor; LOH: loss of heterozygosity; EFS: event-free survival; OS: overall survival; NAC: neoadjuvant chemotherapy; AC: doxorubicin-cyclophosphamide; EC: epirubicin-cyclophosphamide; PM: paclitaxel + nonpegylated liposomal doxorubicin; PO: paclitaxel + olaparib; ctDNA, circulating tumor deoxyribonucleic acid; n.s.: non-significant.

3. Metastatic Breast Cancer (mBC)

In the metastatic setting, fewer data are currently available, especially for patients with metastatic non-TNBC subtypes. Nevertheless, because quality of life is a major concern in the metastatic setting, there is a compelling need for biomarkers that predict sensitivity to drugs such as platinum salts or PARPi. Given that these drugs have a number of side effects, such assays would be helpful to ensure that prescription is pertinent. As in the localized setting, we distinguish *BRCA* mutations from mutations in other genes involved in HR (*BRCA*ness condition).

3.1. Platinum and PARPi in BRCA1/2-Mutated mBC

In 2012, Byrski et al. evaluated the efficacy of cisplatin chemotherapy in *BRCA1* mutation carriers with mBC [93]. In the phase II study, only 20 patients were included: 9 of them had previously been treated for metastatic disease with at least two lines of therapy; 30% were ER+/HER2− and 70% had TNBC. The overall response rate was 80%. Overall survival was 80% at one year, 60% at two years, and 25% at three years, with a median time to progression of 12 months. This study was one of the first to demonstrate the value of platinum in advanced metastatic disease, in the presence of genomic instability represented by the *BRCA1* mutation. Several years later, the phase III TNT trial randomly assigned patients with metastatic TNBC to either docetaxel or carboplatin in the first line of treatment [94]. Results showed that carboplatin was associated with a significantly higher overall response rate (68% vs. 33%, p = 0.03) and improved progression-free survival (6.8 vs. 4.4 months, p = 0.002) for the 43 g*BRCA* mutation carriers enrolled, in contrast to those without *BRCA* mutation.

More recently, PARP inhibitors have also emerged in the treatment of mBC, primarily in g*BRCA*-mutated patients. The OlympiAD trial was designed to compare the efficacy and safety of olaparib versus the standard single-agent chemotherapy of the physician's choice among patients with HER2-negative mBC and a g*BRCA1/2* mutation [80]. Olaparib monotherapy provided a significant benefit over standard therapy; median PFS was 2.8 months longer (7.0 months vs. 4.2 months; HR = 0.58; 95% CI, 0.43 to 0.80) and the risk of disease progression or death was 42% lower with olaparib monotherapy than with standard therapy. The response rate in the olaparib group was approximately twice that of the standard-therapy group (59.9% vs. 28.8%). An exploratory analysis conducted in nearly half of the overall study population showed strong concordance (99%) between g*BRCA* and t*BRCA* mutation. PARPi efficacy was similar, irrespective of HRD score, suggesting that there may be no need for additional tumor testing in case of g*BRCA1/2* mutation in the decision-making process [95]. In the phase II ABRAZO trial, talazoparib also showed promising activity in two cohorts of patients with mBC and g*BRCA1/2* mutation [96]. The response rate was 21% among patients who had previously had response to platinum chemotherapy. Then, in the phase III EMBRACA trial, patients with mBC and g*BRCA1/2* mutation were assigned to receive talazoparib or a standard single-agent chemotherapy of the physician's choice [97]. The risk of disease progression or death was 46% lower in the talazoparib group than in the standard-therapy group (HR = 0.54; 95% CI, 0.41 to 0.71), with a doubling of the response rate (62.6% in the talazoparib group vs. 27.2% in the standard-therapy group). Moreover, clinical benefit obtained with these single PARPi regimens was observed irrespective of g*BRCA* mutation type (g*BRCA1* or g*BRCA2*) or BC subtype (TNBC or ER+). The results of the two phase III trials (OlympiAD and EMBRACA) led to the approval of olaparib and talazoparib for the treatment of mBC with g*BRCA1/2* mutation, and international guidelines now recommend the systematic testing of patients with ER+/HER2− or triple negative mBC, in order to enable early treatment of these patients with PARPi during their metastatic history [98].

Combining DNA-damage therapies was later assessed in BROCADE3, a randomized, phase III trial that tested the association of veliparib with carboplatin and paclitaxel in BRCA-mutated advanced breast cancer [99]. Patients were randomly assigned to carboplatin and paclitaxel plus veliparib (veliparib group) or carboplatin and paclitaxel plus placebo (control group). Median PFS was 14.5 months in the veliparib group versus 12.6 months in the control group (HR = 0.71 [95% CI 0.57–0.88], p = 0.0016). The addition of veliparib to a highly active platinum doublet—with continuation as monotherapy if the doublet were discontinued—resulted in a significant and durable improvement in PFS in patients with gBRCA-mutated advanced HER2-negative breast cancer. These data may indicate the utility of combining platinum and PARP inhibitors in this BRCA-mutated metastatic population, particularly as continuation therapy.

There is therefore a rationale for the use of platinum salts and PARP inhibitors in gBRCA mutated patients early in the course of metastatic disease. However, in the vast majority of these studies, HRD score was not evaluated. Thus, patients with potential genomic instability without gBRCA mutation were not included.

3.2. Platinum and PARPi beyond BRCA-Mutated mBC

In mTNBC treated in first or second line with platinum monotherapy, the TBCRC 009 phase II trial evaluated the objective response rate (ORR) in 86 patients, according to their BRCA and HRD status. In this study, Isakoff et al. reported a response rate of 25.6% in the overall population, and a higher rate (54.5%) in patients with gBRCA1/2 mutations (n = 11) [100]. In patients without BRCA1/2 mutation, exploratory analyses conducted on 32 patients showed higher HRD features (high LST and LOH scores) in responding patients. These pioneering data suggest that some HRD-derived biomarkers may help to preferentially choose a platinum salt early in the disease course; As previously described, beyond BRCA1/2 mutations, many other genomic and epigenetic alterations may explain the inactivation of different HR components, leading to HRD in BRCA-proficient tumors (so-called BRCAness phenotype). However, in the TNT trial, no benefit of carboplatin over docetaxel was observed in mTNBC patients with BRCA 1 methylation, BRCA1 mRNA-low tumors, or in patients whose tumor harbored other HRD features, such as a high HRD score (by the Myriad assay) [94]. Indeed, a high HRD score was associated with an ORR of 44.7% with carboplatin versus 39.6% with docetaxel (p = 0.67). Similarly, no evidence of an increase in median PFS was observed in high-HRD versus non-HRD tumors.

Using the aforementioned HRDetect assay (based on WGS), but in metastatic conditions, Zhao et al. found that an elevated HRDetect score was significantly associated with response to platinum-based chemotherapy in a small series of mBC patients [101]. Thus, although the TNT trial did not find any association between HRD score and response to platinum, Zhao's results re-open the debate in metastatic HRD-high BRCA proficient patients, also regarding the best technique for assessing HRD (commercial tools or WGS). These exploratory results will need to be confirmed in prospective trials.

Galland et al. evaluated response to platinum and survival in 86 patients with mBC of any subtype (50% ER+) [102] and multi-treated (>60% had received three or more prior lines of therapy). Using WES for the determination of the HRD score or the COSMIC signature 3 expression, patients were classified into three groups: BRCA-mutated, BRCA WT HRD-high (or S3 high), and BRCA WT HRD-low (or S3 low). As in Zhao's study mentioned above, Galland et al. were able to identify a subset of BRCA WT mBC harboring high HRD scores ($\geq$42) and a high S3 mutational signature, at levels comparable to those of BRCA1/2 mutated tumors [101]. However, in this study, the mBC patients with high HRD score or high S3 level did not seem to benefit more from platinum-based chemotherapy than the others, in terms of response and/or PFS, regardless of BC molecular subtype and HRD or S3 cut-off. This study was one of the first to look at subtypes other than TNBC for the determination of HRD-associated genomic features. Indeed, these results were also in accordance with recent publications conducted in a large cohort of BC patients with WGS approaches, showing that HRDetect high scores were also observed in ER+

tumors. Similarly, in a recent, large-scale genomic characterization of mBC, Bertucci et al. reported both increased somatic genomic alterations in genes involved in HR pathway, and more HRD features (e.g., increased S3 mutational signature) in mBC, as compared to eBC, particularly in the ER+/HER2− subtype [103]. This highlights the need to look at subtypes other than TNBC in the study of biomarkers of HRD and sensitivity to treatments such as platinum salts.

Trials and studies that have already looked at mBC and response to platinum salts and PARP inhibitors according to the presence of genomic instability are listed in Table 2.

Table 2. Synthesis of trials and studies evaluating genomic instability and response to treatments (platinum salts and PARPi) in mBC (early or advanced metastatic condition).

Clinical Trial						
Trial Name	Stage	Line	Subtype	Treatment	HRD Status or Condition	Main Results
Metastatic platinum regimen						
TBCRC009 [100]	IV	Early metastatic condition (n = 86)	TNBC	Carboplatin or Cisplatin	BRCA1/2 mutation and HRD score (HRD-LST and HRD-LOH)	- Patients with BRCA1/2 mutation : ORR >50% (vs. 25% in total population) - In patients without BRCA1/2 mutation, higher HRD scores in responding patients
TNT [94]	III-IV	Early metastatic condition (n = 376)	TNBC	Carboplatin vs. Docetaxel	BRCA1/2 mutation (germline or somatic) or BRCA1 hypermethylation or HRD score > 42	- Significantly higher ORR and PFS for the gBRCA mutation carriers - No benefit in patients with BRCA1 hypermethylation or in patients whose tumor harbored a high HRD score
Byrski et al. [93]	IV	Advanced metastatic condition (n = 20)	TNBC, ER+/HER2−	Cisplatin	BRCA1 mutation carriers	Interesting platinum salts efficacy in the presence of a BRCA1 mutation
Zhao et al. [101]	IV	Early metastatic condition (n = 33)	TNBC, ER+/HER2− and HER2+	Carboplatin or Cisplatin	HRDetect status (WGS)	Radiographic evidence of clinical improvement, and better survival and treatment duration in patients with high HRDetect and treated with platinum salts
Galland et al. [102]	IV	Early and advanced metastatic condition (n = 86)	TNBC, ER+/HER2− and HER2+	Carboplatin or Cisplatin	HRD score and COSMIC signature 3 (WES)	- Subset of BRCA-proficient tumors with high HRD score or high S3 levels, comparable to BRCA-mutated tumors - However, no better ORR/DCR and PFS in these patients treated with platinum salts than the others
Metastatic platinum-PARPi regimen						
BROCADE3 [99]	III-IV	Early metastatic condition (n = 513)	TNBC	Carboplatin + Paclitaxel vs. Carboplatin + Paclitaxel + veliparib vs. Veliparib	gBRCA1/2 mutation	The addition of veliparib to a highly active platinum doublet resulted in a significant improvement in PFS in patients with gBRCA mutation
Metastatic PARPi regimen						
OlympiAD [80]	IV	Early metastatic condition (n = 302)	TNBC, ER+/HER2−	Olaparib	gBRCA1/2 mutation	- Significant benefit over standard therapy in gBRCA carriers - Benefit irrespective of gBRCA mutation type (gBRCA1 or 2), of BC subtype (TNBC and ER+) and of HRD score

Table 2. Cont.

Clinical Trial Trial Name	Stage	Line	Subtype	Treatment	HRD Status or Condition	Main Results
EMBRACA [97]	IV	Early metastatic condition (n = 431)	TNBC, ER+/HER2−	Talazoparib	gBRCA1/2 mutation	- Significant benefit over standard therapy in gBRCA carriers - Benefit irrespective of gBRCA mutation type (gBRCA1 or 2) and of BC subtype (TNBC and ER+)
TOPACIO [104]	IV	Early and advanced metastatic condition (n = 55)	TNBC	Niraparib + pembrolizumab	gBRCA1/2 mutation or BRCA1/2 WT	- ORR = 25% among the 60 BRCA1/2 WT and ORR = 45% among the 11 BRCA1/2-mutated tumors - Promising antitumor activity, irrespectively of BRCA mutation in mBC
MEDIOLA [105]	IV	Early and advanced metastatic condition (n = 34)	TNBC, ER+/HER2−	Olaparib + durvalumab	gBRCA1/2 mutation	- Promising antitumour activity in gBRCA1/2-mutated mBC
TBCRC 048 [28]	IV	Early and advanced metastatic condition (n = 54)	TNBC, ER+/HER2−	Olaparib	Germline mutations in non-BRCA1/2 HR-related genes or tBRCA1/2 mutations	- gPALB2 : ORR = 82%, tBRCA1/2 : ORR = 50%, no confirmed response among other mutation profiles - Promising antitumour activity beyond gBRCA1/2 mutation
RUBY [106]	IV	Early and advanced metastatic condition (n = 42)	TNBC, ER+/HER2−	Rucaparib	High LOH score or non-gBRCA1/2 mutation	- CBR = 13.5% - Potential benefit among a small subset of patients with high LOH scores without gBRCA1/2 mutation
Gruber et al. [107]	IV	Early and advanced metastatic condition (n = 13)	TNBC, ER+/HER2−	Talazoparib	BRCA WT with mutation in HR-associated gene	- ORR 31% - HRD score correlated with response : driven by gPALB2 mutation - Promising antitumour activity beyond gBRCA1/2 mutation
NCT03685331 (HOPE trial)	III-IV	Early metastatic condition	ER+/HER2−	Palbociclib + Olaparib and Fulvestrant	gBRCA1/2 mutation	In progress (recruiting)
NCT04053322 (DOLAF trial)	III-IV	Early and advanced metastatic condition	ER+/HER2−	Durvalumab + Olaparib and Fulvestrant	g/tBRCA1/2 mutation or HR-defect	In progress (recruiting)
NCT03025035	III-IV	Advanced metastatic condition	TNBC, ER+/HER2− HER2+	Pembrolizumab + Olaparib	gBRCA1/2 mutation or HR-defect	In progress (recruiting)

Trials including platinum salts alone in metastatic conditions are shown in blue, those with PARP inhibitors alone in green, and those with platinum salts and PARP inhibitors in orange. n = number of patients included. HR: homologous recombination, HRD: homologous recombination deficiency, LOH: loss of heterozygosity, TNBC: triple negative breast cancer, gBRCA 1/2 mutation: germline BRCA 1/2 mutation, tBRCA1/2 mutation: tumor BRCA1/2 mutation, BRCA WT: BRCA wild type, ER+: Eostrogen receptor positive cancer, PFS: progression free survival; CBR: clinical benefit rate, ORR: objective response rate, WGS: whole genome sequencing, WES: whole exome sequencing, DCR: disease control rate.

Despite the extensive development of PARP inhibitors, they are not currently authorized for use in breast cancer outside of gBRCA mutations, despite the promising results reported in these patients. For example, in the TBCRC 048 trial, PARPi were shown to be effective in patients with gPALB2 or sBRCA1/2 mutations, significantly expanding the potential target population of patients with BC likely to benefit from PARPi, other than gBRCA1/2 mutation carriers [28]. The RUBY study also suggested that a small subset of patients with high LOH scores without gBRCA1/2 mutation may benefit from PARP inhibitors [106]. Recently, talazoparib demonstrated promising activity in 13 patients pre-treated BRCA WT mBC harboring a HR mutation (11 ER+ and 2 TNBC) with overall response and clinical benefit rates of 31% and 54%, respectively [107]. In this phase II study, higher HRD score was correlated with better response, mainly driven by gPALB 2 carriers. These encouraging results open the way for PARPi treatment beyond gBRCA1/2 mutation. In part for these reasons, Keung et al. studied the inhibitory activity of PARPi on various breast cancer cells, and demonstrated differential inhibitory activities independently of the BRCA status [108]. These results suggest that the status of BRCA is not the only biomarker of response to PARPi. However, many clinical trials recruit patients based on their BRCA mutation status and do not incorporate HRD testing or BRCAness phenotype. Furthermore, in order to expand the potential prescription of PARPi to BRCA WT patients with genomic instability and to better identify patients likely to respond to such treatments, efforts are under way to develop new technologies. McGrail et al. generated a novel predictive algorithm able to predict PARPi response in different cell lines and patient-derived tumor cells [109]. This PARPi sensitivity signature could serve as an important tool to identify patients without BRCA mutation, but with HR defects and BRCAness phenotype. Through the integration of novel HRD biomarkers and scoring systems, the identification of patient populations who may have therapeutic sensitivity to PARPi may be an advantage in mBC. However, this will require confirmation in future clinical trials and is not currently recommended.

Due to the increasing importance of immunotherapy (immune checkpoint inhibitors, ICI) in oncology, there is increasing focus on the rationale for combining immunotherapy and PARP inhibitors in BRCA-mutated tumors, but also in tumors with BRCAness as proposed in the DOLAF study (NCT04053322). This study, which is currently recruiting, aims to evaluate the efficacy of a combination of olaparib, durvalumab, and fulvestrant for the treatment of patients with locally advanced or metastatic breast cancer with BRCA mutation or alterations of genes involved in HRR. Concerning the rationale for adding immunotherapy in case of HR deficiency, Mao et al. demonstrated that tumors with an S3 mutational signature had high expression of certain checkpoint inhibitors of the immune response, such as CTLA-4 or PD-L1 [110]. Teo et al. also suggested that mutations in HR pathways may positively influence response to ICI [111]. Thus, the combination of immunotherapy with PARPi appears attractive and has yielded encouraging initial clinical results in BRCA-mutated tumors. The MEDIOLA trial assessed the efficacy of olaparib in combination with durvalumab in patients with gBRCA-mutated mBC [105]. Patients with BRCA WT tumors were also included, as in the TOPACIO trial, where the combination of niraparib and pembrolizumab provided promising antitumor activity, irrespective of BRCA mutation, with ORRs of 25% and 45% respectively among the 60 BRCA WT and 11 BRCA-mutated tumors [104]. The ORR observed in patients with BRCA-mutated tumors was similar to that reported with olaparib monotherapy in the OlympiAD trial. However, the median PFS of 8.3 months in these patients was nearly 3 months longer than that observed for olaparib (5.6 months) or talazoparib (5.8 months) in patients with gBRCA-mutated TNBC. The few good responses observed among BRCA WT patients raise questions about the presence of other mutations in the homologous recombination pathway. To further elucidate this issue, an ongoing trial (NCT03025035) evaluating the combination of pembrolizumab plus olaparib will focus on this population by including BRCA WT patients with HRD.

In total, the identification of *BRCA*ness status by mutations other than *BRCA*, or the determination of HRD score, could provide benefit to a significant number of patients by enabling the prescription of PARPi and the enrolment in therapeutic trials combining such treatments with immunotherapy. This represents a major challenge for the future.

3.3. Limitations in the Use of HRD Biomarkers in the Metastatic Condition

The current lack of consensus highlights the need for further evaluation of the role of HRD biomarkers, as well as the need for methodological optimization to properly ascertain HRD high tumors. Furthermore, despite the optimization of HRD determination, it is important to take into account that HRD status is likely to change during the course of metastatic disease. This may contribute to the different results observed when studying therapeutic response and survival according to HRD biomarkers in early or advanced stages of metastatic disease.

First, the majority of patients treated in these studies received adjuvant treatment with agents that cause DNA damage, engaging the homologous recombination system. Ter Brugge et al. showed relevant resistance mechanisms to double-strand break DNA drugs (e.g., cisplatin, melphalan, or olaparib) on a cohort of 75 mice carrying *BRCA1*-deficient (mutated or promoter hypermethylation) breast tumors [112]. A number of *BRCA 1*-methylated tumors acquired therapy resistance via re-expression of *BRCA 1* because of the loss of *BRCA1* promoter methylation. It is postulated that *BRCA* methylated tumors treated with adjuvant or neoadjuvant chemotherapy could modify their genetic functionality during treatment since they continue to express the alterations contributing to the HRD score, but drive the tumors towards a soft *BRCA*ness phenotype. An interesting example comes from ovarian cancer, where *BRCA* mutation was found to be related to platinum response, in contrast to tumors with hypermethylation of the *BRCA* promoter [113]. To explore this phenomenon, a tumor biopsy was obtained before and after platinum treatment and showed a reversal of *BRCA 1* methylation in 31% of tumors [114,115]. The genome evolves during the metastatic process and is correlated with an increase in the percentage of genomic scars previously associated with HRD [103]. However, these biological tests, based on the study of genomic scars, do not take into account the potential restoration of functional homologous recombination (which is a resistance mechanism that can appear under therapeutic pressure) [23]. Indeed, a genomic analysis conducted in a *gBRCA1*-mutated patient who had poor response to a NAC platinum-containing regimen with early metastatic relapse and death demonstrated the existence of a reverse *BRCA 1* mutation arising between the original breast tumor and the residual surgical tissue. This led to restored *BRCA 1* function that could have explained the chemoresistance [116]. Moreover, *BRCA* status analysis performed at recurrence found the same mutation on metastatic tissue. In addition, subgroup analyses performed in Olympia [77] for eBC, and in OlympiAD [80] and EMBRACA [97] for mBC, suggest that PARPi may yield less benefit in patients pre-treated with platinum. Altogether, these findings raise questions about the therapeutic sequence with DNA-damage therapies that could give rise to resistance mechanisms, especially when platinum salts are followed by PARPi. It would therefore be useful to incorporate functional biomarkers, such as evaluation of *RAD 51* foci, as a predictive biomarker of functional HR. As previously described, RAD 51 nuclear foci is a surrogate marker of HRR functionality. Cruz et al. reported that the detection of RAD 51 foci in *gBRCA* tumors correlates with PARPi resistance, regardless of the underlying mechanism restoring HRR function [46].

A further question is that of the tissue on which the assessment of homologous recombination functionality is performed; namely, whether it should be on the primary tumor or on metastasis. Indeed, there are biological differences that make it difficult to extrapolate the analysis of homologous recombination from a localized situation to a metastatic situation. These findings suggest that the HRD assay is promising in concept, but whether it can be used to identify somatic or *gBRCA* WT patients who may benefit from PARPi or platinum-based therapy remains to be determined.

Lastly, because of the complexity of the homologous recombination phenomenon and progress in knowledge about it, increasingly complex methods are being used to develop tools and scores likely to predict the effectiveness of treatments targeting DNA. For this reason, the application of WGS, including the HRDetect score for example, in clinical practice is a controversial topic, given the financial costs. Indeed, it is necessary to consider the large number of patients with breast cancer around the world. Moreover, HRD status can vary during the history of a patient's disease, so the question arises of the best timing (localized/early stage metastatic/late stage metastatic), in order to limit potential multiplication of these analyses, and consequently, the costs incurred. In the same manner, acquisition and analysis of WGS-based data calls for large and complex sequence analysis, requiring considerable bioinformatics expertise and associated with technical issues. Altogether, obtaining a HRDetect score represents a limitation to daily clinical practice at the present time. However, the steady drop in the cost of sequencing could make more widespread use of WGS possible in years to come.

4. Conclusions

With the help of next-generation sequencing, the development of biomedical technologies and the use of bioinformatics, it is now possible to identify specific molecular alterations, such as HR deficiencies, which make it possible to consider effective targeted drugs. It appears that the clinical utility of genomic biomarkers assessing HRD in breast cancer is more moderate than in ovarian cancer, with sometimes discordant results, as in metastatic disease. Currently, only the identification of a germline mutation in the *BRCA 1* or *2* gene guides the use of platinum salts (only in the metastatic setting) and PARP inhibitors (both in the adjuvant and metastatic settings), with several clinical approvals (olaparib, talazoparib). The value of mutations in other genes involved in the homologous recombination pathway (e.g., *RAD 51C, PALB 2, RAD 51D*), genomic scar or mutational signatures (e.g., HRD score, COSMIC signature 3, 8), or functional tests (RAD 51 foci) in guiding the use of specific therapies remains debated. Nevertheless, there is growing consensus that it is now possible to identify patients who respond to platinum salts or PARPi using these different scores. For this reason, patients with a *BRCA*ness profile need to be included in greater numbers in future therapeutic trials, with stratification on HRD status. Finally, aside from their potential clinical utility, integrating these scores into daily practice may be challenging, since their routine use will require technical competence and financial resources.

Author Contributions: L.G., N.R. and S.L. contributed to the writing of the manuscript and to the development of figures and tables. L.G., N.R., I.D., D.M., C.K., S.I., A.H., M.R., J.A., L.A., R.B., C.T., F.G. and S.L. contributed to the proofreading and corrections of the manuscript. All authors have read and agreed to the published version of the manuscript.

Funding: This research received no external funding.

Acknowledgments: We wish to thank Fiona Ecarnot (EA3920, University of Franche-Comté, Besançon, France) for English correction and helpful comments.

Conflicts of Interest: The authors declare no conflict of interest.

References

1. Siegel, R.L.; Miller, K.D.; Jemal, A. Cancer Statistics, 2020. *CA Cancer J. Clin.* **2020**, *70*, 7–30. [CrossRef] [PubMed]
2. Tubbs, A.; Nussenzweig, A. Endogenous DNA Damage as a Source of Genomic Instability in Cancer. *Cell* **2017**, *168*, 644–656. [CrossRef] [PubMed]
3. Vilenchik, M.M.; Knudson, A.G. Endogenous DNA Double-Strand Breaks: Production, Fidelity of Repair, and Induction of Cancer. *Proc. Natl. Acad. Sci. USA* **2003**, *100*, 12871–12876. [CrossRef] [PubMed]
4. O'Kane, G.M.; Connor, A.A.; Gallinger, S. Characterization, Detection, and Treatment Approaches for Homologous Recombination Deficiency in Cancer. *Trends Mol. Med.* **2017**, *23*, 1121–1137. [CrossRef] [PubMed]
5. Wright, W.D.; Shah, S.S.; Heyer, W.-D. Homologous Recombination and the Repair of DNA Double-Strand Breaks. *J. Biol. Chem.* **2018**, *293*, 10524–10535. [CrossRef]

6. Lamarche, B.J.; Orazio, N.I.; Weitzman, M.D. The MRN Complex in Double-Strand Break Repair and Telomere Maintenance. *FEBS Lett.* **2010**, *584*, 3682–3695. [CrossRef]
7. Zhao, W.; Steinfeld, J.B.; Liang, F.; Chen, X.; Maranon, D.G.; Ma, C.J.; Kwon, Y.; Rao, T.; Wang, W.; Sheng, C.; et al. BRCA1-BARD1 Promotes RAD51-Mediated Homologous DNA Pairing. *Nature* **2017**, *550*, 360–365. [CrossRef]
8. Mekonnen, N.; Yang, H.; Shin, Y.K. Homologous Recombination Deficiency in Ovarian, Breast, Colorectal, Pancreatic, Non-Small Cell Lung and Prostate Cancers, and the Mechanisms of Resistance to PARP Inhibitors. *Front. Oncol.* **2022**, *12*, 880643. [CrossRef]
9. Harbeck, N.; Penault-Llorca, F.; Cortes, J.; Gnant, M.; Houssami, N.; Poortmans, P.; Ruddy, K.; Tsang, J.; Cardoso, F. Breast Cancer. *Nat. Rev. Dis. Primer* **2019**, *5*, 66. [CrossRef]
10. Gonzalez-Angulo, A.M.; Timms, K.M.; Liu, S.; Chen, H.; Litton, J.K.; Potter, J.; Lanchbury, J.S.; Stemke-Hale, K.; Hennessy, B.T.; Arun, B.K.; et al. Incidence and Outcome of BRCA Mutations in Unselected Patients with Triple Receptor-Negative Breast Cancer. *Clin. Cancer Res. Off. J. Am. Assoc. Cancer Res.* **2011**, *17*, 1082–1089. [CrossRef]
11. Metcalfe, K.; Lynch, H.T.; Foulkes, W.D.; Tung, N.; Olopade, O.I.; Eisen, A.; Lerner-Ellis, J.; Snyder, C.; Kim, S.J.; Sun, P.; et al. Oestrogen Receptor Status and Survival in Women with BRCA2-Associated Breast Cancer. *Br. J. Cancer* **2019**, *120*, 398–403. [CrossRef] [PubMed]
12. Dos Santos, E.S.; Lallemand, F.; Petitalot, A.; Caputo, S.M.; Rouleau, E. HRness in Breast and Ovarian Cancers. *Int. J. Mol. Sci.* **2020**, *21*, 3850. [CrossRef] [PubMed]
13. Turner, N.C. Signatures of DNA-Repair Deficiencies in Breast Cancer. *N. Engl. J. Med.* **2017**, *377*, 2490–2492. [CrossRef]
14. Bryant, H.E.; Schultz, N.; Thomas, H.D.; Parker, K.M.; Flower, D.; Lopez, E.; Kyle, S.; Meuth, M.; Curtin, N.J.; Helleday, T. Specific Killing of BRCA2-Deficient Tumours with Inhibitors of Poly(ADP-Ribose) Polymerase. *Nature* **2005**, *434*, 913–917. [CrossRef] [PubMed]
15. Konstantinopoulos, P.A.; Ceccaldi, R.; Shapiro, G.I.; D'Andrea, A.D. Homologous Recombination Deficiency: Exploiting the Fundamental Vulnerability of Ovarian Cancer. *Cancer Discov.* **2015**, *5*, 1137–1154. [CrossRef]
16. Farmer, H.; McCabe, N.; Lord, C.J.; Tutt, A.N.J.; Johnson, D.A.; Richardson, T.B.; Santarosa, M.; Dillon, K.J.; Hickson, I.; Knights, C.; et al. Targeting the DNA Repair Defect in BRCA Mutant Cells as a Therapeutic Strategy. *Nature* **2005**, *434*, 917–921. [CrossRef]
17. Bradner, W.T.; Rose, W.C.; Huftalen, J.B. Chapter 10—Antitumor Activity of Platinum Analogs. In *Cisplatin*; Prestayko, A.W., Crooke, S.T., Carter, S.K., Eds.; Academic Press: Cambridge, MA, USA, 1980; pp. 171–182. ISBN 978-0-12-565050-2.
18. Rosenberg, B. Chapter 2—Cisplatin: Its History and Possible Mechanisms of Action. In *Cisplatin*; Prestayko, A.W., Crooke, S.T., Carter, S.K., Eds.; Academic Press: Cambridge, MA, USA, 1980; pp. 9–20. ISBN 978-0-12-565050-2.
19. Pommier, Y.; O'Connor, M.J.; de Bono, J. Laying a Trap to Kill Cancer Cells: PARP Inhibitors and Their Mechanisms of Action. *Sci. Transl. Med.* **2016**, *8*, 362ps17. [CrossRef]
20. Rottenberg, S.; Jaspers, J.E.; Kersbergen, A.; van der Burg, E.; Nygren, A.O.H.; Zander, S.A.L.; Derksen, P.W.B.; de Bruin, M.; Zevenhoven, J.; Lau, A.; et al. High Sensitivity of BRCA1-Deficient Mammary Tumors to the PARP Inhibitor AZD2281 Alone and in Combination with Platinum Drugs. *Proc. Natl. Acad. Sci. USA* **2008**, *105*, 17079–17084. [CrossRef]
21. Duarte, A.A.; Gogola, E.; Sachs, N.; Barazas, M.; Annunziato, S.; de Ruiter, J.R.; Velds, A.; Blatter, S.; Houthuijzen, J.M.; van de Ven, M.; et al. BRCA-Deficient Mouse Mammary Tumor Organoids to Study Cancer-Drug Resistance. *Nat. Methods* **2018**, *15*, 134–140. [CrossRef]
22. Pujade-Lauraine, E.; Ledermann, J.A.; Selle, F.; Gebski, V.; Penson, R.T.; Oza, A.M.; Korach, J.; Huzarski, T.; Poveda, A.; Pignata, S.; et al. Olaparib Tablets as Maintenance Therapy in Patients with Platinum-Sensitive, Relapsed Ovarian Cancer and a BRCA1/2 Mutation (SOLO2/ENGOT-Ov21): A Double-Blind, Randomised, Placebo-Controlled, Phase 3 Trial. *Lancet Oncol.* **2017**, *18*, 1274–1284. [CrossRef]
23. Watkins, J.A.; Irshad, S.; Grigoriadis, A.; Tutt, A.N.J. Genomic Scars as Biomarkers of Homologous Recombination Deficiency and Drug Response in Breast and Ovarian Cancers. *Breast Cancer Res. BCR* **2014**, *16*, 211. [CrossRef] [PubMed]
24. Gou, R.; Dong, H.; Lin, B. Application and Reflection of Genomic Scar Assays in Evaluating the Efficacy of Platinum Salts and PARP Inhibitors in Cancer Therapy. *Life Sci.* **2020**, *261*, 118434. [CrossRef] [PubMed]
25. Morice, P.-M.; Coquan, E.; Weiswald, L.-B.; Lambert, B.; Vaur, D.; Poulain, L. Identifying Patients Eligible for PARP Inhibitor Treatment: From NGS-Based Tests to 3D Functional Assays. *Br. J. Cancer* **2021**, *125*, 7–14. [CrossRef] [PubMed]
26. Mateo, J.; Carreira, S.; Sandhu, S.; Miranda, S.; Mossop, H.; Perez-Lopez, R.; Nava Rodrigues, D.; Robinson, D.; Omlin, A.; Tunariu, N.; et al. DNA-Repair Defects and Olaparib in Metastatic Prostate Cancer. *N. Engl. J. Med.* **2015**, *373*, 1697–1708. [CrossRef]
27. Swisher, E.M.; Lin, K.K.; Oza, A.M.; Scott, C.L.; Giordano, H.; Sun, J.; Konecny, G.E.; Coleman, R.L.; Tinker, A.V.; O'Malley, D.M.; et al. Rucaparib in Relapsed, Platinum-Sensitive High-Grade Ovarian Carcinoma (ARIEL2 Part 1): An International, Multicentre, Open-Label, Phase 2 Trial. *Lancet Oncol.* **2017**, *18*, 75–87. [CrossRef]
28. Tung, N.M.; Robson, M.E.; Ventz, S.; Santa-Maria, C.A.; Nanda, R.; Marcom, P.K.; Shah, P.D.; Ballinger, T.J.; Yang, E.S.; Vinayak, S.; et al. TBCRC 048: Phase II Study of Olaparib for Metastatic Breast Cancer and Mutations in Homologous Recombination-Related Genes. *J. Clin. Oncol. Off. J. Am. Soc. Clin. Oncol.* **2020**, *38*, 4274–4282. [CrossRef]
29. Telli, M.L.; Timms, K.M.; Reid, J.; Hennessy, B.; Mills, G.B.; Jensen, K.C.; Szallasi, Z.; Barry, W.T.; Winer, E.P.; Tung, N.M.; et al. Homologous Recombination Deficiency (HRD) Score Predicts Response to Platinum-Containing Neoadjuvant Chemotherapy in Patients with Triple-Negative Breast Cancer. *Clin. Cancer Res. Off. J. Am. Assoc. Cancer Res.* **2016**, *22*, 3764–3773. [CrossRef]

30. Popova, T.; Manié, E.; Rieunier, G.; Caux-Moncoutier, V.; Tirapo, C.; Dubois, T.; Delattre, O.; Sigal-Zafrani, B.; Bollet, M.; Longy, M.; et al. Ploidy and Large-Scale Genomic Instability Consistently Identify Basal-like Breast Carcinomas with BRCA1/2 Inactivation. *Cancer Res.* **2012**, *72*, 5454–5462. [CrossRef]
31. Birkbak, N.J.; Wang, Z.C.; Kim, J.-Y.; Eklund, A.C.; Li, Q.; Tian, R.; Bowman-Colin, C.; Li, Y.; Greene-Colozzi, A.; Iglehart, J.D.; et al. Telomeric Allelic Imbalance Indicates Defective DNA Repair and Sensitivity to DNA-Damaging Agents. *Cancer Discov.* **2012**, *2*, 366–375. [CrossRef]
32. Abkevich, V.; Timms, K.M.; Hennessy, B.T.; Potter, J.; Carey, M.S.; Meyer, L.A.; Smith-McCune, K.; Broaddus, R.; Lu, K.H.; Chen, J.; et al. Patterns of Genomic Loss of Heterozygosity Predict Homologous Recombination Repair Defects in Epithelial Ovarian Cancer. *Br. J. Cancer* **2012**, *107*, 1776–1782. [CrossRef]
33. Timms, K.M.; Abkevich, V.; Hughes, E.; Neff, C.; Reid, J.; Morris, B.; Kalva, S.; Potter, J.; Tran, T.V.; Chen, J.; et al. Association of BRCA1/2 Defects with Genomic Scores Predictive of DNA Damage Repair Deficiency among Breast Cancer Subtypes. *Breast Cancer Res. BCR* **2014**, *16*, 475. [CrossRef] [PubMed]
34. Ladan, M.M.; van Gent, D.C.; Jager, A. Homologous Recombination Deficiency Testing for BRCA-Like Tumors: The Road to Clinical Validation. *Cancers* **2021**, *13*, 1004. [CrossRef] [PubMed]
35. Kondrashova, O.; Nguyen, M.; Shield-Artin, K.; Tinker, A.V.; Teng, N.N.H.; Harrell, M.I.; Kuiper, M.J.; Ho, G.-Y.; Barker, H.; Jasin, M.; et al. Secondary Somatic Mutations Restoring RAD51C and RAD51D Associated with Acquired Resistance to the PARP Inhibitor Rucaparib in High-Grade Ovarian Carcinoma. *Cancer Discov.* **2017**, *7*, 984–998. [CrossRef] [PubMed]
36. Sakai, W.; Swisher, E.M.; Karlan, B.Y.; Agarwal, M.K.; Higgins, J.; Friedman, C.; Villegas, E.; Jacquemont, C.; Farrugia, D.J.; Couch, F.J.; et al. Secondary Mutations as a Mechanism of Cisplatin Resistance in BRCA2-Mutated Cancers. *Nature* **2008**, *451*, 1116–1120. [CrossRef]
37. Alexandrov, L.B.; Nik-Zainal, S.; Wedge, D.C.; Campbell, P.J.; Stratton, M.R. Deciphering Signatures of Mutational Processes Operative in Human Cancer. *Cell Rep.* **2013**, *3*, 246–259. [CrossRef]
38. Alexandrov, L.B.; Nik-Zainal, S.; Wedge, D.C.; Aparicio, S.A.J.R.; Behjati, S.; Biankin, A.V.; Bignell, G.R.; Bolli, N.; Borg, A.; Børresen-Dale, A.-L.; et al. Signatures of Mutational Processes in Human Cancer. *Nature* **2013**, *500*, 415–421. [CrossRef]
39. Helleday, T.; Eshtad, S.; Nik-Zainal, S. Mechanisms Underlying Mutational Signatures in Human Cancers. *Nat. Rev. Genet.* **2014**, *15*, 585–598. [CrossRef]
40. Peng, G.; Chun-Jen Lin, C.; Mo, W.; Dai, H.; Park, Y.-Y.; Kim, S.M.; Peng, Y.; Mo, Q.; Siwko, S.; Hu, R.; et al. Genome-Wide Transcriptome Profiling of Homologous Recombination DNA Repair. *Nat. Commun.* **2014**, *5*, 3361. [CrossRef]
41. Morganella, S.; Alexandrov, L.B.; Glodzik, D.; Zou, X.; Davies, H.; Staaf, J.; Sieuwerts, A.M.; Brinkman, A.B.; Martin, S.; Ramakrishna, M.; et al. The Topography of Mutational Processes in Breast Cancer Genomes. *Nat. Commun.* **2016**, *7*, 11383. [CrossRef]
42. Davies, H.; Glodzik, D.; Morganella, S.; Yates, L.R.; Staaf, J.; Zou, X.; Ramakrishna, M.; Martin, S.; Boyault, S.; Sieuwerts, A.M.; et al. HRDetect Is a Predictor of BRCA1 and BRCA2 Deficiency Based on Mutational Signatures. *Nat. Med.* **2017**, *23*, 517–525. [CrossRef]
43. Nik-Zainal, S.; Davies, H.; Staaf, J.; Ramakrishna, M.; Glodzik, D.; Zou, X.; Martincorena, I.; Alexandrov, L.B.; Martin, S.; Wedge, D.C.; et al. Landscape of Somatic Mutations in 560 Breast Cancer Whole-Genome Sequences. *Nature* **2016**, *534*, 47–54. [CrossRef]
44. Min, A.; Kim, K.; Jeong, K.; Choi, S.; Kim, S.; Suh, K.J.; Lee, K.-H.; Kim, S.; Im, S.-A. Homologous Repair Deficiency Score for Identifying Breast Cancers with Defective DNA Damage Response. *Sci. Rep.* **2020**, *10*, 12506. [CrossRef] [PubMed]
45. Gulhan, D.C.; Lee, J.J.-K.; Melloni, G.E.M.; Cortés-Ciriano, I.; Park, P.J. Detecting the Mutational Signature of Homologous Recombination Deficiency in Clinical Samples. *Nat. Genet.* **2019**, *51*, 912–919. [CrossRef] [PubMed]
46. Cruz, C.; Castroviejo-Bermejo, M.; Gutiérrez-Enríquez, S.; Llop-Guevara, A.; Ibrahim, Y.H.; Gris-Oliver, A.; Bonache, S.; Morancho, B.; Bruna, A.; Rueda, O.M.; et al. RAD51 Foci as a Functional Biomarker of Homologous Recombination Repair and PARP Inhibitor Resistance in Germline BRCA-Mutated Breast Cancer. *Ann. Oncol. Off. J. Eur. Soc. Med. Oncol.* **2018**, *29*, 1203–1210. [CrossRef] [PubMed]
47. Van Wijk, L.M.; Vermeulen, S.; Meijers, M.; van Diest, M.F.; Ter Haar, N.T.; de Jonge, M.M.; Solleveld-Westerink, N.; van Wezel, T.; van Gent, D.C.; Kroep, J.R.; et al. The RECAP Test Rapidly and Reliably Identifies Homologous Recombination-Deficient Ovarian Carcinomas. *Cancers* **2020**, *12*, 2805. [CrossRef]
48. Van Wijk, L.M.; Kramer, C.J.H.; Vermeulen, S.; Ter Haar, N.T.; de Jonge, M.M.; Kroep, J.R.; de Kroon, C.D.; Gaarenstroom, K.N.; Vrieling, H.; Bosse, T.; et al. The RAD51-FFPE Test; Calibration of a Functional Homologous Recombination Deficiency Test on Diagnostic Endometrial and Ovarian Tumor Blocks. *Cancers* **2021**, *13*, 2994. [CrossRef]
49. Meijer, T.G.; Verkaik, N.S.; Sieuwerts, A.M.; van Riet, J.; Naipal, K.A.T.; van Deurzen, C.H.M.; den Bakker, M.A.; Sleddens, H.F.B.M.; Dubbink, H.-J.; den Toom, T.D.; et al. Functional Ex Vivo Assay Reveals Homologous Recombination Deficiency in Breast Cancer Beyond BRCA Gene Defects. *Clin. Cancer Res. Off. J. Am. Assoc. Cancer Res.* **2018**, *24*, 6277–6287. [CrossRef]
50. Naipal, K.A.T.; Verkaik, N.S.; Ameziane, N.; van Deurzen, C.H.M.; Ter Brugge, P.; Meijers, M.; Sieuwerts, A.M.; Martens, J.W.; O'Connor, M.J.; Vrieling, H.; et al. Functional Ex Vivo Assay to Select Homologous Recombination-Deficient Breast Tumors for PARP Inhibitor Treatment. *Clin. Cancer Res. Off. J. Am. Assoc. Cancer Res.* **2014**, *20*, 4816–4826. [CrossRef]
51. Oplustilova, L.; Wolanin, K.; Mistrik, M.; Korinkova, G.; Simkova, D.; Bouchal, J.; Lenobel, R.; Bartkova, J.; Lau, A.; O'Connor, M.J.; et al. Evaluation of Candidate Biomarkers to Predict Cancer Cell Sensitivity or Resistance to PARP-1 Inhibitor Treatment. *Cell Cycle Georget. Tex* **2012**, *11*, 3837–3850. [CrossRef]

52. Tumiati, M.; Hietanen, S.; Hynninen, J.; Pietilä, E.; Färkkilä, A.; Kaipio, K.; Roering, P.; Huhtinen, K.; Alkodsi, A.; Li, Y.; et al. A Functional Homologous Recombination Assay Predicts Primary Chemotherapy Response and Long-Term Survival in Ovarian Cancer Patients. *Clin. Cancer Res. Off. J. Am. Assoc. Cancer Res.* **2018**, *24*, 4482–4493. [CrossRef]
53. Drew, Y.; Mulligan, E.A.; Vong, W.-T.; Thomas, H.D.; Kahn, S.; Kyle, S.; Mukhopadhyay, A.; Los, G.; Hostomsky, Z.; Plummer, E.R.; et al. Therapeutic Potential of Poly(ADP-Ribose) Polymerase Inhibitor AG014699 in Human Cancers with Mutated or Methylated BRCA1 or BRCA2. *J. Natl. Cancer Inst.* **2011**, *103*, 334–346. [CrossRef]
54. Van Wijk, L.M.; Nilas, A.B.; Vrieling, H.; Vreeswijk, M.P.G. RAD51 as a Functional Biomarker for Homologous Recombination Deficiency in Cancer: A Promising Addition to the HRD Toolbox? *Expert Rev. Mol. Diagn.* **2022**, *22*, 185–199. [CrossRef] [PubMed]
55. Castroviejo-Bermejo, M.; Cruz, C.; Llop-Guevara, A.; Gutiérrez-Enríquez, S.; Ducy, M.; Ibrahim, Y.H.; Gris-Oliver, A.; Pellegrino, B.; Bruna, A.; Guzmán, M.; et al. A RAD51 Assay Feasible in Routine Tumor Samples Calls PARP Inhibitor Response beyond BRCA Mutation. *EMBO Mol. Med.* **2018**, *10*, e9172. [CrossRef] [PubMed]
56. Waks, A.G.; Cohen, O.; Kochupurakkal, B.; Kim, D.; Dunn, C.E.; Buendia, J.B.; Wander, S.; Helvie, K.; Lloyd, M.R.; Marini, L.; et al. Reversion and Non-Reversion Mechanisms of Resistance to PARP Inhibitor or Platinum Chemotherapy in BRCA1/2-Mutant Metastatic Breast Cancer. *Ann. Oncol. Off. J. Eur. Soc. Med. Oncol.* **2020**, *31*, 590–598. [CrossRef] [PubMed]
57. Blanc-Durand, F.; Yaniz, E.; Genestie, C.; Rouleau, E.; Berton, D.; Lortholary, A.; Dohollou, N.; Desauw, C.; Fabbro, M.; Malaurie, E.; et al. Evaluation of a RAD51 Functional Assay in Advanced Ovarian Cancer, a GINECO/GINEGEPS Study. *J. Clin. Oncol.* **2021**, *39*, 5513. [CrossRef]
58. Carreira, S.; Porta, N.; Arce-Gallego, S.; Seed, G.; Llop-Guevara, A.; Bianchini, D.; Rescigno, P.; Paschalis, A.; Bertan, C.; Baker, C.; et al. Biomarkers Associating with PARP Inhibitor Benefit in Prostate Cancer in the TOPARP-B Trial. *Cancer Discov.* **2021**, *11*, 2812–2827. [CrossRef]
59. Llop-Guevara, A.; Loibl, S.; Villacampa, G.; Vladimirova, V.; Schneeweiss, A.; Karn, T.; Zahm, D.-M.; Herencia-Ropero, A.; Jank, P.; van Mackelenbergh, M.; et al. Association of RAD51 with Homologous Recombination Deficiency (HRD) and Clinical Outcomes in Untreated Triple-Negative Breast Cancer (TNBC): Analysis of the GeparSixto Randomized Clinical Trial. *Ann. Oncol. Off. J. Eur. Soc. Med. Oncol.* **2021**, *32*, 1590–1596. [CrossRef]
60. Cortazar, P.; Zhang, L.; Untch, M.; Mehta, K.; Costantino, J.P.; Wolmark, N.; Bonnefoi, H.; Cameron, D.; Gianni, L.; Valagussa, P.; et al. Pathological Complete Response and Long-Term Clinical Benefit in Breast Cancer: The CTNeoBC Pooled Analysis. *Lancet* **2014**, *384*, 164–172. [CrossRef]
61. Spring, L.; Greenup, R.; Niemierko, A.; Schapira, L.; Haddad, S.; Jimenez, R.; Coopey, S.; Taghian, A.; Hughes, K.S.; Isakoff, S.J.; et al. Pathologic Complete Response After Neoadjuvant Chemotherapy and Long-Term Outcomes Among Young Women With Breast Cancer. *J. Natl. Compr. Cancer Netw. JNCCN* **2017**, *15*, 1216–1223. [CrossRef]
62. Alba, E.; Chacon, J.I.; Lluch, A.; Anton, A.; Estevez, L.; Cirauqui, B.; Carrasco, E.; Calvo, L.; Segui, M.A.; Ribelles, N.; et al. A Randomized Phase II Trial of Platinum Salts in Basal-like Breast Cancer Patients in the Neoadjuvant Setting. Results from the GEICAM/2006-03, Multicenter Study. *Breast Cancer Res. Treat.* **2012**, *136*, 487–493. [CrossRef]
63. Sikov, W.M.; Berry, D.A.; Perou, C.M.; Singh, B.; Cirrincione, C.T.; Tolaney, S.M.; Kuzma, C.S.; Pluard, T.J.; Somlo, G.; Port, E.R.; et al. Impact of the Addition of Carboplatin and/or Bevacizumab to Neoadjuvant Once-per-Week Paclitaxel Followed by Dose-Dense Doxorubicin and Cyclophosphamide on Pathologic Complete Response Rates in Stage II to III Triple-Negative Breast Cancer: CALGB 40603 (Alliance). *J. Clin. Oncol. Off. J. Am. Soc. Clin. Oncol.* **2015**, *33*, 13–21. [CrossRef]
64. Byrski, T.; Huzarski, T.; Dent, R.; Marczyk, E.; Jasiowka, M.; Gronwald, J.; Jakubowicz, J.; Cybulski, C.; Wisniowski, R.; Godlewski, D.; et al. Pathologic Complete Response to Neoadjuvant Cisplatin in BRCA1-Positive Breast Cancer Patients. *Breast Cancer Res. Treat.* **2014**, *147*, 401–405. [CrossRef] [PubMed]
65. Tung, N.; Arun, B.; Hacker, M.R.; Hofstatter, E.; Toppmeyer, D.L.; Isakoff, S.J.; Borges, V.; Legare, R.D.; Isaacs, C.; Wolff, A.C.; et al. TBCRC 031: Randomized Phase II Study of Neoadjuvant Cisplatin Versus Doxorubicin-Cyclophosphamide in Germline BRCA Carriers With HER2-Negative Breast Cancer (the INFORM Trial). *J. Clin. Oncol. Off. J. Am. Soc. Clin. Oncol.* **2020**, *38*, 1539–1548. [CrossRef] [PubMed]
66. Hahnen, E.; Lederer, B.; Hauke, J.; Loibl, S.; Kröber, S.; Schneeweiss, A.; Denkert, C.; Fasching, P.A.; Blohmer, J.U.; Jackisch, C.; et al. Germline Mutation Status, Pathological Complete Response, and Disease-Free Survival in Triple-Negative Breast Cancer: Secondary Analysis of the GeparSixto Randomized Clinical Trial. *JAMA Oncol.* **2017**, *3*, 1378–1385. [CrossRef] [PubMed]
67. Loibl, S.; O'Shaughnessy, J.; Untch, M.; Sikov, W.M.; Rugo, H.S.; McKee, M.D.; Huober, J.; Golshan, M.; von Minckwitz, G.; Maag, D.; et al. Addition of the PARP Inhibitor Veliparib plus Carboplatin or Carboplatin Alone to Standard Neoadjuvant Chemotherapy in Triple-Negative Breast Cancer (BrighTNess): A Randomised, Phase 3 Trial. *Lancet Oncol.* **2018**, *19*, 497–509. [CrossRef] [PubMed]
68. Metzger-Filho, O.; Collier, K.; Asad, S.; Ansell, P.J.; Watson, M.; Bae, J.; Cherian, M.; O'Shaughnessy, J.; Untch, M.; Rugo, H.S.; et al. Matched Cohort Study of Germline BRCA Mutation Carriers with Triple Negative Breast Cancer in Brightness. *NPJ Breast Cancer* **2021**, *7*, 142. [CrossRef] [PubMed]
69. Wang, C.-J.; Xu, Y.; Lin, Y.; Zhu, H.-J.; Zhou, Y.-D.; Mao, F.; Zhang, X.-H.; Huang, X.; Zhong, Y.; Sun, Q.; et al. Platinum-Based Neoadjuvant Chemotherapy for Breast Cancer With BRCA Mutations: A Meta-Analysis. *Front. Oncol.* **2020**, *10*, 592998. [CrossRef] [PubMed]

70. Sella, T.; Yam, E.N.G.; Levanon, K.; Rotenberg, T.S.; Gadot, M.; Kuchuk, I.; Molho, R.B.; Itai, A.; Modiano, T.M.; Gold, R.; et al. Evaluation of Tolerability and Efficacy of Incorporating Carboplatin in Neoadjuvant Anthracycline and Taxane Based Therapy in a BRCA1 Enriched Triple-Negative Breast Cancer Cohort. *Breast* **2018**, *40*, 141–146. [CrossRef] [PubMed]
71. Audeh, M.W.; Carmichael, J.; Penson, R.T.; Friedlander, M.; Powell, B.; Bell-McGuinn, K.M.; Scott, C.; Weitzel, J.N.; Oaknin, A.; Loman, N.; et al. Oral Poly(ADP-Ribose) Polymerase Inhibitor Olaparib in Patients with BRCA1 or BRCA2 Mutations and Recurrent Ovarian Cancer: A Proof-of-Concept Trial. *Lancet* **2010**, *376*, 245–251. [CrossRef]
72. Kaufman, B.; Shapira-Frommer, R.; Schmutzler, R.K.; Audeh, M.W.; Friedlander, M.; Balmaña, J.; Mitchell, G.; Fried, G.; Stemmer, S.M.; Hubert, A.; et al. Olaparib Monotherapy in Patients with Advanced Cancer and a Germline BRCA1/2 Mutation. *J. Clin. Oncol. Off. J. Am. Soc. Clin. Oncol.* **2015**, *33*, 244–250. [CrossRef] [PubMed]
73. Tutt, A.; Robson, M.; Garber, J.E.; Domchek, S.M.; Audeh, M.W.; Weitzel, J.N.; Friedlander, M.; Arun, B.; Loman, N.; Schmutzler, R.K.; et al. Oral Poly(ADP-Ribose) Polymerase Inhibitor Olaparib in Patients with BRCA1 or BRCA2 Mutations and Advanced Breast Cancer: A Proof-of-Concept Trial. *Lancet* **2010**, *376*, 235–244. [CrossRef] [PubMed]
74. Rugo, H.S.; Olopade, O.I.; DeMichele, A.; Yau, C.; van 't Veer, L.J.; Buxton, M.B.; Hogarth, M.; Hylton, N.M.; Paoloni, M.; Perlmutter, J.; et al. Adaptive Randomization of Veliparib-Carboplatin Treatment in Breast Cancer. *N. Engl. J. Med.* **2016**, *375*, 23–34. [CrossRef]
75. Litton, J.K.; Scoggins, M.E.; Hess, K.R.; Adrada, B.E.; Murthy, R.K.; Damodaran, S.; DeSnyder, S.M.; Brewster, A.M.; Barcenas, C.H.; Valero, V.; et al. Neoadjuvant Talazoparib for Patients With Operable Breast Cancer With a Germline BRCA Pathogenic Variant. *J. Clin. Oncol. Off. J. Am. Soc. Clin. Oncol.* **2020**, *38*, 388–394. [CrossRef] [PubMed]
76. Spring, L.M.; Han, H.; Liu, M.C.; Hamilton, E.; Irie, H.; Santa-Maria, C.A.; Reeves, J.; Pan, P.; Shan, M.; Tang, Y.; et al. Neoadjuvant Study of Niraparib in Patients with HER2-Negative, BRCA-Mutated, Resectable Breast Cancer. *Nat. Cancer* **2022**, *3*, 927–931. [CrossRef] [PubMed]
77. Tutt, A.N.J.; Garber, J.E.; Kaufman, B.; Viale, G.; Fumagalli, D.; Rastogi, P.; Gelber, R.D.; de Azambuja, E.; Fielding, A.; Balmaña, J.; et al. Adjuvant Olaparib for Patients with BRCA1- or BRCA2-Mutated Breast Cancer. *N. Engl. J. Med.* **2021**, *384*, 2394–2405. [CrossRef] [PubMed]
78. OncologyPRO Pre-Specified Event Driven Analysis of Overall Survival (OS) in the OlympiA Phase III Trial of Adjuvant Olaparib (OL) in Germline BRCA1/2 Mutation (GBRCAm) Associated Breast Cancer. Available online: https://oncologypro.esmo.org/meeting-resources/esmo-virtual-plenary-resources/olympia-phase-iii-pre-specified-event-driven-analysis-of-overall-survival-of-olaparib-in-gbrcam-breast-cancer (accessed on 31 October 2022).
79. Zujewski, J.A.; Rubinstein, L. CREATE-X a Role for Capecitabine in Early-Stage Breast Cancer: An Analysis of Available Data. *NPJ Breast Cancer* **2017**, *3*, 27. [CrossRef]
80. Robson, M.; Im, S.-A.; Senkus, E.; Xu, B.; Domchek, S.M.; Masuda, N.; Delaloge, S.; Li, W.; Tung, N.; Armstrong, A.; et al. Olaparib for Metastatic Breast Cancer in Patients with a Germline BRCA Mutation. *N. Engl. J. Med.* **2017**, *377*, 523–533. [CrossRef]
81. Hurvitz, S.A.; Gonçalves, A.; Rugo, H.S.; Lee, K.-H.; Fehrenbacher, L.; Mina, L.A.; Diab, S.; Blum, J.L.; Chakrabarti, J.; Elmeliegy, M.; et al. Talazoparib in Patients with a Germline BRCA-Mutated Advanced Breast Cancer: Detailed Safety Analyses from the Phase III EMBRACA Trial. *Oncologist* **2020**, *25*, e439–e450. [CrossRef]
82. Mayer, E.L.; Abramson, V.; Jankowitz, R.; Falkson, C.; Marcom, P.K.; Traina, T.; Carey, L.; Rimawi, M.; Specht, J.; Miller, K.; et al. TBCRC 030: A Phase II Study of Preoperative Cisplatin versus Paclitaxel in Triple-Negative Breast Cancer: Evaluating the Homologous Recombination Deficiency (HRD) Biomarker. *Ann. Oncol. Off. J. Eur. Soc. Med. Oncol.* **2020**, *31*, 1518–1525. [CrossRef]
83. Telli, M.L.; Metzger, O.; Timms, K.; Evans, B.; Vogel, D.; Wei, H.; Jones, J.T.; Wenstrup, R.J.; McKee, M.D.; Sullivan, D.M.; et al. Evaluation of Homologous Recombination Deficiency (HRD) Status with Pathological Response to Carboplatin +/− Veliparib in BrighTNess, a Randomized Phase 3 Study in Early Stage TNBC. *J. Clin. Oncol.* **2018**, *36*, 519. [CrossRef]
84. Loibl, S.; Weber, K.E.; Timms, K.M.; Elkin, E.P.; Hahnen, E.; Fasching, P.A.; Lederer, B.; Denkert, C.; Schneeweiss, A.; Braun, S.; et al. Survival Analysis of Carboplatin Added to an Anthracycline/Taxane-Based Neoadjuvant Chemotherapy and HRD Score as Predictor of Response-Final Results from GeparSixto. *Ann. Oncol. Off. J. Eur. Soc. Med. Oncol.* **2018**, *29*, 2341–2347. [CrossRef] [PubMed]
85. Fasching, P.A.; Link, T.; Hauke, J.; Seither, F.; Jackisch, C.; Klare, P.; Schmatloch, S.; Hanusch, C.; Huober, J.; Stefek, A.; et al. Neoadjuvant Paclitaxel/Olaparib in Comparison to Paclitaxel/Carboplatinum in Patients with HER2-Negative Breast Cancer and Homologous Recombination Deficiency (GeparOLA Study). *Ann. Oncol. Off. J. Eur. Soc. Med. Oncol.* **2021**, *32*, 49–57. [CrossRef]
86. Chopra, N.; Tovey, H.; Pearson, A.; Cutts, R.; Toms, C.; Proszek, P.; Hubank, M.; Dowsett, M.; Dodson, A.; Daley, F.; et al. Homologous Recombination DNA Repair Deficiency and PARP Inhibition Activity in Primary Triple Negative Breast Cancer. *Nat. Commun.* **2020**, *11*, 2662. [CrossRef] [PubMed]
87. Eikesdal, H.P.; Yndestad, S.; Elzawahry, A.; Llop-Guevara, A.; Gilje, B.; Blix, E.S.; Espelid, H.; Lundgren, S.; Geisler, J.; Vagstad, G.; et al. Olaparib Monotherapy as Primary Treatment in Unselected Triple Negative Breast Cancer. *Ann. Oncol. Off. J. Eur. Soc. Med. Oncol.* **2021**, *32*, 240–249. [CrossRef] [PubMed]
88. Caramelo, O.; Silva, C.; Caramelo, F.; Frutuoso, C.; Almeida-Santos, T. The Effect of Neoadjuvant Platinum-Based Chemotherapy in BRCA Mutated Triple Negative Breast Cancers -Systematic Review and Meta-Analysis. *Hered. Cancer Clin. Pract.* **2019**, *17*, 11. [CrossRef] [PubMed]

89. Chai, Y.; Chen, Y.; Zhang, D.; Wei, Y.; Li, Z.; Li, Q.; Xu, B. Homologous Recombination Deficiency (HRD) and BRCA 1/2 Gene Mutation for Predicting the Effect of Platinum-Based Neoadjuvant Chemotherapy of Early-Stage Triple-Negative Breast Cancer (TNBC): A Systematic Review and Meta-Analysis. *J. Pers. Med.* **2022**, *12*, 323. [CrossRef]
90. Connolly, R.M.; Leal, J.P.; Goetz, M.P.; Zhang, Z.; Zhou, X.C.; Jacobs, L.K.; Mhlanga, J.; Joo, H.O.; Carpenter, J.; Storniolo, A.M.; et al. TBCRC 008: Early Change in 18F-FDG Uptake on PET Predicts Response to Preoperative Systemic Therapy in Human Epidermal Growth Factor Receptor 2-Negative Primary Operable Breast Cancer. *J. Nucl. Med. Off. Publ. Soc. Nucl. Med.* **2015**, *56*, 31–37. [CrossRef]
91. Kaklamani, V.G.; Jeruss, J.S.; Hughes, E.; Siziopikou, K.; Timms, K.M.; Gutin, A.; Abkevich, V.; Sangale, Z.; Solimeno, C.; Brown, K.L.; et al. Phase II Neoadjuvant Clinical Trial of Carboplatin and Eribulin in Women with Triple Negative Early-Stage Breast Cancer (NCT01372579). *Breast Cancer Res. Treat.* **2015**, *151*, 629–638. [CrossRef]
92. Telli, M.L.; Jensen, K.C.; Vinayak, S.; Kurian, A.W.; Lipson, J.A.; Flaherty, P.J.; Timms, K.; Abkevich, V.; Schackmann, E.A.; Wapnir, I.L.; et al. Phase II Study of Gemcitabine, Carboplatin, and Iniparib As Neoadjuvant Therapy for Triple-Negative and BRCA1/2 Mutation-Associated Breast Cancer With Assessment of a Tumor-Based Measure of Genomic Instability: PrECOG 0105. *J. Clin. Oncol. Off. J. Am. Soc. Clin. Oncol.* **2015**, *33*, 1895–1901. [CrossRef]
93. Byrski, T.; Dent, R.; Blecharz, P.; Foszczynska-Kloda, M.; Gronwald, J.; Huzarski, T.; Cybulski, C.; Marczyk, E.; Chrzan, R.; Eisen, A.; et al. Results of a Phase II Open-Label, Non-Randomized Trial of Cisplatin Chemotherapy in Patients with BRCA1-Positive Metastatic Breast Cancer. *Breast Cancer Res. BCR* **2012**, *14*, R110. [CrossRef]
94. Tutt, A.; Tovey, H.; Cheang, M.C.U.; Kernaghan, S.; Kilburn, L.; Gazinska, P.; Owen, J.; Abraham, J.; Barrett, S.; Barrett-Lee, P.; et al. Carboplatin in BRCA1/2-Mutated and Triple-Negative Breast Cancer BRCAness Subgroups: The TNT Trial. *Nat. Med.* **2018**, *24*, 628–637. [CrossRef] [PubMed]
95. Hodgson, D.; Lai, Z.; Dearden, S.; Barrett, J.C.; Harrington, E.A.; Timms, K.; Lanchbury, J.; Wu, W.; Allen, A.; Senkus, E.; et al. Analysis of Mutation Status and Homologous Recombination Deficiency in Tumors of Patients with Germline BRCA1 or BRCA2 Mutations and Metastatic Breast Cancer: OlympiAD. *Ann. Oncol. Off. J. Eur. Soc. Med. Oncol.* **2021**, *32*, 1582–1589. [CrossRef] [PubMed]
96. Turner, N.C.; Telli, M.L.; Rugo, H.S.; Mailliez, A.; Ettl, J.; Grischke, E.-M.; Mina, L.A.; Balmaña, J.; Fasching, P.A.; Hurvitz, S.A.; et al. A Phase II Study of Talazoparib after Platinum or Cytotoxic Nonplatinum Regimens in Patients with Advanced Breast Cancer and Germline BRCA1/2 Mutations (ABRAZO). *Clin. Cancer Res. Off. J. Am. Assoc. Cancer Res.* **2019**, *25*, 2717–2724. [CrossRef] [PubMed]
97. Litton, J.K.; Rugo, H.S.; Ettl, J.; Hurvitz, S.A.; Gonçalves, A.; Lee, K.-H.; Fehrenbacher, L.; Yerushalmi, R.; Mina, L.A.; Martin, M.; et al. Talazoparib in Patients with Advanced Breast Cancer and a Germline BRCA Mutation. *N. Engl. J. Med.* **2018**, *379*, 753–763. [CrossRef] [PubMed]
98. Andre, F.; Filleron, T.; Kamal, M.; Mosele, F.; Arnedos, M.; Dalenc, F.; Sablin, M.-P.; Campone, M.; Bonnefoi, H.; Lefeuvre-Plesse, C.; et al. Genomics to Select Treatment for Patients with Metastatic Breast Cancer. *Nature* **2022**, *610*, 343–348. [CrossRef]
99. Diéras, V.; Han, H.S.; Kaufman, B.; Wildiers, H.; Friedlander, M.; Ayoub, J.-P.; Puhalla, S.L.; Bondarenko, I.; Campone, M.; Jakobsen, E.H.; et al. Veliparib with Carboplatin and Paclitaxel in BRCA-Mutated Advanced Breast Cancer (BROCADE3): A Randomised, Double-Blind, Placebo-Controlled, Phase 3 Trial. *Lancet Oncol.* **2020**, *21*, 1269–1282. [CrossRef] [PubMed]
100. Isakoff, S.J.; Mayer, E.L.; He, L.; Traina, T.A.; Carey, L.A.; Krag, K.J.; Rugo, H.S.; Liu, M.C.; Stearns, V.; Come, S.E.; et al. TBCRC009: A Multicenter Phase II Clinical Trial of Platinum Monotherapy With Biomarker Assessment in Metastatic Triple-Negative Breast Cancer. *J. Clin. Oncol. Off. J. Am. Soc. Clin. Oncol.* **2015**, *33*, 1902–1909. [CrossRef]
101. Zhao, E.Y.; Shen, Y.; Pleasance, E.; Kasaian, K.; Leelakumari, S.; Jones, M.; Bose, P.; Ch'ng, C.; Reisle, C.; Eirew, P.; et al. Homologous Recombination Deficiency and Platinum-Based Therapy Outcomes in Advanced Breast Cancer. *Clin. Cancer Res. Off. J. Am. Assoc. Cancer Res.* **2017**, *23*, 7521–7530. [CrossRef]
102. Galland, L.; Ballot, E.; Mananet, H.; Boidot, R.; Lecuelle, J.; Albuisson, J.; Arnould, L.; Desmoulins, I.; Mayeur, D.; Kaderbhai, C.; et al. Efficacy of Platinum-Based Chemotherapy in Metastatic Breast Cancer and HRD Biomarkers: Utility of Exome Sequencing. *NPJ Breast Cancer* **2022**, *8*, 28. [CrossRef]
103. Bertucci, F.; Ng, C.K.Y.; Patsouris, A.; Droin, N.; Piscuoglio, S.; Carbuccia, N.; Soria, J.C.; Dien, A.T.; Adnani, Y.; Kamal, M.; et al. Genomic Characterization of Metastatic Breast Cancers. *Nature* **2019**, *569*, 560–564. [CrossRef]
104. Vinayak, S.; Tolaney, S.M.; Schwartzberg, L.; Mita, M.; McCann, G.; Tan, A.R.; Wahner-Hendrickson, A.E.; Forero, A.; Anders, C.; Wulf, G.M.; et al. Open-Label Clinical Trial of Niraparib Combined With Pembrolizumab for Treatment of Advanced or Metastatic Triple-Negative Breast Cancer. *JAMA Oncol.* **2019**, *5*, 1132–1140. [CrossRef] [PubMed]
105. Domchek, S.M.; Postel-Vinay, S.; Im, S.-A.; Park, Y.H.; Delord, J.-P.; Italiano, A.; Alexandre, J.; You, B.; Bastian, S.; Krebs, M.G.; et al. Olaparib and Durvalumab in Patients with Germline BRCA-Mutated Metastatic Breast Cancer (MEDIOLA): An Open-Label, Multicentre, Phase 1/2, Basket Study. *Lancet Oncol.* **2020**, *21*, 1155–1164. [CrossRef] [PubMed]
106. Patsouris, A.; Diop, K.; Tredan, O.; Nenciu, D.; Gonçalves, A.; Arnedos, M.; Sablin, M.-P.; Jézéquel, P.; Jimenez, M.; Droin, N.; et al. Rucaparib in Patients Presenting a Metastatic Breast Cancer with Homologous Recombination Deficiency, without Germline BRCA1/2 Mutation. *Eur. J. Cancer* **2021**, *159*, 283–295. [CrossRef] [PubMed]
107. Gruber, J.J.; Afghahi, A.; Timms, K.; DeWees, A.; Gross, W.; Aushev, V.N.; Wu, H.-T.; Balcioglu, M.; Sethi, H.; Scott, D.; et al. A Phase II Study of Talazoparib Monotherapy in Patients with Wild-Type BRCA1 and BRCA2 with a Mutation in Other Homologous Recombination Genes. *Nat. Cancer* **2022**, *3*, 1181–1191. [CrossRef] [PubMed]

108. Keung, M.Y.; Wu, Y.; Badar, F.; Vadgama, J.V. Response of Breast Cancer Cells to PARP Inhibitors Is Independent of BRCA Status. *J. Clin. Med.* **2020**, *9*, 940. [CrossRef]
109. McGrail, D.J.; Lin, C.C.-J.; Garnett, J.; Liu, Q.; Mo, W.; Dai, H.; Lu, Y.; Yu, Q.; Ju, Z.; Yin, J.; et al. Improved Prediction of PARP Inhibitor Response and Identification of Synergizing Agents through Use of a Novel Gene Expression Signature Generation Algorithm. *NPJ Syst. Biol. Appl.* **2017**, *3*, 8. [CrossRef]
110. Mao, Y.; Qu, Q.; Chen, X.; Huang, O.; Wu, J.; Shen, K. The Prognostic Value of Tumor-Infiltrating Lymphocytes in Breast Cancer: A Systematic Review and Meta-Analysis. *PLoS ONE* **2016**, *11*, e0152500. [CrossRef]
111. Teo, M.Y.; Seier, K.; Ostrovnaya, I.; Regazzi, A.M.; Kania, B.E.; Moran, M.M.; Cipolla, C.K.; Bluth, M.J.; Chaim, J.; Al-Ahmadie, H.; et al. Alterations in DNA Damage Response and Repair Genes as Potential Marker of Clinical Benefit From PD-1/PD-L1 Blockade in Advanced Urothelial Cancers. *J. Clin. Oncol. Off. J. Am. Soc. Clin. Oncol.* **2018**, *36*, 1685–1694. [CrossRef]
112. Ter Brugge, P.; Kristel, P.; van der Burg, E.; Boon, U.; de Maaker, M.; Lips, E.; Mulder, L.; de Ruiter, J.; Moutinho, C.; Gevensleben, H.; et al. Mechanisms of Therapy Resistance in Patient-Derived Xenograft Models of BRCA1-Deficient Breast Cancer. *J. Natl. Cancer Inst.* **2016**, *108*, djw148. [CrossRef]
113. Esteller, M.; Silva, J.M.; Dominguez, G.; Bonilla, F.; Matias-Guiu, X.; Lerma, E.; Bussaglia, E.; Prat, J.; Harkes, I.C.; Repasky, E.A.; et al. Promoter Hypermethylation and BRCA1 Inactivation in Sporadic Breast and Ovarian Tumors. *J. Natl. Cancer Inst.* **2000**, *92*, 564–569. [CrossRef]
114. Mickley, L.A.; Spengler, B.A.; Knutsen, T.A.; Biedler, J.L.; Fojo, T. Gene Rearrangement: A Novel Mechanism for MDR-1 Gene Activation. *J. Clin. Investig.* **1997**, *99*, 1947–1957. [CrossRef] [PubMed]
115. Patch, A.-M.; Christie, E.L.; Etemadmoghadam, D.; Garsed, D.W.; George, J.; Fereday, S.; Nones, K.; Cowin, P.; Alsop, K.; Bailey, P.J.; et al. Whole-Genome Characterization of Chemoresistant Ovarian Cancer. *Nature* **2015**, *521*, 489–494. [CrossRef] [PubMed]
116. Afghahi, A.; Timms, K.M.; Vinayak, S.; Jensen, K.C.; Kurian, A.W.; Carlson, R.W.; Chang, P.-J.; Schackmann, E.; Hartman, A.-R.; Ford, J.M.; et al. Tumor BRCA1 Reversion Mutation Arising during Neoadjuvant Platinum-Based Chemotherapy in Triple-Negative Breast Cancer Is Associated with Therapy Resistance. *Clin. Cancer Res. Off. J. Am. Assoc. Cancer Res.* **2017**, *23*, 3365–3370. [CrossRef] [PubMed]

Disclaimer/Publisher's Note: The statements, opinions and data contained in all publications are solely those of the individual author(s) and contributor(s) and not of MDPI and/or the editor(s). MDPI and/or the editor(s) disclaim responsibility for any injury to people or property resulting from any ideas, methods, instructions or products referred to in the content.

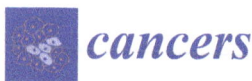

Review

Recent Advances in Optimizing Radiation Therapy Decisions in Early Invasive Breast Cancer

Nazia Riaz [1], Tiffany Jeen [1], Timothy J. Whelan [2,3,†] and Torsten O. Nielsen [1,*,†]

1. Department of Pathology and Laboratory Medicine, University of British Columbia, Vancouver, BC V6T 1Z4, Canada
2. Department of Oncology, McMaster University, Hamilton, ON L8S 4L8, Canada
3. Division of Radiation Oncology, Juravinski Cancer Centre at Hamilton Health Sciences, Hamilton, ON L8V 5C2, Canada
* Correspondence: torsten@mail.ubc.ca
† Co-senior authors.

Simple Summary: Radiation therapy is routinely prescribed for women who undergo breast-sparing surgery for early breast cancers. Over the years, advancements in diagnosis and treatments have dramatically improved breast cancer outcomes, now approaching 100% survival at 5 years for those diagnosed at stage I with favorable clinical and molecular features. In this review, we discuss the investigations that are underway to identify women with low-risk cancers in whom radiation therapy can either be completely avoided or delivered in lower intensities. We also review ongoing clinical trials that are assessing if radiation therapy can increase the capacity of patients' anticancer immune responses and discuss if cancer cells that are shed in the blood can guide radiation decisions.

Abstract: Adjuvant whole breast irradiation after breast-conserving surgery is a well-established treatment standard for early invasive breast cancer. Screening, early diagnosis, refinement in surgical techniques, the knowledge of new and specific molecular prognostic factors, and now the standard use of more effective neo/adjuvant systemic therapies have proven instrumental in reducing the rates of locoregional relapses. This underscores the need for reliably identifying women with such low-risk disease burdens in whom elimination of radiation from the treatment plan would not compromise oncological safety. This review summarizes the current evidence for radiation de-intensification strategies and details ongoing prospective clinical trials investigating the omission of adjuvant whole breast irradiation in molecularly defined low-risk breast cancers and related evidence supporting the potential for radiation de-escalation in HER2+ and triple-negative clinical subtypes. Furthermore, we discuss the current evidence for the de-escalation of regional nodal irradiation after neoadjuvant chemotherapy. Finally, we also detail the current knowledge of the clinical value of stromal tumor-infiltrating lymphocytes and liquid-based biomarkers as prognostic factors for locoregional relapse.

Keywords: breast cancer; breast-conserving surgery; radiation; de-escalation; biomarkers; prognosis

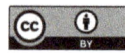

1. Introduction

Breast-conserving surgery consolidated with adjuvant radiation has been the well-established standard of care for women diagnosed with early invasive breast cancer for more than three decades [1–4]. The Early Breast Cancer Trialists' Collaborative Group patient-level meta-analysis of 17 randomized trials, including more than 10,000 women, provides compelling evidence favoring adjuvant radiotherapy over no radiotherapy after breast-conserving surgery for a 10-year absolute risk reduction of 15.7% for any recurrence and a moderate absolute decrease in breast cancer mortality by 3.8% at 15 years [5]. Supplementation with a tumor bed radiation boost further diminishes the relative risk of local recurrence by 50% in high-risk patients [6]. Over the past several decades, screening, early diagnosis, refinements in imaging, surgical techniques, pathological evaluation, improved understanding of tumor biology, and now the standard use of more effective neo/adjuvant systemic therapies have contributed to a steady and substantial improvement in clinical outcomes [7].

Modern radiotherapy techniques incorporating hypofractionation schedules have improved quality of life, decreased hospital stay, and lessened side effects compared to traditional radiotherapy modalities for early breast cancer [8,9]. Furthermore, despite a lack of proven survival benefits in some instances, optimal locoregional control undoubtedly contributes to improved quality of life [8].

Similar to systemic therapy decisions, radiotherapy should be evaluated using an individualized approach to avoid over-treatment for early invasive breast cancer. This need has prompted re-consideration of radiotherapy indications and has initiated investigations to identify any subset of low-risk women with such a negligible burden of residual locoregional disease risk following breast-conserving surgery who could be safely spared radiation therapy. In particular, much attention has been focused lately on elderly early-stage breast cancer patients with favorable prognostic factors [10].

Among these different studies, retrospectively analyzed data by Herskovic et al. has shown an improvement in overall survival with adjuvant radiation in a cohort of >60,000 women > 65 years of age [11]. In contrast, a series of at least seven first-generation clinical trials were conducted between 1981–1998 that evaluated rates for local recurrences and overall survival after breast-conserving surgery with or without radiation. These trials limited the eligibility criteria for patient enrollment to T1–2 node-negative cancers with microscopically clear resection margin status. While no survival benefit was observed, a sufficiently low-risk group in terms of local recurrence could not be identified, signifying the insufficient capacity of standard clinicopathological factors alone in this regard [12]. This, perhaps, was also compounded by less established standards for hormone receptor assessment and variability in the definition of pathologically clear surgical margins at that time.

Among the second generation of relevant phase III clinical trials, noteworthy are the Cancer and Leukemia Group B 9343 cooperative group (CALGB 9343) and the Postoperative Radiotherapy in Minimum-risk Elderly (PRIME II) trials that exercised more stringent eligibility criteria based on age at diagnosis ($\geq$70 years and $\geq$65 years for CALGB 9343 and PRIME II, respectively) and favorable tumor characteristics. For the CALGB 9343 trial, at 10 years, 98% of women randomized to tamoxifen and radiation after breast-conserving surgery, versus 90% of those in the tamoxifen-only arm, remained free from local and regional relapses [13]. PRIME II yielded comparable results at 10 years, showing an ipsilateral breast tumor recurrence rate of 0.9% with and 9.8% without radiation [14,15]. Even with this statistically significant improvement in the risk of locoregional relapses with radiation in both these trials, no prominent impact was noted on survival. The level I evidence thus generated led to a modification in the clinical practice guidelines allowing radiation omission after breast-conserving surgery in women $\geq$ 70 years with T1N0, hormone receptor-positive early breast cancers who are committed to complete a 5-year course of endocrine therapy [16] as low compliance with endocrine therapy is associated with poor locoregional control when radiation therapy is also being omitted from the treatment plan [17].

Regardless of these recommendations, the use of radiation therapy has continued among elderly women, the decision largely influenced by patients' age and physicians' preference [18,19]. Additionally, achieving higher locoregional control with radiation may be the preferred choice of women to avoid the deterioration in quality of life and the financial costs associated with locoregional recurrence, particularly in the presence of poor prognostic factors such as grade 3 histology and positive surgical margins. It has also been reported that elderly women may prefer to receive radiation therapy (that is delivered over weeks) over adjuvant endocrine therapy (delivered over 5 years, with often poor compliance outside clinical trial settings) [17].

Beyond the omission of adjuvant radiation in select indolent tumors in elderly patients, de-intensification strategies have continued to evolve over the past two decades and have positively contributed towards patient convenience and compliance by reducing radiation duration and toxicities without compromising oncological safety.

Despite its undeniable benefits, radiation therapy is linked with the risk of significant morbidities. Radiation dermatitis is the most common early complication of adjuvant radiation following breast-conserving surgery that, if severe, may potentially interrupt the radiation schedule [20,21]. Furthermore, while the risk of acute radiation toxicity is significantly lower with partial breast radiation compared to whole breast radiation, the risk of delayed dermal toxicities, including telangiectasia, fat necrosis, and subcutaneous fibrosis, has been shown to be increased in some studies [22]. Additionally, both early and delayed arm lymphedema remains a debilitating morbidity occurring in every fifth breast cancer survivor, negatively impacting their quality of life and associated with an increased burden on the health care system [23]. In particular, regional radiation therapy is a risk factor contributing to the development of late-onset lymphedema (>12 months) [24] and cardiac and pulmonary complications [25]. However, at least with regard to cardiac toxicity, the use of CT-based radiotherapy planning greatly mitigates this risk [26,27]. Lastly, despite encouraging response rates to pre-operative radiation in early-stage breast cancer, wound-related complications remain a major concern that has prompted further investigations to optimize radiation doses and schedules [28].

In this review, we will summarize the recent advances in hypofractionated and accelerated partial breast irradiation and discuss the ongoing clinical trials that utilize existing validated genomic classifiers and immunohistochemistry-based assays for risk categorization and radiation omission in hormone receptor-positive early breast cancers. We will also provide an overview of the recent literature supporting the potential for radiation de-escalation in HER2-positive and triple-negative subtypes. Next, we will discuss clinical trials underway for the de-escalation of regional nodal radiation after neoadjuvant chemotherapy. Lastly, we will provide an update on current advances in the utilization of immune biomarkers (specifically stromal lymphocytes) and liquid-biopsy-based approaches for prognostication of locoregional risk and prediction of radiation benefit.

2. De-Intensification of Radiation in Early Breast Cancer: Hypofractionation and Accelerated Partial Breast Radiation

Until about a decade ago, the conventional dosage for whole breast irradiation, defined as 45–50 Gy given in 25 fractions of 1.8–2.0 Gy once a day over 5 weeks, with or without a tumor bed boost (suggested as 10 Gy in 4–5 fractions) had been the standard of care [29]. This extended duration of treatment has been associated with acute and late radiation-induced toxicities, poor quality of life, low compliance, increased workload, and high costs incurred by healthcare systems [30,31]. In addition, several factors, including patient age, co-morbidities, income, ethnicity, education attainment, distance to the treatment facility, and the availability of radiation oncologists, have been found to be associated with disparities in the receipt of radiotherapy [32–35]. These barriers contribute to an increased rate of mastectomy among women who might otherwise have chosen breast-conserving surgery with adjuvant radiation [36].

Contrary to the aforementioned conventional radiation, in the hypofractionation approach, a higher dose (>2 Gy) per fraction is delivered in fewer fractions over a shorter duration, such that a lower overall total dose is delivered. The radiobiologic rationale for hypofractionation is based on the concept of fractionation sensitivity (α/β therapeutic ratio) such that if the fractionation sensitivity of the cancer cells is similar to the fractionation sensitivity of irradiated normal cells, a higher dose per fraction can be delivered to achieve tumoricidal effect while limiting toxicities to the normal breast [37].

High-quality, mature follow-up data from multiple phase III randomized clinical trials have consistently demonstrated non-inferiority of moderate hypofractionated radiation (40–42.5 Gy in 15–16 fractions of 2.6–2.7 Gy over 3 weeks) compared to conventional whole breast irradiation, for improving locoregional control, overall survival, and cosmetic outcomes while reducing normal tissue toxicities [38–41]. Based on the level I evidence generated from these clinical trials, guidelines recommend hypofractionation as the standard of care [29]. As a further radiation de-intensification strategy, more recently, the 5-year results from the FAST FORWARD trial have shown the non-inferiority of an ultra-hypofractionation regimen (26 Gy in 5 fractions of 5.2 Gy over 1 week versus standard hypofractionation of 40 Gy in 15 fractions over 3 weeks) for local control of the conserved breast or chest wall without compromising normal breast tissue [42].

Given that most in-breast recurrences occur in the index quadrant [43], Accelerated Partial Breast Irradiation (APBI) is an alternative approach to hypofractionation that delivers targeted radiation (>2 Gy) to the lumpectomy site (and the associated margin) over a period of 2–5 days and has shown promising results for oncological safety and cosmetic outcomes, while decreasing the treatment time to 2–5 days. Methods of APBI delivery include single or multiple catheter brachytherapy [44–48], intraoperative radiotherapy [49–51], and the use of external beam radiation therapy techniques such as three-dimensional conformal radiation therapy [42,52–54] and intensity-modulated radiation therapy [55,56].

One caveat to the use of APBI is the careful selection of eligible patients. This is particularly evident from the phase III NSABP B-39/RTOG 0413 trial, which was unable to demonstrate non-inferiority of APBI compared to whole breast irradiation with regard to the ipsilateral breast tumor recurrence rate. This is likely because the trial included a heterogenous population comprising low-risk as well as high-risk patients with features such as age < 40, invasive lobular carcinomas, multifocality, tumor size > 2 cm, 1–3 positive lymph nodes, or hormone receptor-negative status [57]. However, the absolute difference (1%) in ipsilateral breast tumor recurrence was found to be small and potentially acceptable to some patients.

Variations in APBI fraction size, delivery methods, and radiation schedules are associated with different cosmesis and tissue toxicity results. On the one hand, ABPI (compared to whole breast irradiation) has shown comparable or improved cosmetic outcomes and toxicity profiles [58–61], while on the other hand, some trials have shown contrary results. For example, in the OCOG-RAPID trial, compared to whole breast irradiation, APBI delivered via three-dimensional conformal radiation therapy as 38.5 Gy in 10 fractions twice per day over 5–8 days was associated with a higher rate of delayed radiation toxicity and poor cosmesis [53]. The authors noted that this could be the result of short dosing intervals (daily doses separated by 6–8 h) and that the worse cosmesis could be potentially circumvented by a once-daily dosing regimen. Likewise, the physician reported cosmetic outcomes at 3 years were inferior with APBI compared to whole breast irradiation in NSABP B-39/RTOG 0413, which used a similar fractionation schedule [57].

Intraoperative radiotherapy that delivers a single fraction with electrons or soft X-rays intraoperatively immediately after tumor resection is yet another strategy to decrease the radiotherapy time and has been evaluated in two randomized controlled trials. The European Institute of Oncology's ELIOT trial showed increased local and regional relapse rates associated with intraoperative radiotherapy compared to conventional whole breast radiation at a median follow-up of 12.4 years (11% versus 2%), despite there being no significant difference in the overall survival rate between the two groups. The exploratory analysis identified several factors associated with a significantly increased risk of ipsilateral breast tumor recurrence: tumor size > 2 cm, grade 3, ≥4 positive axillary nodes, Ki-67 > 20%, and luminal B or triple-negative clinical subtype [51]. However, intraoperative radiotherapy as administered in ELIOT may still be an appropriate option for a subset of patients with extremely favorable tumor biology (well-differentiated luminal A cancers < 1 cm in size with Ki-67 < 14%) who experienced a 10-year ipsilateral breast tumor recurrence rate of <1.3% [51]. The second phase III TARGIT-IORT trial found intraoperative radiotherapy to be non-inferior to whole breast radiation in terms of five-year oncological outcomes. In particular, one stratum of the trial was designed to include a risk-adapted approach whereby patients receiving intraoperative radiotherapy, if found to have high-risk features on final pathology, would then receive standard whole breast radiation post-operatively; in those cases, the intraoperative dose was considered as a tumor bed boost [62]. Further detailed analyses have shown the oncological safety of the TARGIT-IORT risk-adapted approach in all relevant subgroups stratified by breast cancer subtype, nodal involvement, tumor size, and grade. Intriguingly, the results also suggest that contrary to standard whole breast radiation, local failures occurring in the TARGIT-IOTR arm are not necessarily associated with poor survival. While the biological mechanisms are not completely understood, this effect could be partly explained by an abscopal effect of intraoperative radiotherapy delivered to a well-vascularized tumor bed [63]. Of note, in the second TARGIT stratum, delayed intraoperative radiotherapy delivered at a median of 37 days at a second surgery failed to demonstrate non-inferiority to standard whole breast irradiation [64]. Although the TARGIT-IORT procedure has been incorporated into clinical practice globally [65], by and large, the intraoperative radiotherapy approach is still regarded as investigational until mature, long-term data becomes available [66,67].

A recently published meta-analysis of 15 clinical trials, including more than 16,000 patients, compared partial breast radiation with whole breast radiation and reported the rates of any ipsilateral breast tumor recurrences as the primary outcome measure. Collectively, partial breast radiation was associated with a higher risk of ipsilateral breast recurrences compared to whole breast radiation (5% versus 2.8%). Of note, after excluding intraoperative radiotherapy trials, the rates of ipsilateral recurrences were 3.3% with partial breast radiation versus 2.6% with whole breast radiation. Another noteworthy observation from this meta-analysis is the higher rate of elsewhere recurrence in the ipsilateral breast with partial breast radiation compared to whole breast radiation. The rates for true/marginal recurrence were, however, comparable between the two treatment modalities. Despite the advantage over whole breast radiation in limiting the risk of acute toxicities, overall partial breast radiation yielded inferior effectiveness [68]. However, these results varied with the delivery techniques such that multi-catheter brachytherapy and external beam radiation approaches with CT planning were associated with higher oncological safety compared to the intraoperative approach.

3. Ongoing Clinical Trials for Guiding Adjuvant Radiation Omission Decisions in Women with Hormone Receptor-Positive Early-Stage Breast Cancers

The clinical utility of validated genomic and immunohistochemistry-based biomarkers for guiding adjuvant radiation omission decisions following breast-conserving surgery in favorable risk invasive breast cancers is under intense prospective investigation (Table 1). The common theme of these third-generation clinical trials is to combine clinical factors with some type of molecular risk assay to identify a low-risk group whose prognosis is so good, at least in the context of adequate endocrine therapy, that radiation could not provide significant additional benefit.

Table 1. Ongoing clinical trials for the omission of adjuvant radiation therapy in molecularly defined low-risk estrogen receptor-positive breast cancers.

Trial Name (NCT ID) & Completion Year	Trial/Study Design (n)	Eligibility Criteria							IHC/Genomic Classifier	Outcome Measures
		Age (yr)	Pathological Stage	Grade	Receptor Status by IHC	Surgery	Margin Status (mm)			
Trials investigating omission of whole breast irradiation in node-negative breast cancers										
LUMINA (NCT01791829) [69] 2024	Prospective, single arm, observational study (n = 501)	≥55	Stage 1 (pT1N0M0)	1–2	ER+/PR+/HER2−	BCS+ SLNB or axillary dissection	≥1		Molecularly defined luminal A by IHC [1]: ER ≥ 1%, PR > 20%, HER2− (by IHC or in situ hybridization) and Ki-67 ≤ 13.25%	Primary: 5-year ipsilateral invasive breast cancer or DCIS recurrence. Secondary: Contralateral breast cancer, RFS based on any recurrence, DFS based on any recurrence, second cancer or death, and OS
PRECISION (NCT02653755) [70] 2026	Phase II prospective cohort study (n = 690)	50–75	Stage I (pT1N0M0) (Axillary nodes with isolated tumor cells permitted)	1–2	ER+/PR+/HER2−	BCS+ SLNB or axillary dissection	No ink on tumor or re-excision with no residual disease		Prosigna ROR	Primary: 5-year risk of ipsilateral LRR. Secondary: 5-year risk of any recurrence, DFS, and OS
IDEA (NCT02400190) [71] 2026	Prospective, single-arm observational study (n = 202)	50–69	Stage I (pT1N0M0) (Axillary nodes with isolated tumor cells permitted)	N/A	ER+/PR+/HER2−	BCS+ SLNB or SLNB→axillary dissection or axillary dissection	≥2		Oncotype Dx RS ≤ 18	Primary: 5-year LRR. Secondary (10 years): Recurrence pattern, subsequent therapy for local recurrences, OS, and BCSS
PRIMETIME (ISRCTN: 41579286) [72] 2027	Case-cohort, prospective study (n = 1500)	≤60	Stage I (pT1N0M0)	1–2	ER+/PR+/HER2− [2]	BCS+ SLNB	≥1		IHC4+C	Primary: 5-year IBTR
DEBRA NCT04852887 [73] 2041	Phase III multicenter randomized trial (n = 1670)	50–70	Stage I (pT1N0M0) (Patients with pathologic staging of pN0(i+) or pN0(mol+) are not permitted)	N/A	ER+/PR+/HER2−	BCS→WBI + ET vs. BCS→ET	No ink on tumor or re-excision with no residual disease		N/A	Primary: 5-year invasive or non-invasive IBTR. Secondary: Percentage of women with an intact index breast, any invasive IBTR, any breast cancer recurrence at a local, regional, or distant site, recurrence or a secondary primary cancer and death

Table 1. Cont.

Trial Name (NCT ID & Completion Year)	Trial/Study Design (n)	Eligibility Criteria							Outcome Measures
		Age (yr)	Pathological Stage	Grade	Receptor Status by IHC	Surgery	Margin Status (mm)	IHC/Genomic Classifier	
EXPERT (NCT02889874) [74] 2023	Randomized phase III clinical trial (n = 1167)	≥50	Stage I (pT1N0M0)	1–2	ER+/PR+/HER2−	BCS+ SLNB or axillary dissection	No ink on margin	PAM50 Luminal A and Prosigna ROR ≤ 60	Primary: 10-year risk of ipsilateral local recurrence Secondary: 10-year LRR, distant recurrence, DFS including DCIS, iDFS, OS, rates of salvage RT or mastectomy, and quality of life-related endpoints such as convenience of care and fear for recurrence
The DBCG RT Natural Trial (NCT03646955) [75] 2035	Randomized phase III clinical trial (n = 926)	≥60	Stage I (pT1N0M0)	1–2	≥10% ER+/HER2−	BCS+ SLNB or axillary dissection	≥2	N/A	Primary: 10-year-invasive local recurrence in ipsilateral breast. Secondary: (10-year) Regional recurrence, distant recurrence, and death.
Trials investigating omission of regional nodal irradiation in node-positive/negative breast cancers									
CCTG MA.39 (TAILOR RT) (NCT03488693) [76] 2027	Randomized phase III, clinical trial (n = 2140)	≥40	Stage 1 T1-3N0-1	N/A	ER+/HER2− (Local testing)	BCS or mastectomy + SLNB and/or axillary dissection	≥1	Oncotype Dx RS < 18	Primary: Breast cancer recurrence-free interval Secondary: DFS, LRR, OS, breast cancer mortality, distant recurrence, toxicity, arm volume, and mobility assessments, patient reported outcomes and cost effectiveness

[1] IHC assay performed in local laboratories as per American Society of Clinical Oncology Guidelines. [2] As per local practice. Abbreviations: ER, estrogen receptor; PR, progesterone receptor; HER2, human epidermal growth factor receptor 2; BCS, breast-conserving surgery; SLNB, sentinel lymph node biopsy; ROR score, risk of recurrence score; RS, recurrence score; LRR, local regional recurrence; DCIS, ductal carcinoma in situ; RFS, relapse-free survival; DFS, disease-free survival; IBTR, ipsilateral breast tumor recurrence; iDFS, invasive disease-free survival; OS, overall survival; BCSS, breast cancer-specific survival; WBI, whole breast irradiation; ET, endocrine therapy; IHC, immunohistochemistry; IHC4+C, immunohistochemistry 4+ clinical.

Amongst these trials, the prespecified 5-year interim analysis of the LUMINA prospective trial was the first to be presented at the 2022 American Society of Clinical Oncology meeting [69]. Briefly, LUMINA is a multicentre, single-arm prospective cohort study investigating the clinical value of clinicopathological characteristics together with Ki-67 immunohistochemistry-based phenotyping for identifying women $\geq$ 55 years with sufficiently low-risk molecularly defined T1N0 luminal A breast cancers (ER $\geq$ 1%, PR > 20%, HER2 negative, and Ki-67 $\leq$ 13.25%) who can be adequately treated with breast-conserving surgery and endocrine therapy alone without compromising oncological outcomes. The primary endpoint is the ipsilateral local recurrence of any invasive or non-invasive breast cancer. Amongst the 501 enrolled patients, the reported 5-year local recurrence rate of 2.3% (90% CI 1.3–3.8) was well below the prespecified boundary of significance (5%), making this a positive study. Moreover, the 5-year rates for contralateral breast cancer, relapse-free, disease-free, and overall survival are 1.9% (90% CI 1.1–3.2), 97.3% (90% CI 95.9–98.4), 89.9% (90% CI 87.5–92.2) and 97.2% (90% CI 95.9–98.4), respectively. While the full analysis is awaited, these 5-year results do provide prospective data supporting the safe omission of adjuvant whole breast radiation in precisely selected luminal A breast cancers with a low Ki-67 index ($\leq$13.25%), quantified using a standardized, validated, decentralized IHC assay [77].

PRECISION (Profiling Early Breast Cancer for Radiotherapy Omission) is a phase II, single-arm prospective cohort study led by the Dana-Faber Cancer Institute that aims to evaluate the 5-year risk of ipsilateral locoregional recurrence following upfront breast-conserving surgery without whole breast radiation. Enrollment criteria comprise women aged 50–75 years with ER+/PR+/HER2−, pT1N0M0, grade 1–2 invasive breast cancers. The tumors from the eligible patients are subjected to central PAM50 transcriptional profiling using the Prosigna assay. Only women whose tumors yield a low risk of Recurrence (ROR) score corresponding to the luminal A subtype qualify to forego radiation to the conserved breast and are offered 5 years of endocrine therapy only [70,78]. At a median follow-up of 26.9 months, 12 events have been recorded among 382 women with a ROR $\leq$ 40 (4, ipsilateral in-breast recurrences; 7, contralateral breast cancers; and 1, unrelated melanoma). No regional-nodal or distant recurrences have been reported thus far. The 2-year cumulative rate of locoregional recurrence is 0.3% (95% CI: 0–1.0%) [79].

IDEA (Individualized Decisions for Endocrine Therapy Alone) is an American, multicentre, single-arm prospective cohort study headed by the University of Michigan Rogel Cancer Centre, enrolling postmenopausal women (50–69 years) with ER+/PR+/HER2−, unifocal, pT1N0M0 breast cancer. This study aims to determine if 5-year locoregional relapse risk remains sufficiently low after breast-conserving surgery and 5 years of endocrine therapy (tamoxifen or aromatase inhibitor) when radiation therapy is withheld from the treatment plan. The characterization of genomically low-risk tumors is based on an Oncotype Dx recurrence score $\leq$ 18 [71].

PRIMETIME is a multicentre UK-based prospective case-cohort study that is evaluating if adjuvant radiation can be safely avoided in very low-risk women $\leq$ 60 years surgically treated with breast conservation followed by standard endocrine therapy. The study's inclusion criteria with regards to clinicopathological tumor characteristics are similar to the PRECISION trial, but the molecular risk eligibility will incorporate the very low-risk category assessed using a validated immunohistochemistry-based prognostic algorithm called IHC4+Clinical (IHC4+C). This recurrence probability score combines the protein expression of triple receptors and Ki-67, along with a Clinical Treatment Score (age, tumor size, nodal status, tumor grade, and endocrine treatment: tamoxifen versus anastrozole) to stratify the residual disease risk into four categories: very low, low, intermediate and high [80,81]. Women whose tumors classify as very low risk qualify for enrollment in PRIMETIME. The primary endpoint is 5-year ipsilateral breast tumor recurrence [72].

De-escalation of Breast Radiation (DEBRA-NRG BR007) is an NRG Oncology-sponsored, multicentre phase III clinical trial that is investigating whether breast-conserving surgery followed by endocrine therapy is non-inferior to breast-conserving surgery followed by endocrine therapy and standard whole breast irradiation. Eligibility criteria include patients aged 50–70 years who are diagnosed with unicentric ER+/PR+/HER2− pT1N0 breast cancer that are also genomically characterized as low-risk by an Oncotype Dx Recurrence Score of ≤ 18. The primary endpoint is invasive or non-invasive in-breast tumor recurrence. The trial is currently recruiting and will accrue 1714 patients enabling a final randomization cohort of 1670 patients (835 per arm). As of 30 June 2022, 169 patients had been screened and 147 randomized [73,82].

The EXPERT trial (EXamining PErsonalised Radiation Therapy for low-risk early breast cancer) is an initiative of Breast Cancer Trials in Australia and New Zealand that also uses PAM50/Prosigna for molecular risk stratification. EXPERT is a randomized phase III trial of adjuvant radiation versus observation, following breast-conserving surgery and endocrine therapy for molecularly defined luminal A breast cancer with a low ROR score (≤ 60) amongst pre or postmenopausal women ≥ 50 years. The clinicopathological factors deemed necessary for inclusion are similar to the PRECISION trial. The primary endpoint is local recurrence at 10 years [74].

The DBCG-RT Natural trial, sponsored by the Danish Breast Cancer Cooperative Group, is a non-inferiority phase III clinical trial designed to compare the 5-year risk of local recurrence between partial breast irradiation versus no irradiation among women ≥ 60 years with unifocal, pT1N0M0, ER+/HER2− invasive ductal carcinomas treated with breast-conserving surgery. This is the only radiation de-escalation trial in which low-risk patient selection is ascertained purely by traditional clinicopathological features [75].

While the above studies are specifically designed for evaluating the safety of omitting whole breast radiation in stage I node-negative breast cancers, the Canadian Cancer Trials Group MA.39 TAILOR RT is a phase III biomarker-directed randomized trial designed to test the non-inferiority of omitting regional nodal irradiation versus regional lymph node irradiation post-lumpectomy and omitting locoregional radiotherapy to the chest wall and regional nodes versus locoregional radiotherapy following mastectomy in women ≥ 35 years. All patients will receive endocrine therapy. The eligibility criteria include ER+, HER2− breast cancers with 1–3 positive axillary lymph nodes, and an Oncotype DX Recurrence score ≤ 25. The primary endpoint will measure any recurrence or death due to breast cancer [76].

4. Evidence for Radiation De-Escalation in HER2-Positive and Triple-Negative Breast Cancers

4.1. HER2+ Early Breast Cancer

About 15–20% of women are diagnosed with HER2+ early breast cancers. The Early Breast Cancer Trialists' Collaborative Group's patient-level meta-analysis of seven randomized clinical trials, including 13,864 women, has confirmed the benefit of adjuvant trastuzumab to chemotherapy in reducing the risk of any invasive breast cancer recurrence and breast cancer-specific mortality by a third in operable breast cancers regardless of the nodal status. In addition, the risk of the first isolated local recurrence was also reduced significantly with trastuzumab treatment [83].

While currently there are no completed clinical trials of radiation omission in HER2+ breast cancer, some insights are gained from observational studies that highlight the value of HER2-targeted therapies in achieving good locoregional control. For instance, Bazan et al. performed a retrospective analysis using the National Cancer Database and identified a cohort of T1N0 HER2+ patients treated with breast conservation, adjuvant chemotherapy, and HER2-targeted therapies. Of these, 6388 patients were treated with adjuvant radiation, while 509 were radiation naïve. Patients in the radiation naïve group experienced a significantly inferior 2-year overall survival compared to those who received adjuvant radiation (88.9% versus 99.2%, respectively). The study has several limitations, including a lack of information on locoregional relapses or cancer-specific survival, short follow-up, and, importantly, non-compliance with systemic therapies that may have contributed to an exaggerated poor overall survival in the radiation naïve group [84].

Some recent trials have investigated the de-intensification of chemotherapies and HER2-targeted therapies in early-stage HER2+ breast cancer, where all patients received radiation as per standard protocol. Encouraging results of these trials highlight the effectiveness of chemotherapies and HER2-targeted therapies for improving the clinical outcomes, including lowering the risk of locoregional relapses. Amongst these, the single-arm, multicentre phase II Adjuvant Paclitaxel and Trastuzumab (APT) trial included patients with T1–2N0–N1mic HER2+ breast cancer treated with upfront surgery followed by radiation therapy (for breast-conserving surgery only). All patients received adjuvant paclitaxel with trastuzumab for 12 weeks, followed by the continuation of trastuzumab for 1 year [85,86]. Only 5 of the 406 patients developed locoregional recurrences, resulting in an impressive 7-year locoregional recurrence-free survival (with radiotherapy) of 98.6% (95% CI 97.4–99.8%) [87].

The phase II ATEMPT trial randomized women with HER2+ T1–2N0–N1mic breast cancer to adjuvant trastuzumab emtansine (T-DM1) versus paclitaxel plus trastuzumab to investigate if the two treatments had comparable efficacy and toxicity profile [88]. A subsequent retrospective-prospective analysis reported at 3 years showed an extremely low rate of isolated local recurrences such that only 2 events were recorded in the group treated with T-DM1 (n = 383) and 4 in the paclitaxel plus trastuzumab arm (n = 114), though it should be noted that the inclusion criteria specified that participants who underwent breast-conserving surgery were required to receive radiation therapy and those who underwent mastectomy were permitted to receive radiation therapy to the chest wall and regional lymph nodes [89]. In the KATHERINE trial, high-risk HER2+ breast cancer patients with residual invasive disease following neoadjuvant chemotherapy and HER2-targeted therapy were randomized to adjuvant T-DM1 versus trastuzumab. Patients received adjuvant radiation therapy as per participating institutional guidelines. The trial yielded positive results showing an impressive 50% relative reduction in the risk of invasive recurrence or mortality favoring the use of T-DM1 [90], leading to subsequent FDA approval [91,92]. Overall, a very low rate of locoregional recurrences was recorded in both the treatment arms (trastuzumab group, n = 743: 4.6%; T-DM1 group, n = 743: 1.1%) in patients who were HER2+ in pre-treatment biopsies but tested negative on the residual disease biopsy [93]. Albeit long-term follow-up from these trials is warranted, the substantially low risk of locoregional relapses is indeed encouraging and may pave the way for future clinical trials investigating radiotherapy de-escalation strategies in stringently selected low-risk early-stage HER2+ breast cancers. In this trial, neither radiation modalities nor the sequence of integration of systemic treatment with radiotherapy are specified. This information could be potentially relevant in future clinical trials.

Considering these encouraging observations, NRG BR008 (HERO) is a phase III randomized clinical trial expected to launch in the first quarter of 2023 that will include women ≥ 40 years diagnosed with early-stage, low-risk HER2-positive invasive breast cancer (those with pT1N0 receiving chemotherapy or those with clinically < 3 cm node-negative cancer achieving pathological complete responses with neoadjuvant chemotherapy and HER2-targeted therapies). The primary endpoint of the trial is recurrence-free interval amongst all patients surgically treated with breast-conserving surgery and randomized to adjuvant radiation versus no radiation. In addition, relevant oncological outcomes, including ipsilateral breast cancer recurrence, locoregional recurrence, disease-free survival, overall survival, and patient-reported outcomes for pain and fear of recurrence, will comprise secondary objectives [94].

4.2. Node-Negative Early-Stage Triple-Negative Breast Cancers

TNBC is a remarkably heterogenous disease entity [95]. Nevertheless, significant progress has recently been made in expanding therapeutic opportunities for both early and advanced stage disease [96,97]. Historically, TNBC has been linked with aggressive disease biology and early locoregional and distant relapses [98]. Hence these cancers are managed aggressively with systemic therapies and adjuvant radiation. Nevertheless, compared to non-TNBC, the magnitude of benefit from adjuvant radiation in TNBC seems limited because in the reported studies, using multivariate analyses, women with TNBC have an increased risk of locoregional relapse, independent of systemic treatments [5,99]. Several retrospective series have shown that adverse clinical outcomes prevail even in small (<2 cm), node-negative TNBC [100,101]; hence it is not surprising that survival gains are evident with the use of adjuvant chemotherapies [102]. Albeit retrospective in nature, data from several study cohorts demonstrate the important observation that a subset of node-negative TNBC not exceeding 1 cm in size experiences exceptionally low rates of locoregional and distant relapses even in the absence of chemotherapy [103,104]. In fact, a patient-level meta-analysis of 12 international cohorts comprising 1835 early-stage chemotherapy naïve TNBC has identified a subset of stage I TNBC with high stromal tumor-infiltrating lymphocytes that display an inherently excellent prognosis, potentially making them suitable candidates for therapeutic de-escalation [105].

Limited studies have addressed the adequacy of locoregional control in small, node-negative TNBC when radiation therapy is omitted from the treatment plan. Eaton et al. queried the Surveillance Epidemiology and End Results database to investigate the influence of radiation after breast-conserving surgery among elderly women ($\geq$70 years) diagnosed with estrogen receptor-negative, T1–2 node-negative breast cancers between 1993–2007. Cumulative incidences of salvage mastectomies (a surrogate for adequacy of local tumor control) and breast cancer-specific deaths were reported for 3432 patients, among whom about 16% were radiation naïve. Their results showed a significantly higher 5-year cumulative incidence of mastectomies (8.3% vs. 4.9%) and breast cancer-specific mortality (24% vs. 10.8%) in the radiation naïve group compared to those that received radiation. However, an exploratory subgroup analysis did find that women $\geq$ 80 years derived somewhat limited benefit from radiation (mastectomy incidence amongst radiation recipients versus radiation naïve group: 3.4% vs. 6.9%, $p = 0.05$) [106]. Another independent analysis of the National Cancer Database cohort compared overall survival with or without adjuvant radiation after breast-conserving surgery for T1N0M0 TNBC among women $\geq$ 70 years and revealed a significantly inferior overall survival in the radiation naïve group compared to the group that received adjuvant radiation. Factors associated with adverse outcomes in the radiation naïve group included re-excision for positive margins, tumor size $\geq$ 2 cm, multiple comorbidities, lower socioeconomic status, and treatment at academic centers [107]. Another study by the same group included data from more than 14,000 non-metastatic pT1–4 node-negative TNBC treated with upfront mastectomy. The authors assessed the factors influencing the use of postmastectomy radiation and showed that pathological tumor size $\leq$ 2 cm with histologically negative margins, advanced age, treatment at academic centers, and omission of chemotherapy showed a positive association with the omission of adjuvant radiation. Importantly, a significant improvement in overall survival was observed only in pT3 tumors treated with radiation, whereas overall survival was similar in pT1–2 and in pT4 tumors regardless of adjuvant radiation [108].

These retrospective observational data, with their inherent limitations, support a pressing need for prospectively addressing if there is a role for escalating or de-escalation adjuvant radiation in T1–2 node-negative TNBC. In this regard, prospective data is far more limited. Wang et al. performed a multicentre prospective randomized clinical trial to investigate if the addition of radiotherapy improved the clinical outcomes in women ($n = 681$) with stage I–II TNBC treated with mastectomy and adjuvant chemotherapy. Their results showed that the omission of radiation was indeed associated with significantly worse relapse-free survival and overall survival [109].

The first analysis of the LUMINA prospective trial for radiation de-escalation in low-risk luminal A breast cancers underscores the capacity for relevant standardized and validated biomarkers of risk distinction being able to identify a group who can safely avoid radiation and several similar trials are underway in women with ER-positive breast cancers (as shown in Table 1). Given the heterogeneity of TNBC [95] and the fact that clinicopathological factors alone are not sufficient to recapitulate this molecular complexity, biomarker-directed approaches will need to be utilized for patient selection in prospectively designed trials to assess if there indeed exists a group of women with TNBC who can safely avoid radiation therapy.

More recent reports have observed very low rates of local recurrence following lumpectomy in patients who have a complete response to neoadjuvant chemotherapy. The Ontario Clinical Oncology Group is mounting a prospective cohort trial similar to LUMINA where patients with T1–3N0 disease who have had a complete response to neoadjuvant chemotherapy following lumpectomy, including triple-negative disease, will not receive RT and be followed.

5. De-Escalation of Adjuvant Locoregional Radiation in Clinically Node-Positive Breast Cancer following Neoadjuvant Chemotherapy

The integration of neoadjuvant chemotherapy into the management of early-stage breast cancer has surged significantly in recent years [110]. Pooled analysis of 33 studies, including 57,531 patients, has demonstrated that axillary pathological complete response (pCR) rates following neoadjuvant chemotherapy with clinically positive axillary nodes vary widely within breast cancer subtypes, with hormone receptor-/HER2+ cancers showing the highest rate (60%) while only 13% of patients with luminal A subtype tumors achieved pCR. The pCR rates for other major subtype definitions are reported as follows: 59% for HER2+, 48% for TNBC, 45% for hormone receptor+/HER2+, 35% for luminal B, and 18% for hormone receptor+/HER2− [111].

An area of much controversy has been the post-neoadjuvant management of patients with clinically positive axillary nodes. Compared to those with residual disease after neoadjuvant chemotherapy, axillary nodal pCR [111] confers a significant survival advantage, with the best prognosis being observed in triple-negative and HER2+ subtypes [112]. This has led to a gradual shift in surgical practice from the routine use of axillary lymph node dissection to less extensive axillary interventions for pathological evaluation, including sentinel lymph node biopsy [113], targeted axillary dissection [114,115], and Marking of the Axilla with Radioactive Iodine (MARI) [116]. The variability of axillary procedures in the post-neoadjuvant setting clearly reflects a current lack of consensus among expert panels on the most accurate axillary staging strategy [3,4,117–119].

With regards to regional nodal irradiation, the current guidelines recommend considering its use in patients, particularly those with risk factors, with clinically node-positive axillae, irrespective of the pathological response to neoadjuvant chemotherapy. Nevertheless, there may be patients who achieve pCR in the axillary lymph nodes and who could be potentially considered as candidates for de-escalation of regional nodal irradiation. Much of this speculation is based on retrospective analyses. Barrio and colleagues investigated the rate of nodal recurrence in a series of consecutive patients with clinically node-positive axillae who received neoadjuvant chemotherapy and standardized sentinel lymph node biopsy alone for axillary staging (without further axillary dissection). All 610 patients with clinically node-positive breast cancer received doxorubicin-based neoadjuvant chemotherapy. About 90% of patients ($n = 555$) were rendered node negative; of these, 42% ($n = 234$) were subjected to sentinel lymph node biopsy with the retrieval of up to three sentinel lymph nodes. Though 70% ($n = 164$) of these patients received regional nodal radiation in this cohort, only a single patient developed locoregional recurrence (rate = 0.4%) at a median follow-up of 35 months, supporting the oncological safety of standardized sentinel lymph biopsy alone [120]. Likewise, European Institute of Oncology authors have reported an axillary failure rate of 1.8% when the axillary evaluation was limited to the removal of a single sentinel lymph node after primary chemotherapy in a cohort of patients with clinically node-positive or node-negative axillae. Only 11% of breast-conservation surgery and 38% of mastectomy patients with clinically node-positive axillae received regional nodal irradiation [121].

Haffty and colleagues retrospectively analyzed locoregional recurrence rates among women with T0–T4, N1–N2, M0 breast cancer treated with neoadjuvant chemotherapy and radiation therapy in the ACOSOG Z1071 trial. The decisions about adjuvant radiation in this trial were made by the treating radiation oncologists' best judgment rather than being prescribed by protocol. The reported overall locoregional recurrence risk was 6% after a mean follow-up of 5.9 years. Subgroup analysis of patients with axillary pCR revealed that omission of postmastectomy radiation and regional nodal radiation after breast-conserving surgery did not adversely influence the locoregional relapse risk [122]. Contrary to these data, some studies have instead reported significantly poor locoregional control with the omission of radiation [123,124]. These estimates are based on retrospective analyses and are possibly susceptible to biases due to confounding factors and selection.

The question of de-escalating regional nodal irradiation after neoadjuvant chemotherapy has been recently addressed in a multicentre Dutch prospective registry cohort (RAPCHEM; BOOG 2010-03) that included 838 patients diagnosed with breast cancers measuring up to 5 cm with 1–3 positive axillary lymph nodes, who received neoadjuvant chemotherapy followed by surgery [125]. The primary endpoint was the 5-year locoregional recurrence rate. As per study protocol, a clinically positive axillary status required the presence of up to three radiologically suspicious axillary nodes with pathological confirmation of metastasis in at least one. In contrast to the ACOSOG Z1071 trial protocol [122], the recommendation for regional nodal irradiation after neoadjuvant chemotherapy was based on three prespecified locoregional recurrence risk categories [(low-risk, ypN0 (i.e., complete pathological response with no residual disease in axillary lymph nodes based on axillary lymph node dissection or sentinel lymph node biopsy); intermediate-risk, ypN1 (i.e., partial pathological response with residual disease in 1–3 axillary lymph nodes based on axillary lymph node dissection); high-risk, ypN2–3 (i.e., residual disease in ≥ 4 nodes based on axillary dissection)]. For the full study cohort, the 5-year locoregional recurrence rate was 2.2%, supporting the oncological safety of omitting regional nodal irradiation in low- and intermediate-risk groups, i.e., those with pre-treatment clinically positive axillae that downstage to either no residual disease or up to 1–3 positive lymph nodes [125].

Individualization for optimal locoregional management of node-positive patients receiving neoadjuvant chemotherapy is being investigated in two ongoing clinical trials. NSABP B51/Radiation Therapy Oncology Group 1304 is a phase III multicentre randomized clinical trial that is investigating if the addition of regional nodal irradiation to postmastectomy chest wall radiation or whole breast radiation after breast-conserving surgery will significantly reduce the event rate for invasive breast cancer recurrence, in patients diagnosed with breast cancers more than 5 cm in size with up to 3 positive axillary lymph nodes (pathologically confirmed by fine needle aspiration cytology or core biopsy) that convert to pathologically negative axillary nodes following primary chemotherapy. A total of 1636 patients are enrolled. The trial was activated in 2013 and is expected to complete in 2028 (NCT01872975) [126]. Alliance 011202 is a phase III non-inferiority clinical trial in which women with breast cancers more than 5 cm in size with up to 3 positive axillary lymph nodes, who have a residual positive sentinel lymph node following neoadjuvant chemotherapy, are subsequently randomized to axillary lymph node dissection with nodal irradiation or to nodal irradiation alone (NCT01901094). The primary endpoint is invasive breast cancer recurrence-free interval. It is important to note that while both these trials include patients unselected with regards to ER, PR, and HER2 status, responses to neoadjuvant chemotherapies will vary with molecular subtype [111]. Hence incorporation of correlative biomarker studies is imperative to draw the most meaningful conclusions for individualizing critical therapeutic decisions that can be effectively generalized and implemented beyond the setting of this clinical trial.

6. Immune Responses in Early Breast Cancer: Ongoing Clinical Trials of Preoperative Radiotherapy and Evidence from Prospective-Retrospective Translational Studies

Tumor-infiltrating lymphocytes (TILs) are populations of mononuclear host immune cells that display phenotypic and functional heterogeneity. A pro-inflammatory, anti-tumoral role is predominantly mediated by CD8+ cytotoxic T cells, natural killer cells, dendritic cells, and M1 macrophages. In contrast, CD4+ regulatory T cells, CD4+ Th2 cells, M2 macrophages, and myeloid-derived suppressor cells promote an immune inhibitory, protumoral milieu [127]. The level of lymphocytic infiltration, as assessed simply and inexpensively by light microscopy on standard hematoxylin and eosin (H&E) stained sections, has evolved as a promising surrogate biomarker of a pre-existing host adaptive immune response portending favorable prognosis and has attained level 1B evidence for clinical utility in early-stage TNBC [128]. Furthermore, stromal TILs have also shown potential for identifying such intrinsically low-risk TNBCs that chemotherapy de-escalation could be considered as a potentially safe choice [129,130]. The clinical relevance of TILs for predicting response to adjuvant [131,132] or neoadjuvant systemic therapies [133–135] alone or in combination with immune checkpoint inhibitors is gaining momentum [136,137]. However, the value of immune biomarkers in relation to radiation responses and clinical outcomes in early breast cancer is much less well explored.

Ionizing radiation promotes several alterations in the targeted malignant cells and their associated microenvironmental niche that may impact the immunogenicity of the irradiated tumor. On the one hand, radiation elicits DNA damage leading to immunogenic cell death of the cancer cells, which in turn activates adaptive and innate immune responses that boost anti-tumoral effector functions of cytotoxic T cells. On the other hand, radiation-induced rebound immune suppression is fostered through the recruitment of protumorigenic macrophages, increased expression of immune checkpoints on tumor cells, and TGF-β stimulated accumulation of regulatory FOXP3+ T cells that suppress adaptive immune responses [138,139].

Compared to TNBC, ER+ breast cancers are generally regarded as less immunogenic as they are associated with low levels of lymphocytic infiltrates, immune checkpoint activation, and tumor mutation burden [140]. Hence the immune priming potential of radiation provides at least a theoretical opportunity for switching these immunologically cold tumors to an inflamed phenotype [141] and is being actively investigated in ongoing clinical trials (Table 2). The initial results are available for one of these trials. The SPORT trial (Single Pre-Operative Radiation Therapy for low-risk breast cancer) investigated residual disease burden and immunological responses following single-dose preoperative radiotherapy in women $\geq$ 60 years with ER+/HER2− T1N0 breast cancers surgically treated with partial mastectomy and sentinel lymph node biopsy. While no complete pathological responses were seen, a partial response was seen in patients undergoing delayed surgery (11–13 weeks) but not in those operated on within 24–72 h after radiation. No significant enrichment in lymphocytic infiltrates was observed at the ablative dose of 20 Gy. No recurrences have been recorded up to 11 months in the follow-up period [142].

Multi-omic profiling has identified an immune-hot subset corresponding to an immunomodulatory subtype of TNBC which is considered most likely to respond to immune checkpoint inhibitor therapy [143]. The comparatively high frequency of this TNBC subtype perhaps explains the relative success of recent trials evaluating the combination of immune checkpoint inhibitors and chemotherapy in the neoadjuvant setting in unselected TNBC, where a pathological complete response is achieved in up to 65% of cases [136,144]. In this context, it remains an outstanding question as to whether radiation-induced immune augmentation could improve therapeutic responses in some TNBCs. Table 2 summarizes the ongoing trials evaluating preoperative radiotherapy alone or in combination with immune checkpoint inhibitors in early-stage disease. Of these, BreastVAX is a phase 1b/2 trial investigating the feasibility and efficacy of combining a single dose infusion of pembrolizumab with radiation boost (delivered as a single fraction of 7 Gy) in patients with operable breast cancers, including TNBC and hormone receptor-positive/HER2 negative tumors [145,146]. The inclusion criteria, however, do not require evaluation of baseline tumoral immune profile. Feasibility and tolerability were evaluated as primary endpoints, and secondary endpoints include pathological complete responses and percentage change in tumor-infiltrating lymphocytes in pre- versus post-treatment samples. The preliminary results have shown major pathological complete responses (<10% viable tumor) in 3 of 9 TNBCs. Compared to the pre-treatment specimens, a significant increase in the density of tumor-infiltrating lymphocytes was seen in the post-treatment tissues of TNBC cases (only). Results of detailed correlative science studies involving digital spatial profiling to identify relevant biomarkers in responsive tumors are pending [147].

Table 2. Ongoing clinical trials investigating preoperative radiation therapy in early-stage invasive breast cancer.

Trial Identifier (n)	Study Description	Tumor Characteristics	Preoperative Radiation Regime +/− other Therapeutic Agents	Adjuvant Treatments	Endpoints	Prespecified/Exploratory Translational Studies	Estimated Study Completion Year
			Preoperative Radiation (single fraction)				
NCT01717261 Single Pre-Operative Radiation Therapy (SPORT) for Low-Risk Breast Cancer (SPORT) Phase I (n = 13) [142,148]	To investigate the tolerability of a Single Pre-Operative Radiation Therapy (SPORT)	Age ≥ 60 years cT1N0M0 ER+, HER2− unifocal, invasive ductal cancers	Single fraction of preoperative partial breast radiation dose: 20 Gy	Surgery: Early group (within 24–72 h) Late group (11–13 weeks)	Primary: Acute toxicity Secondary: Chronic toxicity and cosmetic outcome, IBTR	Pre/post analysis for Ki-67 and TILs	2020
NCT02482376 Phase II (n = 68) [149]	Preoperative single-fraction radiotherapy	Age ≥ 50 years T1N0M0 ER+/HER2+ Invasive ductal histology, DCIS Oncotype RS < 18 (for invasive ductal carcinoma)	Stereotactic Body Radiotherapy: Single fraction of 21 Gy.	BCS	Primary: Physician reported cosmetic outcomes Secondary: Patient reported cosmetic outcomes, rates of local control compared to the historic controls	Analysis for pre/post Ki-67 and gene expression analysis. Analysis of cfDNA for assessment of radiation response	2032
NCT03520894 Radiotherapy in Preoperative Setting with CyberKnife for Breast Cancer (ROCK) (n = 25) [150]	Preoperative radiotherapy with CyberKnife	Age ≥ 50 years T1N0M0, ER+/PR+ (≥10%)/HER2−, No LVI	Single fraction of 21 Gy	BCS	Primary: Acute skin toxicities Secondary: (3-years): pCR, rate of complete resection with <1 cm margin, LRR, metastasis progression-free survival, cause-specific survival OS, chronic cutaneous and extra-cutaneous toxicities	Radiogenomic analysis using validated signatures. Quantitative immunological analyses using fresh biopsies. IHC-based analysis for pericytes and assessment of vascularization. Serial biochemical analysis of peripheral blood and urine for biomarkers of oxidative stress	2024
NCT02212860 Stereotactic Image-Guided Neoadjuvant Ablative Radiation Then Lumpectomy (SIGNAL 2) (n = 139) [151]	Randomized trial to investigate 1 vs. 3 doses of preoperative stereotactic radiation therapy.	Age ≥ 50 years T < 3 cm, node-negative ER+/HER2−	Volumetric modulated arc therapy will be used to deliver: Single fraction of 21 Gy versus 3 fractions of 10 Gy	Surgery after 3 weeks	Primary: Biomarker assessment for immune priming, angiogenesis, hypoxia, proliferation, apoptosis, and invasion. Secondary: Cosmesis, DFS, mastectomy-free survival, and OS	Specified as primary endpoints	2023

Table 2. Cont.

Trial Identifier (n)	Study Description	Tumor Characteristics	Preoperative Radiation Regime +/− other Therapeutic Agents	Adjuvant Treatments	Endpoints	Prespecified/Exploratory Translational Studies	Estimated Study Completion Year
			Preoperative Radiotherapy (more than a single fraction)				
NCT04360330 Study for Selected Early-Stage Breast Cancer (SABER) Phase 1b (n = 18) [152]	To determine the most effective dose of preoperative radiation therapy that can be delivered in shorter duration before standard partial mastectomy/axillary surgery	Age ≥ 50 years Unifocal T1N0M0 ER+/PR+/HER2− (Oncotype MammaPrint required)	4 prespecified levels: (35 Gy, 40 Gy, 45 Gy, 50 Gy) in 5 fractions given on non-consecutive days, spanning 2 weeks	Partial mastectomy/axillary surgery 4–6 weeks after preoperative SABER. Standard of care adjuvant systemic therapy	Primary: Establish the most effective preoperative SABER dose. Secondary: Toxicity, pCR, cosmesis, and quality of life	Blood and tissue-based biomarkers Multiparametric MRI studies for assessment of radiation response	2025
NCT04224386 Phase 1b (n = 50) [153]	To determine safe and effective dose of pre-operative radiation delivered by FDA approved GammaPod device	Age ≥ 45 years T < 3 cm, N0, ER+/HER2− unifocal, ductal histology, no LVI	Delivery of focussed radiation using GammaPod: 4 prespecified doses: (21 Gy, 24 Gy, 27 Gy, 30 Gy)	BCS	Primary: Establish the most effective single-fraction radiation dose Dose-limiting toxicities Secondary: (5-years) Acute and late toxicities, surgical complications, cosmesis, quality of life, pCR and 5-year IBTR	Not stated	2028
NCT03624478 Phase II (n = 25) [154]	Hypofractionated radiotherapy to the whole breast alone before surgery	T0–2, N0 ≥18 years	Hypofractionated radiation therapy daily for 5 days.	Breast-conserving surgery 4–16 weeks after preoperative radiation	Primary: pCR. Secondary: Acute and late toxicities, LRR, distant recurrence, cause-specific survival, DFS, OS	Pre/post-treatment tumor mutation signatures	2022
NCT03043794 Phase II (n = 40) [155]	Single fraction Stereotactic Body Radiotherapy to the intact breast		Stereotactic Body Radiation: 21 Gy	Surgery	Primary endpoint: RCB 4–6 weeks after radiation prior to surgery Secondary: Toxicities, local recurrence, cosmesis, quality of life.	Not stated	2026

Table 2. Cont.

Trial Identifier (n)	Study Description	Tumor Characteristics	Preoperative Radiation Regime +/− other Therapeutic Agents	Adjuvant Treatments	Endpoints	Prespecified/Exploratory Translational Studies	Estimated Study Completion Year
Preoperative Radiotherapy and Immune Check Point Inhibitors							
NCT04454528 Radiation Boost to Enhance Immune Checkpoint Blockade Therapy (BreastVAX) Phase Ib/2 (n = 27) [146,147]	To investigate feasibility and efficacy of preoperative pembrolizumab +/− tumor-directed radiotherapy fraction	Age ≥ 18 years T1-2, N0–1M0 TNBC, hormone receptor+/HER2−, Hormone receptor +/− and HER2+	Single dose pembrolizumab +/− Hypofractionated (single fraction of radiation boost: 7 Gy)	Standard of care surgery	Primary: Feasibility of experimental treatment with no delay in surgery. Clinical response (physical exam, breast ultrasound, and histological evaluation)	Comparison of pre/post-treatment immune response on blood and tissue samples	2024
NCT03366844 Phase I/II (n = 60) [156]	Preoperative pembrolizumab and radiation boost	First cohort: ER+/HER2− with high-risk features (T1) Second cohort: TNBC T1	Pembrolizumab × single dose followed by second dose of pembrolizumab with radiation boost (24 Gy in 3 fractions)	Surgery and/or chemotherapy (within 8 weeks of enrollment) followed by standard radiation	Primary: Feasibility of experimental treatment with no delay in surgery Secondary: Treatment toxicities, iDFS, pCR	Change in TIL counts	2023
NCT03875573 Neo-CheckRay Phase II (n = 147) [157]	Neo-adjuvant chemotherapy combined with stereotactic body radiotherapy +/− durvalumab, +/− oleclumab (Neo-CheckRay) in luminal B breast cancers	Luminal B breast cancer patients randomized to: 1. paclitaxel→ddAC+preoperative radiation boost 2. Arm 1 + durvalumab 3. Arm 2 + antiCD73 antibody		Surgery 2–6 weeks after completion ddAC	Primary: Toxicities, Feasibility of surgery, Pathological evaluation for RCB Secondary: iDFS and cosmetic outcomes	Not stated	2026

Abbreviations: ER, estrogen receptor; HER2, human epidermal growth factor receptor 2; pCR, pathological complete response; RCB, residual cancer burden; DFS, disease-free survival; OS, overall survival; LRR, locoregional recurrence; iDFS, invasive disease-free survival; IBTR, ipsilateral breast tumor recurrence; TILs, tumor-infiltrating lymphocytes; IHC, immunohistochemistry; BCS, breast-conserving surgery; DCIS, ductal carcinoma in situ; RS, recurrence score; cfDNA, cell-free deoxyribonucleic acid; pCR, pathological complete response; ddAC, dose-dense doxorubicin, and cyclophosphamide.

While mature results from these ongoing trials are awaited, archival materials from completed randomized trials linked with long-term follow-up data can provide a valuable resource to investigate the impact of pre-treatment immune cell composition on prognosis and radiation response prediction.

Kovacs et al. [158] investigated the clinical value of stromal TILs on H&E stained sections prepared from pre-treatment primary tumor specimens of patients diagnosed with node-negative, stage I–II early breast cancers who were randomized to breast-conserving surgery with or without whole breast irradiation in the SweBCG91RT clinical trial [159,160]. Their results showed that among patients assigned to the radiation arm, high stromal TILs ($\geq$10%) were positively associated with a significantly lower probability of ipsilateral breast tumor recurrence in multivariate analysis. Patients whose tumors exhibited low stromal TILs (<10%) derived significant benefits from radiation as opposed to those with high stromal TILs, though the interaction test between radiation and TILs was not significant [158]. The authors expanded on their translational study by characterizing CD8 and FOXP3 expressing T lymphocytes by immunohistochemistry. They found that in contrast to immune-depleted tumors ($CD8^{low}/FOXP3^{low}$), immune-rich tumors ($CD8^{high}/FOXP3^{low}$) showed significantly reduced hazards for ipsilateral breast tumor recurrence or for any recurrence amongst unirradiated patients, perhaps instantiating the antitumoral attributes of the cytotoxic T cells. Additionally, the immune-depleted phenotype appeared to be of benefit from radiation. However, no such advantage was evident in the immune-rich tumors [161]. The relationship between the stromal TIL density and prognostic versus predictive value is rather counterintuitive in the translational studies by Tullberg and colleagues. This may be partly explained by an intrinsically favorable tumor biology indicated by a high stromal TIL density at baseline that translates into satisfactory local control. It is conceivable that these tumors may have an excellent outcome regardless of radiation. Alternatively, or in addition, radiation therapy may kill off activated, proliferating immune cells (a detrimental form of "collateral damage"). On the other hand, tumors with low stromal TILs are perhaps immunologically muted with a higher baseline risk, where radiation therapy appears to be useful in achieving optimal local control by potentially inducing antitumoral immune responses, perhaps through the release of neoantigens from tumor cells killed by radiotherapy (an abscopal effect).

The value of pre-treatment immune infiltrates has been recently examined in the Canadian MA.20 phase III clinical trial in which women undergoing breast-conserving surgery for T1–2, node-positive or node-negative breast cancer with poor risk features were randomized to standard irradiation with or without regional nodal radiation [162]. The results have shown that both CD8+ and H&E assessed stromal TILs informed favorable clinical outcomes when quantified as a continuous variable. Only CD8+ stromal TILs as a continuous parameter predicted response from regional nodal irradiation [163].

Taking advantage of the randomized design of the Danish Breast Cancer Cooperative Group 82bc clinical trial [164,165], Tramm and colleagues investigated the value of stromal TILs for predicting response from post-mastectomy irradiation. They reported that in the full cohort, high TILs ($\geq$30%) were favorably associated with overall survival and risk of distant metastasis. However, no prognostic value of TILs was found with regard to locoregional relapse risk. High stromal TILs were predictive for benefit in the group randomized to radiation for the endpoint of overall survival. Stratification according to ER status showed that ER-negative tumors with high TILs derived greater benefit from post-mastectomy radiation, whereas no such benefit was observed in ER-negative cases with low TIL counts. The improvement in the locoregional recurrence was independent of the immune infiltration [166].

Building on the abundance of clinical evidence supporting the role of immune biomarkers in risk stratification and guiding decisions for chemotherapy and immune checkpoint inhibitors, analogous data with respect to radiation therapy in early breast cancers is only beginning to emerge from prospective-retrospective studies. Since these trials were not originally designed for subtype-based translational studies, the lack of statistical power remains a major shortcoming in generating consistent results. Hence prospective validation in biomarker-directed studies is imperative. Testing the immune priming potential of radiation in combination with chemotherapy and/or immune checkpoint inhibitors provides an ideal opportunity to induce immune modulation in breast cancers which are largely considered to be poorly immunogenic. It is expected that accompanying, preplanned correlative studies will allow for an in-depth assessment of immunological responses (or lack thereof) in the primary tumor and draining lymph nodes that can inform future definitive clinical trials.

7. Biomarkers to Guide Adjuvant Radiation Decisions

Over the years, several groups have invested significant efforts to develop radiation-specific genomic classifiers for prognostication of locoregional relapse risk and prediction of response to radiation therapy. These classifiers have been reviewed in detail in previous publications [167,168], and those with the potential for clinical development are summarized in Table 3. To date, none of these classifiers have progressed to stages of analytical and clinical validity which is critical before these genomic assays can be tested for their clinical utility in phase III randomized trials [169–171].

Here we will focus on liquid biopsy-based approaches and review the recent investigations into the role of disseminated tumor cells and circulating tumor cells as prognostic biomarkers for locoregional relapse risk.

Table 3. Radiation Specific Genomic Classifiers.

Genomic Classifier	Description of the Classifier	Breast Cancer Cohort/Trial Characteristics	Prognostic Value	Predictive Value
Radiation Sensitivity Index (RSI) [172–174]	- Systems biology-based pan cancer radiosensitivity classifier of 10 hub genes that are involved in regulating radiation signaling pathways. - Developed by modeling the survival fraction of 48 human cancer cell lines at 2 Gy as a measure of cellular radiation responsiveness such that RSI index is directly proportional to radioresistance. - Validated in rectal, esophageal, and head and neck cancers treated with chemoradiation. - RSI is measured as a continuous score and categorized into 3 categories as: (a) RSI radioresistant subtype: Top 25th percentile of RSI scores, (b) RSI radiosensitive subtype: Lower 25th percentile of RSI scores, (c) RSI-intermediate subtype: RSI scores between the 25th–75th percentile	FIRST PUBLICATION COHORTS [173] (I) Karolinska prospective cohort: segmentectomy/mastectomy +RT (n = 77); mastectomy only (n = 82) (II) Erasmus cohort: BCS+RT (n = 219) MRM (n = 67) SECOND PUBLICATION COHORTS [174]: 4 Dutch + 1 French cohorts (n = 343) BCS+SLNB/Axillary dissection → WBI+/− RNI (Integration of RSI index with breast cancer molecular subtype)	RSI is a radiation-specific signature that has shown prognostic value in RT treated group but not in the no-RT group. FIRST PUBLICATION [173] Karolinska cohort: Compared to radioresistant patients, radiosensitive patients had improved 5-year RFS. Erasmus cohort: Compared to radioresistant patients, radiosensitive patients had improved 5-year DMFS. Multivariate analysis: Independent prognostic variable associated with outcome in RT-treated patients in both cohorts and in RT-treated ER+ subset in the Erasmus cohort. SECOND PUBLICATION [174]: -RSI index was not prognostic in the full cohort. - In patients with triple-negative subtype, RSI-resistant tumors were associated with higher risk of local relapse compared to those with RSI-sensitive/intermediate categories.	No
Radiation Sensitivity Signature (RSS) and Immune Signature (IMS) [175]	Gene signatures are based on intrinsic radiation sensitivity and antitumor immunity. RSS: 34 gene classifier was derived from MSigDB. IMS: comprised of 119 genes involved in antigen presentation and processing pathways curated from the Immunology Database and Analysis Portal. Four genes (ADRM1, MICB, PSMD13, RFXANK) showed significant interaction with radiotherapy. Immune-effective: IMS score > −3.8 Immune defective: IMSscore < −3.8	Model training cohort for RSS: GSE30682 cohort (n = 343) treated with BCS+RT. Endpoint: LRFS Model training cohort for IMS: E-TABM-158 RI: n = 66, No RI: n = 63. Endpoint: DSS Validation of ISS and IMS: METABRIC cohort (n = 1981)	In the METABRIC cohort: For radiation-sensitive group, patients who received radiotherapy experienced an improved DSS than those who did not. For immune-effective group, patients treated with radiotherapy had significantly better DSS compared with those without radiation therapy. Combined ISS and IMS were validated in the METABRIC cohort. Patients were categorized into four groups: -Concordant group: immune-sensitive/immune effective group treated with radiation had significantly better DSS. -Concordant group: immune-resistant/immune defective treated with radiation had significantly poor DSS. No significant prognostic associations were found in the two discordant groups.	When evaluated independently, both RSS and IMS predicted benefit from radiation in the RI-treated cohort for the endpoint of DSS. Integration of RSS and IMS stratified patients into groups. Benefit from radiation is seen in the radiation-sensitive/immune effective group treated with radiotherapy. Radiation resistant/immune defective group did not derive benefit from radiation.

Table 3. Cont.

Genomic Classifier	Description of the Classifier	Breast Cancer Cohort/Trial Characteristics	Prognostic Value	Predictive Value
DBCG-RT Profile [176]	7 gene classifiers (HLA-DQA, RCS1, DNAL11, hCG2023290, IGKC, OR8G2, and ADH1B) developed on the fresh frozen tissues from the training cohort. The classifier stratified the training cohort into high- and low-risk groups for locoregional relapse. The final signature consisted of 4 genes (IGKC, RCS1, ADH1B, and DNAL11) as the remaining 3 genes failed quality control during transfer to formalin fixed paraffin embedded tissues.	DBCG82b/c randomized clinical trial: 3083 women (<70 years) with high-risk disease randomized PMRT+RNI or not. All post-menopausal women received tamoxifen (82c) and premenopausal women (82b) received CMF. Training set = 191 Validation set: 112	Prognostic value was assessed in the non-irradiated group of training set who received systemic treatments and stratified the population into two groups: low LRR risk and high LRR risk, which demonstrated low- and high-risk for locoregional failures, respectively. Multivariate analysis: DBCG-RT profile provided independent prognostic information for locoregional relapse risk.	Predictive value was demonstrated in both training and validation cohorts. DBCG-RT profile predicted benefit from PMRT in patients classified as high-risk-LRR. No benefit was derived from PMRT in DBCG-RT low-risk category.
Radiation Sensitivity Signature (RSS) [177]	Clonogenic survival assays were performed on a panel of 16 breast cancer cell lines to identify the surviving fraction at 2 Gy, which represents the intrinsic radiosensitivity or radioresistance of the breast cancer cells. The classifier was trained and cross-validated from 147 to 51 genes enriched in cell cycle, DNA damage, and DNA repair pathways. The classifier was independent of breast cancer molecular subtypes.	Training cohort (n = 343) treated with BCS + RT for which locoregional recurrence data were available. Validation cohort (n = 228) treated with mastectomy or BCT and radiation if indicated.	RSS provided prognostic information for overall survival of locoregional recurrences and stratifies patients unlikely to develop local recurrence after radiation from those at high risk of recurrence despite receiving standard radiation.	No
Adjuvant Radiotherapy Intensification Classifier (ARTIC) [178]	Clinicogenomic classifier comprising of 27 genes and age.	Training cohort: 3 publicly available data sets with gene expression data: Servant (n = 343) van de Vijver (n = 228) Lund fresh frozen (n = 102) Validation cohort: SweBCG91-RT phase III trial cohort (n = 748) in which patients were treated with BCS with or without radiation.	ARTIC provided prognostic information for locoregional recurrence in both the treatment arms (with or without radiation).	Patients with low ARTIC scores derived significant benefits from radiation for the endpoint of locoregional recurrence compared to patients with high ARTIC scores who gained less from radiation.
Profile for the Omission of Local Adjuvant Radiotherapy (POLAR) [179]	Transcriptome-wide profiling of tumors was performed using the Affymetrix Human Exon 1.0 ST microarray. A 16-gene signature (proliferation and immune response) was trained in the training set of patients who did not receive radiation.	SweBCG91-RT cohort was divided into a training set (n = 243) and validation set (n = 354)	Tumors with POLAR low-risk had a 10-year locoregional recurrence rate of 7% in the absence of radiation. POLAR high-risk had a significantly decreased risk of locoregional recurrence when treated with radiation.	Independent external validation for predictive performance was performed in 623 patients from three randomized clinical trials (SweBCG91-RT, n = 354; Scottish Conservation Trial; n = 137 and trial from Princess Margaret Hospital, Canada, n = 132). High POLAR score was predictive of benefits from radiation with significant reduction in the local recurrence rate [180,181].

Abbreviations: MRM, modified radical mastectomy; BCT, breast-conserving therapy; RT, radiation therapy; SLNB, sentinel lymph node biopsy; RFS, relapse-free survival; PMRT, post-mastectomy radiation therapy; RNI, regional nodal irradiation; DMFS, distant metastasis-free survival; LRR, locoregional recurrence; DFS, disease-specific survival; CMF, cyclophosphamide methotrexate fluorouracil.

7.1. Disseminated Tumor Cells

Disseminated tumor cells (DTCs) are isolated cancer cells that, upon physical detachment from the primary tumor, escape the circulation, extravasate into distant sites such as bone marrow, and are capable of survival in a hostile host niche, reversible quiescence, and therapeutic resistance. DTCs detected via bone marrow aspiration are found in approximately 40% of women with stage I–III breast cancers who do not have any clinical or histological evidence of overt metastatic disease at initial presentation. A substantial body of evidence from clinical studies has demonstrated that compared to patients without DTCs, those with DTC positivity have features of aggressive tumor biology, including larger tumor size, higher grade, axillary lymph node metastasis, estrogen/progesterone receptor negativity, and HER2 positivity [182,183]. An earlier pooled analysis of 9 studies comprising 4703 patients with operable breast cancer (enrolled before 2002) provided evidence for a strong association of DTCs with significant adverse outcomes [182]. These findings have been further confirmed in a recently published patient-level meta-analysis comprising 10,307 early breast cancer patients from 11 centers with a median follow-up of 7.6 years [183].

Only a few studies have investigated the impact of bone marrow occult metastasis on locoregional relapses, showing either no association [183–185] or a significantly increased risk of locoregional failures. In a single centre prospective cohort of more than 3000 stage I–III treatment naïve breast cancers, Hartkopf and colleagues demonstrated bone marrow DTCs in 24% of patients at the time of initial surgical intervention. DTC positivity was independently associated with locoregional failures. Their results further revealed that, of the available biopsy samples from patients with isolated local relapses, the 55 subjected to a repeat bone marrow aspiration showed a DTC detection rate of 35% [186]. Bidard et al. investigated the relationship between locoregional relapse-free survival and bone marrow DTCs in a prospective cohort of 621 patients from Institute Curie's Breast Cancer Micrometastasis Project for a median follow-up of 4.6 years. In this cohort, 15% of patients had detectable DTCs in the bone marrow. Overall, 18/621 patients experienced a locoregional relapse, among whom 44% had evidence of DTCs at their initial evaluation. Amongst patients with DTC positivity, a longer locoregional relapse-free survival was observed in patients who received endocrine therapy and radiation to supraclavicular/internal mammary lymph nodes [187]. These results remained consistent at an updated median follow-up of 11.7 years, where there was a 10-year locoregional relapse rate of 20% in patients with DTC-positive status compared to 10% in those without, supporting the capacity of DTCs as a biomarker predictive of benefit from regional nodal irradiation [188]. The biological basis of locoregional relapse in patients with bone marrow micrometastasis is not completely understood. However, preclinical studies using mouse models suggest that DTCs may transition into circulating tumor cells, a fraction of which have the potential to re-colonize the primary tumor site [189]. It is conceivable that irradiating regional lymph nodes in patients with DTC-positive status may eradicate subclinical micrometastases and may serve as a candidate predictive biomarker for optimizing patient selection for regional nodal irradiation. This may be potentially relevant in the context of selecting patients who may benefit most from irradiation of regional lymph nodes [162,190–192].

7.2. Circulating Tumor Cells

Circulating tumor cells (CTCs) are occult malignant cells that exit from the primary tumor into the circulation and are associated with enhanced metastatic potential [193]. When examined prior to any treatment (neoadjuvant chemotherapy or upfront surgery) by utilizing CellSearch®, an FDA-approved standardized assay, the prevalence of CTCs has been found to be 25% in an international meta-analysis including 2156 patients from 21 studies. After eliminating T4 tumors from analysis, CTC positivity did not have a statistically prominent association with clinicopathological factors or pathological complete response. However, CTC presence prior to initiation of neoadjuvant therapy was indicative of shortened disease-free survival, overall survival, and locoregional relapse-free interval in univariate and multivariate analyses. Moreover, the inclusion of baseline CTC counts significantly improved the prognostic capacity of the clinicopathological model [194].

Goodman and colleagues have reported on the association between CTCs and response to adjuvant radiation in patients with pT1–T2, N0–1 early breast cancer utilizing patients' clinical and CTC data from the National Cancer Database (n = 1697) and validated their findings in a cohort from the German SUCCESS trial [195,196] (n = 1516). CTC positivity was associated with the benefit from adjuvant radiation with a significant increase in overall survival in the National Cancer Database cohort and in disease-free-, overall, and locoregional relapse-free survival in the SUCCESS cohort. In addition, an improvement in overall survival was seen in CTC+ patients undergoing breast-conserving surgery with standard adjuvant radiation but not in CTC- patients. When stratified by CTC status, the benefit of radiation was not evident in patients treated with mastectomy. These results should be interpreted carefully in light of the existing evidence [5,197], as adjuvant radiation was not the randomization criteria in either of the evaluated cohorts. Nevertheless, these encouraging results support value for CTCs as a potential biomarker for guiding radiotherapy decisions, requiring prospective validation to analyze the benefit of adjuvant radiation therapy in low-risk patients with CTC positivity who otherwise might otherwise be considered for radiation omission.

BreastImmune03 is a randomized phase II clinical trial designed to assess the clinical benefit of post-surgery adjuvant radiotherapy + immunotherapy with nivolumab + ipilimumab, versus radiotherapy + capecitabine in TNBC patients with residual disease after neoadjuvant chemotherapy. Evaluation of CTC will be performed as a secondary outcome measure for immune monitoring at cycles 1, 2, 5, and 2 years post-randomization or in the event of a relapse [198].

8. Summary

Adjuvant radiotherapy is an integral component of early breast cancer management, with proven efficacy for preventing locoregional and distant failures. Over the years, traditional whole breast irradiation approaches have evolved considerably, such that the less intensive option of whole breast hypofractionated radiation has now become the preferred standard, yielding improved compliance, cosmetic outcomes, and quality of life. More recent data have shown the comparable efficacy and safety of an ultra-hypofractionation regimen that is delivered as five fractions in less than a week. Equivalence of accelerated partial breast radiation delivered by external beam has been demonstrated in several clinical trials and endorsed for women with tumors with favorable biology, and together with ultra-hypofractionation, may be an attractive option in resource-restricted regions. Investigations for further de-intensifying radiation schedules using ultra-accelerated partial breast radiation as a single fraction are being planned to be tested against accelerated partial breast radiation + endocrine therapy [199,200].

The encouraging results of the LUMINA trial support the safe omission of adjuvant radiation following breast-conserving surgery when selection criteria are strictly limited to low-risk cancers (T1N0, grade 1 or 2) with luminal A phenotype with a Ki-67 index of $\leq$ 13.25%. This and the other ongoing trials of radiation omission underscore the significance of biomarker-driven risk stratification for critical decisions involving radiation de-escalation. These trials are a step forward in personalizing options for radiation, the integration of which into clinical practice has lagged behind analogous de-escalation protocols in systemic therapy.

Recognizing the immune-modulatory potential of radiation, the ongoing clinical trials of pre-operative radiotherapy will provide opportunities to investigate combinatorial therapies in early-stage settings. Nevertheless, critical to the success of immune priming approaches will be the understanding of the biological interactions of host immunity with key factors that influence immune-modulating properties of radiotherapy, such as radiation dose, quality, fractionation schedules, and sequence of the therapies [201].

Ultimately, the actively evolving scientific understanding of breast cancer biology is driving clinical trials that are providing radiation oncologists and women with breast cancer with the information they need to make personalized choices that both protect them from recurrences and from unwarranted treatment morbidity. In view of the evolving evidence, therapeutic strategies incorporating tumor and patient characteristics, as well as patient preferences, should be discussed in a multidisciplinary tumor board to tailor the treatment for the patient [10].

Author Contributions: Conceptualization: N.R. and T.O.N.; methodology: N.R., T.J., T.J.W. and T.O.N.; investigation: N.R., T.J., T.J.W. and T.O.N.; resources, T.J.W. and T.O.N.; writing—original draft preparation: N.R., T.J. and T.O.N.; writing—review and editing: N.R., T.J., T.J.W. and T.O.N.; supervision: T.J.W. and T.O.N. All authors have read and agreed to the published version of the manuscript.

Funding: This research was funded by the grants awarded by the Canadian Cancer Society (706768) and the Cancer Research Society (944513).

Conflicts of Interest: T.O.N. reports grants from the Canadian Cancer Society and the Cancer Research Society; personal fees from Bioclassifier LLC and NanoString Technologies outside the submitted work; In addition, Nielsen has a patent gene expression profile to predict breast cancer outcomes with royalties paid by licensee Veracyte. Other authors have nothing to disclose.

References

1. Fisher, B.; Anderson, S.; Bryant, J.; Margolese, R.G.; Deutsch, M.; Fisher, E.R.; Jeong, J.H.; Wolmark, N. Twenty-year follow-up of a randomized trial comparing total mastectomy, lumpectomy, and lumpectomy plus irradiation for the treatment of invasive breast cancer. *N. Engl. J. Med.* **2002**, *347*, 1233–1241. [CrossRef] [PubMed]
2. Veronesi, U.; Cascinelli, N.; Mariani, L.; Greco, M.; Saccozzi, R.; Luini, A.; Aguilar, M.; Marubini, E. Twenty-year follow-up of a randomized study comparing breast-conserving surgery with radical mastectomy for early breast cancer. *N. Engl. J. Med.* **2002**, *347*, 1227–1232. [CrossRef] [PubMed]
3. Cardoso, F.; Kyriakides, S.; Ohno, S.; Penault-Llorca, F.; Poortmans, P.; Rubio, I.T.; Zackrisson, S.; Senkus, E.; Committee, E.G. Early breast cancer: ESMO Clinical Practice Guidelines for diagnosis, treatment and follow-up. *Ann. Oncol.* **2019**, *30*, 1674. [CrossRef] [PubMed]
4. Gradishar, W.J.; Moran, M.S.; Abraham, J.; Aft, R.; Agnese, D.; Allison, K.H.; Anderson, B.; Burstein, H.J.; Chew, H.; Dang, C.; et al. Breast Cancer, Version 3.2022, NCCN Clinical Practice Guidelines in Oncology. *J. Natl. Compr. Cancer Netw.* **2022**, *20*, 691–722. [CrossRef] [PubMed]
5. Early Breast Cancer Trialists' Collaborative, G.; Darby, S.; McGale, P.; Correa, C.; Taylor, C.; Arriagada, R.; Clarke, M.; Cutter, D.; Davies, C.; Ewertz, M.; et al. Effect of radiotherapy after breast-conserving surgery on 10-year recurrence and 15-year breast cancer death: Meta-analysis of individual patient data for 10,801 women in 17 randomised trials. *Lancet* **2011**, *378*, 1707–1716. [CrossRef]
6. Kindts, I.; Laenen, A.; Depuydt, T.; Weltens, C. Tumour bed boost radiotherapy for women after breast-conserving surgery. *Cochrane Database Syst. Rev.* **2017**, *11*, CD011987. [CrossRef] [PubMed]
7. Miller, K.D.; Nogueira, L.; Devasia, T.; Mariotto, A.B.; Yabroff, K.R.; Jemal, A.; Kramer, J.; Siegel, R.L. Cancer treatment and survivorship statistics, 2022. *CA Cancer J. Clin.* **2022**, *72*, 409–436. [CrossRef]
8. Marta, G.N.; Riera, R.; Pacheco, R.L.; Cabrera Martimbianco, A.L.; Meattini, I.; Kaidar-Person, O.; Poortmans, P. Moderately hypofractionated post-operative radiation therapy for breast cancer: Systematic review and meta-analysis of randomized clinical trials. *Breast* **2022**, *62*, 84–92. [CrossRef]
9. Whelan, T.J.; Kim, D.H.; Sussman, J. Clinical experience using hypofractionated radiation schedules in breast cancer. *Semin. Radiat. Oncol.* **2008**, *18*, 257–264. [CrossRef]
10. Palumbo, I.; Borghesi, S.; Gregucci, F.; Falivene, S.; Fontana, A.; Aristei, C.; Ciabattoni, A. Omission of adjuvant radiotherapy for older adults with early-stage breast cancer particularly in the COVID era: A literature review (on the behalf of Italian Association of Radiotherapy and Clinical Oncology). *J. Geriatr. Oncol.* **2021**, *12*, 1130–1135. [CrossRef]
11. Herskovic, A.C.; Wu, X.; Christos, P.J.; Nagar, H. Omission of Adjuvant Radiotherapy in the Elderly Breast Cancer Patient: Missed Opportunity? *Clin. Breast Cancer* **2018**, *18*, 418–431. [CrossRef] [PubMed]
12. Franco, P.; De Rose, F.; De Santis, M.C.; Pasinetti, N.; Lancellotta, V.; Meduri, B.; Meattini, I.; Clinical Oncology Breast Cancer Group, I. Omission of postoperative radiation after breast conserving surgery: A progressive paradigm shift towards precision medicine. *Clin. Transl. Radiat. Oncol.* **2020**, *21*, 112–119. [CrossRef] [PubMed]
13. Hughes, K.S.; Schnaper, L.A.; Bellon, J.R.; Cirrincione, C.T.; Berry, D.A.; McCormick, B.; Muss, H.B.; Smith, B.L.; Hudis, C.A.; Winer, E.P.; et al. Lumpectomy plus tamoxifen with or without irradiation in women age 70 years or older with early breast cancer: Long-term follow-up of CALGB 9343. *J. Clin. Oncol.* **2013**, *31*, 2382–2387. [CrossRef] [PubMed]

14. Kunkler, I.H.; Williams, L.J.; Jack, W.; Cameron, D.A.; Dixon, M. Abstract GS2-03: Prime 2 randomised trial (postoperative radiotherapy in minimum-risk elderly): Wide local excision and adjuvant hormonal therapy +/− whole breast irradiation in women =/> 65 years with early invasive breast cancer: 10 year results. *Cancer Res.* **2021**, *81*, GS2-03. [CrossRef]
15. Kunkler, I.H.; Williams, L.J.; Jack, W.J.; Cameron, D.A.; Dixon, J.M.; Investigators, P.I. Breast-conserving surgery with or without irradiation in women aged 65 years or older with early breast cancer (PRIME II): A randomised controlled trial. *Lancet Oncol.* **2015**, *16*, 266–273. [CrossRef] [PubMed]
16. National Comprehensive Cancer Network, B.C.V. Breast Cancer Version 4. 2022. Available online: https://www.nccn.org/professionals/physician_gls/pdf/breast.pdf (accessed on 1 December 2022).
17. Matar, R.; Sevilimedu, V.; Gemignani, M.L.; Morrow, M. Impact of Endocrine Therapy Adherence on Outcomes in Elderly Women with Early-Stage Breast Cancer Undergoing Lumpectomy Without Radiotherapy. *Ann. Surg. Oncol.* **2022**, *29*, 4753–4760. [CrossRef] [PubMed]
18. Downs-Canner, S.; Zabor, E.C.; Wind, T.; Cobovic, A.; McCormick, B.; Morrow, M.; Heerdt, A. Radiation Therapy After Breast-Conserving Surgery in Women 70 Years of Age and Older: How Wisely Do We Choose? *Ann. Surg. Oncol.* **2019**, *26*, 969–975. [CrossRef]
19. Squeo, G.; Malpass, J.K.; Meneveau, M.; Balkrishnan, R.; Desai, R.P.; Lattimore, C.; Anderson, R.T.; Showalter, S.L. Long-term Impact of CALGB 9343 on Radiation Utilization. *J. Surg. Res.* **2020**, *256*, 577–583. [CrossRef]
20. Xie, Y.; Wang, Q.; Hu, T.; Chen, R.; Wang, J.; Chang, H.; Cheng, J. Risk Factors Related to Acute Radiation Dermatitis in Breast Cancer Patients After Radiotherapy: A Systematic Review and Meta-Analysis. *Front. Oncol.* **2021**, *11*, 738851. [CrossRef]
21. Ramseier, J.Y.; Ferreira, M.N.; Leventhal, J.S. Dermatologic toxicities associated with radiation therapy in women with breast cancer. *Int. J. Women's Dermatol.* **2020**, *6*, 349–356. [CrossRef]
22. Hickey, B.E.; Lehman, M. Partial breast irradiation versus whole breast radiotherapy for early breast cancer. *Cochrane Database Syst. Rev.* **2021**, *8*, CD007077. [CrossRef] [PubMed]
23. DiSipio, T.; Rye, S.; Newman, B.; Hayes, S. Incidence of unilateral arm lymphoedema after breast cancer: A systematic review and meta-analysis. *Lancet Oncol.* **2013**, *14*, 500–515. [CrossRef] [PubMed]
24. McDuff, S.G.R.; Mina, A.I.; Brunelle, C.L.; Salama, L.; Warren, L.E.G.; Abouegylah, M.; Swaroop, M.; Skolny, M.N.; Asdourian, M.; Gillespie, T.; et al. Timing of Lymphedema After Treatment for Breast Cancer: When Are Patients Most At Risk? *Int. J. Radiat. Oncol. Biol. Phys.* **2019**, *103*, 62–70. [CrossRef] [PubMed]
25. Poortmans, P.M.; Struikmans, H.; De Brouwer, P.; Weltens, C.; Fortpied, C.; Kirkove, C.; Budach, V.; Peignaux-Casasnovas, K.; van der Leij, F.; Vonk, E.; et al. Side Effects 15 Years After Lymph Node Irradiation in Breast Cancer: Randomized EORTC Trial 22922/10925. *J. Natl. Cancer Inst.* **2021**, *113*, 1360–1368. [CrossRef] [PubMed]
26. Milo, M.L.H.; Thorsen, L.B.J.; Johnsen, S.P.; Nielsen, K.M.; Valentin, J.B.; Alsner, J.; Offersen, B.V. Risk of coronary artery disease after adjuvant radiotherapy in 29,662 early breast cancer patients: A population-based Danish Breast Cancer Group study. *Radiother. Oncol.* **2021**, *157*, 106–113. [CrossRef] [PubMed]
27. Yit, L.F.N.; Ng, C.T.; Wong, F.Y.; Master, Z.; Zhou, S.; Ng, W.L. Modern-era radiotherapy and ischaemic heart disease-related mortality outcomes in Asian breast-cancer patients. *Contemp. Oncol.* **2022**, *26*, 59–68. [CrossRef] [PubMed]
28. Mulliez, T.; Miedema, G.; Van Parijs, H.; Hottat, N.; Vassilieff, M.; Gillet, E.; Baeyens, L.; Voordeckers, M.; Coelmont, J.; Besse-Hammer, T.; et al. Pre-OPerative accelerated radiotherapy for early stage breast cancer patients (POPART): A feasibility study. *Radiother. Oncol.* **2022**, *170*, 118–121. [CrossRef]
29. Smith, B.D.; Bellon, J.R.; Blitzblau, R.; Freedman, G.; Haffty, B.; Hahn, C.; Halberg, F.; Hoffman, K.; Horst, K.; Moran, J.; et al. Radiation therapy for the whole breast: Executive summary of an American Society for Radiation Oncology (ASTRO) evidence-based guideline. *Pract. Radiat. Oncol.* **2018**, *8*, 145–152. [CrossRef]
30. Deshmukh, A.A.; Shirvani, S.M.; Lal, L.; Swint, J.M.; Cantor, S.B.; Smith, B.D.; Likhacheva, A. Cost-effectiveness Analysis Comparing Conventional, Hypofractionated, and Intraoperative Radiotherapy for Early-Stage Breast Cancer. *J. Natl. Cancer Inst.* **2017**, *109*, djx068. [CrossRef]
31. Whelan, T.J.; Levine, M.; Julian, J.; Kirkbride, P.; Skingley, P. The effects of radiation therapy on quality of life of women with breast carcinoma: Results of a randomized trial. Ontario Clinical Oncology Group. *Cancer* **2000**, *88*, 2260–2266. [CrossRef]
32. Lautner, M.; Lin, H.; Shen, Y.; Parker, C.; Kuerer, H.; Shaitelman, S.; Babiera, G.; Bedrosian, I. Disparities in the Use of Breast-Conserving Therapy Among Patients With Early-Stage Breast Cancer. *JAMA Surg.* **2015**, *150*, 778–786. [CrossRef]
33. Parekh, A.; Fu, W.; Hu, C.; Shen, C.J.; Alcorn, S.; Rao, A.D.; Asrari, F.; Camp, M.S.; Wright, J.L. Impact of race, ethnicity, and socioeconomic factors on receipt of radiation after breast conservation surgery: Analysis of the national cancer database. *Breast Cancer Res. Treat.* **2018**, *172*, 201–208. [CrossRef] [PubMed]
34. Pan, I.W.; Smith, B.D.; Shih, Y.C. Factors contributing to underuse of radiation among younger women with breast cancer. *J. Natl. Cancer Inst.* **2014**, *106*, djt340. [CrossRef]
35. Lam, J.; Cook, T.; Foster, S.; Poon, R.; Milross, C.; Sundaresan, P. Examining Determinants of Radiotherapy Access: Do Cost and Radiotherapy Inconvenience Affect Uptake of Breast-conserving Treatment for Early Breast Cancer? *Clin. Oncol.* **2015**, *27*, 465–471. [CrossRef] [PubMed]
36. Gu, J.; Groot, G.; Boden, C.; Busch, A.; Holtslander, L.; Lim, H. Review of Factors Influencing Women's Choice of Mastectomy Versus Breast Conserving Therapy in Early Stage Breast Cancer: A Systematic Review. *Clin. Breast Cancer* **2018**, *18*, e539–e554. [CrossRef] [PubMed]

37. Yarnold, J.; Bentzen, S.M.; Coles, C.; Haviland, J. Hypofractionated whole-breast radiotherapy for women with early breast cancer: Myths and realities. *Int. J. Radiat. Oncol. Biol. Phys.* **2011**, *79*, 1–9. [CrossRef]
38. Whelan, T.J.; Pignol, J.P.; Levine, M.N.; Julian, J.A.; MacKenzie, R.; Parpia, S.; Shelley, W.; Grimard, L.; Bowen, J.; Lukka, H.; et al. Long-term results of hypofractionated radiation therapy for breast cancer. *N. Engl. J. Med.* **2010**, *362*, 513–520. [CrossRef]
39. Offersen, B.V.; Alsner, J.; Nielsen, H.M.; Jakobsen, E.H.; Nielsen, M.H.; Krause, M.; Stenbygaard, L.; Mjaaland, I.; Schreiber, A.; Kasti, U.M.; et al. Hypofractionated Versus Standard Fractionated Radiotherapy in Patients With Early Breast Cancer or Ductal Carcinoma In Situ in a Randomized Phase III Trial: The DBCG HYPO Trial. *J. Clin. Oncol.* **2020**, *38*, 3615–3625. [CrossRef]
40. Haviland, J.S.; Owen, J.R.; Dewar, J.A.; Agrawal, R.K.; Barrett, J.; Barrett-Lee, P.J.; Dobbs, H.J.; Hopwood, P.; Lawton, P.A.; Magee, B.J.; et al. The UK Standardisation of Breast Radiotherapy (START) trials of radiotherapy hypofractionation for treatment of early breast cancer: 10-year follow-up results of two randomised controlled trials. *Lancet Oncol.* **2013**, *14*, 1086–1094. [CrossRef]
41. Brunt, A.M.; Haviland, J.S.; Sydenham, M.; Agrawal, R.K.; Algurafi, H.; Alhasso, A.; Barrett-Lee, P.; Bliss, P.; Bloomfield, D.; Bowen, J.; et al. Ten-Year Results of FAST: A Randomized Controlled Trial of 5-Fraction Whole-Breast Radiotherapy for Early Breast Cancer. *J. Clin. Oncol.* **2020**, *38*, 3261–3272. [CrossRef]
42. Murray Brunt, A.; Haviland, J.S.; Wheatley, D.A.; Sydenham, M.A.; Alhasso, A.; Bloomfield, D.J.; Chan, C.; Churn, M.; Cleator, S.; Coles, C.E.; et al. Hypofractionated breast radiotherapy for 1 week versus 3 weeks (FAST-Forward): 5-year efficacy and late normal tissue effects results from a multicentre, non-inferiority, randomised, phase 3 trial. *Lancet* **2020**, *395*, 1613–1626. [CrossRef] [PubMed]
43. Freedman, G.M.; Anderson, P.R.; Hanlon, A.L.; Eisenberg, D.F.; Nicolaou, N. Pattern of local recurrence after conservative surgery and whole-breast irradiation. *Int. J. Radiat. Oncol. Biol. Phys.* **2005**, *61*, 1328–1336. [CrossRef] [PubMed]
44. Strnad, V.; Ott, O.J.; Hildebrandt, G.; Kauer-Dorner, D.; Knauerhase, H.; Major, T.; Lyczek, J.; Guinot, J.L.; Dunst, J.; Gutierrez Miguelez, C.; et al. 5-year results of accelerated partial breast irradiation using sole interstitial multicatheter brachytherapy versus whole-breast irradiation with boost after breast-conserving surgery for low-risk invasive and in-situ carcinoma of the female breast: A randomised, phase 3, non-inferiority trial. *Lancet* **2016**, *387*, 229–238. [CrossRef] [PubMed]
45. Polgar, C.; Ott, O.J.; Hildebrandt, G.; Kauer-Dorner, D.; Knauerhase, H.; Major, T.; Lyczek, J.; Guinot, J.L.; Dunst, J.; Miguelez, C.G.; et al. Late side-effects and cosmetic results of accelerated partial breast irradiation with interstitial brachytherapy versus whole-breast irradiation after breast-conserving surgery for low-risk invasive and in-situ carcinoma of the female breast: 5-year results of a randomised, controlled, phase 3 trial. *Lancet Oncol.* **2017**, *18*, 259–268. [CrossRef]
46. Shah, C.; Badiyan, S.; Ben Wilkinson, J.; Vicini, F.; Beitsch, P.; Keisch, M.; Arthur, D.; Lyden, M. Treatment efficacy with accelerated partial breast irradiation (APBI): Final analysis of the American Society of Breast Surgeons MammoSite((R)) breast brachytherapy registry trial. *Ann. Surg. Oncol.* **2013**, *20*, 3279–3285. [CrossRef]
47. Polgar, C.; Fodor, J.; Major, T.; Sulyok, Z.; Kasler, M. Breast-conserving therapy with partial or whole breast irradiation: Ten-year results of the Budapest randomized trial. *Radiother. Oncol.* **2013**, *108*, 197–202. [CrossRef]
48. Shah, C.; Khwaja, S.; Badiyan, S.; Wilkinson, J.B.; Vicini, F.A.; Beitsch, P.; Keisch, M.; Arthur, D.; Lyden, M. Brachytherapy-based partial breast irradiation is associated with low rates of complications and excellent cosmesis. *Brachytherapy* **2013**, *12*, 278–284. [CrossRef]
49. Vaidya, J.S.; Wenz, F.; Bulsara, M.; Tobias, J.S.; Joseph, D.J.; Keshtgar, M.; Flyger, H.L.; Massarut, S.; Alvarado, M.; Saunders, C.; et al. Risk-adapted targeted intraoperative radiotherapy versus whole-breast radiotherapy for breast cancer: 5-year results for local control and overall survival from the TARGIT-A randomised trial. *Lancet* **2014**, *383*, 603–613. [CrossRef]
50. Veronesi, U.; Orecchia, R.; Maisonneuve, P.; Viale, G.; Rotmensz, N.; Sangalli, C.; Luini, A.; Veronesi, P.; Galimberti, V.; Zurrida, S.; et al. Intraoperative radiotherapy versus external radiotherapy for early breast cancer (ELIOT): A randomised controlled equivalence trial. *Lancet Oncol.* **2013**, *14*, 1269–1277. [CrossRef]
51. Orecchia, R.; Veronesi, U.; Maisonneuve, P.; Galimberti, V.E.; Lazzari, R.; Veronesi, P.; Jereczek-Fossa, B.A.; Cattani, F.; Sangalli, C.; Luini, A.; et al. Intraoperative irradiation for early breast cancer (ELIOT): Long-term recurrence and survival outcomes from a single-centre, randomised, phase 3 equivalence trial. *Lancet Oncol.* **2021**, *22*, 597–608. [CrossRef]
52. Coles, C.E.; Griffin, C.L.; Kirby, A.M.; Titley, J.; Agrawal, R.K.; Alhasso, A.; Bhattacharya, I.S.; Brunt, A.M.; Ciurlionis, L.; Chan, C.; et al. Partial-breast radiotherapy after breast conservation surgery for patients with early breast cancer (UK IMPORT LOW trial): 5-year results from a multicentre, randomised, controlled, phase 3, non-inferiority trial. *Lancet* **2017**, *390*, 1048–1060. [CrossRef] [PubMed]
53. Whelan, T.J.; Julian, J.A.; Berrang, T.S.; Kim, D.H.; Germain, I.; Nichol, A.M.; Akra, M.; Lavertu, S.; Germain, F.; Fyles, A.; et al. External beam accelerated partial breast irradiation versus whole breast irradiation after breast conserving surgery in women with ductal carcinoma in situ and node-negative early breast cancer (RAPID): A randomised controlled trial. *Lancet* **2019**, *394*, 2165–2172. [CrossRef] [PubMed]
54. Li, X.; Sanz, J.; Foro, P.; Martinez, A.; Zhao, M.; Reig, A.; Liu, F.; Huang, Y.; Membrive, I.; Algara, M.; et al. Long-term results of a randomized partial irradiation trial compared to whole breast irradiation in the early stage and low-risk breast cancer patients after conservative surgery. *Clin. Transl. Oncol.* **2021**, *23*, 2127–2132. [CrossRef] [PubMed]
55. Livi, L.; Meattini, I.; Marrazzo, L.; Simontacchi, G.; Pallotta, S.; Saieva, C.; Paiar, F.; Scotti, V.; De Luca Cardillo, C.; Bastiani, P.; et al. Accelerated partial breast irradiation using intensity-modulated radiotherapy versus whole breast irradiation: 5-year survival analysis of a phase 3 randomised controlled trial. *Eur. J. Cancer* **2015**, *51*, 451–463. [CrossRef]

56. Meattini, I.; Marrazzo, L.; Saieva, C.; Desideri, I.; Scotti, V.; Simontacchi, G.; Bonomo, P.; Greto, D.; Mangoni, M.; Scoccianti, S.; et al. Accelerated Partial-Breast Irradiation Compared With Whole-Breast Irradiation for Early Breast Cancer: Long-Term Results of the Randomized Phase III APBI-IMRT-Florence Trial. *J. Clin. Oncol.* **2020**, *38*, 4175–4183. [CrossRef]
57. Vicini, F.A.; Cecchini, R.S.; White, J.R.; Arthur, D.W.; Julian, T.B.; Rabinovitch, R.A.; Kuske, R.R.; Ganz, P.A.; Parda, D.S.; Scheier, M.F.; et al. Long-term primary results of accelerated partial breast irradiation after breast-conserving surgery for early-stage breast cancer: A randomised, phase 3, equivalence trial. *Lancet* **2019**, *394*, 2155–2164. [CrossRef]
58. Polgar, C.; Major, T.; Takacsi-Nagy, Z.; Fodor, J. Breast-Conserving Surgery Followed by Partial or Whole Breast Irradiation: Twenty-Year Results of a Phase 3 Clinical Study. *Int. J. Radiat. Oncol. Biol. Phys.* **2021**, *109*, 998–1006. [CrossRef]
59. Schafer, R.; Strnad, V.; Polgar, C.; Uter, W.; Hildebrandt, G.; Ott, O.J.; Kauer-Dorner, D.; Knauerhase, H.; Major, T.; Lyczek, J.; et al. Quality-of-life results for accelerated partial breast irradiation with interstitial brachytherapy versus whole-breast irradiation in early breast cancer after breast-conserving surgery (GEC-ESTRO): 5-year results of a randomised, phase 3 trial. *Lancet Oncol.* **2018**, *19*, 834–844. [CrossRef]
60. Bhattacharya, I.S.; Haviland, J.S.; Kirby, A.M.; Kirwan, C.C.; Hopwood, P.; Yarnold, J.R.; Bliss, J.M.; Coles, C.E.; Trialists, I. Patient-Reported Outcomes Over 5 Years After Whole- or Partial-Breast Radiotherapy: Longitudinal Analysis of the IMPORT LOW (CRUK/06/003) Phase III Randomized Controlled Trial. *J. Clin. Oncol.* **2019**, *37*, 305–317. [CrossRef]
61. Meattini, I.; Saieva, C.; Miccinesi, G.; Desideri, I.; Francolini, G.; Scotti, V.; Marrazzo, L.; Pallotta, S.; Meacci, F.; Muntoni, C.; et al. Accelerated partial breast irradiation using intensity modulated radiotherapy versus whole breast irradiation: Health-related quality of life final analysis from the Florence phase 3 trial. *Eur. J. Cancer* **2017**, *76*, 17–26. [CrossRef]
62. Vaidya, J.S.; Bulsara, M.; Baum, M.; Wenz, F.; Massarut, S.; Pigorsch, S.; Alvarado, M.; Douek, M.; Saunders, C.; Flyger, H.L.; et al. Long term survival and local control outcomes from single dose targeted intraoperative radiotherapy during lumpectomy (TARGIT-IORT) for early breast cancer: TARGIT-A randomised clinical trial. *BMJ* **2020**, *370*, m2836. [CrossRef] [PubMed]
63. Vaidya, J.S.; Bulsara, M.; Baum, M.; Wenz, F.; Massarut, S.; Pigorsch, S.; Alvarado, M.; Douek, M.; Saunders, C.; Flyger, H.; et al. New clinical and biological insights from the international TARGIT-A randomised trial of targeted intraoperative radiotherapy during lumpectomy for breast cancer. *Br. J. Cancer* **2021**, *125*, 380–389. [CrossRef] [PubMed]
64. Vaidya, J.S.; Bulsara, M.; Saunders, C.; Flyger, H.; Tobias, J.S.; Corica, T.; Massarut, S.; Wenz, F.; Pigorsch, S.; Alvarado, M.; et al. Effect of Delayed Targeted Intraoperative Radiotherapy vs Whole-Breast Radiotherapy on Local Recurrence and Survival: Long-term Results From the TARGIT-A Randomized Clinical Trial in Early Breast Cancer. *JAMA Oncol.* **2020**, *6*, e200249. [CrossRef] [PubMed]
65. Vaidya, J.S.; Vaidya, U.J.; Baum, M.; Bulsara, M.K.; Joseph, D.; Tobias, J.S. Global adoption of single-shot targeted intraoperative radiotherapy (TARGIT-IORT) for breast cancer-better for patients, better for healthcare systems. *Front. Oncol.* **2022**, *12*, 786515. [CrossRef]
66. Halima, A.; Parker, S.M.; Asha, W.; Mayo, Z.S.; Kilic, S.S.; Obi, E.; Kim, S.; Gentle, C.; Valente, S.; Cherian, S.; et al. Accelerated Partial Breast Irradiation vs. Intraoperative Radiation Therapy for Early-Stage Breast Cancer and Ductal Carcinoma In Situ. *Int. J. Radiat. Oncol. Biol. Phys.* **2022**, *114*, e16. [CrossRef]
67. Shah, C. Intraoperative Radiation Therapy for Breast Cancer: Are We There Yet? *Ann. Surg. Oncol.* **2021**, *28*, 20–21. [CrossRef]
68. Goldberg, M.; Bridhikitti, J.; Khan, A.J.; McGale, P.; Whelan, T.J. A Meta-Analysis of Trials of Partial Breast Irradiation. *Int. J. Radiat. Oncol. Biol. Phys.* **2023**, *115*, 60–72. [CrossRef]
69. Whelan, T.J.; Smith, S.; Nielsen, T.O.; Parpia, S.; Fyles, A.W.; Bane, A.; Liu, F.-F.; Grimard, L.; Stevens, C.; Bowen, J.; et al. LUMINA: A prospective trial omitting radiotherapy (RT) following breast conserving surgery (BCS) in T1N0 luminal A breast cancer (BC). *J. Clin. Oncol.* **2022**, *40*, LBA501. [CrossRef]
70. The PRECISION Trial (Profiling Early Breast Cancer for Radiotherapy Omission): A Phase II Study of Breast-Conserving Surgery Without Adjuvant Radiotherapy for Favorable-Risk Breast Cancer. Available online: https://www.clinicaltrials.gov/ct2/show/NCT02653755 (accessed on 1 December 2022).
71. The IDEA Study (Individualized Decisions for Endocrine Therapy Alone). Available online: https://clinicaltrials.gov/ct2/show/NCT02400190 (accessed on 1 December 2022).
72. Kirwan, C.C.; Coles, C.E.; Bliss, J.; Group, P.P.W.; Group, P.P.W. It's PRIMETIME. Postoperative Avoidance of Radiotherapy: Biomarker Selection of Women at Very Low Risk of Local Recurrence. *Clin. Oncol.* **2016**, *28*, 594–596. [CrossRef]
73. De-Escalation of Breast Radiation Trial for Hormone Sensitive, HER-2 Negative, Oncotype Recurrence Score Less Than or Equal to 18 Breast Cancer (DEBRA). Available online: https://www.clinicaltrials.gov/ct2/show/NCT04852887 (accessed on 1 December 2022).
74. EXamining PErsonalised Radiation Therapy for Low-risk Early Breast Cancer (EXPERT). Available online: https://clinicaltrials.gov/ct2/show/NCT02889874 (accessed on 1 December 2022).
75. Partial Breast Versus no Irradiation for Women With Early Breast Cancer. Available online: https://www.clinicaltrials.gov/ct2/show/NCT03646955 (accessed on 1 December 2022).
76. Parulekar, W.R.; Berrang, T.; Kong, I.; Rakovitch, E.; Theberge, V.; Gelmon, K.A.; Chia, S.K.L.; Bellon, J.R.; Jagsi, R.; Ho, A.Y.; et al. CCTG MA.39 tailor RT: A randomized trial of regional radiotherapy in biomarker low-risk node-positive breast cancer (NCT03488693). *J. Clin. Oncol.* **2019**, *37*, TPS602. [CrossRef]

77. Nielsen, T.O.; Leung, S.C.; Riaz, N.; Kos, Z.; Bane, A.; Whelan, T.J. P6-04-02: Ki67 Assessment Protocol: Companion Diagnostic Biomarker for LUMINA Prospective Cohort Study. In Proceedings of the Presented at the San Antonio Breast Cancer Symposium, San Antonio, TX, USA, 6–10 December 2022.
78. Patel, M.A.; Dillon, D.A.; Digiovanni, G.; Chen, Y.-H.; Catalano, P.; Perez, C.; Wazer, D.; Wright, J.; Jimenez, R.; Winer, E.; et al. Abstract CT271: PRECISION (Profiling early breast cancer for radiotherapy omission): A phase II study of breast-conserving surgery without adjuvant radiotherapy for favorable-risk breast cancer. *Cancer Res.* **2020**, *80*, CT271. [CrossRef]
79. Braunstein, L.Z.; Wong, J.; Dillon, D.A.; Chen, Y.-H.; Catalano, P.; Cahlon, O.; El-Tamer, M.B.; Jimenez, R.; Khan, A.; Perez, C.; et al. OT1-12-02-Preliminary report of the PRECISION Trial (Profiling Early Breast Cancer for Radiotherapy Omission): A Phase II Study of Breast-Conserving Surgery Without Adjuvant Radiotherapy for Favorable-Risk Breast Cancer. In Proceedings of the Presented at San Antonio Breast Cancer Symposium, San Antonio, TX, USA, 6–10 December 2022.
80. Cuzick, J.; Dowsett, M.; Pineda, S.; Wale, C.; Salter, J.; Quinn, E.; Zabaglo, L.; Mallon, E.; Green, A.R.; Ellis, I.O.; et al. Prognostic value of a combined estrogen receptor, progesterone receptor, Ki-67, and human epidermal growth factor receptor 2 immunohistochemical score and comparison with the Genomic Health recurrence score in early breast cancer. *J. Clin. Oncol.* **2011**, *29*, 4273–4278. [CrossRef] [PubMed]
81. Dowsett, M.; Sestak, I.; Lopez-Knowles, E.; Sidhu, K.; Dunbier, A.K.; Cowens, J.W.; Ferree, S.; Storhoff, J.; Schaper, C.; Cuzick, J. Comparison of PAM50 risk of recurrence score with oncotype DX and IHC4 for predicting risk of distant recurrence after endocrine therapy. *J. Clin. Oncol.* **2013**, *31*, 2783–2790. [CrossRef] [PubMed]
82. White, J.; Cecchini, R.S.; Harris, E.E.; Mamounas, E.T.; Daniel Stover, D.; Ganz, P.A.; Jagsi, R.; Bergom, C.; Théberge, V.; El-Tamer, M.B.; et al. OT1-12-01: A phase III trial evaluating De-escalation of Breast Radiation (DEBRA) following breast-conserving surgery (BCS) of stage 1, HR+, HER2−, RS ≤ 18 breast cancer: NRG-BR007. In Proceedings of the Presented at San Antonio Breast Cancer Symposium, San Antonio, TX, USA, 6–10 December 2022.
83. Early Breast Cancer Trialists' Collaborative, g. Trastuzumab for early-stage, HER2-positive breast cancer: A meta-analysis of 13 864 women in seven randomised trials. *Lancet Oncol.* **2021**, *22*, 1139–1150. [CrossRef]
84. Bazan, J.G.; Jhawar, S.R.; Stover, D.; Park, K.U.; Beyer, S.; Healy, E.; White, J.R. De-escalation of radiation therapy in patients with stage I, node-negative, HER2-positive breast cancer. *NPJ Breast Cancer* **2021**, *7*, 33. [CrossRef]
85. Tolaney, S.M.; Barry, W.T.; Dang, C.T.; Yardley, D.A.; Moy, B.; Marcom, P.K.; Albain, K.S.; Rugo, H.S.; Ellis, M.; Shapira, I.; et al. Adjuvant paclitaxel and trastuzumab for node-negative, HER2-positive breast cancer. *N. Engl. J. Med.* **2015**, *372*, 134–141. [CrossRef]
86. Tolaney, S.M.; Guo, H.; Pernas, S.; Barry, W.T.; Dillon, D.A.; Ritterhouse, L.; Schneider, B.P.; Shen, F.; Fuhrman, K.; Baltay, M.; et al. Seven-Year Follow-Up Analysis of Adjuvant Paclitaxel and Trastuzumab Trial for Node-Negative, Human Epidermal Growth Factor Receptor 2-Positive Breast Cancer. *J. Clin. Oncol.* **2019**, *37*, 1868–1875. [CrossRef]
87. Bellon, J.R.; Guo, H.; Barry, W.T.; Dang, C.T.; Yardley, D.A.; Moy, B.; Marcom, P.K.; Albain, K.S.; Rugo, H.S.; Ellis, M.; et al. Local-regional recurrence in women with small node-negative, HER2-positive breast cancer: Results from a prospective multi-institutional study (the APT trial). *Breast Cancer Res. Treat.* **2019**, *176*, 303–310. [CrossRef]
88. Tolaney, S.M.; Tayob, N.; Dang, C.; Yardley, D.A.; Isakoff, S.J.; Valero, V.; Faggen, M.; Mulvey, T.; Bose, R.; Hu, J.; et al. Adjuvant Trastuzumab Emtansine Versus Paclitaxel in Combination With Trastuzumab for Stage I HER2-Positive Breast Cancer (ATEMPT): A Randomized Clinical Trial. *J. Clin. Oncol.* **2021**, *39*, 2375–2385. [CrossRef]
89. Bellon, J.R.; Tayob, N.; Yang, D.D.; Tralins, J.; Dang, C.T.; Isakoff, S.J.; DeMeo, M.; Burstein, H.J.; Partridge, A.H.; Winer, E.P.; et al. Local Therapy Outcomes and Toxicity From the ATEMPT Trial (TBCRC 033): A Phase II Randomized Trial of Adjuvant Trastuzumab Emtansine Versus Paclitaxel in Combination With Trastuzumab in Women With Stage I HER2-Positive Breast Cancer. *Int. J. Radiat. Oncol. Biol. Phys.* **2022**, *113*, 117–124. [CrossRef]
90. von Minckwitz, G.; Huang, C.S.; Mano, M.S.; Loibl, S.; Mamounas, E.P.; Untch, M.; Wolmark, N.; Rastogi, P.; Schneeweiss, A.; Redondo, A.; et al. Trastuzumab Emtansine for Residual Invasive HER2-Positive Breast Cancer. *N. Engl. J. Med.* **2019**, *380*, 617–628. [CrossRef] [PubMed]
91. FDA Approves Ado-Trastuzumab Emtansine for Early Breast Cancer. Available online: https://www.fda.gov/drugs/resources-information-approved-drugs/fda-approves-ado-trastuzumab-emtansine-early-breast-cancer (accessed on 1 December 2022).
92. Denduluri, N.; Somerfield, M.R.; Chavez-MacGregor, M.; Comander, A.H.; Dayao, Z.; Eisen, A.; Freedman, R.A.; Gopalakrishnan, R.; Graff, S.L.; Hassett, M.J.; et al. Selection of Optimal Adjuvant Chemotherapy and Targeted Therapy for Early Breast Cancer: ASCO Guideline Update. *J. Clin. Oncol.* **2021**, *39*, 685–693. [CrossRef] [PubMed]
93. Loibl, S.; Huang, C.S.; Mano, M.S.; Mamounas, E.P.; Geyer, C.E., Jr.; Untch, M.; Thery, J.C.; Schwaner, I.; Limentani, S.; Loman, N.; et al. Adjuvant trastuzumab emtansine in HER2-positive breast cancer patients with HER2-negative residual invasive disease in KATHERINE. *NPJ Breast Cancer* **2022**, *8*, 106. [CrossRef] [PubMed]
94. NRG-BR008 ("HERO"): A Phase III Randomized Trial Seeking to Optimize Use of Radiotherapy in Patients with Early-Stage, Low Risk, HER2-Positive Breast Cancer. Available online: https://www.nrgoncology.org/Home/News/Post/nrg-br008-hero-a-phase-iii-randomized-trial-seeking-to-optimize-use-of-radiotherapy-in-patients-with-early-stage-low-risk-her2-positive-breast-cancer (accessed on 1 December 2022).
95. Asleh, K.; Riaz, N.; Nielsen, T.O. Heterogeneity of triple negative breast cancer: Current advances in subtyping and treatment implications. *J. Exp. Clin. Cancer Res.* **2022**, *41*, 265. [CrossRef]

96. Bianchini, G.; De Angelis, C.; Licata, L.; Gianni, L. Treatment landscape of triple-negative breast cancer—Expanded options, evolving needs. *Nat. Rev. Clin. Oncol.* **2022**, *19*, 91–113. [CrossRef]
97. Abdou, Y.; Goudarzi, A.; Yu, J.X.; Upadhaya, S.; Vincent, B.; Carey, L.A. Immunotherapy in triple negative breast cancer: Beyond checkpoint inhibitors. *NPJ Breast Cancer* **2022**, *8*, 121. [CrossRef]
98. Dent, R.; Trudeau, M.; Pritchard, K.I.; Hanna, W.M.; Kahn, H.K.; Sawka, C.A.; Lickley, L.A.; Rawlinson, E.; Sun, P.; Narod, S.A. Triple-negative breast cancer: Clinical features and patterns of recurrence. *Clin. Cancer Res.* **2007**, *13*, 4429–4434. [CrossRef]
99. Nguyen, P.L.; Taghian, A.G.; Katz, M.S.; Niemierko, A.; Abi Raad, R.F.; Boon, W.L.; Bellon, J.R.; Wong, J.S.; Smith, B.L.; Harris, J.R. Breast cancer subtype approximated by estrogen receptor, progesterone receptor, and HER-2 is associated with local and distant recurrence after breast-conserving therapy. *J. Clin. Oncol.* **2008**, *26*, 2373–2378. [CrossRef]
100. Cancello, G.; Maisonneuve, P.; Rotmensz, N.; Viale, G.; Mastropasqua, M.G.; Pruneri, G.; Montagna, E.; Dellapasqua, S.; Iorfida, M.; Cardillo, A.; et al. Prognosis in women with small (T1mic,T1a,T1b) node-negative operable breast cancer by immunohistochemically selected subtypes. *Breast Cancer Res. Treat.* **2011**, *127*, 713–720. [CrossRef]
101. Rask, G.; Nazemroaya, A.; Jansson, M.; Wadsten, C.; Nilsson, G.; Blomqvist, C.; Holmberg, L.; Warnberg, F.; Sund, M. Correlation of tumour subtype with long-term outcome in small breast carcinomas: A Swedish population-based retrospective cohort study. *Breast Cancer Res. Treat.* **2022**, *195*, 367–377. [CrossRef]
102. An, X.; Lei, X.; Huang, R.; Luo, R.; Li, H.; Xu, F.; Yuan, Z.; Wang, S.; de Nonneville, A.; Goncalves, A.; et al. Adjuvant chemotherapy for small, lymph node-negative, triple-negative breast cancer: A single-center study and a meta-analysis of the published literature. *Cancer* **2020**, *126* (Suppl. S16), 3837–3846. [CrossRef] [PubMed]
103. Vaz-Luis, I.; Ottesen, R.A.; Hughes, M.E.; Mamet, R.; Burstein, H.J.; Edge, S.B.; Gonzalez-Angulo, A.M.; Moy, B.; Rugo, H.S.; Theriault, R.L.; et al. Outcomes by tumor subtype and treatment pattern in women with small, node-negative breast cancer: A multi-institutional study. *J. Clin. Oncol.* **2014**, *32*, 2142–2150. [CrossRef] [PubMed]
104. Ho, A.Y.; Gupta, G.; King, T.A.; Perez, C.A.; Patil, S.M.; Rogers, K.H.; Wen, Y.H.; Brogi, E.; Morrow, M.; Hudis, C.A.; et al. Favorable prognosis in patients with T1a/T1bN0 triple-negative breast cancers treated with multimodality therapy. *Cancer* **2012**, *118*, 4944–4952. [CrossRef] [PubMed]
105. Leon-Ferre, R.A.; Flora Jonas, S.F.; Salgado, R.; Loi, S.; De Jong, V.; Carter, J.M.; Nielson, T.; Leung, S.; Riaz, N.; Curigliano, G.; et al. PD9-05 Stromal tumor-infiltrating lymphocytes identify early-stage triple-negative breast cancer patients with favorable outcomes at 10-year follow-up in the absence of systemic therapy: A pooled analysis of 1835 patients. In Proceedings of the Presented at San Antonio Breast Cancer Symposium, San Antonio, TX, USA, 1 December 2022.
106. Eaton, B.R.; Jiang, R.; Torres, M.A.; Kahn, S.T.; Godette, K.; Lash, T.L.; Ward, K.C. Benefit of adjuvant radiotherapy after breast-conserving therapy among elderly women with T1-T2N0 estrogen receptor-negative breast cancer. *Cancer* **2016**, *122*, 3059–3068. [CrossRef]
107. Haque, W.; Verma, V.; Hsiao, K.Y.; Hatch, S.; Arentz, C.; Szeja, S.; Schwartz, M.; Niravath, P.; Bonefas, E.; Miltenburg, D.; et al. Omission of radiation therapy following breast conservation in older (>/=70 years) women with T1-2N0 triple-negative breast cancer. *Breast J.* **2019**, *25*, 1126–1133. [CrossRef]
108. Haque, W.; Verma, V.; Farach, A.; Brian Butler, E.; Teh, B.S. Postmastectomy radiation therapy for triple negative, node-negative breast cancer. *Radiother. Oncol.* **2019**, *132*, 48–54. [CrossRef]
109. Wang, J.; Shi, M.; Ling, R.; Xia, Y.; Luo, S.; Fu, X.; Xiao, F.; Li, J.; Long, X.; Wang, J.; et al. Adjuvant chemotherapy and radiotherapy in triple-negative breast carcinoma: A prospective randomized controlled multi-center trial. *Radiother. Oncol.* **2011**, *100*, 200–204. [CrossRef]
110. Spring, L.M.; Bar, Y.; Isakoff, S.J. The Evolving Role of Neoadjuvant Therapy for Operable Breast Cancer. *J. Natl. Compr. Cancer Netw.* **2022**, *20*, 723–734. [CrossRef]
111. Samiei, S.; Simons, J.M.; Engelen, S.M.E.; Beets-Tan, R.G.H.; Classe, J.M.; Smidt, M.L.; Group, E. Axillary Pathologic Complete Response After Neoadjuvant Systemic Therapy by Breast Cancer Subtype in Patients With Initially Clinically Node-Positive Disease: A Systematic Review and Meta-analysis. *JAMA Surg.* **2021**, *156*, e210891. [CrossRef]
112. Cortazar, P.; Zhang, L.; Untch, M.; Mehta, K.; Costantino, J.P.; Wolmark, N.; Bonnefoi, H.; Cameron, D.; Gianni, L.; Valagussa, P.; et al. Pathological complete response and long-term clinical benefit in breast cancer: The CTNeoBC pooled analysis. *Lancet* **2014**, *384*, 164–172. [CrossRef]
113. Tee, S.R.; Devane, L.A.; Evoy, D.; Rothwell, J.; Geraghty, J.; Prichard, R.S.; McDermott, E.W. Meta-analysis of sentinel lymph node biopsy after neoadjuvant chemotherapy in patients with initial biopsy-proven node-positive breast cancer. *Br. J. Surg.* **2018**, *105*, 1541–1552. [CrossRef] [PubMed]
114. Boughey, J.C.; Ballman, K.V.; Le-Petross, H.T.; McCall, L.M.; Mittendorf, E.A.; Ahrendt, G.M.; Wilke, L.G.; Taback, B.; Feliberti, E.C.; Hunt, K.K. Identification and Resection of Clipped Node Decreases the False-negative Rate of Sentinel Lymph Node Surgery in Patients Presenting With Node-positive Breast Cancer (T0-T4, N1-N2) Who Receive Neoadjuvant Chemotherapy: Results From ACOSOG Z1071 (Alliance). *Ann. Surg.* **2016**, *263*, 802–807. [CrossRef] [PubMed]
115. Caudle, A.S.; Yang, W.T.; Krishnamurthy, S.; Mittendorf, E.A.; Black, D.M.; Gilcrease, M.Z.; Bedrosian, I.; Hobbs, B.P.; DeSnyder, S.M.; Hwang, R.F.; et al. Improved Axillary Evaluation Following Neoadjuvant Therapy for Patients With Node-Positive Breast Cancer Using Selective Evaluation of Clipped Nodes: Implementation of Targeted Axillary Dissection. *J. Clin. Oncol.* **2016**, *34*, 1072–1078. [CrossRef] [PubMed]

116. Simons, J.M.; van Nijnatten, T.J.A.; van der Pol, C.C.; van Diest, P.J.; Jager, A.; van Klaveren, D.; Kam, B.L.R.; Lobbes, M.B.I.; de Boer, M.; Verhoef, C.; et al. Diagnostic Accuracy of Radioactive Iodine Seed Placement in the Axilla With Sentinel Lymph Node Biopsy After Neoadjuvant Chemotherapy in Node-Positive Breast Cancer. *JAMA Surg.* **2022**, *157*, 991–999. [CrossRef] [PubMed]
117. Ditsch, N.; Kolberg-Liedtke, C.; Friedrich, M.; Jackisch, C.; Albert, U.S.; Banys-Paluchowski, M.; Bauerfeind, I.; Blohmer, J.U.; Budach, W.; Dall, P.; et al. AGO Recommendations for the Diagnosis and Treatment of Patients with Early Breast Cancer: Update 2021. *Breast Care* **2021**, *16*, 214–227. [CrossRef] [PubMed]
118. Ayala de la Pena, F.; Andres, R.; Garcia-Saenz, J.A.; Manso, L.; Margeli, M.; Dalmau, E.; Pernas, S.; Prat, A.; Servitja, S.; Ciruelos, E. SEOM clinical guidelines in early stage breast cancer (2018). *Clin. Transl. Oncol.* **2019**, *21*, 18–30. [CrossRef]
119. Consensus Guideline on the Management of the Axilla in Patients with Invasive/In-Situ Breast Cancer. The American Society of Breast Surgeons. Available online: https://www.breastsurgeons.org/docs/statements/Consensus-Guideline-on-the-Management-of-the-Axilla-Concise-Overview.pdf (accessed on 26 November 2022).
120. Barrio, A.V.; Montagna, G.; Mamtani, A.; Sevilimedu, V.; Edelweiss, M.; Capko, D.; Cody, H.S., 3rd; El-Tamer, M.; Gemignani, M.L.; Heerdt, A.; et al. Nodal Recurrence in Patients With Node-Positive Breast Cancer Treated With Sentinel Node Biopsy Alone After Neoadjuvant Chemotherapy-A Rare Event. *JAMA Oncol.* **2021**, *7*, 1851–1855. [CrossRef]
121. Kahler-Ribeiro-Fontana, S.; Pagan, E.; Magnoni, F.; Vicini, E.; Morigi, C.; Corso, G.; Intra, M.; Canegallo, F.; Ratini, S.; Leonardi, M.C.; et al. Long-term standard sentinel node biopsy after neoadjuvant treatment in breast cancer: A single institution ten-year follow-up. *Eur. J. Surg. Oncol.* **2021**, *47*, 804–812. [CrossRef]
122. Haffty, B.G.; McCall, L.M.; Ballman, K.V.; Buchholz, T.A.; Hunt, K.K.; Boughey, J.C. Impact of Radiation on Locoregional Control in Women with Node-Positive Breast Cancer Treated with Neoadjuvant Chemotherapy and Axillary Lymph Node Dissection: Results from ACOSOG Z1071 Clinical Trial. *Int. J. Radiat. Oncol. Biol. Phys.* **2019**, *105*, 174–182. [CrossRef]
123. Krug, D.; Lederer, B.; Seither, F.; Nekljudova, V.; Ataseven, B.; Blohmer, J.U.; Costa, S.D.; Denkert, C.; Ditsch, N.; Gerber, B.; et al. Post-Mastectomy Radiotherapy After Neoadjuvant Chemotherapy in Breast Cancer: A Pooled Retrospective Analysis of Three Prospective Randomized Trials. *Ann. Surg. Oncol.* **2019**, *26*, 3892–3901. [CrossRef]
124. Stecklein, S.R.; Park, M.; Liu, D.D.; Valle Goffin, J.J.; Caudle, A.S.; Mittendorf, E.A.; Barcenas, C.H.; Mougalian, S.; Woodward, W.A.; Valero, V.; et al. Long-Term Impact of Regional Nodal Irradiation in Patients With Node-Positive Breast Cancer Treated With Neoadjuvant Systemic Therapy. *Int. J. Radiat. Oncol. Biol. Phys.* **2018**, *102*, 568–577. [CrossRef] [PubMed]
125. De Wild, S.R.; de Munck, L.; Simons, J.M.; Verloop, J.; van Dalen, T.; Elkhuizen, P.H.M.; Houben, R.M.A.; van Leeuwen, A.E.; Linn, S.C.; Pijnappel, R.M.; et al. De-escalation of radiotherapy after primary chemotherapy in cT1-2N1 breast cancer (RAPCHEM; BOOG 2010-03): 5-year follow-up results of a Dutch, prospective, registry study. *Lancet Oncol.* **2022**, *23*, 1201–1210. [CrossRef] [PubMed]
126. Mamounas, E.P.; Bandos, H.; White, J.R.; Julian, T.B.; Khan, A.J.; Shaitelman, S.F.; Torres, M.A.; Vicini, F.; Ganz, P.A.; McCloskey, S.A.; et al. NRG Oncology/NSABP B-51/RTOG 1304: Phase III trial to determine if chest wall and regional nodal radiotherapy (CWRNRT) post mastectomy (Mx) or the addition of RNRT to whole breast RT post breast-conserving surgery (BCS) reduces invasive breast cancer recurrence-free interval (IBCR-FI) in patients (pts) with pathologically positive axillary (PPAx) nodes who are ypN0 after neoadjuvant chemotherapy (NC). *J. Clin. Oncol.* **2019**, *37*, TPS600. [CrossRef]
127. Kushekhar, K.; Chellappa, S.; Aandahl, E.M.; Taskén, K. Role of Lymphocytes in Cancer Immunity and Immune Evasion Mechanisms. In *Biomarkers of the Tumor Microenvironment*, 2nd ed.; Akslen, L.A., Watnick, R.S., Eds.; Springer Nature Switzerland AG: Cham, Switzerland, 2022; pp. 159–182.
128. El Bairi, K.; Haynes, H.R.; Blackley, E.; Fineberg, S.; Shear, J.; Turner, J.; de Freitas, J.R.; Sur, D.; Amendola, L.C.; Gharib, M.; et al. The tale of TILs in breast cancer: A report from The International Immuno-Oncology Biomarker Working Group. *NPJ Breast Cancer* **2021**, *7*, 150. [CrossRef]
129. De Jong, V.M.T.; Wang, Y.; Ter Hoeve, N.D.; Opdam, M.; Stathonikos, N.; Jozwiak, K.; Hauptmann, M.; Cornelissen, S.; Vreuls, W.; Rosenberg, E.H.; et al. Prognostic Value of Stromal Tumor-Infiltrating Lymphocytes in Young, Node-Negative, Triple-Negative Breast Cancer Patients Who Did Not Receive (neo)Adjuvant Systemic Therapy. *J. Clin. Oncol.* **2022**, *40*, 2361–2374. [CrossRef]
130. Park, J.H.; Jonas, S.F.; Bataillon, G.; Criscitiello, C.; Salgado, R.; Loi, S.; Viale, G.; Lee, H.J.; Dieci, M.V.; Kim, S.B.; et al. Prognostic value of tumor-infiltrating lymphocytes in patients with early-stage triple-negative breast cancers (TNBC) who did not receive adjuvant chemotherapy. *Ann. Oncol.* **2019**, *30*, 1941–1949. [CrossRef]
131. Shenasa, E.; Stovgaard, E.S.; Jensen, M.B.; Asleh, K.; Riaz, N.; Gao, D.; Leung, S.; Ejlertsen, B.; Laenkholm, A.V.; Nielsen, T.O. Neither Tumor-Infiltrating Lymphocytes nor Cytotoxic T Cells Predict Enhanced Benefit from Chemotherapy in the DBCG77B Phase III Clinical Trial. *Cancers* **2022**, *14*, 3808. [CrossRef]
132. Dieci, M.V.; Mathieu, M.C.; Guarneri, V.; Conte, P.; Delaloge, S.; Andre, F.; Goubar, A. Prognostic and predictive value of tumor-infiltrating lymphocytes in two phase III randomized adjuvant breast cancer trials. *Ann. Oncol.* **2015**, *26*, 1698–1704. [CrossRef]
133. Denkert, C.; von Minckwitz, G.; Darb-Esfahani, S.; Lederer, B.; Heppner, B.I.; Weber, K.E.; Budczies, J.; Huober, J.; Klauschen, F.; Furlanetto, J.; et al. Tumour-infiltrating lymphocytes and prognosis in different subtypes of breast cancer: A pooled analysis of 3771 patients treated with neoadjuvant therapy. *Lancet Oncol.* **2018**, *19*, 40–50. [CrossRef]
134. Denkert, C.; von Minckwitz, G.; Brase, J.C.; Sinn, B.V.; Gade, S.; Kronenwett, R.; Pfitzner, B.M.; Salat, C.; Loi, S.; Schmitt, W.D.; et al. Tumor-infiltrating lymphocytes and response to neoadjuvant chemotherapy with or without carboplatin in human epidermal growth factor receptor 2-positive and triple-negative primary breast cancers. *J. Clin. Oncol.* **2015**, *33*, 983–991. [CrossRef]

135. Solinas, C.; Ceppi, M.; Lambertini, M.; Scartozzi, M.; Buisseret, L.; Garaud, S.; Fumagalli, D.; de Azambuja, E.; Salgado, R.; Sotiriou, C.; et al. Tumor-infiltrating lymphocytes in patients with HER2-positive breast cancer treated with neoadjuvant chemotherapy plus trastuzumab, lapatinib or their combination: A meta-analysis of randomized controlled trials. *Cancer Treat. Rev.* **2017**, *57*, 8–15. [CrossRef] [PubMed]
136. Schmid, P.; Salgado, R.; Park, Y.H.; Munoz-Couselo, E.; Kim, S.B.; Sohn, J.; Im, S.A.; Foukakis, T.; Kuemmel, S.; Dent, R.; et al. Pembrolizumab plus chemotherapy as neoadjuvant treatment of high-risk, early-stage triple-negative breast cancer: Results from the phase 1b open-label, multicohort KEYNOTE-173 study. *Ann. Oncol.* **2020**, *31*, 569–581. [CrossRef] [PubMed]
137. Sharma, P.; Stecklein, S.R.; Yoder, R.; Staley, J.M.; Schwensen, K.; O'Dea, A.; Nye, L.E.; Elia, M.; Satelli, D.; Crane, G.; et al. Clinical and biomarker results of neoadjuvant phase II study of pembrolizumab and carboplatin plus docetaxel in triple-negative breast cancer (TNBC) (NeoPACT). *J. Clin. Oncol.* **2022**, *40*, 513. [CrossRef]
138. Cytlak, U.M.; Dyer, D.P.; Honeychurch, J.; Williams, K.J.; Travis, M.A.; Illidge, T.M. Immunomodulation by radiotherapy in tumour control and normal tissue toxicity. *Nat. Rev. Immunol.* **2022**, *22*, 124–138. [CrossRef] [PubMed]
139. Monjazeb, A.M.; Schalper, K.A.; Villarroel-Espindola, F.; Nguyen, A.; Shiao, S.L.; Young, K. Effects of Radiation on the Tumor Microenvironment. *Semin. Radiat. Oncol.* **2020**, *30*, 145–157. [CrossRef]
140. Goldberg, J.; Pastorello, R.G.; Vallius, T.; Davis, J.; Cui, Y.X.; Agudo, J.; Waks, A.G.; Keenan, T.; McAllister, S.S.; Tolaney, S.M.; et al. The Immunology of Hormone Receptor Positive Breast Cancer. *Front. Immunol.* **2021**, *12*, 674192. [CrossRef]
141. Bates, A.M.; O'Leary, K.A.; Emma, S.; Nystuen, E.; Sumiec, E.G.; Schuler, L.A.; Morris, Z.S. Abstract 2255: Enhancing immunogenicity in immunologically cold ER+ breast cancer using estrogen receptor blockade and radiation therapy. *Cancer Res.* **2020**, *80*, 2255. [CrossRef]
142. Ngo, M.-H.; Tiberi, D.; Vavassis, P.; Nguyen, D.; Fortin, B.; Gervais, M.-K.; Sideris, L.; Dubé, P.; Leblanc, G.; Dufresne, M.-P.; et al. Abstract P4-12-07: Single pre-operative radiation therapy (SPORT) trial for low risk breast cancer: A phase 1 study comparing pathological findings in immediate versus delayed surgery. *Cancer Res.* **2020**, *80*, P4-12-07. [CrossRef]
143. Xiao, Y.; Ma, D.; Zhao, S.; Suo, C.; Shi, J.; Xue, M.Z.; Ruan, M.; Wang, H.; Zhao, J.; Li, Q.; et al. Multi-Omics Profiling Reveals Distinct Microenvironment Characterization and Suggests Immune Escape Mechanisms of Triple-Negative Breast Cancer. *Clin. Cancer Res.* **2019**, *25*, 5002–5014. [CrossRef]
144. Mittendorf, E.A.; Zhang, H.; Barrios, C.H.; Saji, S.; Jung, K.H.; Hegg, R.; Koehler, A.; Sohn, J.; Iwata, H.; Telli, M.L.; et al. Neoadjuvant atezolizumab in combination with sequential nab-paclitaxel and anthracycline-based chemotherapy versus placebo and chemotherapy in patients with early-stage triple-negative breast cancer (IMpassion031): A randomised, double-blind, phase 3 trial. *Lancet* **2020**, *396*, 1090–1100. [CrossRef]
145. Verbus, E.A.; Rossi, A.J.; Clark, A.S.; Taunk, N.K.; Nayak, A.; Hernandez, J.M.; Tchou, J.C. Preoperative Use of a Radiation Boost to Enhance Effectiveness of Immune Checkpoint Blockade Therapy in Operable Breast Cancer. *Ann. Surg. Oncol.* **2022**, *29*, 1530–1532. [CrossRef] [PubMed]
146. BreastVAX: Radiation Boost to Enhance Immune Checkpoint Blockade Therapy (BreastVAX). Available online: https://clinicaltrials.gov/ct2/show/NCT04454528 (accessed on 1 December 2022).
147. Tchou, J.; Clark, A.; Taunk, N.; Freedman, G.; Xu, N.; Minn, A.; Bradbury, A.; Gross, A.D.; Domchek, S.; Knollman, H.; et al. 644 Major pathologic response after a single radiotherapy fraction + a single pembrolizumab dose given preoperatively in patients with cT1N0 triple negative breast cancer (TNBC)—Preliminary results of a phase 1b/2 study (NCT04454528). *J. ImmunoTherapy Cancer* **2022**, *10*, A674. [CrossRef]
148. Single Pre-Operative Radiation Therapy (SPORT) for Low Risk Breast Cancer (SPORT). Available online: https://clinicaltrials.gov/ct2/show/NCT01717261 (accessed on 1 December 2022).
149. Preoperative Single-Fraction Radiotherapy in Early Stage Breast Cancer. Available online: https://clinicaltrials.gov/ct2/show/NCT02482376 (accessed on 1 December 2022).
150. Radiotherapy in Preoperative Setting With CyberKnife for Breast Cancer (ROCK). Available online: https://clinicaltrials.gov/ct2/show/NCT03520894 (accessed on 1 December 2022).
151. Stereotactic Image-Guided Neoadjuvant Ablative Radiation Then Lumpectomy (SIGNAL 2). Available online: https://clinicaltrials.gov/ct2/show/NCT02212860 (accessed on 1 December 2022).
152. SABER Study for Selected Early Stage Breast Cancer (SABER). Available online: https://clinicaltrials.gov/ct2/show/NCT04360330 (accessed on 1 December 2022).
153. GammaPod Dose Escalation Radiation for Early Stage Breast Cancer. Available online: https://clinicaltrials.gov/ct2/show/NCT04234386 (accessed on 1 December 2022).
154. Hypofractionated Radiation Therapy in Treating Participants With Breast Cancer Before Surgery. Available online: https://clinicaltrials.gov/ct2/show/NCT03624478 (accessed on 1 December 2022).
155. Study of Stereotactic Radiotherapy for Breast Cancer. Available online: https://clinicaltrials.gov/ct2/show/NCT03043794 (accessed on 1 December 2022).
156. Breast Cancer Study of Preoperative Pembrolizumab + Radiation. Available online: https://clinicaltrials.gov/ct2/show/NCT03366844 (accessed on 1 December 2022).
157. Neo-adjuvant Chemotherapy Combined With Stereotactic Body Radiotherapy to the Primary Tumour +/- Durvalumab, +/- Oleclumab in Luminal B Breast Cancer: (Neo-CheckRay). Available online: https://www.clinicaltrials.gov/ct2/show/NCT03875573 (accessed on 1 December 2022).

158. Kovacs, A.; Stenmark Tullberg, A.; Werner Ronnerman, E.; Holmberg, E.; Hartman, L.; Sjostrom, M.; Lundstedt, D.; Malmstrom, P.; Ferno, M.; Karlsson, P. Effect of Radiotherapy After Breast-Conserving Surgery Depending on the Presence of Tumor-Infiltrating Lymphocytes: A Long-Term Follow-Up of the SweBCG91RT Randomized Trial. *J. Clin. Oncol.* **2019**, *37*, 1179–1187. [CrossRef] [PubMed]
159. Malmstrom, P.; Holmberg, L.; Anderson, H.; Mattsson, J.; Jonsson, P.E.; Tennvall-Nittby, L.; Balldin, G.; Loven, L.; Svensson, J.H.; Ingvar, C.; et al. Breast conservation surgery, with and without radiotherapy, in women with lymph node-negative breast cancer: A randomised clinical trial in a population with access to public mammography screening. *Eur. J. Cancer* **2003**, *39*, 1690–1697. [CrossRef]
160. Killander, F.; Karlsson, P.; Anderson, H.; Mattsson, J.; Holmberg, E.; Lundstedt, D.; Holmberg, L.; Malmstrom, P. No breast cancer subgroup can be spared postoperative radiotherapy after breast-conserving surgery. Fifteen-year results from the Swedish Breast Cancer Group randomised trial, SweBCG 91 RT. *Eur. J. Cancer* **2016**, *67*, 57–65. [CrossRef]
161. Stenmark Tullberg, A.; Puttonen, H.A.J.; Sjostrom, M.; Holmberg, E.; Chang, S.L.; Feng, F.Y.; Speers, C.; Pierce, L.J.; Lundstedt, D.; Killander, F.; et al. Immune Infiltrate in the Primary Tumor Predicts Effect of Adjuvant Radiotherapy in Breast Cancer; Results from the Randomized SweBCG91RT Trial. *Clin. Cancer Res.* **2021**, *27*, 749–758. [CrossRef]
162. Whelan, T.J.; Olivotto, I.A.; Parulekar, W.R.; Ackerman, I.; Chua, B.H.; Nabid, A.; Vallis, K.A.; White, J.R.; Rousseau, P.; Fortin, A.; et al. Regional Nodal Irradiation in Early-Stage Breast Cancer. *N. Engl. J. Med.* **2015**, *373*, 307–316. [CrossRef]
163. Riaz, N.; E.Chen, B.; Bane, A.; Gao, D.; Stovgaard, E.S.; Kos, Z.; Leung, S.C.; Shenasa, E.; Parulekar, W.; Chambers, S.; et al. P4-02-16: Prognostic and Predictive Capacity of Tumor Infiltrating Lymphocytes in the MA.20 regional radiotherapy trial. In Proceedings of the Poster Presentation at San Antonio Breast Cancer Symposium, San Antonio, TX, USA, 6–10 December 2022.
164. Overgaard, M.; Hansen, P.S.; Overgaard, J.; Rose, C.; Andersson, M.; Bach, F.; Kjaer, M.; Gadeberg, C.C.; Mouridsen, H.T.; Jensen, M.B.; et al. Postoperative radiotherapy in high-risk premenopausal women with breast cancer who receive adjuvant chemotherapy. Danish Breast Cancer Cooperative Group 82b Trial. *N. Engl. J. Med.* **1997**, *337*, 949–955. [CrossRef]
165. Overgaard, M.; Jensen, M.B.; Overgaard, J.; Hansen, P.S.; Rose, C.; Andersson, M.; Kamby, C.; Kjaer, M.; Gadeberg, C.C.; Rasmussen, B.B.; et al. Postoperative radiotherapy in high-risk postmenopausal breast-cancer patients given adjuvant tamoxifen: Danish Breast Cancer Cooperative Group DBCG 82c randomised trial. *Lancet* **1999**, *353*, 1641–1648. [CrossRef]
166. Tramm, T.; Vinter, H.; Vahl, P.; Ozcan, D.; Alsner, J.; Overgaard, J. Tumor-infiltrating lymphocytes predict improved overall survival after post-mastectomy radiotherapy: A study of the randomized DBCG82bc cohort. *Acta Oncol.* **2022**, *61*, 153–162. [CrossRef]
167. Liveringhouse, C.L.; Washington, I.R.; Diaz, R.; Jimenez, R.B.; Harris, E.E.; Rabinovitch, R.; Woodward, W.A.; Torres-Roca, J.F.; Ahmed, K.A. Genomically Guided Breast Radiation Therapy: A Review of the Current Data and Future Directions. *Adv. Radiat. Oncol.* **2021**, *6*, 100731. [CrossRef] [PubMed]
168. Allen, S.G.; Speers, C.; Jagsi, R. Tailoring the Omission of Radiotherapy for Early-Stage Breast Cancer Based on Tumor Biology. *Semin. Radiat. Oncol.* **2022**, *32*, 198–206. [CrossRef] [PubMed]
169. Committee on the Review of Omics-Based Tests for Predicting Patient Outcomes in Clinical Trials; Board on Health Care Services; Board on Health Sciences Policy; Institute of Medicine. *Evolution of Translational Omics: Lessons Learned and the Path Forward*; National Academic Press: Washington, DC, USA, 2012.
170. Simon, R.M.; Paik, S.; Hayes, D.F. Use of archived specimens in evaluation of prognostic and predictive biomarkers. *J. Natl. Cancer Inst.* **2009**, *101*, 1446–1452. [CrossRef] [PubMed]
171. Jennings, L.; Van Deerlin, V.M.; Gulley, M.L. College of American Pathologists Molecular Pathology Resource C: Recommended principles and practices for validating clinical molecular pathology tests. *Arch. Pathol. Lab. Med.* **2009**, *133*, 743–755. [CrossRef]
172. Eschrich, S.A.; Pramana, J.; Zhang, H.; Zhao, H.; Boulware, D.; Lee, J.H.; Bloom, G.; Rocha-Lima, C.; Kelley, S.; Calvin, D.P.; et al. A gene expression model of intrinsic tumor radiosensitivity: Prediction of response and prognosis after chemoradiation. *Int. J. Radiat. Oncol. Biol. Phys.* **2009**, *75*, 489–496. [CrossRef]
173. Eschrich, S.A.; Fulp, W.J.; Pawitan, Y.; Foekens, J.A.; Smid, M.; Martens, J.W.; Echevarria, M.; Kamath, V.; Lee, J.H.; Harris, E.E.; et al. Validation of a radiosensitivity molecular signature in breast cancer. *Clin. Cancer Res.* **2012**, *18*, 5134–5143. [CrossRef]
174. Torres-Roca, J.F.; Fulp, W.J.; Caudell, J.J.; Servant, N.; Bollet, M.A.; van de Vijver, M.; Naghavi, A.O.; Harris, E.E.; Eschrich, S.A. Integration of a Radiosensitivity Molecular Signature Into the Assessment of Local Recurrence Risk in Breast Cancer. *Int. J. Radiat. Oncol. Biol. Phys.* **2015**, *93*, 631–638. [CrossRef]
175. Cui, Y.; Li, B.; Pollom, E.L.; Horst, K.C.; Li, R. Integrating Radiosensitivity and Immune Gene Signatures for Predicting Benefit of Radiotherapy in Breast Cancer. *Clin. Cancer Res.* **2018**, *24*, 4754–4762. [CrossRef]
176. Tramm, T.; Mohammed, H.; Myhre, S.; Kyndi, M.; Alsner, J.; Børresen-Dale, A.-L.; Sørlie, T.; Frigessi, A.; Overgaard, J. Development and validation of a gene profile predicting benefit of postmastectomy radiotherapy in patients with high-risk breast cancer: A study of gene expression in the DBCG82bc cohort. *Clin. Cancer Res.* **2014**, *20*, 5272–5280. [CrossRef]
177. Speers, C.; Zhao, S.; Liu, M.; Bartelink, H.; Pierce, L.J.; Feng, F.Y. Development and Validation of a Novel Radiosensitivity Signature in Human Breast Cancer. *Clin. Cancer Res.* **2015**, *21*, 3667–3677. [CrossRef]
178. Sjostrom, M.; Chang, S.L.; Fishbane, N.; Davicioni, E.; Zhao, S.G.; Hartman, L.; Holmberg, E.; Feng, F.Y.; Speers, C.W.; Pierce, L.J.; et al. Clinicogenomic Radiotherapy Classifier Predicting the Need for Intensified Locoregional Treatment After Breast-Conserving Surgery for Early-Stage Breast Cancer. *J. Clin. Oncol.* **2019**, *37*, 3340–3349. [CrossRef] [PubMed]

179. Sjöström, M.; Chang, S.L.; Hartman, L.; Holmberg, E.; Feng, F.Y.; Speers, C.W.; Pierce, L.J.; Malmström, P.; Fernö, M.; Karlsson, P. Discovery and validation of a genomic signature to identify women with early-stage invasive breast cancer who may safely omit adjuvant radiotherapy after breast-conserving surgery. *J. Clin. Oncol.* **2021**, *39*, 512. [CrossRef]
180. Taylor, K.J.; Bartlett, J.M.S.; Bennett, J.; Chang, S.L.; Arrick, B.; Baehner, F.; Loane, J.F.; Piper, T.; Mallon, E.; Dunlop, J.; et al. Abstract: Validation of Profile for the Omission of Local Adjuvant Radiotherapy (POLAR) in early stage invasive breast cancer patients of the Scottish Conservation Trial. In Proceedings of the Presented at San Antonio Breast Cancer Symposium, San Antonio, TX, USA, 6–10 December 2022.
181. Sjostrom, M.; Fyles, A.; Liu, F.F.; McCready, D.; Shi, W.; Rey-McIntyre, K.; Chang, S.L.; Feng, F.Y.; Speers, C.W.; Pierce, L.J.; et al. Development and Validation of a Genomic Profile for the Omission of Local Adjuvant Radiation in Breast Cancer. *J. Clin. Oncol.* **2023**, JCO2200655. [CrossRef]
182. Braun, S.; Vogl, F.D.; Naume, B.; Janni, W.; Osborne, M.P.; Coombes, R.C.; Schlimok, G.; Diel, I.J.; Gerber, B.; Gebauer, G.; et al. A pooled analysis of bone marrow micrometastasis in breast cancer. *N. Engl. J. Med.* **2005**, *353*, 793–802. [CrossRef] [PubMed]
183. Hartkopf, A.D.; Brucker, S.Y.; Taran, F.A.; Harbeck, N.; von Au, A.; Naume, B.; Pierga, J.Y.; Hoffmann, O.; Beckmann, M.W.; Ryden, L.; et al. Disseminated tumour cells from the bone marrow of early breast cancer patients: Results from an international pooled analysis. *Eur. J. Cancer* **2021**, *154*, 128–137. [CrossRef] [PubMed]
184. Wiedswang, G.; Borgen, E.; Karesen, R.; Kvalheim, G.; Nesland, J.M.; Qvist, H.; Schlichting, E.; Sauer, T.; Janbu, J.; Harbitz, T.; et al. Detection of isolated tumor cells in bone marrow is an independent prognostic factor in breast cancer. *J. Clin. Oncol.* **2003**, *21*, 3469–3478. [CrossRef]
185. Braun, S.; Pantel, K.; Muller, P.; Janni, W.; Hepp, F.; Kentenich, C.R.; Gastroph, S.; Wischnik, A.; Dimpfl, T.; Kindermann, G.; et al. Cytokeratin-positive cells in the bone marrow and survival of patients with stage I, II, or III breast cancer. *N. Engl. J. Med.* **2000**, *342*, 525–533. [CrossRef] [PubMed]
186. Hartkopf, A.D.; Wallwiener, M.; Fehm, T.N.; Hahn, M.; Walter, C.B.; Gruber, I.; Brucker, S.Y.; Taran, F.A. Disseminated tumor cells from the bone marrow of patients with nonmetastatic primary breast cancer are predictive of locoregional relapse. *Ann. Oncol.* **2015**, *26*, 1155–1160. [CrossRef]
187. Bidard, F.C.; Kirova, Y.M.; Vincent-Salomon, A.; Alran, S.; de Rycke, Y.; Sigal-Zafrani, B.; Sastre-Garau, X.; Mignot, L.; Fourquet, A.; Pierga, J.Y. Disseminated tumor cells and the risk of locoregional recurrence in nonmetastatic breast cancer. *Ann. Oncol.* **2009**, *20*, 1836–1841. [CrossRef]
188. Mignot, F.; Loirat, D.; Dureau, S.; Bataillon, G.; Caly, M.; Vincent-Salomon, A.; Berger, F.; Fourquet, A.; Pierga, J.Y.; Kirova, Y.M.; et al. Disseminated Tumor Cells Predict Efficacy of Regional Nodal Irradiation in Early Stage Breast Cancer. *Int. J. Radiat. Oncol. Biol. Phys.* **2019**, *103*, 389–396. [CrossRef]
189. Kim, M.Y.; Oskarsson, T.; Acharyya, S.; Nguyen, D.X.; Zhang, X.H.; Norton, L.; Massague, J. Tumor self-seeding by circulating cancer cells. *Cell* **2009**, *139*, 1315–1326. [CrossRef] [PubMed]
190. Thorsen, L.B.J.; Overgaard, J.; Matthiessen, L.W.; Berg, M.; Stenbygaard, L.; Pedersen, A.N.; Nielsen, M.H.; Overgaard, M.; Offersen, B.V.; Committee, D.R. Internal Mammary Node Irradiation in Patients With Node-Positive Early Breast Cancer: Fifteen-Year Results From the Danish Breast Cancer Group Internal Mammary Node Study. *J. Clin. Oncol.* **2022**, *40*, 4198–4206. [CrossRef] [PubMed]
191. Kim, Y.B.; Byun, H.K.; Kim, D.Y.; Ahn, S.J.; Lee, H.S.; Park, W.; Kim, S.S.; Kim, J.H.; Lee, K.C.; Lee, I.J.; et al. Effect of Elective Internal Mammary Node Irradiation on Disease-Free Survival in Women With Node-Positive Breast Cancer: A Randomized Phase 3 Clinical Trial. *JAMA Oncol.* **2022**, *8*, 96–105. [CrossRef] [PubMed]
192. Poortmans, P.M.; Weltens, C.; Fortpied, C.; Kirkove, C.; Peignaux-Casasnovas, K.; Budach, V.; van der Leij, F.; Vonk, E.; Weidner, N.; Rivera, S.; et al. Internal mammary and medial supraclavicular lymph node chain irradiation in stage I-III breast cancer (EORTC 22922/10925): 15-year results of a randomised, phase 3 trial. *Lancet Oncol.* **2020**, *21*, 1602–1610. [CrossRef] [PubMed]
193. Deng, Z.; Wu, S.; Wang, Y.; Shi, D. Circulating tumor cell isolation for cancer diagnosis and prognosis. *EBioMedicine* **2022**, *83*, 104237. [CrossRef]
194. Bidard, F.C.; Michiels, S.; Riethdorf, S.; Mueller, V.; Esserman, L.J.; Lucci, A.; Naume, B.; Horiguchi, J.; Gisbert-Criado, R.; Sleijfer, S.; et al. Circulating Tumor Cells in Breast Cancer Patients Treated by Neoadjuvant Chemotherapy: A Meta-analysis. *J. Natl. Cancer Inst.* **2018**, *110*, 560–567. [CrossRef]
195. Rack, B.; Schindlbeck, C.; Juckstock, J.; Andergassen, U.; Hepp, P.; Zwingers, T.; Friedl, T.W.; Lorenz, R.; Tesch, H.; Fasching, P.A.; et al. Circulating tumor cells predict survival in early average-to-high risk breast cancer patients. *J. Natl. Cancer Inst.* **2014**, *106*, dju066. [CrossRef]
196. Trapp, E.K.; Fasching, P.A.; Fehm, T.; Schneeweiss, A.; Mueller, V.; Harbeck, N.; Lorenz, R.; Schumacher, C.; Heinrich, G.; Schochter, F.; et al. Does the Presence of Circulating Tumor Cells in High-Risk Early Breast Cancer Patients Predict the Site of First Metastasis-Results from the Adjuvant SUCCESS A Trial. *Cancers* **2022**, *14*, 3949. [CrossRef]
197. Early Breast Cancer Trialists' Collaborative, G.; McGale, P.; Taylor, C.; Correa, C.; Cutter, D.; Duane, F.; Ewertz, M.; Gray, R.; Mannu, G.; Peto, R.; et al. Effect of radiotherapy after mastectomy and axillary surgery on 10-year recurrence and 20-year breast cancer mortality: Meta-analysis of individual patient data for 8135 women in 22 randomised trials. *Lancet* **2014**, *383*, 2127–2135. [CrossRef]

198. Evaluate the Clinical Benefit of a Post-operative Treatment Associating Radiotherapy + Nivolumab + Ipilimumab Versus Radiotherapy + Capecitabine for Triple Negative Breast Cancer Patients With Residual Disease (BreastImmune03). Available online: https://clinicaltrials.gov/ct2/show/NCT03818685 (accessed on 1 December 2022).
199. Hannoun-Levi, J.M.; Montagne, L.; Sumodhee, S.; Schiappa, R.; Boulahssass, R.; Gautier, M.; Gal, J.; Chand, M.E. APBI Versus Ultra-APBI in the Elderly With Low-Risk Breast Cancer: A Comparative Analysis of Oncological Outcome and Late Toxicity. *Int. J. Radiat. Oncol. Biol. Phys.* **2021**, *111*, 56–67. [CrossRef]
200. Hannoun-Levi, J.M.; Chamorey, E.; Boulahssass, R.; Polgar, C.; Strnad, V. Endocrine therapy with accelerated Partial breast irradiatiOn or exclusive ultra-accelerated Partial breast irradiation for women aged >/= 60 years with Early-stage breast cancer (EPOPE): The rationale for a GEC-ESTRO randomized phase III-controlled trial. *Clin. Transl. Radiat. Oncol.* **2021**, *29*, 1–8. [CrossRef] [PubMed]
201. Zhang, Z.; Liu, X.; Chen, D.; Yu, J. Radiotherapy combined with immunotherapy: The dawn of cancer treatment. *Signal Transduct. Target. Ther.* **2022**, *7*, 258. [CrossRef] [PubMed]

Disclaimer/Publisher's Note: The statements, opinions and data contained in all publications are solely those of the individual author(s) and contributor(s) and not of MDPI and/or the editor(s). MDPI and/or the editor(s) disclaim responsibility for any injury to people or property resulting from any ideas, methods, instructions or products referred to in the content.

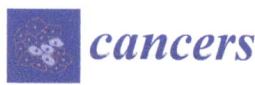

Review

Current Biological, Pathological and Clinical Landscape of HER2-Low Breast Cancer

Huina Zhang [1,*] and Yan Peng [2,*]

[1] Department of Pathology, University of Rochester Medical Center, Rochester, NY 14642, USA
[2] Department of Pathology and Simmons Comprehensive Cancer Center, University of Texas Southwestern Medical Center, Dallas, TX 75390, USA
* Correspondence: huina_zhang@urmc.rochester.edu (H.Z.); yan.peng@utsouthwestern.edu (Y.P.); Tel.: +1-585-276-5499 (H.Z.)

Simple Summary: The breakthrough in developing novel HER2-targeting antibody drug conjugates and identifying their clinical benefits in HER2-low breast cancer will dramatically revolutionize the clinical treatment landscape of HER2 negative breast cancers, as well as the pathologic evaluation of HER2 status in breast cancers. This review updates the current biological, pathological and clinical landscape of HER2-low breast cancer and proposes the future directions on clinical management, pathology practice, and translational research in this subset of breast cancer.

Abstract: HER2-low breast cancer (BC) is a newly defined subset of HER2-negative BC that has HER2 immunohistochemical (IHC) score of 1+ or score of 2+/in situ hybridization (ISH) negative phenotype. Recent clinical trials have demonstrated significant clinical benefits of novel HER2 directing antibody-drug conjugates (ADCs) in treating this group of tumors. Trastuzumab-deruxtecan (T-Dxd), a HER2-directing ADC was recently approved by the U.S. Food and Drug Administration as the first targeted therapy to treat HER2-low BC. However, HER2-low BC is still not well characterized clinically and pathologically. This review aims to update the current biological, pathological and clinical landscape of HER2-low BC based on the English literature published in the past two years and to propose the future directions on clinical management, pathology practice, and translational research in this subset of BC. We hope it would help better understand the tumor biology of HER2-low BC and the current efforts for identifying and treating this newly recognized targetable group of BC.

Keywords: HER2; breast cancer; HER2-low; antibody-drug conjugate; trastuzumab-deruxtecan; T-Dxd

Citation: Zhang, H.; Peng, Y. Current Biological, Pathological and Clinical Landscape of HER2-Low Breast Cancer. *Cancers* 2023, 15, 126. https://doi.org/10.3390/cancers15010126

Academic Editors: Filippo Pesapane and Enrico Cassano

Received: 24 November 2022
Revised: 21 December 2022
Accepted: 21 December 2022
Published: 25 December 2022

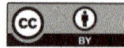

Copyright: © 2022 by the authors. Licensee MDPI, Basel, Switzerland. This article is an open access article distributed under the terms and conditions of the Creative Commons Attribution (CC BY) license (https://creativecommons.org/licenses/by/4.0/).

1. The Natural History of HER2-Low Breast Cancer

Human epidermal growth factor receptor 2 (HER2) is an important prognostic and predicative biomarker in breast cancer (BC) and all patients with newly diagnosed primary or metastatic BCs should be tested for HER2 protein expression by immunohistochemistry (IHC) and/or gene expression by in situ hybridization (ISH) to guide the clinical management [1–3]. BCs are currently classified as HER2 positive when HER2 expression is scored 3+ by IHC or an IHC score of 2+ with HER2 gene amplification tested by ISH. Patients with HER2-positive tumors are eligible for HER2-pathway blockade agents including anti-HER2 monoclonal antibodies (trastuzumab, pertuzumab and margetuximab), anti-HER2 antibody drug conjugates (ADCs) [trastuzumab emtansine (T-DM1) and trastuzumab deruxtecan (T-Dxd)] and tyrosine kinase inhibitors (tucatinib, lapatinib and neratinib). These HER2-targeted agents have dramatically improved the clinical outcomes of HER2-positive BCs [4]. On the contrary, BCs with HER2 IHC score of 0 or 1+, or an IHC score of 2+ without gene amplification are considered as HER2-negative and these tumors lack a significant clinical benefit from these traditional HER2-pathway blockade agents.

Among HER2-negative BCs, hormonal receptor (HR)-negative tumor (triple negative, TNBC) is a biologically aggressive subtype of BC with a poor prognosis and limited treatment options. Currently, the mainstay treatment for TNBCs is cytotoxic chemotherapy, although other therapies including immunotherapy are expanding [5,6]. In a recent meta-analysis, Li et al. reported median overall survival (OS) of 17.5 and 8.1 months and median progression-free survival (PFS) of 5.4 months and 2.9 months in patients with metastatic TNBCs after first-line chemotherapy and later lines of treatment, respectively [7]. In addition, although HR positive, HER2-negative BCs have overall relatively favorable prognosis, most advanced/metastatic HR positive/HER2 negative BCs remain incurable with a median overall survival of 24.8 months [8]. Up to 40% of advanced/metastatic HR positive/HER2-negative BCs respond to the first line treatment, but eventually develop endocrine therapy resistance and options are limited for later line of therapy [8]. The limited activity and associated unfavorable toxicity profiles of chemotherapies in treating high risk or advanced HER2 negative BCs highlight a considerable unmet need for improved therapeutic options.

Promising results of recent clinical trials opened the door for treating a subset of HER2 negative BCs with HER2-targting ADCs. Banerji et al. first published a phase I clinical trial results of trastuzumab duocarmazine, a new HER2-targeting ADC in patients who had advanced BCs with HER2 IHC scores of 1+ or 2+/negative ISH. Treatment with trastuzumab duocarmazine achieved objective response in 28% (9/32) of HR positive tumors and in 40% (6/16) of patients with HR negative tumors [9]. Modi et al. subsequently reported the results of another phase Ib clinical trial which showed patients with advanced BCs and HER2 IHC scores of 1+ or 2+/ISH negative results achieved an objective response rate (ORR) of 37% after the administration of T-Dxd, a previously FDA-approved HER2-targeting ADC for metastatic HER2 positive BCs [10]. Based on these promising clinical trial results, in 2020, Tarantino et al. first proposed the concept of "HER2 low" in BC which refers to BC with HER2 IHC score of 1+ or 2+/ISH negative result [11]. Figure 1 illustrates the changes of HER2 scoring in BC from the current two-tier to three-tier scoring system with the addition of HER2-low category.

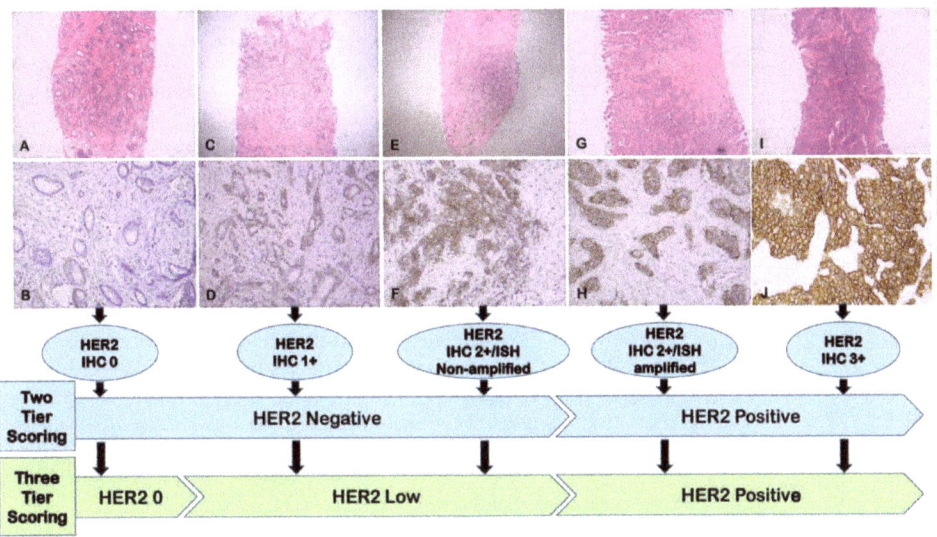

Figure 1. The changes of HER2 scoring in BC from the current two-tier to three-tier scoring system with the addition of HER2-low category. (**A,C,E,G,I**): Hematoxylin & eosin staining of breast cancer, ×40; (**B,D,F,H,J**): Corresponding HER2 IHC, ×200. Abbreviations: HER2: Human epidermal growth factor receptor 2; IHC: Immunohistochemistry; ISH: In situ hybridization.

The result of phase 3 clinical trial (DESTINY Breast-04, DB-04) of T-Dxd in previously heavily-treated HER2-low advanced BC was published in June 2022 and it showed T-Dxd significantly improved survival in patients with HER2-low advanced BC, compared to chemotherapy of physician choice [12]. In August 2022, the U.S. Food and Drug Administration (FDA) approved T-Dxd as the first targeted therapy for the treatment of patients with unresectable or metastatic HER2-low BC [13]. The breakthrough in developing novel HER2-targeting ADCs and identifying their clinical benefits in HER2-low BC will dramatically revolutionize the clinical treatment landscape of BC, as well as the pathologic evaluation of HER2 status in BC. Figure 2 lists the key publications and timeline in the natural history of HER2-low BC.

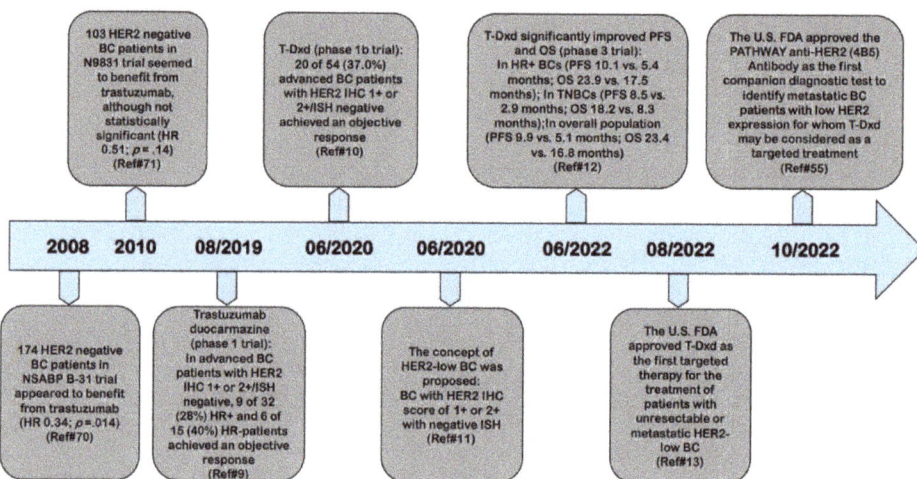

Figure 2. Key publications and timeline in the natural history of HER2-low BC. BC: Breast cancer; DFS: Disease-free survival; FDA: Food and Drug Administration; HER2: Human epidermal growth factor receptor 2; HR: Hazard ratio; HR: Hormonal receptor; IHC: Immunohistochemistry; ISH: In situ hybridization; OS: Overall survival; PFS: Progression-free survival; T-Dxd: Trastuzumab deruxtecan; TNBC: Triple negative breast cancer.

2. Current Biological Landscape of HER2-Low Breast Cancer

2.1. The Incidence of HER2-Low Breast Cancer

HER2-low BC is estimated to account for approximately 45–55% of BCs; however, this estimation is based on studies using variable HER2 scoring criteria [11,14,15]. After the introduction of "HER2-low" in BC in 2020, few studies have reported the incidence of HER2-low BC was between 31% and 51% [16–19]. HER2-low BC is more common in HR+ positive BCs (ranges: 43.5–67.6%) than TNBCs (ranges:15.7–53.6%) [20]. More specifically, in the advanced BCs, the reported incidence of HER2-low BC ranged from 35.2–63.2% [19,21,22].

2.2. The Biology of HER2-Low Breast Cancer

Currently, the knowledge on the biology of HER2-low BC is still limited and it appears to represent a group of breast tumors with significant biological heterogeneity. Both pooled-analysis of large cohorts and smaller single-institutional studies have revealed that most of HER2-low tumors are luminal molecular subtypes (Luminal A: 29.3–65.5%; Luminal B: 22.8–50.5%; HER2-enriched: 1.1–4.1%; Basal: 4.6–7.7%) [16,18,23,24], are enriched in HR positive BCs [16,19,25–32], have a lower Ki-67 proliferation index [17,18,25–27,32], and are less responsive to neoadjuvant chemotherapy (NAC) with a pCR rate between 9.8% and 36.3% [17,25,26,32–38].

Whether HER2-low BC represents a distinct biologic/clinical group and the HER2-low expression has prognostic significance in BC, especially when compared to HER2-0 BC (BC with HER2 IHC score of 0), remain controversial in the current literature [17,26,28,31,33,39,40]. In a large cohort study by Denkert et al., HER2-low BC appeared to be a distinct biological subtype in HER2-negative BCs because this group of tumors had different clinicopathologic characteristics, less responsive to NAC, and relatively-better survival in therapy-resistant HR-negative BCs [17]. On the contrary, in another large cohort study of 5235 patients with HER2-negative BCs, Tarantino et al. [31] found that most of clinicopathologic differences between HER2-0 and HER2-low BCs were associated with HR status. Compared to HER2-0 BC, HER2-low BC had no prognostic significance when adjusting to HR status. The results of that study failed to support the interpretation of HER2-low as a distinct biologic subtype of BC [31]. Likewise, the superior prognosis in HER2-low than HER2-0 tumors has been reported in several studies [17,28,30,41]; while, other studies have failed to demonstrate any prognostic values of HER2-low status in BCs [16,19,29,31,38,39,42–44]. Based on these conflicting results, no clear conclusions can be drawn at present time on both the prognostic value of HER2-low expression and the distinct biologic/clinical entity of HER2-low BC, and this is likely due to differences in the studied patient population, the HR status, the study design/endpoint, and/or follow-up duration. More studies, especially prospective studies which include HR status and treatment protocols may be helpful to better understand the biology of this group of BCs.

The dynamic change associated with HER2-low BC in both primary BCs and matched local recurrences/distant metastases or post-NAC tumors has also been reported. Both Miglietta et al. [22] and Tarantino et al. [45] reported that HER2-low expression was highly unstable during disease progression, and there was a significant discordance (38% and 66%) in HER2-low expression between primary tumors and matched advanced stage tumors, with enrichment of HER2-low carcinomas in the advanced setting. It was also demonstrated that 26.4% of patients had discordant HER2 expression between pre- and post-NAC treatments, mostly seen in cases converting either from HER2-low (14.8%) or to HER2-low (8.9%) expression [46].

2.3. The Molecular Basis of HER2-Low Breast Cancer

Compared to HER2-0 BC, HER2-low BC has been reported to have a higher *ERBB2* mRNA expression [16,47], increased prevalence of *PIK3CA* mutation [17,26,48] and reduced *TP53* mutation [17,48]. A higher prevalence of *FGFR1* amplification (defined as $\geq$10 copy number gain) in the HER2-low group (12% vs. 1.8%) compared to HER2-0 carcinomas was reported [48].

To gain insights into the molecular basis of HER2-low BC, Berrino et al. performed high-throughput molecular analysis on 99 HER2-low BC tissue samples and compared the mutation rates and gene expression profiles of HER2-low BC with those of HER2-negative and HER2-positive BCs in a Memorial Sloan-Kettering Cancer Center BC cohort [24]. The results showed that the most common mutations in HER2-low BC were *PIK3CA* (31/99, 31%), *GATA3* (18/99, 18%), *TP53* (17/99, 17%), and *ERBB2* (8/99, 8%). In addition, the RNA-based class discovery analysis also unveiled four subsets in the HER2-low tumors using LAURA classification: 1) lymphocyte activation, 2) unique enrichment in HER2-related features, 3) stromal remodeling alterations, and 4) actionability of *PIK3CA* mutations. Tumor mutational burden was significantly higher in HER2-low BC with IHC score 1+ compared to those with IHC score 2+, HER2/CEP17 ratio < 2 and copy number between 4 and 6 (p = 0.04). Comparison of mutation spectra revealed that HER2-low BC was different from both HER2-0 and HER2-positive BCs, with score 1+ tumors resembling more the HER2-0 tumors and score 2+/ISH negative tumors more related to the HER2-positive tumors. Intra-group gene expressions also demonstrated overlapping features between IHC score 1+ tumors and HER2-0 BCs, whereas tumors with IHC score 2+, HER2 HER2/CEP17 ratio <2 and copy number between 4 and 6 showed the highest diversity [24]. van den Ende et al. studied the gene expressions in 429 HER2-0 and 100 HER2-low

BCs. HER2-low tumors were found to have higher Era Like 12S Mitochondrial RRNA Chaperone 1 (*ERAL1*), Mediator Complex Subunit 24 (*MED24*) and Post-GPI Attachment to Proteins Phospholipase 3 (*PGAP3*) gene expression, likely due to the amplification of a common chromosomal region. In addition, HER2-low BC was associated with a limited immune response compared to HER2-0 BC, as demonstrated by the gene-expression data in the ER-positive tumors and the tumor infiltrating lymphocytes-score in the ER-negative cohort [47].

2.4. Factors may Contribute to the HER2-Low Expression in Breast Cancer

Although BCs have been scored as HER2 0, 1+, 2+ or 3+ by IHC, the numbers of HER2 receptor molecule in human breast cancer cells are continuously distributed, ranging from approximately 20,000 per cell in normal breast epithelium and HER2 IHC 0 BCs to approximately 2,300,000 per cell in HER2 IHC 3+ BCs [49]. Several factors have been speculated to contribute to the HER2-low expression in BC including the bi-directional crosstalk between ER and HER2, the modification effect by endocrine therapy, and the activation of NF-kB pathway by chemotherapy and radiation therapy [11]. It is well-documented that the presence of complex bi-directional molecular crosstalk between the ER and HER2 pathways in BC plays a significant role in the development of tumor resistance to endocrine or HER2-targeted therapies, since treatment strategies targeting either pathway result in the upregulation of the other one [50,51]. In the recently published literature, it has been consistently demonstrated that HER2-low BC is enriched in HR+ tumors and majority of HER2-low tumors are ER+ [16,19,25–31], indicating ER signaling contributes significantly to the HER2-low expression and related tumor biology. In addition, the dynamic changes of HER2 expression in HER2-low tumors between primary and metastatic/recurrent/NAC BCs further support the roles of endocrine therapy, chemotherapy and radiation therapy in shaping the HER2-low expression in BC [22,45,46].

3. Current Pathological Landscape of HER2-Low Breast Cancer

3.1. The Fundamental Challenge in the Pathological Landscape of HER2-Low Breast Cancer: Accurate Definition

Due to lack of clinical benefits from the HER2-pathway blockade agents, HER2-low expressing BC has long been disregarded as an epiphenomenon without clinical implication of considering HER2-targted therapy. The American Society of Clinical Oncology (ASCO)/College of American Pathologists (CAP) HER2 testing guidelines in BC, initially published in 2007, and updated in 2013 and 2018, have been focusing on separating patients with HER2 positive tumors who are eligible for HER2-targeted therapy, from those with HER2 negative tumors [1–3].

There is no formal definition for HER2-low BC up to this point and this is a fundamental challenge in the current pathological landscape of this newly recognized, targetable tumor group, especially for developing an accurate testing method. The widely used HER2 IHC 1+ or 2+ with negative ISH result for defining HER2-low in BC is based on the inclusion criteria of those clinical trials. In the DB-04 study, the PFS benefit of T-Dxd was consistently observed in patients with HER2 IHC 1+ (10.3 months) and IHC 2+/ISH-negative disease (10.1 months) [12], indicating the number of HER2 receptor molecules in the IHC 1+ tumor cell membrane (~100,000 molecules) reached the threshold for the unique bystander killing effect of T-Dxd in HER2-low expressing tumors. However, the current definition for HER2-low BC may not be an adequate representation of the target population for these novel ADCs and how to decide the lower end of HER2 expression to define HER2-low BC is still evolving. Preliminary results from a phase II clinical trial demonstrated similar response rates to T-Dxd treatment between advanced BC patients with HER2 IHC score of 0+ (30.6%) and HER2-low (33.3%) [52]. In the ongoing DB-06 trial (NCT04494425), which is designed to evaluate the efficacy of T-Dxd in metastatic HER2-low/HR-positive metastatic BC patients with disease progression on endocrine therapy, BC patients with both HER2-low and HER2 IHC expression of >0 and <1+ (currently considered as HER2-0, or ultra-low) are included. Hopefully the results of this trial will provide more evidence on defining the threshold levels /lower limits of HER2 expression required to benefit from an ADC therapeutic approach, such as T-Dxd, and determining the clinical significance of distinguishing HER2-low BC from HER2-0 tumor by using current testing methods.

3.2. IHC Testing as the Primary Method for Identifying HER2-Low Breast Cancer

Under the current definition, the identification of HER2-low BC relies on the IHC testing protocol and scoring system as laid out in the ASCO/CAP guidelines [1–3]. In the DB-04 study, the VENTANA anti-HER2/neu (4B5) IUO Assay system (with ISH testing when applicable) was used to identify patients with HER2-low status, which suggested that a conventional IHC test can accurately identify patients who may benefit from T-Dxd [12]. However, as a semi-quantitative test, HER2 IHC testing was primarily developed to help separate high levels of HER2 expression [~2 millions of molecules per cell, corresponding to HER2 IHC score 3+] from lower level HER2 expression (~20,000–500,000 molecules per cell, corresponding to HER2 IHC 0–2+) and may not be an ideal method for detecting HER2-low BC. The pre-analytic, analytic and post-analytic variables of IHC testing also significantly affect the interpretation of HER2 status. We have previously emphasized the limitations and challenges of IHC as the primary testing method for identifying HER2-low BC in detail, including the notable inter-observer and inter-antibody variability in HER2 IHC scoring, especially in the HER2-low expressing tumors [15,53,54]. Since it was used in the DB-04 trial, the U.S. FDA recently approved the VENTANA PATHWAY anti-HER2/neu (4B5) Rabbit Monoclonal Primary Antibody as the first companion diagnostic test to identify metastatic BC patients with low HER2 expression for whom T-Dxd may be considered as a targeted treatment [55]. This approval would have a significant impact on the pathology practice, especially in those pathology laboratories which do not have the VENTANA platform. In addition, although it has demonstrated that HER2-low BC is targetable group of tumor in the clinical trials, those clinical trials do not necessarily serve as the platform for validating the assay of the vendor used in the trial [56]. Further efforts to address whether other commonly used, FDA-approved HER2 IHC testing methods could reliably identify appropriate patients for T-Dxd treatment are needed.

3.3. Current Developments in More Accurate and Reliable Methods for Identifying HER2-Low Expressing Tumors

Due to the limitations of IHC method as the primary testing for identifying patients with HER2-low tumors, more accurate and reproducible methods are urgently needed for an accurate prediction of efficacy of the novel HER2-targeting ADCs used to treat HER2-low BC. The scientific community and industry are currently making efforts to develop more accurate and reliable methods to facilitate the identification of patients with HER2-low BC.

After investigating 363 BCs with HER2 IHC scores 0, 1+ and 2+ without HER2 gene amplification, with the aid of an artificial neural network model and the correlated HER2 mRNA levels, Atallah et al. proposed a refined HER2-low definition in BC [57]. More specifically, the proposed definition for HER2 IHC score 1+ in this study was membranous staining in invasive tumor cells as either (1) faint intensity in $\geq$20% of cells regardless the circumferential completeness; (2) weak complete staining in $\leq$10%; (3) weak incomplete staining in >10% or (4) moderate incomplete staining in $\leq$10%. It has showed that this refined definition reached high intra-observer agreement (kappa value of 0.8) and inter-observer agreement (kappa value of 0.9) [57].

Deep learning-based technology plays an increasingly significant role in the pathology field, especially in the image analysis and quantitative evaluations. With the assistance of artificial intelligence (AI), it is feasible to develop computer algorithms to analyze HER2 IHC images and provide more objective, reproducible scoring results [58–62]. Gustavson et al. used deep learning-based image analysis and generated a novel HER2 Quantitative Continuous Score (QCS). The HER2 QCS was largely consistent with pathologist's HER2 scoring, and could potentially enhance prediction of patient outcome with T-Dxd by increasing sensitivity and specificity of response, especially in the HER2-low population [63]. A study from China accessed the role of AI in the accurate interpretation of HER2 IHC 0 and 1+ in 246 BCs and found the interpretation accuracy was significantly increased with AI assistance (Accuracy 0.93 vs. 0.80), as well as the evaluation precision of HER2 0 and 1+. The AI algorithm also improved the total consistency (ICC = 0.542 to 0.812), especially in HER2 1+ cases, as well as the accuracy in cases with heterogeneity (Accuracy 0.68 to 0.89) [64]. Recently, PAIGE, an AI-based company announced CE-IVD and UKCA designations of its new digital biomarker assay, HER2Complete, to identify patients with HER2-low BC, but this software has not been approved for diagnostic procedure in the U.S. [65].

Developing accurate and quantitative methods to facilitate the identification of HER2-low BC is also under active investigation. Moutafi et al. recently developed a quantitative immunofluorescence coupled with a mass spectrometry standardized HER2 array to measure absolute amounts of HER2 protein on conventional histology sections. It showed the assay was linear between 2–20 attomols/mm^2 which was within the range of expression in normal breast epithelium, but below the levels seen in the HER2 amplified cell lines or tumors, indicating it may allow for objective and quantitative low HER2 assessment [66]. Kennedy et al. also reported that an immunoaffinity-enrichment coupled to multiple reaction monitoring-mass spectrometry (immuno-MRM-MS) had acceptable analytical characteristics, high concordance with predicate assays, even at low HER2 expression levels [67]. In addition, a study by Xu et al. suggested that molecular method such as mRNA may better serve on defining HER2-low cancer for the treatment decision needs due to its relatively broader dynamic range [68]; while, a recent study found neither IHC nor HER2 mRNA measured by qRT-PCR method would be optimal to quantify HER2-low expression, especially for HER2 1+ BC [69].

These exciting results in the quantitative measurement of HER2 protein expression have opened the doors, but efforts are largely needed in developing cost-effective and easily-implemented methods for facilitating patient selection in the HER2-low era. Furthermore, as we mentioned previously [15], any of new quantitative methods on HER2 protein detection will need to undergo extensive analytic and clinical validation to demonstrate level 1 evidence of clinical utility before approval for the use in clinical practice.

3.4. HER2 Evaluation and Reporting in Breast Cancer in the New HER2-Low Era

Until more accurate and reliable quantitative methods are available for identifying HER2-low BC in routine clinical practice, IHC stays as the primary method to select patients with HER2-low expressing BCs who may benefit from the newly approved HER2-targeted agent. It is important for the pathologist to be familiar with the concept and definition of HER2-low BC and be aware of any changes in the ASCO/CAP HER2 testing guidelines. When evaluating HER2 status in BC, we should adhere strictly to the most updated ASCO/CAP HER2 testing guidelines and carefully evaluate HER2 IHC slide, especially at 400×. Pursuing consensus opinion among pathologists on challenging/borderline cases, and repeating HER2 IHC on the same or different block as well as communicating with clinical team can be helpful. Additional training may be necessary for the accurate and reproducible evaluation of HER2-low phenotype. In addition, revising the pathology report to include the HER2 IHC score and the staining patterns would provide valuable information for the clinical team to decide whether patient is eligible for T-Dxd treatment.

4. Current Clinical Landscape of HER2-Low Breast Cancer: Role of HER2-Targeted Agents

4.1. Limited Activity of Anti-HER2 Monoclonal Antibodies in HER2-Low Breast Cancer

In the retrospective subgroup analysis of two landmark adjuvant trastuzumab trials (NSABP B-31 and N9831), 174 tumors in NSABP B-31 trial and 103 tumors in N9831 trial were reclassified from HER2 positive to negative after central review, and these patients appeared possibly to benefit from additional trastuzumab therapy [70,71]. However, the recent NSABP B-47/NRG oncology phase III trial demonstrated the unequivocal evidence that the addition of trastuzumab to adjuvant chemotherapy did not benefit women with high-risk HER2-low BCs [72]. With a median follow-up of 46 months, the addition of trastuzumab to the standard adjuvant chemotherapy did not improve DFS (89.8% vs. 89.2%; hazard ratio, 0.98; p = 0.85), distant recurrence-free interval (92.7% vs. 93.6%; hazard ratio, 1.10; p = 0.55), or OS (94.8% vs. 96.3%; hazard ratio, 1.33; p = 0.15). Similarly, pertuzumab has limited activity in patient with HER2-low metastatic BCs, with only 4.9% (2/78) of patients achieved partial response as monotherapy, or very narrow therapeutic window with high incidence of diarrhea when combined with pertuzumab and paclitaxel [73,74]. It has been reported that margetuximab showed anti-tumor activity against HER2-low expressing cell lines in an in vitro study [75], and a phase 2 clinical trial on the activity of margetuximab in relapsed or refractory advanced BC with HER2-low expression (NCT01828021) was not completed due to lack of efficacy in 17 patients (68%), adverse effect in 2 patients (20%) and withdrawal in 1 patient (4%) [76].

4.2. Limited Activity of First Generation of HER2-Targeted ADC in HER2-Low Breast Cancer

ADC is a novel class of anticancer agents, which consists of a recombinant monoclonal antibody (mAbs), a cytotoxic drug (payload) and a synthetic linker. By targeting the antigen in the cell membrane by the mAb, the payload will be delivered into the targeted cells more specifically, thus improving the efficacy of payload and significantly reducing the systemic toxicities. T-DM1 is the first HER2-targeted ADC that received the U.S. FDA approval as second or beyond-line for HER2-positive BC and as adjuvant treatment for HER2 positive patients with residual disease after NAC. Currently, there is no formal clinical trial on evaluating T-DM1 in HER2-low BC. In an exploratory analysis of two phase 2 trials designed for HER2-positive BC (TDM4258 g and TDM4374 g), T-DM1 showed a lower ORR (4.8 vs. 33.8% in 4258 g, and 20 vs. 41.3% in 4374 g) and PFS (2.6 vs. 8.2 months in 4258 g, and 2.8 vs. 7.3 months in 4374 g) for HER2-negative than HER2-positive BCs [77,78].

4.3. Significant Clinical Benefit of New HER2-Targeted ADC in HER2-Low BCs

T-Dxd is the 2nd U.S. FDA-approved HER2-targeted ADC in metastatic HER2-positive BC and the first HER2-targeted agent in metastatic or inoperable HER2-low BC. It is composed of an anti-HER2 immunoglobulin G1 antibody, a tetrapeptide-based cleavable linker and a membrane permeable topoisomerase I inhibitor payload with a drug-to-antibody ratio of 8:1. A randomized phrase III, DB-04 trial evaluated T-Dxd in 557 patients (494 HR positive and 63 TNBCs) with HER2-low unresectable or metastatic BC previously treated with one or two lines chemotherapy [12]. Treatment with T-Dxd (5.4 mg/kg, every 3 weeks), in addition to chemotherapy of physician's choice, resulted in a confirmed objective response rate of 52.6% in HR-positive patients and 52.3% in the overall study population compared to chemotherapy of physicians' choice (16.3%). Compared to the chemotherapy of physician's choices, T-Dxd significantly improved PFS in HR-positive patients (10.1 vs. 5.4 months, hazard ratio 0.51, p < 0.001) and in the overall population (9.9 vs. 5.1 months, hazard ratio 0.50, p < 0.001). OS was also improved by T-Dxd treatment among HR-positive patients (23.9 vs. 17.5 months, hazard ratio 0.64, p = 0.003) and the overall population (23.4 vs. 16.8 months, hazard ratio 0.64, p = 0.001). Similarly, in an exploratory analysis in a small number of patients with TNBCs, T-Dxd also improved PFS (8.5 vs. 2.9 months, hazard ratio 0.46) and OS (18.2 vs. 8.3 months, hazard ratio 0.48) [12].

In contrast to other anti-HER2 agents, the unique clinical benefits of T-Dxd in HER2-low BC might be achieved by the so-called "bystander killing" mechanisms due to the highly membrane-permeable payload, high drug-to-antibody ratio and cleavable linker. An in vitro study has demonstrated that T-Dxd could induce a potent "bystander killing" effect on cells in close proximity to targeted HER2-expressing tumor cells by transferring the released payload into the neighboring cells, regardless of their HER2 status [79]. It appears that in HER2-low BC, HER2 molecules on the tumor cell surface primarily function as a means for delivering antibody conjugated drugs, instead of direct inhibition of HER2 dimerization or the blockade of downstream signaling [15].

T-Dxd has generally manageable and tolerable safety profile with gastrointestinal disturbances, myelotoxicity, and alopecia being most common adverse effects. Approximately 28% of patients developed adverse reactions, and 16% of patients had to stop receiving the drug permanently during the clinical trial [80]. Interstitial lung disease (ILD)/pneumonitis is the most concerning adverse event associated with T-Dxd treatment. In a recent pooled analysis of 1150 patients who received one or more dose of ≥5.4 mg/kg T-Dxd monotherapy from nine phase I and II clinical trials, T-Dxd-related ILD/pneumonitis was found in 15.4% of patients, and most were low grade (77.4%, grade 1 or 2; 3.4% grade 3 and above) and occurred in the first 12 months of treatment [81]. Age <65 years, enrollment in Japan, T-Dxd dose >6.4 mg/kg, oxygen saturation <95%, moderate/severe renal impairment, presence of lung comorbidities, and time since initial diagnosis >4 years are the factors of interest associated with any-grade adjudicated drug-related ILD/pneumonitis [81,82]. It needs to be mentioned that with the implementation of updated guidelines for the management of toxic effects in 2019, in the DB-04 trial, the numerical incidence of high-grade events (grade 3 and above) decreased to 2.1% [12]. The specific mechanism of lung injury by T-Dxd is not clear, although it was hypothesized that the ADC-induced alveolar damage is likely due to the target-independent uptake of the conjugated payload by immune cells [82,83]. During T-Dxd treatment, if patients develop dry cough, dyspnea, fever or other new or worsening respiratory symptoms, prompt clinical and imaging evaluation of potential ILD/pneumonitis is warranted [82,84], and permanent discontinuation of T-Dxd in patients with grade 2 or higher ILD/pneumonitis should be considered. Further work is needed to better understand the pathophysiology of T-Dxd-associated ILD/pneumonitis along with the delineation of risk factors, prevention, and treatment measures, ultimately to improve the safety profile of T-Dxd for treating HER2-low BC.

4.4. Other Clinical Development of Agents in the Setting of HER2-Low Breast Cancer

Currently, there are several other agents under clinical development for treating HER2-low BC, including T-Dxd combined with nivolumab, T-Dxd combined with Durvalumab, trastuzumab duocarmazine, disitamab vedotin (RC-48), ARX788, A166, FS-1502 and zenocutuzumab [20].

5. Future Directions

Compared to 2 years ago when the concept of "HER2-low" in BC was first introduced, our understanding of HER2-low BC has significantly advanced, especially on the tumor biology. Nevertheless, there are still challenges and unanswered questions that need to be addressed, including pathology practice, translational research and clinical management in this subset of BCs. We herein propose the following future directions on the topic of HER2-low BC:

1. What is the most appropriate/accurate assay to use for identifying HER2-low BC in the clinical practice;
2. How to best incorporate this new classification of BC into scoring approaches and what changes are needed in terms of test implementation, validation and quality control measures;
3. To establish a more accurate and reproducible definition of HER2-low BC;
4. To further address whether HER2-low tumor represents a distinct clinical entity and whether HER2-low expression has prognostic value, especially prospective studies that include HR status and treatment protocols;
5. Real-world experience with large multicenter case series on the treatment pattern and efficacy of T-Dxd in HER2-low BC;
6. How should T-Dxd be sequenced with other treatment options for treating HER2-low BC and further evaluation of treatment combination strategies of T-Dxd with other drugs;

7. To investigate the pathophysiology of ADC-associated adverse events especially ILD/pneumonitis along with the delineation of risk factors, prevention, and treatment measures, ultimately to improve the safety profile of these ADCs for treating HER2-low BC.

6. Conclusions

The development of novel HER2-targeting ADCs and identification of their significant clinical benefits in HER2-low BC, currently defined as BC with HER2 IHC 1+ or 2+/ISH negative phenotype, will dramatically revolutionize the clinical treatment landscape of HER2 negative BCs. Although our understanding of HER2-low BC has significantly advanced in the past 2 years, further efforts including basic and translational research as well as clinical studies in this newly recognized targetable group of BC are still largely needed. Figure 3 summarizes the current biological, pathological and clinical treatment landscape of HER2-low BC and our proposal for future directions on clinical management, pathology practice, and translational research in this subset of BC.

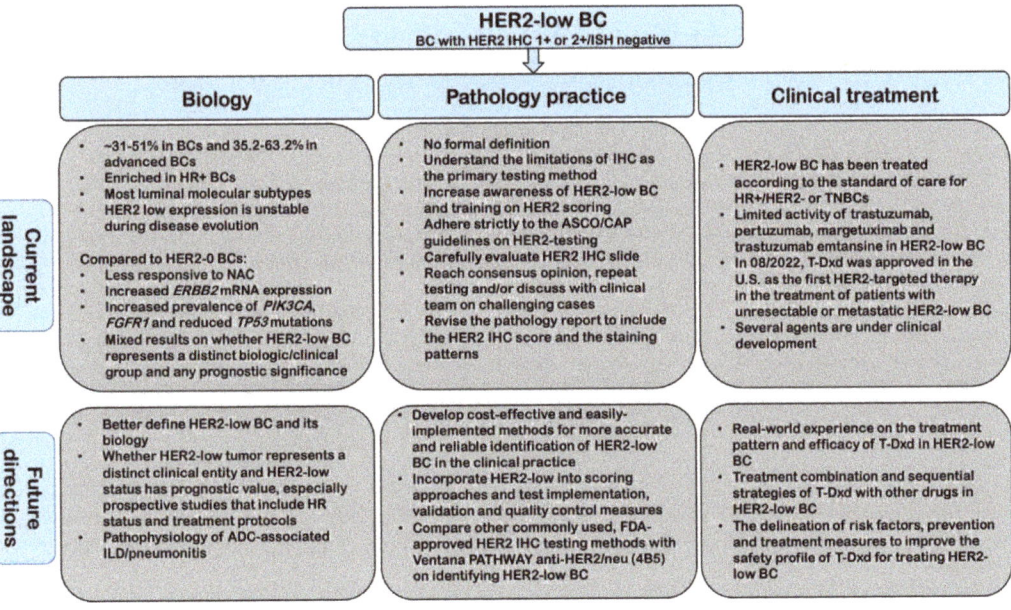

Figure 3. Summary of the current biological, pathological and clinical treatment landscape of HER2-low BC and our proposal for future directions on clinical management, pathology practice, and translational research in this subset of BC. Abbreviations: ADC: Antibody-drug conjugate; ASCO/CAP: The American Society of Clinical Oncology (ASCO)/College of American Pathologists (CAP); BC: Breast cancer; HER2: Human epidermal growth factor receptor 2; IHC: Immunohistochemistry; HR: Hormonal receptor; ILD: Interstitial lung disease; NAC: Neoadjuvant chemotherapy.

Author Contributions: Conceptualization: H.Z. and Y.P. Writing—Original draft preparation: H.Z.; Writing—Reivew & Editing: Y.P. All authors have read and agreed to the published version of the manuscript.

Funding: This research received no external funding.

Conflicts of Interest: The authors declare no conflict of interest.

References

1. Wolff, A.C.; Hammond, M.E.; Schwartz, J.N.; Hagerty, K.L.; Allred, D.C.; Cote, R.J.; Dowsett, M.; Fitzgibbons, P.L.; Hanna, W.M.; Langer, A.; et al. American Society of Clinical Oncology; College of American Pathologists. American Society of Clinical Oncology/College of American Pathologists guideline recommendations for human epidermal growth factor receptor 2 testing in breast cancer. *J. Clin. Oncol.* **2007**, *25*, 118–145. [CrossRef] [PubMed]
2. Wolff, A.C.; Hammond, M.E.; Hicks, D.G.; Dowsett, M.; McShane, L.M.; Allison, K.H.; Allred, D.C.; Bartlett, J.M.; Bilous, M.; Fitzgibbons, P.; et al. Recommendations for human epidermal growth factor receptor 2 testing in breast cancer: American Society of Clinical Oncology/College of American Pathologists clinical practice guideline update. *J. Clin. Oncol.* **2013**, *31*, 3997–4013. [CrossRef] [PubMed]
3. Wolff, A.C.; Hammond, M.E.; Allison, K.H.; Harvey, B.E.; Mangu, P.B.; Bartlett, J.M.; Bilous, M.; Ellis, I.O.; Fitzgibbons, P.; Hanna, W.; et al. Human epidermal growth factor receptor 2 testing in breast cancer:American Society of Clinical Oncology/College of American Pathologists clinical practice guideline focused update. *J. Clin. Oncol.* **2018**, *36*, 2105–2122. [CrossRef]
4. Martínez-Sáez, O.; Prat, A. Current and Future Management of HER2-Positive Metastatic Breast Cancer. *JCO Oncol. Pract.* **2021**, *17*, 594–604. [CrossRef] [PubMed]
5. Sakach, E.; O'Regan, R.; Meisel, J.; Li, X. Molecular Classification of Triple Negative Breast Cancer and the Emergence of Targeted Therapies. *Clin. Breast Cancer* **2021**, *21*, 509–520. [CrossRef]
6. Schettini, F.; Venturini, S.; Giuliano, M.; Lambertini, M.; Pinato, D.J.; Onesti, C.E.; Vidal-Sicart, S.; Ganau, S.; Cebrecos, I.; Brasó-Maristany, F.; et al. Multiple Bayesian network meta-analyses to establish therapeutic algorithms for metastatic triple negative breast cancer. *Cancer Treat. Rev.* **2022**, *111*, 102468. [CrossRef] [PubMed]
7. Li, C.H.; Karantza, V.; Aktan, G.; Lala, M. Current treatment landscape for patients with locally recurrent inoperable or metastatic triple-negative breast cancer: A systematic literature review. *Breast Cancer Res.* **2019**, *21*, 143. [CrossRef]
8. Başaran, G.A.; Twelves, C.; Diéras, V.; Cortés, J.; Awada, A. Ongoing unmet needs in treating estrogen receptor-positive/HER2-negative metastatic breast cancer. *Cancer Treat. Rev.* **2018**, *63*, 144–155. [CrossRef]
9. Banerji, U.; van Herpen, C.M.L.; Saura, C.; Thistlethwaite, F.; Lord, S.; Moreno, V.; Macpherson, I.R.; Boni, V.; Rolfo, C.; de Vries, E.G.E.; et al. Trastuzumab duocarmazine in locally advanced and metastatic solid tumours and HER2-expressing breast cancer: A phase 1 dose-escalation and dose-expansion study. *Lancet Oncol.* **2019**, *20*, 1124–1135. [CrossRef]
10. Modi, S.; Park, H.; Murthy, R.K.; Iwata, H.; Tamura, K.; Tsurutani, J.; Moreno-Aspitia, A.; Doi, T.; Sagara, Y.; Redfern, C.; et al. Antitumor activity and safety of trastuzumab deruxtecan in patients with HER2-low-expressing advanced breast cancer: Results from a phase Ib study. *J. Clin. Oncol.* **2020**, *38*, 1887–1896. [CrossRef]
11. Tarantino, P.; Hamilton, E.; Tolaney, S.M.; Cortes, J.; Morganti, S.; Ferraro, E.; Marra, A.; Viale, G.; Trapani, D.; Cardoso, F.; et al. HER2-Low Breast Cancer: Pathological and Clinical Landscape. *J. Clin. Oncol.* **2020**, *38*, 1951–1962. [CrossRef] [PubMed]
12. Modi, S.; Jacot, W.; Yamashita, T.; Sohn, J.; Vidal, M.; Tokunaga, E.; Tsurutani, J.; Ueno, N.T.; Prat, A.; Chae, Y.S.; et al. Trastuzumab deruxtecan in previously treated HER2-low advanced breast cancer. *N. Engl. J. Med* **2022**, *387*, 9–20. [CrossRef] [PubMed]
13. FDA approves fam-trastuzumab deruxtecan-nxki for HER2-low breast cancer. Available online: https://www.fda.gov/drugs/resources-information-approved-drugs/fda-approves-fam-trastuzumab-deruxtecan-nxki-her2-low-breast-cancer (accessed on 21 October 2022).
14. Marchiò, C.; Annaratone, L.; Marques, A.; Casorzo, L.; Berrino, E.; Sapino, A. Evolving concepts in HER2 evaluation in breast cancer: Heterogeneity, HER2-low carcinomas and beyond. *Semin. Cancer Biol.* **2021**, *72*, 123–135. [CrossRef] [PubMed]
15. Zhang, H.; Katerji, H.; Turner, B.M.; Hicks, D.G. HER2-Low Breast Cancers: New opportunities and challenges. *Am. J. Clin. Pathol.* **2022**, *157*, 328–336. [CrossRef]
16. Agostinetto, E.; Rediti, M.; Fimereli, D.; Debien, V.; Piccart, M.; Aftimos, P.; Sotiriou, C.; de Azambuja, E. HER2-low breast cancer: Molecular characteristics and prognosis. *Cancers* **2021**, *13*, 2824. [CrossRef]
17. Denkert, C.; Seither, F.; Schneeweiss, A.; Link, T.; Blohmer, J.U.; Just, M.; Wimberger, P.; Forberger, A.; Tesch, H.; Jackisch, C.; et al. Clinical and molecular characteristics of HER2-low-positive breast cancer: Pooled analysis of individual patient data from four prospective, neoadjuvant clinical trials. *Lancet Oncol.* **2021**, *22*, 1151–1161. [CrossRef]
18. Zhang, H.; Katerji, H.; Turner, B.M.; Audeh, W.; Hicks, D.G. HER2-low breast cancers: Incidence, HER2 staining patterns, clinicopathologic features, MammaPrint and BluePrint genomic profiles. *Mod. Pathol.* **2022**, *35*, 1075–1082. [CrossRef]
19. Gampenrieder, S.P.; Rinnerthaler, G.; Tinchon, C.; Petzer, A.; Balic, M.; Heibl, S.; Schmitt, C.; Zabernigg, A.F.; Egle, D.; Sandholzer, M.; et al. Landscape of HER2-low metastatic breast cancer (MBC): Results from the Austrian AGMT_MBC-Registry. *Breast Cancer Res.* **2021**, *23*, 112. [CrossRef]
20. Prat, A.; Bardia, A.; Curigliano, G.; Hammond, M.E.H.; Loibl, S.; Tolaney, S.M.; Viale, G. An Overview of Clinical Development of Agents for Metastatic or Advanced Breast Cancer Without ERBB2 Amplification (HER2-Low). *JAMA Oncol.* **2022**, *8*, 1676–1687. [CrossRef]
21. Viale, G.; Niikura, N.; Tokunaga, E.; Aleynikova, O.; Hayashi, N.; Sohn, J.; O'Brien, C.; Higgins, G.; Varghese, D.; James, G.D.; et al. Retrospective study to estimate the prevalence of HER2-low breast cancer (BC) and describe its clinicopathological characteristics. *J. Clin. Oncol.* **2022**, *40* (Suppl. 16), 1087. [CrossRef]
22. Miglietta, F.; Griguolo, G.; Bottosso, M.; Giarratano, T.; Lo Mele, M.; Fassan, M.; Cacciatore, M.; Genovesi, E.; De Bartolo, D.; Vernaci, G.; et al. Evolution of HER2-low expression from primary to recurrent breast cancer. *NPJ Breast Cancer* **2021**, *7*, 137. [CrossRef] [PubMed]

23. Schettini, F.; Chic, N.; Brasó-Maristany, F.; Paré, L.; Pascual, T.; Conte, B.; Martínez-Sáez, O.; Adamo, B.; Vidal, M.; Barnadas, E.; et al. Clinical, pathological, and PAM50 gene expression features of HER2-low breast cancer. *NPJ Breast Cancer* **2021**, *7*, 1. [CrossRef]
24. Berrino, E.; Annaratone, L.; Bellomo, S.E.; Ferrero, G.; Gagliardi, A.; Bragoni, A.; Grassini, D.; Guarrera, S.; Parlato, C.; Casorzo, L.; et al. Integrative genomic and transcriptomic analyses illuminate the ontology of HER2-low breast carcinomas. *Genome Med.* **2022**, *14*, 98. [CrossRef] [PubMed]
25. Alves, F.R.; Gil, L.; Vasconcelos de Matos, L.; Baleiras, A.; Vasques, C.; Neves, M.T.; Ferreira, A.; Fontes-Sousa, M.; Miranda, H.; Martins, A. Impact of human epidermal growth factor receptor 2 (HER2) low status in response to neoadjuvant chemotherapy in early breast cancer. *Cureus* **2022**, *14*, e22330. [CrossRef] [PubMed]
26. Zhang, G.; Ren, C.; Li, C.; Wang, Y.; Cheng, B.; Wen, L.; Jia, M.; Li, K.; Mok, H.; Cal, L.; et al. Distinct clinical and somatic mutational features of breast tumors with high-, low-, or non-expressing human epidermal growth factor receptor 2 status. *BMC Med.* **2022**, *20*, 142. [CrossRef] [PubMed]
27. Won, H.S.; Ahn, J.; Kim, Y.; Kim, J.S.; Song, J.Y.; Kim, H.K.; Lee, J.; Park, H.K.; Kim, Y.S. Clinical significance of HER2-low expression in early breast cancer: A nationwide study from the Korean breast cancer society. *Breast Cancer Res.* **2022**, *24*, 22. [CrossRef] [PubMed]
28. Li, Y.; Abudureheiyimu, N.; Mo, H.; Guan, X.; Lin, S.; Wang, Z.; Chen, Y.; Chen, S.; Li, Q.; Cai, R.; et al. In real life, low-level HER2 expression may be associated with better outcome in HER2-negative breast cancer: A study of the national cancer center. China. *Front. Oncol.* **2022**, *11*, 774577. [CrossRef]
29. Chen, M.; Chen, W.; Liu, D.; Chen, W.; Shen, K.; Wu, J.; Zhu, L. Prognostic values of clinical and molecular features in HER2 low-breast cancer with hormonal receptor overexpression: Features of HER2- low breast cancer. *Breast Cancer* **2022**, *29*, 844–853. [CrossRef]
30. Rosso, C.; Voutsadakis, I.A. Characteristics, clinical differences and outcomes of breast cancer patients with negative or low HER2 expression. *Clin. Breast Cancer* **2022**, *22*, 391–397. [CrossRef]
31. Tarantino, P.; Jin, Q.; Tayob, N.; Jeselsohn, R.M.; Schnitt, S.J.; Vincuilla, J.; Parker, T.; Tyekucheva, S.; Li, T.; Lin, N.U.; et al. Prognostic and Biologic Significance of ERBB2-Low Expression in Early-Stage Breast Cancer. *JAMA Oncol.* **2022**, *8*, 1177–1183. [CrossRef]
32. Di Cosimo, S.; La Rocca, E.; Ljevar, S.; De Santis, M.C.; Bini, M.; Cappelletti, V.; Valenti, M.; Baili, P.; de Braud, F.G.; Folli, S.; et al. Moving HER2-low breast cancer predictive and prognostic data from clinical trials into the real world. *Front. Mol. Biosci.* **2022**, *9*, 996434. [CrossRef] [PubMed]
33. de Moura Leite, L.; Cesca, M.G.; Tavares, M.C.; Santana, D.M.; Saldanha, E.F.; Guimarães, P.T.; Sá, D.D.S.; Simões, M.F.E.; Viana, R.L.; Rocha, F.G.; et al. HER2-low status and response to neoadjuvant chemotherapy in HER2 negative early breast cancer. *Breast Cancer Res. Treat* **2021**, *190*, 155–163. [CrossRef]
34. Cherifi, F.; Da Silva, A.; Johnson, A.; Blanc-Fournier, C.; Abramovici, O.; Broyelle, A.; Levy, C.; Allouache, D.; Hrab, I.; Segura, C.; et al. HELENA: HER2-Low as a predictive factor of response to Neoadjuvant chemotherapy in early breast cancer. *BMC Cancer* **2022**, *22*, 1081. [CrossRef] [PubMed]
35. de Nonneville, A.; Houvenaeghel, G.; Cohen, M.; Sabiani, L.; Bannier, M.; Viret, F.; Gonçalves, A.; Bertucci, F. Pathological complete response rate and disease-free survival after neoadjuvant chemotherapy in patients with HER2-low and HER2-0 breast cancers. *Eur. J. Cancer* **2022**, *176*, 181–188. [CrossRef] [PubMed]
36. Kang, S.; Lee, S.H.; Lee, H.J.; Jeong, H.; Jeong, J.H.; Kim, J.E.; Ahn, J.H.; Jung, K.H.; Gong, G.; Kim, H.H.; et al. Pathological complete response, long-term outcomes, and recurrence patterns in HER2-low versus HER2-zero breast cancer after neoadjuvant chemotherapy. *Eur. J. Cancer* **2022**, *176*, 30–40. [CrossRef]
37. Shao, Y.; Yu, Y.; Luo, Z.; Guan, H.; Zhu, F.; He, Y.; Chen, Q.; Liu, C.; Nie, B.; Liu, H. Clinical, Pathological Complete Response, and Prognosis Characteristics of HER2-Low Breast Cancer in the Neoadjuvant Chemotherapy Setting: A Retrospective Analysis. *Ann. Surg. Oncol.* **2022**, *29*, 8026–8034. [CrossRef]
38. Domergue, C.; Martin, E.; Lemarié, C.; Jézéquel, P.; Frenel, J.S.; Augereau, P.; Campone, M.; Patsouris, A. Impact of HER2 Status on Pathological Response after Neoadjuvant Chemotherapy in Early Triple-Negative Breast Cancer. *Cancers* **2022**, *14*, 2509. [CrossRef]
39. Carlino, F.; Diana, A.; Ventriglia, A.; Piccolo, A.; Mocerino, C.; Riccardi, F.; Bilancia, D.; Giotta, F.; Antoniol, G.; Famiglietti, V.; et al. HER2-Low Status Does Not Affect Survival Outcomes of Patients with Metastatic Breast Cancer (MBC) Undergoing First-Line Treatment with Endocrine Therapy plus Palbociclib: Results of a Multicenter, Retrospective Cohort Study. *Cancers* **2022**, *14*, 4981. [CrossRef]
40. Almstedt, K.; Heimes, A.S.; Kappenberg, F.; Battista, M.J.; Lehr, H.A.; Krajnak, S.; Lebrecht, A.; Gehrmann, M.; Stewen, K.; Brenner, W.; et al. Long-term prognostic significance of HER2-low and HER2-zero in node-negative breast cancer. *Eur. J. Cancer* **2022**, *173*, 10–19. [CrossRef]
41. Tan, R.S.Y.C.; Ong, W.S.; Lee, K.H.; Lim, A.H.; Park, S.; Park, Y.H.; Lin, C.H.; Lu, Y.S.; Ono, M.; Ueno, T.; et al. HER2 expression, copy number variation and survival outcomes in HER2-low non-metastatic breast cancer: An international multicentre cohort study and TCGA-METABRIC analysis. *BMC Med.* **2022**, *20*, 105. [CrossRef]

42. Douganiotis, G.; Kontovinis, L.; Markopoulou, E.; Ainali, A.; Zarampoukas, T.; Natsiopoulos, I.; Papazisis, K. Prognostic Significance of Low HER2 Expression in Patients With Early Hormone Receptor Positive Breast Cancer. *Cancer Diagn. Progn.* **2022**, *2*, 316–323. [CrossRef] [PubMed]
43. Horisawa, N.; Adachi, Y.; Takatsuka, D.; Nozawa, K.; Endo, Y.; Ozaki, Y.; Sugino, K.; Kataoka, A.; Kotani, H.; Yoshimura, A.; et al. The frequency of low HER2 expression in breast cancer and a comparison of prognosis between patients with HER2-low and HER2-negative breast cancer by HR status. *Breast Cancer* **2022**, *29*, 234–241. [CrossRef] [PubMed]
44. Jacot, W.; Maran-Gonzalez, A.; Massol, O.; Sorbs, C.; Mollevi, C.; Guiu, S.; Boissière-Michot, F.; Ramos, J. Prognostic Value of HER2-Low Expression in Non-Metastatic Triple-Negative Breast Cancer and Correlation with Other Biomarkers. *Cancers* **2021**, *13*, 6059. [CrossRef] [PubMed]
45. Tarantino, P.; Gandini, S.; Nicolò, E.; Trillo, P.; Giugliano, F.; Zagami, P.; Vivanet, G.; Bellerba, F.; Trapani, D.; Marra, A.; et al. Evolution of low HER2 expression between early and advanced-stage breast cancer. *Eur. J. Cancer* **2022**, *163*, 35–43. [CrossRef] [PubMed]
46. Miglietta, F.; Griguolo, G.; Bottosso, M.; Giarratano, T.; Lo Mele, M.; Fassan, M.; Cacciatore, M.; Genovesi, E.; De Bartolo, D.; Vernaci, G.; et al. HER2-low-positive breast cancer: Evolution from primary tumor to residual disease after neoadjuvant treatment. *NPJ Breast Cancer* **2022**, *8*, 66. [CrossRef]
47. van den Ende, N.S.; Smid, M.; Timmermans, A.; van Brakel, J.B.; Hansum, T.; Foekens, R.; Trapman, A.M.A.C.; Heemskerk-Gerritsen, B.A.M.; Jager, A.; Martens, J.W.M.; et al. HER2-low breast cancer shows a lower immune response compared to HER2-negative cases. *Sci. Rep.* **2022**, *12*, 12974. [CrossRef]
48. Bayona, R.S.; Luna, A.M.; Tolosa, P.; De Torre, A.S.; Castelo, A.; Marín, M.; García, C.; Boni, V.; Hertfelder, E.B.; Vega, E.; et al. HER2-low vs HER2-zero metastatic breast carcinoma: A clinical and genomic descriptive analysis. *Ann. Oncol.* **2021**, *32* (Suppl. 2), S29–S30. [CrossRef]
49. Ross, J.S.; Fletcher, J.A.; Linette, G.P.; Stec, J.; Clark, E.; Ayers, M.; Symmans, W.F.; Pusztai, L.; Bloom, K.J. The Her-2/neu gene and protein in breast cancer 2003: Biomarker and target of therapy. *Oncologist* **2003**, *8*, 307–325. [CrossRef]
50. Giuliano, M.; Trivedi, M.V.; Schiff, R. Bidirectional Crosstalk between the Estrogen Receptor and Human Epidermal Growth Factor Receptor 2 Signaling Pathways in Breast Cancer: Molecular Basis and Clinical Implications. *Breast Care* **2013**, *8*, 256–262. [CrossRef]
51. Lousberg, L.; Collignon, J.; Jerusalem, G. Resistance to therapy in estrogen receptor positive and human epidermal growth factor 2 positive breast cancers: Progress with latest therapeutic strategies. *Ther. Adv. Med. Oncol.* **2016**, *8*, 429–449. [CrossRef]
52. Diéras, V.; Deluche, E.; Lusque, A.; Pistilli, B.; Bachelot, T.; Pierga, J.Y.; Viret, F.; Levy, C.; Salabert, L.; Le Du, F.; et al. Trastuzumab deruxtecan (T-DXd) for advanced breast cancer patients (ABC), regardless HER2 status: A phase II study with biomarkers analysis (DAISY) (meeting abstract). *Cancer Res.* **2022**, *82* (Suppl. 4), PD8-02. [CrossRef]
53. Zhang, H.; Karakas, C.; Tyburski, H.; Turner, B.M.; Peng, Y.; Wang, X.; Katerji, H.; Schiffhauer, L.; Hicks, D.G. HER2-low breast cancers: Current insights and future directions. *Semin. Diagn. Pathol.* **2022**, *39*, 305–312. [CrossRef] [PubMed]
54. Karakas, C.; Tyburski, H.; Turner, B.M.; Wang, X.; Schiffhauer, L.; Katerji, M.; Hicks, D.G.; Zhang, H. Inter-observer and Inter-antibody Reproducibility of HER2 Immunohistochemical Scoring in a HER2-low Expressing Breast Cancer Enriched Cohort. *Am. J. Clin. Pathol.* **2023**; *in press*.
55. Roche receives FDA approval for first companion diagnostic to identify patients with HER2 low metastatic breast cancer eligible for Enhertu. Available online: https://diagnostics.roche.com/global/en/news-listing/2022/roche-receives-fda-approval-for-first-companion-diagnostic-to-id.html. (accessed on 2 November 2022).
56. Baez-Navarro, X.; Salgado, R.; Denkert, C.; Lennerz, J.K.; Penault-Llorca, F.; Viale, G.; Bartlett, J.M.S.; van Deurzen, C.H.M. Selecting patients with HER2-low breast cancer: Getting out of the tangle. *Eur. J. Cancer* **2022**, *175*, 187–192. [CrossRef] [PubMed]
57. Atallah, N.M.; Toss, M.S.; Green, A.R.; Mongan, N.P.; Ball, G.; Rakha, E.A. Refining the definition of HER2-low class in invasive breast cancer. *Histopathology* **2022**, *81*, 770–785. [CrossRef]
58. Farahmand, S.; Fernandez, A.I.; Ahmed, F.S.; Rimm, D.L.; Chuang, J.H.; Reisenbichler, E.; Zarringhalam, K. Deep learning trained on hematoxylin and eosin tumor region of Interest predicts HER2 status and trastuzumab treatment response in HER2 + breast cancer. *Mod. Pathol.* **2022**, *35*, 44–51. [CrossRef]
59. Qaiser, T.; Mukherjee, A.; Reddy, P.C.; Munugoti, S.D.; Tallam, V.; Pitkaaho, T.; Lehtimäki, T.; Naughton, T.; Berseth, M.; Pedraza, A.; et al. HER2 challenge contest: A detailed assessment of automated HER2 scoring algorithms in whole slide images of breast cancer tissues. *Histopathology* **2018**, *72*, 227–238. [CrossRef]
60. Helin, H.O.; Tuominen, V.J.; Ylinen, O.; Helin, H.J.; Isola, J. Free digital image analysis software helps to resolve equivocal scores in HER2 immunohistochemistry. *Virchows Arch.* **2016**, *468*, 191–198. [CrossRef]
61. Tuominen, V.J.; Tolonen, T.T.; Isola, J. ImmunoMembrane: A publicly available web application for digital image analysis of HER2 immunohistochemistry. *Histopathology* **2012**, *60*, 758–767. [CrossRef]
62. Laurinaviciene, A.; Dasevicius, D.; Ostapenko, V.; Jarmalaite, S.; Lazutka, J.; Laurinavicius, A. Membrane connectivity estimated by digital image analysis of HER2 immunohistochemistry is concordant with visual scoring and fluorescence in situ hybridization results: Algorithm evaluation on breast cancer tissue microarrays. *Diagn. Pathol.* **2012**, *7*, 27. [CrossRef]

63. Gustavson, M.; Haneder, S.; Spitzmueller, A.; Kapil, A.; Schneider, K.; Cecchi, F.; Sridhar, S.; Schmidt, G.; Lakis, S.; Teichert, R.; et al. Novel approach to HER2 quantification: Digital pathology coupled with AI-based image and data analysis delivers objective and quantitative HER2 expression analysis for enrichment of responders to trastuzumab deruxtecan (T-DXd; DS-8201), specifically in HER2-low patients (meeting abstract). *Cancer Res.* **2021**, *81* (Suppl. 4), PD6-01.
64. Wu, S.; Yue, M.; Zhang, J.; Li, X.; Li, Z.; Zhang, H.; Wang, X.; Han, X.; Cai, L.; Shang, J.; et al. The role of artificial intelligence in accurate interpretation of HER2 IHC 0 and 1+ in breast cancers. *Mod. Pathol.* **2023**; *in press*.
65. Paige Answers Call to Better Identify Breast Cancer Patients with Low Expression of HER2-Paige. Available online: https://www.businesswire.com/news/home/20220623005253/en/Paige-Answers-Call-to-Better-Identify-Breast-Cancer-Patients-with-Low-Expression-of-HER2 (accessed on 2 November 2022).
66. Moutafi, M.; Robbins, C.J.; Yaghoobi, V.; Fernandez, A.I.; Martinez-Morilla, S.; Xirou, V.; Bai, Y.; Song, Y.; Gaule, P.; Krueger, J.; et al. Quantitative measurement of HER2 expression to subclassify ERBB2 unamplified breast cancer. *Lab. Invest* **2022**, *102*, 1101–1108. [CrossRef] [PubMed]
67. Kennedy, J.J.; Whiteaker, J.R.; Kennedy, L.C.; Bosch, D.E.; Lerch, M.L.; Schoenherr, R.M.; Zhao, L.; Lin, C.; Chowdhury, S.; Kilgore, M.R.; et al. Quantification of Human Epidermal Growth Factor Receptor 2 by Immunopeptide Enrichment and Targeted Mass Spectrometry in Formalin-Fixed Paraffin-Embedded and Frozen Breast Cancer Tissues. *Clin. Chem.* **2021**, *67*, 1008–1018. [CrossRef]
68. Xu, K.; Bayani, J.; Mallon, E.; Pond, G.R.; Piper, T.; Hasenburg, A.; Markopoulos, C.J.; Dirix, L.; Seynaeve, C.M.; van de Velde, C.J.H.; et al. Discordance between Immunohistochemistry and ERBB2 mRNA to Determine HER2 Low Status for Breast Cancer. *J. Mol. Diagn* **2022**, *24*, 775–783. [CrossRef]
69. Shu, L.; Tong, Y.; Li, Z.; Chen, X.; Shen, K. Can HER2 1+ Breast Cancer Be Considered as HER2-Low Tumor? A Comparison of Clinicopathological Features, Quantitative HER2 mRNA Levels, and Prognosis among HER2-Negative Breast Cancer. *Cancers* **2022**, *14*, 4250. [CrossRef]
70. Paik, S.; Kim, C.; Wolmark, N. HER2 status and benefit from adjuvant trastuzumab in breast cancer. *N. Engl. J. Med.* **2008**, *358*, 1409–1411. [CrossRef]
71. Perez, E.A.; Reinholz, M.M.; Hillman, D.W.; Tenner, K.S.; Schroeder, M.J.; Davidson, N.E.; Martino, S.; Sledge, G.W.; Harris, L.N.; Gralow, J.R.; et al. HER2 and chromosome 17 effect on patient outcome in the N9831 adjuvant trastuzumab trial. *J. Clin. Oncol.* **2010**, *28*, 4307–4315. [CrossRef]
72. Fehrenbacher, L.; Cecchini, R.S.; Geyer, C.E., Jr.; Rastogi, P.; Costantino, J.P.; Atkins, J.N.; Crown, J.P.; Polikoff, J.; Boileau, J.F.; Provencher, L.; et al. NSABP B-47/NRG oncology phase III randomized trial comparing adjuvant chemotherapy with or without trastuzumab in high-risk invasive breast cancer negative for HER2 by FISH and with IHC 1+ or 2+. *J. Clin. Oncol.* **2020**, *38*, 444–453. [CrossRef]
73. Gianni, L.; Lladó, A.; Bianchi, G.; Cortes, J.; Kellokumpu-Lehtinen, P.L.; Cameron, D.A.; Miles, D.; Salvagni, S.; Wardley, A.; Goeminne, J.C.; et al. Open-label, phase II, multicenter, randomized study of the efficacy and safety of two dose levels of Pertuzumab, a human epidermal growth factor receptor 2 dimerization inhibitor, in patients with human epidermal growth factor receptor 2-negative metastatic breast cancer. *J. Clin. Oncol.* **2010**, *28*, 1131–1137. [CrossRef]
74. Schneeweiss, A.; Park-Simon, T.W.; Albanell, J.; Lassen, U.; Cortés, J.; Dieras, V.; May, M.; Schindler, C.; Marmé, F.; Cejalvo, J.M.; et al. Phase Ib study evaluating safety and clinical activity of the anti-HER3 antibody lumretuzumab combined with Schneethe anti-HER2 antibody pertuzumab and paclitaxel in HER3-positive, HER2-low metastatic breast cancer. *Invest. New Drugs* **2018**, *36*, 848–859. [CrossRef] [PubMed]
75. Nordstrom, J.L.; Gorlatov, S.; Zhang, W.; Yang, Y.; Huang, L.; Burke, S.; Li, H.; Ciccarone, V.; Zhang, T.; Stavenhagen, J.; et al. Anti-tumor activity and toxicokinetics analysis of MGAH22, an anti-HER2 monoclonal antibody with enhanced Fcγ receptor binding properties. *Breast Cancer Res.* **2011**, *13*, R123. [CrossRef] [PubMed]
76. Phase 2 Study of the Monoclonal Antibody MGAH22 (Margetuximab) in Patients with Relapsed or Refractory Advanced Breast Cancer—Study Results. Available online: https://clinicaltrials.gov/ (accessed on 2 November 2022).
77. Burris, H.A., 3rd; Rugo, H.S.; Vukelja, S.J.; Vogel, C.L.; Borson, R.A.; Limentani, S.; Tan-Chiu, E.; Krop, I.E.; Michaelson, R.A.; Girish, S.; et al. Phase II study of the antibody drug conjugate trastuzumab-DM1 for the treatment of human epidermal growth factor receptor 2 (HER2)-positive breast cancer after prior HER2-directed therapy. *J. Clin. Oncol.* **2011**, *29*, 398–405. [CrossRef] [PubMed]
78. Krop, I.E.; LoRusso, P.; Miller, K.D.; Modi, S.; Yardley, D.; Rodriguez, G.; Guardino, E.; Lu, M.; Zheng, M.; Girish, S.; et al. A Phase II Study of Trastuzumab Emtansine in Patients with Human Epidermal Growth Factor Receptor 2-positive Metastatic Breast Cancer Who Were Previously Treated with Trastuzumab, Lapatinib, an Anthracycline, a Taxane, and Capecitabine. *J. Clin. Oncol.* **2012**, *30*, 3234–3241. [CrossRef]
79. Ogitani, Y.; Hagihara, K.; Oitate, M.; Naito, H.; Agatsuma, T. Bystander killing effect of DS-8201a, a novel anti-human epidermal growth factor receptor 2 antibody-drug conjugate, in tumors with human epidermal growth factor receptor 2 heterogeneity. *Cancer Sci.* **2016**, *107*, 1039–1046. [CrossRef]
80. Siddiqui, T.; Rani, P.; Ashraf, T.; Ellahi, A. Enhertu (Fam-trastuzumab-deruxtecan-nxki)—Revolutionizing treatment paradigm for HER2-Low breast cancer. *Ann. Med. Surg* **2022**, *82*, 104665. [CrossRef]

81. Powell, C.A.; Modi, S.; Iwata, H.; Takahashi, S.; Smit, E.F.; Siena, S.; Chang, D.Y.; Macpherson, E.; Qin, A.; Singh, J.; et al. Pooled analysis of drug-related interstitial lung disease and/or pneumonitis in nine trastuzumab deruxtecan monotherapy studies. *ESMO Open* **2022**, *7*, 100554. [CrossRef]
82. Tarantino, P.; Modi, S.; Tolaney, S.M.; Cortés, J.; Hamilton, E.P.; Kim, S.B.; Toi, M.; Andrè, F.; Curigliano, G. Interstitial Lung Disease Induced by Anti-ERBB2 Antibody-Drug Conjugates: A Review. *JAMA Oncol.* **2021**, *7*, 1873–1881. [CrossRef]
83. Kumagai, K.; Aida, T.; Tsuchiya, Y.; Kishino, Y.; Kai, K.; Mori, K. Interstitial pneumonitis related to trastuzumab deruxtecan, a human epidermal growth factor receptor 2-targeting Ab-drug conjugate, in monkeys. *Cancer Sci.* **2020**, *111*, 4636–4645. [CrossRef]
84. Adams, E.; Wildiers, H.; Neven, P.; Punie, K. Sacituzumab govitecan and trastuzumab deruxtecan: Two new antibody-drug conjugates in the breast cancer treatment landscape. *ESMO Open* **2021**, *6*, 100204. [CrossRef]

Disclaimer/Publisher's Note: The statements, opinions and data contained in all publications are solely those of the individual author(s) and contributor(s) and not of MDPI and/or the editor(s). MDPI and/or the editor(s) disclaim responsibility for any injury to people or property resulting from any ideas, methods, instructions or products referred to in the content.

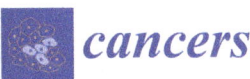

Review

The Role of the Aryl Hydrocarbon Receptor (AhR) and Its Ligands in Breast Cancer

Stephen Safe * and Lei Zhang

Department of Veterinary Physiology and Pharmacology, College of Veterinary Medicine and Biomedical Sciences, Texas A&M University, College Station, TX 77843, USA
* Correspondence: ssafe@cvm.tamu.edu; Tel.: +1-(979)-845-5988; Fax: +1-(979)-862-4929

Simple Summary: The aryl hydrocarbon receptor (AhR) is expressed in breast cancer cells and tumors and in some studies, the AhR is a negative prognostic factor for patient survival. Structurally diverse AhR ligands have been extensively investigated as anticancer agents in breast cancer cells and tumors and show efficacy in both estrogen receptor (ER)-positive and ER -negative breast cancer cells. Moreover, synthetic AhR ligands are being developed and have been in clinical trials for treating breast cancer. In contrast, other reports show that AhR ligands enhance mammary carcinogenesis and in a few studies opposite results are observed for the same AhR ligands in comparable breast cancer cells lines. This paper attempts to provide an extensive, unbiased review of the contrasting effects of AhR ligands in breast cancer and points out that future research will be required to resolve these conflicting results.

Abstract: Breast cancer is a complex disease which is defined by numerous cellular and molecular markers that can be used to develop more targeted and successful therapies. The aryl hydrocarbon receptor (AhR) is overexpressed in many breast tumor sub-types, including estrogen receptor-positive (ER+) tumors; however, the prognostic value of the AhR for breast cancer patient survival is not consistent between studies. Moreover, the functional role of the AhR in various breast cancer cell lines is also variable and exhibits both tumor promoter- and tumor suppressor- like activity and the AhR is expressed in both ER-positive and ER-negative cells/tumors. There is strong evidence demonstrating inhibitory AhR-Rα crosstalk where various AhR ligands induce ER degradation. It has also been reported that different structural classes of AhR ligands, including halogenated aromatics, polynuclear aromatics, synthetic drugs and other pharmaceuticals, health promoting phytochemical-derived natural products and endogenous AhR-active compounds inhibit one or more of breast cancer cell proliferation, survival, migration/invasion, and metastasis. AhR–dependent mechanisms for the inhibition of breast cancer by AhR agonists are variable and include the downregulation of multiple genes/gene products such as CXCR4, MMPs, CXCL12, SOX4 and the modulation of microRNA levels. Some AhR ligands, such as aminoflavone, have been investigated in clinical trials for their anticancer activity against breast cancer. In contrast, several publications have reported that AhR agonists and antagonists enhance and inhibit mammary carcinogenesis, respectively, and differences between the anticancer activities of AhR agonists in breast cancer may be due in part to cell context and ligand structure. However, there are reports showing that the same AhR ligand in the same breast cancer cell line gives opposite results. These differences need to be resolved in order to further develop and take advantage of promising agents that inhibit mammary carcinogenesis by targeting the AhR.

Keywords: AhR; breast cancer; agonist; ligand; TCDD

1. Introduction

The aryl hydrocarbon receptor (AhR) is a basic helix-loop-helix protein that binds the environmental toxicant 2,3,7,8-tetrachlorodibenzo-p-dioxin (TCDD) with high affinity and mediates the toxic and biologic effects induced by this compound and structurally-related halogenated aromatics [1–5]. The classical mechanism of AhR-mediated gene expression and functions involves the ligand-dependent formation of the AhR and the AhR nuclear translocator (ARNT) protein as a heterodimer, which in turn binds cognate cis elements in target gene promoters [6]. The cis elements or xenobiotic response elements (XREs) contain a core GCGTG pentanucleotide sequence and variable flanking nucleotides [6–8]. This classical mechanism of action of the AHR:ARNT complex which targets sequence-specific cis-elements is similar to that described for many members of the nuclear receptor (NR) superfamily of intracellular receptors such as estrogen receptors (ERs, ESR1) [9–11].

Among all intracellular receptors, the AhR is the only receptor identified in molecular toxicology studies focused on determining the mechanism of action of TCDD and structurally related compounds [1,2]. The discovery of the AhR as a "toxicant" receptor has subsequently been a significant hindrance in development and clinical applications of AhR ligands for the treatment of multiple diseases. Overcoming the concerns regarding the potential toxicity of AhR ligands was due to several factors, including the development of AhR knockout (AhRKO) mouse models [12–14] and discoveries showing that many AhR ligands are "health promoting" compounds [15–19]. Differences in AhR ligand persistence may be related to their dioxin-like toxicities. In this review article, the role of the AhR and its ligands as inhibitors of breast cancer in cellular and in vivo models will be investigated. Several studies support a role for AhR ligands as inhibitors of breast cancer and this includes some studies in this laboratory on TCDD and related compounds as antiestrogens associated with ligand-dependent inhibitory AhR-ERα crosstalk [20–22]. There is extensive support from cell culture and in vivo studies indicating that the AhR is a target for breast cancer therapy [23] and human clinical trials using the AhR ligand "aminoflavone" have been carried out for treating breast and other cancers [24–27]. Moreover, studies from several laboratories show that many structural classes of AhR ligands also inhibit some aspects of mammary carcinogenesis [23]. In contrast, there are also reports showing that AhR ligands enhance breast cancer growth and development [28–31] and there are other examples of AhR/AhR ligands exhibiting both tumor suppressive and tumor promoter-like activities for specific cancers [32–36]. Some of these differences are irreconcilable. However, in breast cancer there are several factors that can contribute differences in the role of the AhR/AhR ligands in breast cancer and this includes the following:

1. breast cancer cell context which includes differential expression of the ER and other as yet unidentified factors,
2. breast cancer complexity associated with multiple classifications of tumors based on differences in their histopathology, gene expression, and other clinical parameters,
3. ligand structure and the fact that selective AhR modulators (SAhRMs) exhibit tissue/cell-specific AhR agonist or antagonist activity,
4. other mechanisms of action of the AhR which involve altered genomic and non-genomic (e.g., cell membrane) pathways that may be differentially be affected by AhR ligands some of which also activate more than one receptor. An example of dual receptor ligands are the polyaromatic hydrocarbons (PAHs) and other compounds which bind both the AhR and ER [36–39].

2. Selective AhR Modulators (SAhRMs)

Initial studies on the AhR and the steroid hormone NRs identified exogenous (e.g.,: TCDD) or endogenous (e.g., steroid hormones) ligands that act primarily as receptor agonists. However, for the AhR and other nuclear receptors, it was soon recognized that many different structural classes of ligands also bound the receptor and could act as tissue/cell-and even gene specific agonists, antagonists or partial agonists/antagonists. For example, the AhR binds structurally diverse industrial and synthetic compounds, PAHs, pharmaceuticals, mycotoxins, multiple classes of health promoting phytochemicals including flavonoids, polyphenolics, heteroaromatics such as indole-3-carbinol (I3C), microbial metabolites, and 1,4-dihyroxy-2-naphthoic acid (DHNA) [15–19] (Figures 1 and 2).

In addition, some endogenous compounds, including 6-formyl (3,2-b) carbazole (FICZ), 2-(1′-H-indole-3-carbonyl) thiazole-4-carboxylic acid methyl ester (ITE), tryptophan metabolites such as kynurenine and other gut microbial products, and leukotrienes may play a role as endogenous ligands for the AhR [40–45].

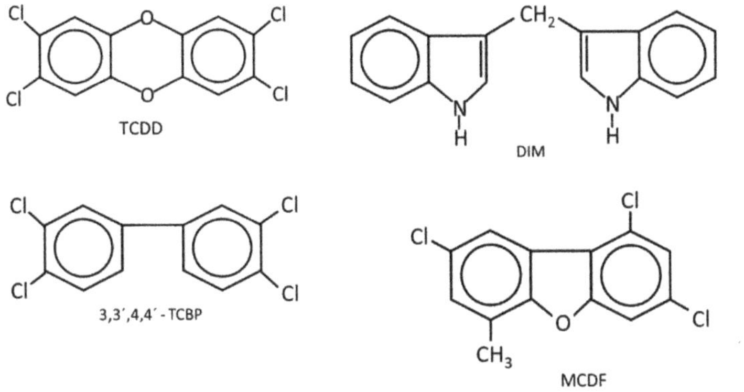

Figure 1. The structures of AhR ligands that inhibit DMBA-induced mammary cancer growth in female Sprague Dawley rats [46–51] using the Huggins model [52].

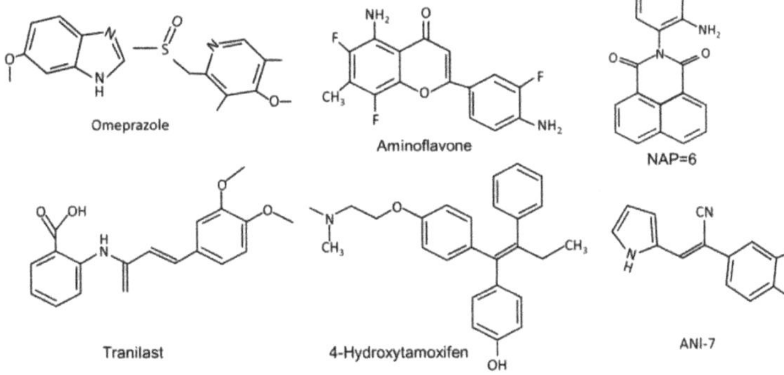

Figure 2. The structures of synthetic compounds, including pharmaceuticals that are AhR ligands.

The selectivity of AhR ligands in terms of their tissue-specific agonist or antagonist activity has been reported in breast and other cancer cell lines and also has been recently reviewed [15]. It is striking that the RNAseq analysis of TCDD and related toxicants are highly variable with respect to their differentially expressed genes. A landmark study of 596 drug-related compounds identified a sub-set of 147 compounds that were evaluated in several Ah-responsive assays, including receptor binding, reporter gene activation and CYP1A1 gene expression [53]. They observed multiple differences among these pharmaceutical compounds to activate putative Ah-responsive endpoints. For example, 59% (81/137) of the compounds induced hepatic CYP1A1 mRNA in mice but did not bind or activate the AhR in vitro. Only nine of these compounds exhibited both in vitro and in vivo activity as AhR agonists in the complete panel of assays which included cytochrome P450 induction in mouse cancer cell lines and liver (in vivo). The selectivity of these AhR-active pharmaceuticals has been further investigated in our laboratory in breast and pancreatic cancer cells [54–56].

The pharmaceutical-derived AhR agonists identified in the screening study [54], including flutamide, leflunomide, mexiletine hydrochloride, nimodipine, omeprazole, sulindac and tranilast were investigated in breast cancer cells. Their activity as inducers of CYP1A1 and CYP1B1 in MDA-MB-468 and BT474 breast cancer cells was structure, response and cell type-specific. Compared to TCDD, induction of CYP1A1 was more robust in BT474 than MDA-MB-468 cells, whereas for most of these compounds the reverse was true for the induction of CYP1B1. 4-Hydroxytamoxifen induced minimal (<25% of maximal induction observed for 10 nM TCDD) CYP1A1 and CYP1B1 expression in both cell lines and with the exception of induction of CYP1B1 (50% of maximal induction observed for 10 nM TCDD), tranilast was also a weak inducer of CYP1A1 and CYP1B1 [54]. The pattern of CYP1A1/CYP1B1 induction in MDA-MB-231 cells also differed from that observed in MDA-MB-468 and BT474 cells. The selectivity was also observed for the effects of these pharmaceuticals on the invasion (Boyden chamber) of MDA-MB-231 cells. TCDD (minimal), omeprazole and tranilast inhibited invasion at sub-toxic concentrations, whereas no effects were observed for 4-hydroxytamoxifen, flutamide, leflunomide, mexiletine, nimodipine, and sulindac [55]. Using omeprazole as a model, it was also shown that inhibition of MDA-MB-231 cell invasion by omeprazole was reversed by AhR antagonists and AhR knockdown (siAhR) and inhibition of invasion was primarily due to AhR-dependent down-regulation of CXCR4, which was observed both in vitro and in vivo [55]. These highly variable ligand-dependent results in breast cancer cells were observed for pharmaceuticals that were all AhR-active in liver and liver cancer cells, demonstrating that these compounds are SAhRMs. Moreover, there is evidence for SAhRM-like activity for many other structural classes of AhR ligands [15,16].

3. AhR in Breast Cancer: Prognostic Significance

There are multiple genes/gene products expressed in breast cancer and other tumors that can predict overall survival or recurrence of disease and they also may be useful for selecting appropriate treatment regimens [57]. These markers, which include receptors, may or may not be indicative of their functional activity or predict effects of therapeutic regimens. There were some differences in the nuclear and extranuclear distribution of AhR protein in non-pathological breast ductal epithelial cells and invasive ductal carcinoma and AhR overexpression was associated with better prognosis of ER-negative and ER-positive invasive ductal carcinoma patients [58]. In another study on 436 breast cancer cases, it was concluded "that AhR expression is not a prognostic factor in breast cancer" [59]. There were correlations between AhR, and levels of several genes associated with inflammation and high levels of AhR repressor (AhRR) mRNA which predicted enhanced patient survival. This might suggest that since AhRR inhibits AhR function due to competition for ARNT, then high AhR levels would be negative prognostic factors; however, this was not observed in a prospective study of 1116 patients where correlations between multiple prognostic factors and their combination with AhR expression were evaluated for their prognostic value. Low cytosolic AhR levels and positive aromatase were associated with more aggressive ER negative (ER$^-$) tumors; however, AhR tumor genotypes did not correlate with AhR protein levels [60]. Another report indicated that the predictive value of the AhR was dependent on the lymph node status of the patient and concluded "that AhR is a marker of poor prognosis for patients with LN-negative luminal-like BCs" [61]. The results suggest that the prognostic value of AhR levels (mRNA and protein), intracellular location and AhR polymorphisms with respect to patient survival/disease recurrence is complex and dependent on many other factors, including prior patient treatment protocols [58–61].

4. Role of the AhR and Its Ligands as Inhibitors Breast Cancer in Cellular and Rodent Models

(i) **Long-term feeding and Huggins model:** Knockdown of the AhR in mice results in lesions in multiple tissues and immune function abnormalities [62–65]. However, the loss of this receptor and development of murine mammary tumorigenesis has not been reported. Studies on the potential effects of TCDD on the development of mammary cancer in rodent models were initially investigated as part of the risk assessment of TCDD, and there is also evidence for impacts of this toxicant on mammary gland development [66–68]. A long-term feeding study in female Sprague Dawley rats showed that TCDD decreased benign mammary tumor formation in one study [69] but this response was minimal in another chronic toxicity feeding study [70]. Another breast cancer model involves 7,12-dimethylbenz[a]anthracene (DMBA)-induced mammary cancer in female Sprague Dawley rats which can then be subsequently treated to identify potential antitumor agents. This model developed by Huggins and coworkers [52] depends on the administration of DMBA to 50 day-old rats and appropriate metabolic activation of DMBA which produces a maximal mammary tumor response. The prenatal administration of TCDD altered mammary gland development [66–68] and enhanced DMBA-induced mammary cancer formation, whereas AhR activation during pregnancy decreased DMBA-induced tumor promotion [71,72]. The Huggins protocol has been used to determine the anticancer activities of AhR ligands. The results show that several AhR agonists, including TCDD, $3,3^1,4,4^1$-tetrachlorobiphenyl (TCBP), diindolylmethane (DIM) and substituted DIM analogs, and 6-methyl-1,3,8-trichlorodibenzofuran (MCDF) inhibit the formation and growth of mammary tumors [46–51]. These studies are consistent with the antiestrogenic effects of AhR ligands, resulting in antitumorigenic activity.

(ii) **AhR Function:** In many tumor types, the AhR alone exhibits tumor promoter or tumor suppressor like activity (Table 1) [73–89], and this can be observed in animals or cells after knockdown or overexpression studies [33,34]. Although the loss of AhR in mice does not affect mammary tumorigenesis, studies in breast cancer cell lines give variable results. For example, knockdown of the AhR by RNA interference increased or did not affect proliferation in BT474 and MDA-MB-468 cells, respectively [73]. In MCF-7 breast cancer cells in a mouse xenograft model, AhR expression was not required for mammary tumorigenesis [74]. In another study, the loss of AhR did not affect the growth of MCF-7 cells; however, TCDD inhibited the growth of AhR-expressing and AhR-KO cells [75]. Another report showed that overexpression of the AhR enhanced MCF-7 cell growth [76,77]. AhR knockdown in ER-negative, MDA-MB-231 cells decreased proliferation and wound healing but induced apoptosis and inhibited tumor growth in an athymic nude mouse xenograft model. [78]. In contrast, knockdown of the AhR in MDA-MB-231 and SKBR3 cells increased invasion [79], whereas other studies gave variable results [55,80]. Stable AhRKO MDA-MB-231 cells were analyzed in a 3-dimensional microfluidic invasion assay that examined both functional and genomic differences with respect to loss of the AhR. MDA-MB-231-AhRKO cells exhibited enhanced invasion characteristics and transient AhR expression in these cells' decreased invasion, confirming that the AhR inhibited invasion. In contrast, the loss of AhR in these cells decreased proliferation and proliferation-related genes, indicating that the receptor played a role in cell proliferation, which was in contrast to its effect as an inhibitor of invasion [81]. Thus, the role of the AhR alone in breast cancer is variable and is breast cancer cell type-dependent; current evidence favors a pro-oncogenic phenotype for the AhR, but this needs to be further investigated in multiple breast cancer cell lines. Nevertheless, the expression of the AhR in breast cancer and in breast cancer cell lines offers the opportunity for investigating the potential for AhR ligands as chemotherapeutic agents for treating breast cancer.

(iii) **Synthetic halogenated aromatic AhR ligands:** Confirmation that the AhR is a target for developing anticancer drugs for treating breast cancer has been extensively investigated using different structural classes of AhR ligands and an array of breast cancer cell lines, including ER-positive (T47D, MCF-7 and ZR-75), ER-negative (MDA-MB-231, MDA-MB-468, MDA-MB-436, MDA-MB-157, MDA-MB435, BT26, CRL2335, BT20, BT549, BT479, HS5787, HCC38, mouse 4T1) and HER-2/ErbB2 positive (BT474, SKBR3 and MDA-MB-453) cells. AhR-active ligands have primarily been used in these studies, but it is also possible that some of these compounds also target other receptors and proteins. AhR specificity is confirmed in many studies by results from AhR knockdown (KO) or cotreating with AhR antagonists. Many of these studies investigate the effects of AhR ligands on one or more of cell proliferation/cell cycle progression, survival/apoptosis invasion/migration, metastasis, inflammation, changes in mRNA and microRNA expression, and as SAhRMs most AhR ligands selectively modulate responses.

Table 1. TCDD and halogenated aromatics as inhibitors of mammary carcinogenesis.

Compounds	Responses	Cell	KO	In Vivo	Reference
TCDD	multiple	MDA-MB-231 MDA-MB-436 MDA-MB-157 MDA-MB-435 and BT474	✓		[73]
2,3,7,8-TCDF	multiple	MDA-MB-231 MDA-MB-436 MDA-MB-157 MDA-MB-435 and BT474	✓		[73]
2,3,4,7,8-PeCDD	multiple	MDA-MB-231 MDA-MB-436 MDA-MB-157 MDA-MB-435 and BT474	✓		[73]
1,2,3,7,8-PeCDD	multiple	MDA-MB-231 MDA-MB-436 MDA-MB-157 MDA-MB-435 and BT474	✓		[73]
3,3′4,4′,5-PeCB	multiple	MDA-MB-231 MDA-MB-436 MDA-MB-157 MDA-MB-435 and BT474	✓		[73]
TCDD	cell cycle prog.	MCF-7	-	-	[82]
TCDD	gr.	MDA-MB-468	-	✓	[83]
TCDD	gr.	MCF-7	-	-	[84]
TCDD	CXCR4/CXCL12	Multiple			[85]
TCDD	Inv	MDA-MB-231, SKBR3	✓	-	[79]
TCDD	Inv	MDA-MB-231, SKBR3	✓	-	[79]
TCDD	Inv	MDA-MB-231, T47D	✓	-	[86]
TCDD	Inv	MDA-MB-231 and BT474	✓	-	[87]
TCDD	gr	MCF-7	-	✓	[88]
TCDD	met	4T-1	-	✓	[89]

Inv = invasion; met = metastasis; gr = growth.

Table 1 summarizes the effects of TCDD and structurally related halogenated aromatics as AhR agonists in breast cancer cells (Figure 1). One study used 5 different ligands and 6 different breast cancer cell lines to show that these AhR ligands inhibited breast cancer cell growth, and this was supported by limited KO studies in which loss of the AhR resulted in loss of AhR ligand-dependent growth inhibition [73]. Moreover, it was also shown that TCDD inhibited tumor growth in an athymic nude mouse xenograft model bearing MDA-MB-468 cells [83]. Several other studies reported that TCDD inhibited growth or invasiveness, decreasing pro-invasion genes (CXCR4 and MMP-9) in breast cancer cells [83–86] and 2,3,7,8-tetrachlorodibenzofuran (TCDF) also inhibited invasion of MDA-MB-431 and T47D cells [86] and BT474 cells [87]. Another early study using MCF-7 cells showed that TCDD inhibited early tumor growth, but this effect was lost during the later stages of the experiment [88]. Wang and coworkers used a syngeneic immune competent mouse xenograft study with mouse mammary cancer 4T-1 cells and showed that TCDD inhibited lung metastasis and metastasis from the primary tumor site but did not affect growth of the primary tumor [89]. In addition, TCDD and DIM suppressed metastasis by targeting SOX4 via microRNAs [86]. Thus, results obtained using TCDD and related AhR ligands indicate that these compounds inhibit some pro-oncogenic functions of breast cancer.

(iv) Synthetic AhR ligands including pharmaceuticals (Figure 2): Initial studies in this laboratory identified MCDF as a partial AhR antagonist which inhibited induction of CYP1A1 by TCDD in cell culture, whereas MCDF exhibited AhR-dependent antiestrogenic activity in the mouse uterus and breast cancer cells. Table 2 summarizes the inhibitory effects of MCDF on the growth and invasion of breast cancer cells [73,87] and this compound also inhibited growth of tumors in an athymic nude mouse model bearing MDA-MB-231 cells [87]. Synthetic aminoflavone [5-amino-2-(4-amino-3-fluorophenyl)-6,8-difluoro-7-methyl-4H-1-benzopyran-4-one; NSC-688228] and its prodrug conjugate are AhR ligands that have been in clinical trials for breast cancer chemotherapy [24–27,90–94]. In contrast to most other AhR ligands, aminoflavone and some related synthetic aromatic amines require AhR-dependent activation of CYP1A1 and other drug metabolizing enzymes. The induced enzymes result in metabolic activation of the pro-drug, which causes downstream cellular damage and pathways leading to cell killing. Two aminobenzothiazole derivatives, namely 2-(4-amino-3-methylphenyl)benzothiazole (DF-203) and 2-(4-amino-3-methlyphenyl)-5 fluorobenzothiazole (SF-203) are AhR ligands that have also been in clinic trials for treating breast cancer [95–103]. These compounds are similar to aminoflavones, undergo metabolic activation and induce cytotoxic downstream pathways, including oxidative stress. Some ER-negative cell lines which exhibit low CYP induction were relatively insensitive to the cytotoxic effects of the aminobenzothiazoles. Several other AhR ligands, including a novel naphthylamide (2-(2-aminophenyl) -H-benzo [d,e]isquinoline-1,3 [2H]-dione) (NAP6) and related compounds [104,105] and N,2-dimethyl-N-[1,2-dimethylindol-5-yl] quinazoline-5-amine ([#]12), [106] also inhibit breast cancer cell/tumor growth. Both AhR ligands may act in part via metabolic activation and #12 also inhibits microtubule polymerization. (Z)-2 (3,4-dichlorophenyl)-3-(1H -pyrrol-2-yl) acrylonitrile (ANI-7) and related compounds are AhR ligands that exhibit antitumor activity in breast cancer and there is some evidence that metabolic activation also contributes to their effects [107–109]. CGS-15943 is an aminoglycoside identified in a screen for inhibitors of multidrug resistance plasmid [110] that was also identified as an AhR ligand that exhibits anticancer activity [111]. This compound induced apoptosis in MDA-MB-468 cells and its activity as a SAhRM was confirmed primarily in liver cancer cell lines. A recent study also showed that carbidopa, a drug used in treating Parkinson's disease, inhibited breast cancer cell and tumor growth through the AhR-dependent degradation of ER [112], and this pathway has also been observed for TCDD [20].

Hu and coworkers [54] investigated 596 pharmaceuticals for their AhR activity and identified only 9 compounds that were active in vitro in mouse liver and in mouse hepatoma cells. As indicated above, some of these AhR active compounds were subsequently screened for their activity in breast cancer cells. Among the AhR -active (liver) pharmaceuticals 4-hydroxytamoxifen mexiletine, flutamide, leflunomide, nimodipine omeprazole, sulindac and tranilast, all but 4-hydroxytamoxifen and mexiletine inhibited migration of MDA-MB-468 cells [55]. In contrast, only nimodipine and omeprazole inhibited MDA-MB-231 cell invasion, and for omeprazole, this response was reversed after knockdown of AhR [87]. Tranilast has also been investigated in mouse 4T1 cancer cells and inhibits cell growth and invasion and migration, as well as tumor growth and metastasis in a syngeneic mouse model [113]. Tranilast was also anticarcinogenic in BT474 and MDA-MB-231 human breast cancer cell lines [114,115]. Beta-Naphthoflavone is a well-known "non-toxic" AhR ligand which inhibits MCF-7 but not MDA-MB-231 cell proliferation, cell cycle progression and related genes [116]. Both raloxifene and 4-hydroxytamoxifen are two antiestrogens that are also AhR ligands that inhibit apoptosis and differentiation of breast cancer cells [117,118] and they are part of a group of compounds that are dual AhR-ER and ligands. Results summarized in Table 2 demonstrate that structurally diverse ligands inhibit mammary carcinogenesis in multiple breast cancer cell lines and in vivo xenograft models. The specific responses observed are ligand structure- and cell context-dependent and this includes compounds such as aminoflavone that have been in clinical trials for breast cancer and other cancers. A role for the AhR in mediating these responses has been confirmed in cell cultures and in vivo studies; however, contributions from the drug acting on its traditional target cannot be excluded.

Table 2. Synthetic and pharmaceutical AhR ligands as inhibitors of mammary carcinogenesis.

Compounds	Responses	Cells	KO	In Vivo	Reference
MCDF	gr	MDA-MB-453, MDA-MB-436, HCC-38, MDA-MB-435, BT-474, MDA-MB-157	✓		[73]
MCDF	inv	MDA-MB-231 and BT474	✓	✓	[87]
MCDF	gr	MDA-MB-468	–	✓	[83]
Aminoflavone	gr, DNA damage cytotoxicity, ROS apoptosis	MCF-7, MDA-MB-231, T47D. ZR-75, MDA-MB-468	–	✓	[24–26,90–95]
Aminobenzothiazoles (DF-203 and SF-203)	gr, ROS, DNA damage	MCF-7, MDA-MB-468, CRL2335, MDA-MB-435	–	✓	[96–103]
Naphthylamide der-invatives (NAP6)	gr	MCF-7, MDA-MB-231, BT26, BT474, MDA-MB-468	–	✓	[104,105]
#12 (quinazoline derivative)	gr, apoptosis, MMP, ROS	MCF-7	–	✓	[106]
ANI -7 (acrylo-nitriles)	gr	MCF-7, T47D, ZR-75 SKBR3, MDA-MB-468, BT20, and BT474	✓	–	[107–109]
Aminoglycoside CG3-15943		MDA-MB-468	✓	–	[110,111]
Flutamide	migr.	MDA-MB-468	–	–	[54]
Leflunomide	migr.	MDA-MB-468	–	–	[54]
Nimodipine	migr.	MDA-MB-468	–	–	[54]
Omeprazole	migr.	MDA-MB-468	–	–	[54]
Sulindac	migr.	MDA-MB-468	–	–	[54]
Sulindac	migr	MDA-MB-468	–	–	[54]
Tranilast	inv, migr, gr, met	MDA-MB-468, 4T1	–	✓	[54,113–115]
β-Naphthoflavone	gr	MCF-7, MDA-MB-231	✓	–	[116]
Raloxifene	Apoptosis	MDA-MB-231	✓	–	[117]
Carbidopa	multiple	MCF-7, MDA-MB-231	–	✓	[112]
4-Hydroxytamoxifen	diff	MCF-7	–	–	[118]

gr = growth; inv = invasion; diff = differentiation; migr = migration; met = metastasis; ROS = reactive oxygen species; MMP = mitochondrial membrane potential.

(v) **Natural products and endogenous AhR ligands**: Natural products such as the polyphenolics are also AhR ligands; however, many of these compounds bind multiple receptors or have other activities which contribute to their anticancer activities in breast and other cancers (Figure 3). 1, 1-Bis (3^1-indolyl) methane (DIM), the dimeric metabolite of indole-3-carbinol (I3C) binds the AhR and several studies confirm the activity of this compound as an inhibitor of breast cancer cell and tumor growth [48,85,119–122]. DIM inhibits growth of ER$^+$ and ER$^+$ cancer cell lines and inhibits growth of carcinogen induced mammary tumors in both orthotopic and syngeneic mouse models. These effects have been associated with CXCR4/CXCL12 downregulation and induction of miR-212/132 [86].

The antiestrogenic activity of DIM was also reported in a human nutritional intervention study with healthy women that express BRCA [122]. I3C also binds the AhR with lower affinity than DIM and I3C inhibits breast cancer cell growth and migration [123–126]; some of this activity may be due to the facile conversion of I3C into DIM. Indolo-[3,2b]-carbazole is another AhR-active metabolite of I3C that inhibits breast cancer cell migration [125]. Although many flavonoids have been characterized as AhR ligands [127,128], very few have been investigated for their effects on breast cancer. Luteolin was particularly effective against MD-MB-231 cells [129] and the prenylflavone icaritin exhibited dose-dependent antiestrogenic activity but also inhibited the growth of MCF-7 cells in culture and in a xenograft model in vivo [130]. Icaritin also downregulated ER expression and this was presumed to be a major pathway for mediating cell growth inhibition. 3,4,5-Trihydroxy-6-methylphthaldehyde (Flavipin) is a fungal metabolite that inhibits T47D, and MDA-MB-231 cell growth, invasion and migration and these responses are blunted after AhR knockdown [131]. Glyceollins (Figure 3) are soybean phytoalexins that are AhR ligands and both glyceollin I and glyceollin II inhibit migration of MDA-MB-231 cells [132]. Camalexin, an indole phytoalexin, 2-hydroxy-6-tridecylbenzoic acid and the polyphenolic gallic acid, are also phytochemical AhR ligands that exhibit anticancer activity in breast cancer [133,134]. Gallic acid inhibits tumor growth in athymic mouse xenograft models bearing MDA-MB-231 and T47D cells, and also inhibited growth, migration, and invasion in cell culture [135].

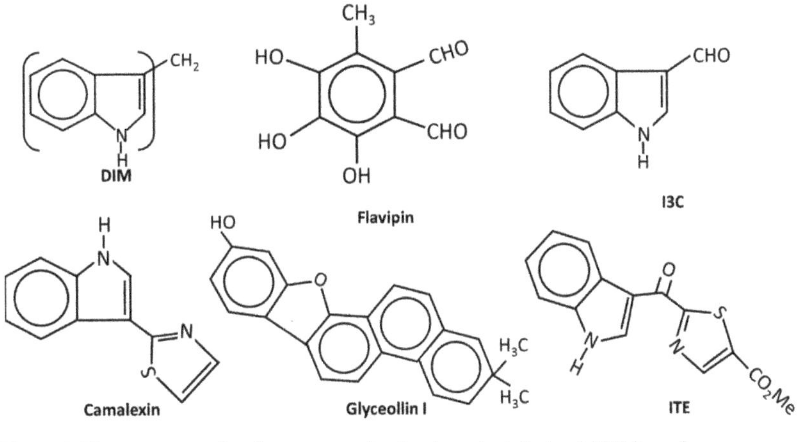

Figure 3. The structures of endogenous and natural product-derived AhR ligands.

FICZ and ITE are endogenous AhR ligands that may play a role in AhR function and both compounds are inhibitory in breast cancer cells [136,137]. ITE inhibits growth, migration, and invasion of MDA-MB-231 but not MCF-7 cells, and this may be related in part to decreased JAG1 and NOTCH signaling. In contrast, the antiproliferative and antimigration effects of FICZ in MCF-7 cells are associated with several miRs. The tryptophan metabolites indoxyl sulfate and indole propionic acid are AhR ligands and inhibited 4T1 cell and tumor growth (syngeneic mouse model) and EMT and induced oxidative stress [138,139]. The results observed with the natural products and potential endogenous AhR ligands clearly show that these compounds exhibit anticancer activity in breast cancer cells (Figure 4). However, it is also apparent that this activity is response and cell context dependent, which is typically observed for SAhRMs.

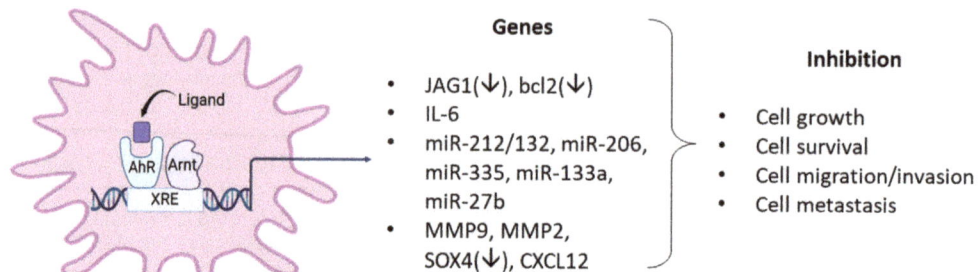

Figure 4. Examples of AhR ligand-activated pathways/genes that result in anticancer activity in breast cancer cells.

5. AhR and AhR Ligands Enhance Mammary Carcinogenesis

Although endogenous expression and function of the AhR in breast cancer cells is variable, the effects of structurally diverse AhR ligands (Tables 1–3) are primarily associated with selective inhibition of pro-oncogenic responses. This was observed in cells in which AhR knockdown exhibited increased or decreased proliferation, survival, or migration/invasion (Figure 5). Studies by Sherr and colleagues contrast with results summarized in Tables 1–3. It was initially reported that the AhR and RelA cooperatively activated cMyc expression in Hs578T cells and thereby enhanced cMyc-dependent tumorigenesis [140]. In a subsequent study in Hs578T cells, it was reported that the constitutive AhR suppressed cMyc expression and was activated by the AhR repressor (AhRR) but not TCDD [30]. These studies, which focused primarily on the role of constitutive AhR, gave variable results; however, subsequent reports show that in ER-negative Hs578T and SUM149 breast cancer cells that AhR ligands enhance tumorigenesis (Table 4) (Figure 5) and contrast with results summarized in Tables 1–3. For example, the tryptophan metabolites kynurenine, xanthurenic, acid (XA) FICZ, and benzol(a)pyrene (BaP) enhance SUM149 cell migration and the AhR antagonist CH223191 inhibited these responses for the former two compounds [141]. Moreover, a newly identified AhR antagonist (CB7993113) [142] and CH223191 also inhibited migration in Hs578T and SUM149 cells, and this is supported by a study showing that the AhR antagonist galangin decreased growth promoting genes in Hs578T cells [143]. Similar results were observed in SUM149, Hs578T and MCF-7 cells where the AhR and its agonists were associated with inducing cancer stem cell characteristics [144]. Suspended ER negative BT549, MDA-MB-231 and SUM159 breast cancers cells express higher AhR levels and AhR inhibition or loss decreased pro-oncogenic pathways. AhR agonists DIM and TCDD enhanced migration of Hs578T and SUM149 cells and complementary results were observed in a zebrafish model [31]. TCDD also induced the inflammatory precursor gene COX-2 and in MCF7-cells DIM inhibited the induction by TCDD [145]. In contrast, it has also been reported that the AhR agonist DIM inhibits mammary carcinogenesis (Table 2). In a study on interactions between tryptophan-2.3-dioxygenase (TD02) and AhR signaling [146], it was observed that cells in suspension exhibited an enhanced response that was associated with expression of higher AhR levels. Knockdown of AhR or treatment with CH223191 decreased MDA-MB-231 and BT549 cell growth and colony formation and kynurenine decreased apoptosis in BT479 cells [146]. Knockdown of the AhR in BT549 and MDA-MB-231 cells in suspension induced apoptosis, which has also been observed in MDA-MB-231 cells treated with AhR ligands that inhibit mammary carcinogenesis (Tables 1–3), and these differences need to be resolved. BaP was used as an AhR ligand and it was shown that it induced migration of MDA-MB-231 cells and this response was inhibited by CH223191 [147]. This inhibitory interaction between an AhR ligand and an AhR antagonist is expected but the results showing that the AhR ligand BaP induced migration of MDA-MB-231 cells contrast with the effects of other AhR ligand in this and other cells lines, as summarized in Tables 1–3.

Table 3. Endogenous and natural product AhR ligands as inhibitors of mammary carcinogenesis.

Compounds	Responses	Cells	KO	In vivo	Reference
DIM	gr, invasion, met	MDA-MB-231, MCF-7, 4T-1	✓	✓	[78,86,119–122]
I3C	gr, migr. apoptosis	MIF-7, MDA-MB-231, MDA-MB-468, T47D	–	–	[123–126]
ICZ	migr	MCF-7, MDA-MB-231,	–	–	[125]
Luteolin	inv, gr, met	MDA-MB-231	–	–	[129]
Icaritin MIR-212/132	gr	MCF-7	✓	✓	[130]
Flavipin	gr, inv, migr	MDA-MB-231, T47D	✓	✓	[131]
Glyceollins CI and II	migr	MDA-MB-231	–	–	[132]
Camalexin	gr, migr (mammosphere)	MCF-7, T47D	–	✓	[133]
2-Hydroxy-6-tridecylbenzone acia	gr	MDA-MB-231	–	–	[134]
Gallic acid	apoptosis, migr, inv, gr	T47D, MDA-MB-231			[135]
ITE		MCF7, MDA-MB-231. MDA-MB-157	✓	–	[136]
FICZ	gr, migr	MCF-7	✓	–	[137]
Indoxylsulfate	ROS, met, migr	4T1	✓	–	[138]
Indolepropionic acid	gr, ROS, met	4T1, SKBR3	✓	–	[139]

gr = growth; migr = migration; inv = invasion; met = metastasis; ROS = reactive oxygen species.

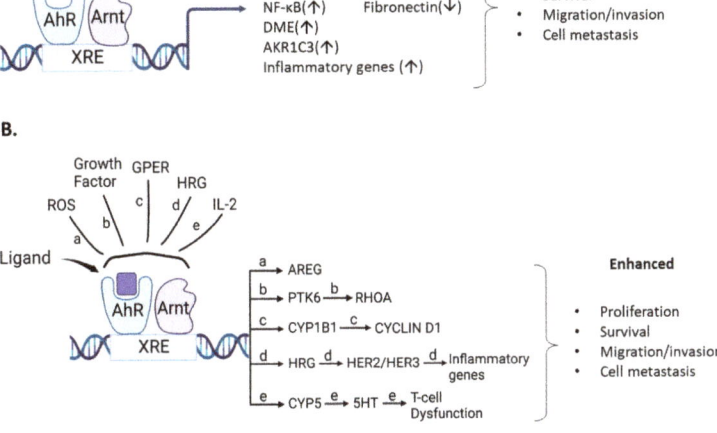

Figure 5. Ligand/AhR-mediated pro-oncogenic activities. (A). AhR ligands metabolically activate pro-oncogenic genes/pathways that are inhibited by AhR loss or AhR antagonists. (B). Role of AhR in pro-oncogenic pathways that involve other factors resulting in activation of downstream pro-oncogenic pathways.

Table 4. AhR/AhR ligands enhancing mammary carcinogenesis.

Compound	Responses/Pathway	Cells	KO	In Vivo	Reference
TCDD	gr, Myc/Rel-AhR	Hs5787	–	–	[30,140]
FICZ, BaP, TCDD, XA, Kyn	migr/AhR-TDO-Kyn	SUM149, Hs578T	✓	✓	[141]
CB7993113 DMBA	migr, inv, tox	BP1, Hs5787	✓	–	[142]
FICZ, BaP, TCDD	migr/AhR-SOX2	Hs578T, MCF-7, SUM149	✓	–	[144]
Galangin, NF, MC	gr/genes	Hs5787	✓	–	[143]
DIM, TCDD	colony form, migr	BP1, Hs578T, SUM149, MDA-MB-231	✓	–	[31,145]
Kyn	colonies, inv met/AhR-TDO-KYN, NFkB	BT59, SUM159, MDA-MB-231	✓	–	[146]
BaP	inv, gr, migr	MDA-MB-231	✓	–	[147]
Phthalates	migr, inv/HDAC6	MCF-7, MDA-MB-231	✓	–	[148–150]
TCDD, Kyn	surv, infl/COX2, NFkB	MDA-MB-231, SKBR3, others	✓	–	[151]
MC	cytotox/AKR1C3	MDA-MB-231	✓	–	[152]
TCDD	apoptosis, gr, AhRR	MDA-MB-231, MCF-7, others	✓	–	[153]
CH223191	Proangiogenic/AhR-AREG-ROS	multiple	✓	✓	[154]
CH223191	met, migr, motility	MDA-MB-231, Hs578T Others	✓	✓	[155]
MC	gr/AhR-GPER	SKBR3	✓	–	[156]
TCDD, BaP	infl, IL6	MCF-7	✓	–	[157]
MC	migr/HRG-AhR	MCF-7	✓	–	[158]
5-Hydroxtryptophan	IL-2-CD8 +T cell exhaustion	4T1	✓	✓	[159]

migr = migration; gr = growth; inv = invasion; form = formation; surv = survival; infl = inflammation; met = metastasis; ROS = reactive oxygen species.

There are also studies where the AhR and other ligands or cellular factors play a pro-oncogenic role in breast cancer. For example, several phthalates activate the extranuclear AhR in MDA-MB-231 cells via activation of histone deacetylase 6 (HDAC6) and downstream induction of cMyc [148]. A subsequent study by this group focused on other factors involved in phthalate-AhR interactions in MCF-7 and MDA-MB-231 cells and their data suggest some phthalates may directly activate the AhR-dependent metabolic genes and enhance doxorubicin metabolism [149]. A third study [149] showed that TCDD induced migration of MCF7 cells, which also contrasted with results of previous studies with TCDD and other AhR ligands (Tables 1–3). Moreover, they observed that mono 2-ethylhexylphthalate (MEHP) induced MCF7 cell migration that was inhibited after cotreatment with TCDD. The phthalate/AhR/AhR ligand interactions gave some conflicting results [148–150] and warrant further investigation due to the importance of environmental/dietary exposures to phthalates. The effects of AhR ligands on drug-induced responses, such as apoptosis in breast cancer, have also been investigated in several cancer cell lines, including MDA-MB-231 and SKBR3 cells treated with doxorubicin, lapatinib and paclitaxel [151]. Cotreatment with TCDD decreased drug induced apoptosis, which was partially reversed by the AhR antagonist 3^1-methoxy-4^1-nitroflavone. A complementary study [152] showed that the AhR blunted the effects of doxorubicin on cell viability in MDA-MB-231 cells and this was due in part to AhR regulation of aldo-ketoreductase 1C3. The AhRR decreases availability of functional AhR by competing for ARNT, and using transgenic mice overexpressing AhRR, it was shown that AhRR suppresses mammary tumor development and AhR-dependent growth and the inflammatory gene COX2 (±TCDD) [153]. Similar results were observed in MCF-7 and MDA-MB-231 cells treated with etoposide and doxorubicin; both drugs induced the percentage of apoptotic cells which was further enhanced after cotransfection with an AhRR expression plasmid. These results are also consistent with a role for the AhR in blunting the effects of drug induced cytotoxic responses in breast cancer.

There is also evidence that the AhR plays a pro-oncogenic role in other models of breast cancer. One study reported that ROS levels in BRCA1 and basal-like breast cancer correlated with AhR expression and this increased expression of amphiregulin (AREG), a ligand for the epidermal growth factor receptor (EGFR) [154]. The AhR antagonist CH223191 inhibited AREG expression in HCC1937 and MDA-MB-468 cells and synergistically interacted with the kinase inhibitor erlotinib in BT20, MDA-MB-468 and HCC1937 cells but not MDA-MB-231 cells (due to low EGFR expression). These results demonstrating growth inhibition of MDA-MB-468 cells by the AhR antagonist CH223191 contrasts with previous reports showing that TCDD, MCDF, I3C and other AhR agonists inhibit MDA-MB-468 cell growth (Tables 1–3). Protein kinase 6 (PTK6) is also overexpressed in many breast tumors and plays a role in lung metastasis and cell motility in triple negative breast cancer cells [155]. Mechanistic studies show a relationship between PTK6, RhOA and the AhR and AhR activities require the PTK6SH2 domain. In SKBR3 cells, it has also been shown that the AhR agonist 3-methylcholanthrene (MC) binds and integrates the AhR and the G protein estrogen receptor (GPER) [156]. This results in induction of CYP1B1 in cancer-associate fibroblasts and SKBR3 cells. Cyclin D1 was also increased and was inhibited not only by CH223191, but also mithramycin (Sp1 inhibitor), G15 (GPER inhibitor) and TMS (CYP1B1) inhibitor. Endogenous growth of SKBR3 cells was not affected by CH223191, suggesting that MC may be acting as a dual AhR/ER ligand [37,39,40,153], and this system needs to be further investigated.

Several studies have also linked expression of the AhR with inflammatory response pathways in breast cancer cells. For example, phorbol ester, (PMA) alone induced interleukin-8 (IL-8) and IL-6 in MCF-7 cells and PMA in combination with TCDD synergistically enhanced Il-6 but not IL-8 mRNA levels [157]. Similar interactions of PMA and interleukin-1β with other AhR ligands enhanced IL-6 levels. Another report showed that heregulin enhanced AhR levels, IL-6 and IL-8 expression and also increased invasion in a HER2 overexpressing breast cancer cell line. Loss of AhR decreased invasion, IL-6 and IL-eight levels [157]. IL-2 plays an important role in the development of T cell exhaustion [159] and this compromises the effects of the CD8 + T cell dependent-immune response to tumors and infection. IL-2 also enhances AhR expression and metabolism of tryptophan to 5-hydroxytryptophan, an AhR ligand which enhances markers of CD8 + T cell exhaustion [159]. Evidence for the IL-2-AhR-5HTP-dependent activation of T cell exhaustion is supported by human and laboratory animal studies, and this pro-oncogenic role for the AhR and 5HTP suggests that targeting the AhR to inhibit IL-2-dependent initiation of CD8 + T cell exhaustion may be feasible for treating breast cancer. It will also be important to resolve potential differences between this and other studies using a syngeneic mouse model and mouse cancer 4T-1 cells. For example, tumors derived from this cell line exhibit T cell exhaustion and two AhR-active tryptophan -related metabolites, indoxyl sulfate and indole propionic acid inhibited tumor growth [138,139].

6. Conclusions

In this review, there is strong evidence that in a large number of breast cancer cell lines the AhR alone exhibits both pro-and anti-oncogenic activity or minimal activity based on results of knockdown experiments. In these cell lines and in some animal models, structurally diverse synthetic, pharmaceutical, natural product and endogenous AhR ligands exhibit pro-oncogenic activity and inhibit one or more of cell/tumor proliferation survival migration/invasion and metastasis (Tables 1–3) (Figure 4). In some studies, these responses are reversed by AhR knockdown or AhR antagonists. Moreover, many of these ligands have been tested in clinical trials for breast cancer chemotherapy. Not surprisingly, the mechanisms associated with the anticancer activity of these SAhRMs exhibit selectivity and are dependent on ligand structure and cell context, and for some compounds this includes their differential effects in ER-positive and ER negative cell lines. However, results illustrated in Figure 4 summarize a number of the key genes/pathways that have been characterized, and these include CXCR4, CXCL12, MMP-9, SOX4, and several microRNAs.

In contrast, the treatment of some cell lines such as the inflammatory Hs578T and SUM149 cells, AhR ligands inhibit AhR-dependent pro-oncogenic genes and signaling pathways. Moreover, several in vitro and in vivo studies show that the AhR plays a pro-oncogenic and pro-inflammatory role in mammary carcinogenesis; AhR agonists enhance these responses, while AhR antagonists inhibit them, as outlined in Figure 5. However, in some cases, effects of AhR ligands in the same cell line gave opposite responses and these differences need to be resolved. However, it is clear that AhR ligands effect some AhR-dependent genes and pathways to promote mammary cancer (Figure 5), whereas there is also strong evidence that AhR agonists are potential drugs for clinical application in breast cancer therapy (Tables 1–3).

It will be important in the future to identify factors that are responsible for these differences in the anticancer activities of AhR ligands (cell context) in order to use AhR-active compounds as "precision" therapeutics for treating breast cancer.

Author Contributions: Writing—original draft preparation, S.S.; writing—review and editing, S.S and L.Z.; visualization, L.Z. All authors have read and agreed to the published version of the manuscript.

Funding: This research was funded by the National Institutes of Health (P30-ES029067) and the Syd Kyle Chair.

Acknowledgments: The financial assistance of the Syd Kyle Chair endowment and the National Institutes of Health (P30-ES029067) are acknowledged. The assistance of Donna Lewis and Weston Porter are gratefully appreciated.

Conflicts of Interest: The authors declare no conflict of interest. The funders had no role in the design of the study; in the collection, analyses, or interpretation of data; in the writing of the manuscript, or in the decision to publish the results.

Abbreviations

AhR repressor, AhRR; amphiregulin, AREG; AhR nuclear translocator ARNT; AhR knockout, AhRKO; Aryl Hydrocarbon Receptor, AhR; 1,4-dihydroxy-2-naphthoic acid, DHNA; diindolylmethane, DIM; 7,12-dimethylbenz[a]anthracene, DMBA; epidermal growth factor receptor, EGFR; estrogen receptor, ER; 6-formyl (3,2-b) carbazole, FICZ; G protein estrogen receptor, GPER; histone deacetylase 6, HDAC6; indole-3-carbinol, I3C; 2-(1′-H-indole-3-carbonyl) thiazole-4-carboxylic acid methyl ester (ITE); 6-methyl-1,3,8-trichlorodibenzofuran, MCDF; Nuclear receptor, NR; Nuclear Receptor 4A1, NR4A1; polyaromatic hydrocarbons, PAHs; Protein kinase 6, PTK6; selective AhR modulators, SAhRMs; $3,3^{1},4,4^{1}$-tetrachlorobiphenyl, TCBP; 2,3,7,8-tetrachlorodibenzo-p-dioxin, TCDD; xenobiotic response elements, XREs.

References

1. Poland, A.; Glover, E.; Kende, A.S. Stereospecific, high affinity binding of 2,3,7,8-tetrachlorodibenzo-p-dioxin by hepatic cytosol: Evidence that the binding species is receptor for induction of aryl hydrocarbon hydroxylase. *J. Biol. Chem.* **1976**, *251*, 4936–4946. [CrossRef]
2. Poland, A.; Knutson, J.C. 2,3,7,8-tetrachlorodibenzo-p-dioxin and related halogenated aromatic hydrocarbons: Examination of the mechanism of toxicity. *Annu. Rev. Pharmacol. Toxicol.* **1982**, *22*, 517–554. [CrossRef] [PubMed]
3. Avilla, M.N.; Malecki, K.M.C.; Hahn, M.E.; Wilson, R.H.; Bradfield, C.A. The Ah Receptor: Adaptive Metabolism, Ligand Diversity, and the Xenokine Model. *Chem. Res. Toxicol.* **2020**, *33*, 860–879. [CrossRef]
4. Schmidt, J.V.; Bradfield, C.A. Ah receptor signaling pathways. *Annu. Rev. Cell Dev. Biol.* **1996**, *12*, 55–89. [CrossRef]

5. Beischlag, T.V.; Luis Morales, J.; Hollingshead, B.D.; Perdew, G.H. The aryl hydrocarbon receptor complex and the control of gene expression. *Crit. Rev. Eukaryot. Gene Expr.* **2008**, *18*, 207–250. [CrossRef]
6. Whitlock, J.P., Jr.; Okino, S.T.; Dong, L.; Ko, H.P.; Clarke-Katzenberg, R.; Ma, Q.; Li, H. Cytochromes P450 5: Induction of cytochrome P4501A1: A model for analyzing mammalian gene transcription. *FASEB J.* **1996**, *10*, 809–818. [CrossRef]
7. Whitlock Jr, J.P. Genetic and molecular aspects of 2, 3, 7, 8-tetrachlorodibenzo-p-dioxin action. *Annu. Rev. Pharmacol. Toxicol.* **1990**, *30*, 251–277. [CrossRef]
8. Hankinson, O. The aryl hydrocarbon receptor complex. *Annu. Rev. Pharmacol. Toxicol.* **1995**, *35*, 307–340. [CrossRef]
9. Evans, R.M. The nuclear receptor superfamily: A rosetta stone for physiology. *Mol. Endocrinol.* **2005**, *19*, 1429–1438. [CrossRef]
10. Chambon, P. The nuclear receptor superfamily: A personal retrospect on the first two decades. *Mol. Endocrinol.* **2005**, *19*, 1418–1428. [CrossRef] [PubMed]
11. Simpson, E.; Santen, R.J. Celebrating 75 years of oestradiol. *J. Mol. Endocrinol.* **2015**, *55*, T1–T20. [CrossRef]
12. Schmidt, J.V.; Su, G.H.; Reddy, J.K.; Simon, M.C.; Bradfield, C.A. Characterization of a murine AhR null allele: Involvement of the Ah receptor in hepatic growth and development. *Proc. Natl. Acad. Sci. USA* **1996**, *93*, 6731–6736. [CrossRef]
13. Mimura, J.; Yamashita, K.; Nakamura, K.; Morita, M.; Takagi, T.N.; Nakao, K.; Ema, M.; Sogawa, K.; Yasuda, M.; Katsuki, M.; et al. Loss of teratogenic response to 2,3,7,8-tetrachlorodibenzo-p-dioxin (TCDD) in mice lacking the Ah (dioxin) receptor. *Genes Cells* **1997**, *2*, 645–654. [CrossRef] [PubMed]
14. Gonzalez, F.J.; Fernandez-Salguero, P. The aryl hydrocarbon receptor: Studies using the AHR-null mice. *Drug Metab Dispos.* **1998**, *26*, 1194–1198.
15. Safe, S.; Jin, U.H.; Park, H.; Chapkin, R.S.; Jayaraman, A. Aryl Hydrocarbon Receptor (AHR) Ligands as Selective AHR Modulators (SAhRMs). *Int. J. Mol. Sci.* **2020**, *21*, 6654. [CrossRef]
16. Safe, S.; Han, H.; Goldsby, J.; Mohankumar, K.; Chapkin, R.S. Aryl Hydrocarbon Receptor (AhR) Ligands as Selective AhR Modulators: Genomic Studies. *Curr. Opin. Toxicol.* **2018**, *11–12*, 10–20. [CrossRef]
17. Denison, M.S.; Nagy, S.R. Activation of the aryl hydrocarbon receptor by structurally diverse exogenous and endogenous chemicals. *Annu. Rev. Pharmacol. Toxicol.* **2003**, *43*, 309–334. [CrossRef]
18. Denison, M.S.; Seidel, S.D.; Rogers, W.J.; Ziccardi, M.H.; Winter, G.M.; Heath-Pagliuso, S. Natural and synthetic ligands for the Ah receptor. In *Molecular Bioloy Approaches to Toxicology*; Puga, A., Kendall, K.B., Eds.; Taylor and Francis: London, UK, 1998; pp. 3–33.
19. Safe, S. Selective Ah receptor modulators (SAhRMs): Progress towards development of a new class of inhibitors of breast cancer growth. *J. Women's Cancer* **2001**, *3*, 37–45.
20. Wormke, M.; Stoner, M.; Saville, B.; Walker, K.; Abdelrahim, M.; Burghardt, R.; Safe, S. The aryl hydrocarbon receptor mediates degradation of estrogen receptor alpha through activation of proteasomes. *Mol. Cell Biol.* **2003**, *23*, 1843–1855. [CrossRef] [PubMed]
21. Krishnan, V.; Porter, W.; Santostefano, M.; Wang, X.; Safe, S. Molecular mechanism of inhibition of estrogen-induced cathepsin D gene expression by 2,3,7,8-tetrachlorodibenzo-p-dioxin (TCDD) in MCF-7 cells. *Mol. Cell Biol.* **1995**, *15*, 6710–6719. [CrossRef] [PubMed]
22. Safe, S.; Wormke, M. Inhibitory aryl hydrocarbon receptor-estrogen receptor alpha cross-talk and mechanisms of action. *Chem. Res. Toxicol.* **2003**, *16*, 807–816. [CrossRef]
23. Baker, J.R.; Sakoff, J.A.; McCluskey, A. The aryl hydrocarbon receptor (AhR) as a breast cancer drug target. *Med. Res. Rev.* **2020**, *40*, 972–1001. [CrossRef] [PubMed]
24. Meng, L.-h.; Kohlhagen, G.; Liao, Z.-y.; Antony, S.; Sausville, E.; Pommier, Y. DNA-protein cross-links and replication-dependent histone H2AX phosphorylation induced by aminoflavone (NSC 686288), a novel anticancer agent active against human breast cancer cells. *Cancer Res.* **2005**, *65*, 5337–5343. [CrossRef]
25. Terzuoli, E.; Puppo, M.; Rapisarda, A.; Uranchimeg, B.; Cao, L.; Burger, A.M.; Ziche, M.; Melillo, G. Aminoflavone, a ligand of the aryl hydrocarbon receptor, inhibits HIF-1α expression in an AhR-independent fashion. *Cancer Res.* **2010**, *70*, 6837–6848. [CrossRef] [PubMed]
26. Callero, M.A.; Suarez, G.V.; Luzzani, G.; Itkin, B.; Nguyen, B.; Loaiza-Perez, A.I. Aryl hydrocarbon receptor activation by aminoflavone: New molecular target for renal cancer treatment. *Int. J. Oncol.* **2012**, *41*, 125–134. [CrossRef] [PubMed]
27. Kuffel, M.J.; Schroeder, J.C.; Pobst, L.J.; Naylor, S.; Reid, J.M.; Kaufmann, S.H.; Ames, M.M. Activation of the antitumor agent aminoflavone (NSC 686288) is mediated by induction of tumor cell cytochrome P450 1A1/1A2. *Mol. Pharmacol.* **2002**, *62*, 143–153. [CrossRef]
28. Guarnieri, T. Aryl Hydrocarbon Receptor Connects Inflammation to Breast Cancer. *Int. J. Mol. Sci.* **2020**, *21*, 5264. [CrossRef]
29. Schlezinger, J.J.; Liu, D.; Farago, M.; Seldin, D.C.; Belguise, K.; Sonenshein, G.E.; Sherr, D.H. A role for the aryl hydrocarbon receptor in mammary gland tumorigenesis. *Biol. Chem.* **2006**, *387*, 1175–1187. [CrossRef]
30. Yang, X.; Liu, D.; Murray, T.J.; Mitchell, G.C.; Hesterman, E.V.; Karchner, S.I.; Merson, R.R.; Hahn, M.E.; Sherr, D.H. The aryl hydrocarbon receptor constitutively represses c-myc transcription in human mammary tumor cells. *Oncogene* **2005**, *24*, 7869–7881. [CrossRef]
31. Narasimhan, S.; Stanford Zulick, E.; Novikov, O.; Parks, A.J.; Schlezinger, J.J.; Wang, Z.; Laroche, F.; Feng, H.; Mulas, F.; Monti, S.; et al. Towards Resolving the Pro- and Anti-Tumor Effects of the Aryl Hydrocarbon Receptor. *Int. J. Mol. Sci.* **2018**, *19*, 1388. [CrossRef]

32. Murray, I.A.; Patterson, A.D.; Perdew, G.H. Aryl hydrocarbon receptor ligands in cancer: Friend and foe. *Nat. Rev. Cancer* **2014**, *14*, 801–814. [CrossRef]
33. Kolluri, S.K.; Jin, U.H.; Safe, S. Role of the aryl hydrocarbon receptor in carcinogenesis and potential as an anti-cancer drug target. *Arch. Toxicol.* **2017**, *91*, 2497–2513. [CrossRef] [PubMed]
34. Jin, U.-H.; Karki, K.; Cheng, Y.; Michelhaugh, S.K.; Mittal, S.; Safe, S. The aryl hydrocarbon receptor is a tumor suppressor–like gene in glioblastoma. *J. Biol. Chem.* **2019**, *294*, 11342–11353. [CrossRef]
35. Opitz, C.A.; Litzenburger, U.M.; Sahm, F.; Ott, M.; Tritschler, I.; Trump, S.; Schumacher, T.; Jestaedt, L.; Schrenk, D.; Weller, M.; et al. An endogenous tumour-promoting ligand of the human aryl hydrocarbon receptor. *Nature* **2011**, *478*, 197–203. [CrossRef]
36. Abdelrahim, M.; Ariazi, E.; Kim, K.; Khan, S.; Barhoumi, R.; Burghardt, R.; Liu, S.; Hill, D.; Finnell, R.; Wlodarczyk, B. 3-Methylcholanthrene and other aryl hydrocarbon receptor agonists directly activate estrogen receptor α. *Cancer Res.* **2006**, *66*, 2459–2467. [CrossRef] [PubMed]
37. Liu, S.; Abdelrahim, M.; Khan, S.; Ariazi, E.; Jordan, V.C.; Safe, S. Aryl hydrocarbon receptor agonists directly activate estrogen receptor alpha in MCF-7 breast cancer cells. *Biol. Chem.* **2006**, *387*, 1209–1213. [CrossRef]
38. Shipley, J.M.; Waxman, D.J. Aryl hydrocarbon receptor-independent activation of estrogen receptor-dependent transcription by 3-methycholanthrene. *Toxicol. Appl. Pharmacol.* **2006**, *213*, 87–97. [CrossRef]
39. Swedenborg, E.; Rüegg, J.; Hillenweck, A.; Rehnmark, S.; Faulds, M.H.; Zalko, D.; Pongratz, I.; Pettersson, K. 3-Methylcholanthrene displays dual effects on estrogen receptor (ER) α and ERβ signaling in a cell-type specific fashion. *Mol. Pharmacol.* **2008**, *73*, 575–586. [CrossRef] [PubMed]
40. Rannug, A.; Rannug, U.; Rosenkranz, H.S.; Winqvist, L.; Westerholm, R.; Agurell, E.; Grafstrom, A.K. Certain photooxidized derivatives of tryptophan bind with very high affinity to the Ah receptor and are likely to be endogenous signal substances. *J. Biol. Chem.* **1987**, *262*, 15422–15427. [CrossRef]
41. Song, J.; Clagett-Dame, M.; Peterson, R.E.; Hahn, M.E.; Westler, W.M.; Sicinski, R.R.; DeLuca, H.F. A ligand for the aryl hydrocarbon receptor isolated from lung. *Proc. Natl. Acad. Sci. USA* **2002**, *99*, 14694–14699. [CrossRef] [PubMed]
42. Chiaro, C.R.; Morales, J.L.; Prabhu, K.S.; Perdew, G.H. Leukotriene A4 metabolites are endogenous ligands for the Ah receptor. *Biochemistry* **2008**, *47*, 8445–8455. [CrossRef] [PubMed]
43. Zelante, T.; Iannitti, R.G.; Cunha, C.; De Luca, A.; Giovannini, G.; Pieraccini, G.; Zecchi, R.; D'Angelo, C.; Massi-Benedetti, C.; Fallarino, F.; et al. Tryptophan catabolites from microbiota engage aryl hydrocarbon receptor and balance mucosal reactivity via interleukin-22. *Immunity* **2013**, *39*, 372–385. [CrossRef] [PubMed]
44. Fukumoto, S.; Toshimitsu, T.; Matsuoka, S.; Maruyama, A.; Oh-Oka, K.; Takamura, T.; Nakamura, Y.; Ishimaru, K.; Fujii-Kuriyama, Y.; Ikegami, S.; et al. Identification of a probiotic bacteria-derived activator of the aryl hydrocarbon receptor that inhibits colitis. *Immunol. Cell Biol.* **2014**, *92*, 460–465. [CrossRef] [PubMed]
45. Mexia, N.; Gaitanis, G.; Velegraki, A.; Soshilov, A.; Denison, M.S.; Magiatis, P. Pityriazepin and other potent AhR ligands isolated from Malassezia furfur yeast. *Arch. Biochem. Biophys.* **2015**, *571*, 16–20. [CrossRef] [PubMed]
46. Holcomb, M.; Safe, S. Inhibition of 7,12-dimethylbenzanthracene-induced rat mammary tumor growth by 2,3,7,8-tetrachlorodibenzo-p-dioxin. *Cancer Lett.* **1994**, *82*, 43–47. [CrossRef]
47. Ramamoorthy, K.; Gupta, M.S.; Sun, G.; McDougal, A.; Safe, S. 3,3′,4,4′-Tetrachlorobiphenyl exhibits antiestrogenic and antitumorigenic activity in the rodent uterus and mammary and in human breast cancer cells. *Carcinogenesis* **1999**, *20*, 115–123. [CrossRef]
48. Chen, I.; McDougal, A.; Wang, F.; Safe, S. Aryl hydrocarbon receptor-mediated antiestrogenic and antitumorigenic activity of diindolylmethane. *Carcinogenesis* **1998**, *19*, 1631–1639. [CrossRef]
49. McDougal, A.; Wilson, C.; Safe, S. Inhibition of 7,12-dimethylbenz[a]anthracene-induced rat mammary tumor growth by aryl hydrocarbon receptor agonists. *Cancer Lett.* **1997**, *120*, 53–63. [CrossRef]
50. McDougal, A.; Sethi Gupta, M.; Ramamoorthy, K.; Sun, G.; Safe, S.H. Inhibition of carcinogen-induced rat mammary tumor growth and other estrogen-dependent responses by symmetrical dihalo-substituted analogs of diindolylmethane. *Cancer Lett.* **2000**, *151*, 169–179. [CrossRef]
51. McDougal, A.; Wormke, M.; Calvin, J.; Safe, S. Tamoxifen-induced antitumorigenic/antiestrogenic action synergized by a selective aryl hydrocarbon receptor modulator. *Cancer Res.* **2001**, *61*, 3902–3907.
52. Huggins, C.B. Selective induction of hormone-dependent mammary adenocarcinoma in the rat. *J. Lab. Clin. Med.* **1987**, *109*, 262–266. [PubMed]
53. Hu, W.; Sorrentino, C.; Denison, M.S.; Kolaja, K.; Fielden, M.R. Induction of cyp1a1 is a nonspecific biomarker of aryl hydrocarbon receptor activation: Results of large scale screening of pharmaceuticals and toxicants in vivo and in vitro. *Mol. Pharmacol.* **2007**, *71*, 1475–1486. [CrossRef] [PubMed]
54. Jin, U.H.; Lee, S.O.; Safe, S. Aryl hydrocarbon receptor (AHR)-active pharmaceuticals are selective AHR modulators in MDA-MB-468 and BT474 breast cancer cells. *J. Pharm. Exp.* **2012**, *343*, 333–341. [CrossRef] [PubMed]
55. Jin, U.H.; Lee, S.O.; Pfent, C.; Safe, S. The aryl hydrocarbon receptor ligand omeprazole inhibits breast cancer cell invasion and metastasis. *BMC Cancer* **2014**, *14*, 498. [CrossRef] [PubMed]
56. Jin, U.H.; Kim, S.B.; Safe, S. Omeprazole Inhibits Pancreatic Cancer Cell Invasion through a Nongenomic Aryl Hydrocarbon Receptor Pathway. *Chem. Res. Toxicol.* **2015**, *28*, 907–918. [CrossRef]

57. Saito, R.; Miki, Y.; Hata, S.; Takagi, K.; Iida, S.; Oba, Y.; Ono, K.; Ishida, T.; Suzuki, T.; Ohuchi, N. Aryl hydrocarbon receptor in breast cancer—A newly defined prognostic marker. *Horm. Cancer* **2014**, *5*, 11–21. [CrossRef]
58. Vacher, S.; Castagnet, P.; Chemlali, W.; Lallemand, F.; Meseure, D.; Pocard, M.; Bieche, I.; Perrot-Applanat, M. High AHR expression in breast tumors correlates with expression of genes from several signaling pathways namely inflammation and endogenous tryptophan metabolism. *PLoS ONE* **2018**, *13*, e0190619. [CrossRef]
59. Tryggvadottir, H.; Sandén, E.; Björner, S.; Bressan, A.; Ygland Rödström, M.; Khazaei, S.; Edwards, D.P.; Nodin, B.; Jirström, K.; Isaksson, K. The Prognostic Impact of Intratumoral Aryl Hydrocarbon Receptor in Primary Breast Cancer Depends on the Type of Endocrine Therapy: A Population-Based Cohort Study. *Front. Oncol.* **2021**, *11*, 1671. [CrossRef]
60. Jeschke, U.; Zhang, X.; Kuhn, C.; Jalaguier, S.; Colinge, J.; Pfender, K.; Mayr, D.; Ditsch, N.; Harbeck, N.; Mahner, S. The prognostic impact of the aryl hydrocarbon receptor (AhR) in primary breast cancer depends on the lymph node status. *Int. J. Mol. Sci.* **2019**, *20*, 1016. [CrossRef]
61. Li, Y.; Qin, H.Z.; Song, Q.; Wu, X.D.; Zhu, J.H. Lack of association between the aryl hydrocarbon receptor rs2066853 polymorphism and breast cancer: A meta-analysis on Ahr polymorphism and breast cancer. *Genet. Mol. Res.* **2015**, *14*, 16162–16168. [CrossRef]
62. Marshall, N.B.; Kerkvliet, N.I. Dioxin and immune regulation: Emerging role of aryl hydrocarbon receptor in the generation of regulatory T cells. *Ann. N. Y. Acad. Sci.* **2010**, *1183*, 25–37. [CrossRef]
63. Gutierrez-Vazquez, C.; Quintana, F.J. Regulation of the Immune Response by the Aryl Hydrocarbon Receptor. *Immunity* **2018**, *48*, 19–33. [CrossRef]
64. Esser, C.; Rannug, A. The aryl hydrocarbon receptor in barrier organ physiology, immunology, and toxicology. *Pharm. Rev.* **2015**, *67*, 259–279. [CrossRef]
65. Stockinger, B.; Di Meglio, P.; Gialitakis, M.; Duarte, J.H. The aryl hydrocarbon receptor: Multitasking in the immune system. *Annu. Rev. Immunol.* **2014**, *32*, 403–432. [CrossRef] [PubMed]
66. Lewis, B.C.; Hudgins, S.; Lewis, A.; Schorr, K.; Sommer, R.; Peterson, R.E.; Flaws, J.A.; Furth, P.A. In utero and lactational treatment with 2,3,7,8-tetrachlorodibenzo-p-dioxin impairs mammary gland differentiation but does not block the response to exogenous estrogen in the postpubertal female rat. *Toxicol. Sci.* **2001**, *62*, 46–53. [CrossRef] [PubMed]
67. Lew, B.J.; Collins, L.L.; O'Reilly, M.A.; Lawrence, B.P. Activation of the aryl hydrocarbon receptor during different critical windows in pregnancy alters mammary epithelial cell proliferation and differentiation. *Toxicol. Sci.* **2009**, *111*, 151–162. [CrossRef]
68. Vorderstrasse, B.A.; Fenton, S.E.; Bohn, A.A.; Cundiff, J.A.; Lawrence, B.P. A novel effect of dioxin: Exposure during pregnancy severely impairs mammary gland differentiation. *Toxicol. Sci.* **2004**, *78*, 248–257. [CrossRef]
69. Kociba, R.J.; Keyes, D.G.; Beyer, J.E.; Carreon, R.M.; Wade, C.E.; Dittenber, D.A.; Kalnins, R.P.; Frauson, L.E.; Park, C.L.; Barnard, S.D.; et al. Results of a 2-year chronic toxicity and oncogenicity study of 2,3,7,8-tetrachlorodibenzo-p-dioxin (TCDD) in rats. *Toxicol. Appl. Pharmacol.* **1978**, *46*, 279–303. [CrossRef]
70. Walker, N.J.; Wyde, M.E.; Fischer, L.J.; Nyska, A.; Bucher, J.R. Comparison of chronic toxicity and carcinogenicity of 2,3,7,8-tetrachlorodibenzo-p-dioxin (TCDD) in 2-year bioassays in female Sprague-Dawley rats. *Mol. Nutr. Food Res.* **2006**, *50*, 934–944. [CrossRef] [PubMed]
71. Jenkins, S.; Rowell, C.; Wang, J.; Lamartiniere, C.A. Prenatal TCDD exposure predisposes for mammary cancer in rats. *Reprod. Toxicol.* **2007**, *23*, 391–396. [CrossRef]
72. Wang, T.; Gavin, H.M.; Arlt, V.M.; Lawrence, B.P.; Fenton, S.E.; Medina, D.; Vorderstrasse, B.A. Aryl hydrocarbon receptor activation during pregnancy, and in adult nulliparous mice, delays the subsequent development of DMBA-induced mammary tumors. *Int. J. Cancer* **2011**, *128*, 1509–1523. [CrossRef]
73. Zhang, S.; Lei, P.; Liu, X.; Li, X.; Walker, K.; Kotha, L.; Rowlands, C.; Safe, S. The aryl hydrocarbon receptor as a target for estrogen receptor-negative breast cancer chemotherapy. *Endocr. Relat. Cancer* **2009**, *16*, 835–844. [CrossRef] [PubMed]
74. Spink, B.C.; Bennett, J.A.; Lostritto, N.; Cole, J.R.; Spink, D.C. Expression of the aryl hydrocarbon receptor is not required for the proliferation, migration, invasion, or estrogen-dependent tumorigenesis of MCF-7 breast cancer cells. *Mol. Carcinog.* **2013**, *52*, 544–554. [CrossRef] [PubMed]
75. Yoshioka, H.; Hiromori, Y.; Aoki, A.; Kimura, T.; Fujii-Kuriyama, Y.; Nagase, H.; Nakanishi, T. Possible aryl hydrocarbon receptor-independent pathway of 2,3,7,8-tetrachlorodibenzo-p-dioxin-induced antiproliferative response in human breast cancer cells. *Toxicol. Lett.* **2012**, *211*, 257–265. [CrossRef] [PubMed]
76. Li, E.-Y.; Huang, W.-Y.; Chang, Y.-C.; Tsai, M.-H.; Chuang, E.Y.; Kuok, Q.-Y.; Bai, S.-T.; Chao, L.-Y.; Sher, Y.-P.; Lai, L.-C. Aryl hydrocarbon receptor activates NDRG1 transcription under hypoxia in breast cancer cells. *Sci. Rep.* **2016**, *6*, 1–13. [CrossRef]
77. Luecke-Johansson, S.; Gralla, M.; Rundqvist, H.; Ho, J.C.; Johnson, R.S.; Gradin, K.; Poellinger, L. A Molecular Mechanism To Switch the Aryl Hydrocarbon Receptor from a Transcription Factor to an E3 Ubiquitin Ligase. *Mol. Cell Biol.* **2017**, *37*, e00630-16. [CrossRef] [PubMed]
78. Goode, G.; Pratap, S.; Eltom, S.E. Depletion of the aryl hydrocarbon receptor in MDA-MB-231 human breast cancer cells altered the expression of genes in key regulatory pathways of cancer. *PLoS ONE* **2014**, *9*, e100103. [CrossRef]
79. Hall, J.M.; Barhoover, M.A.; Kazmin, D.; McDonnell, D.P.; Greenlee, W.F.; Thomas, R.S. Activation of the aryl-hydrocarbon receptor inhibits invasive and metastatic features of human breast cancer cells and promotes breast cancer cell differentiation. *Mol. Endocrinol.* **2010**, *24*, 359–369. [CrossRef]

80. Goode, G.D.; Ballard, B.R.; Manning, H.C.; Freeman, M.L.; Kang, Y.; Eltom, S.E. Knockdown of aberrantly upregulated aryl hydrocarbon receptor reduces tumor growth and metastasis of MDA-MB-231 human breast cancer cell line. *Int. J. Cancer.* **2013**, *133*, 2769–2780. [CrossRef]
81. Li, B.B.; Scott, E.Y.; Olafsen, N.E.; Matthews, J.; Wheeler, A.R. Analysis of the effects of aryl hydrocarbon receptor expression on cancer cell invasion via three-dimensional microfluidic invasion assays. *Lab A Chip* **2022**, *22*, 313–325. [CrossRef]
82. Barhoover, M.A.; Hall, J.M.; Greenlee, W.F.; Thomas, R.S. Aryl hydrocarbon receptor regulates cell cycle progression in human breast cancer cells via a functional interaction with cyclin-dependent kinase 4. *Mol. Pharmacol.* **2010**, *77*, 195–201. [CrossRef] [PubMed]
83. Wang, W.L.; Porter, W.; Burghardt, R.; Safe, S.H. Mechanism of inhibition of MDA-MB-468 breast cancer cell growth by 2,3,7,8-tetrachlorodibenzo-p-dioxin. *Carcinogenesis* **1997**, *18*, 925–933. [CrossRef] [PubMed]
84. Vogel, C.; Abel, J. Effect of 2,3,7,8-tetrachlorodibenzo-p-dioxin on growth factor expression in the human breast cancer cell line MCF-7. *Arch. Toxicol.* **1995**, *69*, 259–265. [CrossRef] [PubMed]
85. Hsu, E.L.; Yoon, D.; Choi, H.H.; Wang, F.; Taylor, R.T.; Chen, N.; Zhang, R.; Hankinson, O. A proposed mechanism for the protective effect of dioxin against breast cancer. *Toxicol. Sci. Off. J. Soc. Toxicol.* **2007**, *98*, 436–444. [CrossRef] [PubMed]
86. Hanieh, H. Aryl hydrocarbon receptor-microRNA-212/132 axis in human breast cancer suppresses metastasis by targeting SOX4. *Mol. Cancer* **2015**, *14*, 172. [CrossRef] [PubMed]
87. Zhang, S.; Kim, K.; Jin, U.H.; Pfent, C.; Cao, H.; Amendt, B.; Liu, X.; Wilson-Robles, H.; Safe, S. Aryl hydrocarbon receptor agonists induce microRNA-335 expression and inhibit lung metastasis of estrogen receptor negative breast cancer cells. *Mol. Cancer* **2012**, *11*, 108–118. [CrossRef]
88. Gierthy, J.F.; Bennett, J.A.; Bradley, L.M.; Cutler, D.S. Correlation of in vitro and in vivo growth suppression of MCF-7 human breast cancer by 2,3,7,8-tetrachlorodibenzo-p-dioxin. *Cancer Res.* **1993**, *53*, 3149–3153.
89. Wang, T.; Wyrick, K.L.; Meadows, G.G.; Wills, T.B.; Vorderstrasse, B.A. Activation of the aryl hydrocarbon receptor by TCDD inhibits mammary tumor metastasis in a syngeneic mouse model of breast cancer. *Toxicol. Sci.* **2011**, *124*, 291–298. [CrossRef] [PubMed]
90. Loaiza-Perez, A.I.; Kenney, S.; Boswell, J.; Hollingshead, M.; Alley, M.C.; Hose, C.; Ciolino, H.P.; Yeh, G.C.; Trepel, J.B.; Vistica, D.T.; et al. Aryl hydrocarbon receptor activation of an antitumor aminoflavone: Basis of selective toxicity for MCF-7 breast tumor cells. *Mol. Cancer* **2004**, *3*, 715–725. [CrossRef]
91. Callero, M.A.; Loaiza-Pérez, A.I. The role of aryl hydrocarbon receptor and crosstalk with estrogen receptor in response of breast cancer cells to the novel antitumor agents benzothiazoles and aminoflavone. *Int. J. Breast Cancer* **2011**, *2011*, 923250. [CrossRef]
92. McLean, L.; Soto, U.; Agama, K.; Francis, J.; Jimenez, R.; Pommier, Y.; Sowers, L.; Brantley, E. Aminoflavone induces oxidative DNA damage and reactive oxidative species-mediated apoptosis in breast cancer cells. *Int. J. Cancer* **2008**, *122*, 1665–1674. [CrossRef] [PubMed]
93. Campbell, P.S.; Mavingire, N.; Khan, S.; Rowland, L.K.; Wooten, J.V.; Opoku-Agyeman, A.; Guevara, A.; Soto, U.; Cavalli, F.; Loaiza-Pérez, A.I. AhR ligand aminoflavone suppresses α6-integrin–Src-Akt signaling to attenuate tamoxifen resistance in breast cancer cells. *J. Cell. Physiol.* **2019**, *234*, 108–121. [CrossRef]
94. Brantley, E.; Callero, M.A.; Berardi, D.E.; Campbell, P.; Rowland, L.; Zylstra, D.; Amis, L.; Yee, M.; Simian, M.; Todaro, L. AhR ligand Aminoflavone inhibits α6-integrin expression and breast cancer sphere-initiating capacity. *Cancer Lett.* **2016**, *376*, 53–61. [CrossRef]
95. Callero, M.A.; Rodriguez, C.E.; Sólimo, A.; Bal de Kier Joffé, E.; Loaiza Perez, A.I. The immune system as a new possible cell target for AFP 464 in a spontaneous mammary cancer mouse model. *J. Cell. Biochem.* **2017**, *118*, 2841–2849. [CrossRef] [PubMed]
96. Loaiza-Perez, A.I.; Trapani, V.; Hose, C.; Singh, S.S.; Trepel, J.B.; Stevens, M.F.; Bradshaw, T.D.; Sausville, E.A. Aryl hydrocarbon receptor mediates sensitivity of MCF-7 breast cancer cells to antitumor agent 2-(4-amino-3-methylphenyl) benzothiazole. *Mol. Pharmacol.* **2002**, *61*, 13–19. [CrossRef] [PubMed]
97. Chua, M.-S.; Kashiyama, E.; Bradshaw, T.D.; Stinson, S.F.; Brantley, E.; Sausville, E.A.; Stevens, M.F. Role of CYP1A1 in modulation of antitumor properties of the novel agent 2-(4-amino-3-methylphenyl) benzothiazole (DF 203, NSC 674495) in human breast cancer cells. *Cancer Res.* **2000**, *60*, 5196–5203.
98. McLean, L.S.; Watkins, C.N.; Campbell, P.; Zylstra, D.; Rowland, L.; Amis, L.H.; Scott, L.; Babb, C.E.; Livingston, W.J.; Darwanto, A. Aryl hydrocarbon receptor ligand 5F 203 induces oxidative stress that triggers DNA damage in human breast cancer cells. *Chem. Res. Toxicol.* **2015**, *28*, 855–871. [CrossRef] [PubMed]
99. Stone, E.L.; Citossi, F.; Singh, R.; Kaur, B.; Gaskell, M.; Farmer, P.B.; Monks, A.; Hose, C.; Stevens, M.F.; Leong, C.-O. Antitumour benzothiazoles. Part 32: DNA adducts and double strand breaks correlate with activity; synthesis of 5F203 hydrogels for local delivery. *Bioorganic Med. Chem.* **2015**, *23*, 6891–6899. [CrossRef]
100. Trapani, V.; Patel, V.; Leong, C.; Ciolino, H.; Yeh, G.; Hose, C.; Trepel, J.; Stevens, M.; Sausville, E.; Loaiza-Perez, A. DNA damage and cell cycle arrest induced by 2-(4-amino-3-methylphenyl)-5-fluorobenzothiazole (5F 203, NSC 703786) is attenuated in aryl hydrocarbon receptor deficient MCF-7 cells. *Br. J. Cancer* **2003**, *88*, 599–605. [CrossRef]
101. Bradshaw, T.D.; Bibby, M.C.; Double, J.A.; Fichtner, I.; Cooper, P.A.; Alley, M.C.; Donohue, S.; Stinson, S.F.; Tomaszewjski, J.E.; Sausville, E.A. Preclinical evaluation of amino acid prodrugs of novel antitumor 2-(4-amino-3-methylphenyl) benzothiazoles. *Mol. Cancer Ther.* **2002**, *1*, 239–246. [PubMed]

102. Brantley, E.; Antony, S.; Kohlhagen, G.; Meng, L.; Agama, K.; Stinson, S.F.; Sausville, E.A.; Pommier, Y. Anti-tumor drug candidate 2-(4-amino-3-methylphenyl)-5-fluorobenzothiazole induces single-strand breaks and DNA-protein cross-links in sensitive MCF-7 breast cancer cells. *Cancer Chemother. Pharmacol.* **2006**, *58*, 62–72. [CrossRef]
103. Leong, C.O.; Gaskell, M.; Martin, E.A.; Heydon, R.T.; Farmer, P.B.; Bibby, M.C.; Cooper, P.A.; Double, J.A.; Bradshaw, T.D.; Stevens, M.F. Antitumour 2-(4-aminophenyl)benzothiazoles generate DNA adducts in sensitive tumour cells in vitro and in vivo. *Br. J. Cancer* **2003**, *88*, 470–477. [CrossRef] [PubMed]
104. Gilbert, J.; De Iuliis, G.N.; McCluskey, A.; Sakoff, J.A. A novel naphthalimide that selectively targets breast cancer via the arylhydrocarbon receptor pathway. *Sci. Rep.* **2020**, *10*, 13978. [CrossRef] [PubMed]
105. Baker, J.R.; Pollard, B.L.; Lin, A.J.S.; Gilbert, J.; Paula, S.; Zhu, X.; Sakoff, J.A.; McCluskey, A. Modelling and Phenotypic Screening of NAP-6 and 10-Cl-BBQ, AhR Ligands Displaying Selective Breast Cancer Cytotoxicity in Vitro. *ChemMedChem* **2021**, *16*, 1499–1512. [CrossRef] [PubMed]
106. Wang, K.; Zhong, H.; Li, N.; Yu, N.; Wang, Y.; Chen, L.; Sun, J. Discovery of Novel Anti-Breast-Cancer Inhibitors by Synergistically Antagonizing Microtubule Polymerization and Aryl Hydrocarbon Receptor Expression. *J. Med. Chem.* **2021**, *64*, 12964–12977. [CrossRef]
107. Gilbert, J.; De Iuliis, G.N.; Tarleton, M.; McCluskey, A.; Sakoff, J.A. (Z)-2-(3,4-Dichlorophenyl)-3-(1H-Pyrrol-2-yl)Acrylonitrile Exhibits Selective Antitumor Activity in Breast Cancer Cell Lines via the Aryl Hydrocarbon Receptor Pathway. *Mol. Pharmacol.* **2018**, *93*, 168–177. [CrossRef]
108. Baker, J.R.; Russell, C.C.; Gilbert, J.; McCluskey, A.; Sakoff, J.A. Amino alcohol acrylonitriles as broad spectrum and tumour selective cytotoxic agents. *RSC Med. Chem.* **2021**, *12*, 929–942. [CrossRef]
109. Stanton, D.T.; Baker, J.R.; McCluskey, A.; Paula, S. Development and interpretation of a QSAR model for in vitro breast cancer (MCF-7) cytotoxicity of 2-phenylacrylonitriles. *J. Comput. Aided. Mol. Des.* **2021**, *35*, 613–628. [CrossRef]
110. Zulauf, K.E.; Kirby, J.E. Discovery of small-molecule inhibitors of multidrug-resistance plasmid maintenance using a high-throughput screening approach. *Proc. Natl. Acad. Sci. USA* **2020**, *117*, 29839–29850. [CrossRef]
111. O'Donnell, E.F., 3rd; Jang, H.S.; Liefwalker, D.F.; Kerkvliet, N.I.; Kolluri, S.K. Discovery and Mechanistic Characterization of a Select Modulator of AhR-regulated Transcription (SMAhRT) with Anti-cancer Effects. *Apoptosis* **2021**, *26*, 307–322. [CrossRef]
112. Chen, Z.; Xia, X.; Chen, H.; Huang, H.; An, X.; Sun, M.; Yao, Q.; Kim, K.; Zhang, H.; Chu, M.; et al. Carbidopa suppresses estrogen receptor-positive breast cancer via AhR-mediated proteasomal degradation of ERalpha. *Investig. New Drugs*, 2022; Online ahead of print. [CrossRef]
113. Chakrabarti, R.; Subramaniam, V.; Abdalla, S.; Jothy, S.; Prud'homme, G.J. Tranilast inhibits the growth and metastasis of mammary carcinoma. *Anticancer Drugs* **2009**, *20*, 334–345. [CrossRef] [PubMed]
114. Subramaniam, V.; Chakrabarti, R.; Prud'homme, G.J.; Jothy, S. Tranilast inhibits cell proliferation and migration and promotes apoptosis in murine breast cancer. *Anticancer Drugs* **2010**, *21*, 351–361. [CrossRef] [PubMed]
115. Subramaniam, V.; Ace, O.; Prud'homme, G.J.; Jothy, S. Tranilast treatment decreases cell growth, migration and inhibits colony formation of human breast cancer cells. *Exp. Mol. Pathol.* **2011**, *90*, 116–122. [CrossRef] [PubMed]
116. Wang, C.; Xu, C.X.; Bu, Y.; Bottum, K.M.; Tischkau, S.A. Beta-naphthoflavone (DB06732) mediates estrogen receptor-positive breast cancer cell cycle arrest through AhR-dependent regulation of PI3K/AKT and MAPK/ERK signaling. *Carcinogenesis* **2014**, *35*, 703–713. [CrossRef] [PubMed]
117. O'Donnell, E.F.; Koch, D.C.; Bisson, W.H.; Jang, H.S.; Kolluri, S.K. The aryl hydrocarbon receptor mediates raloxifene-induced apoptosis in estrogen receptor-negative hepatoma and breast cancer cells. *Cell Death Dis.* **2014**, *5*, e1038. [CrossRef]
118. DuSell, C.D.; Nelson, E.R.; Wittmann, B.M.; Fretz, J.A.; Kazmin, D.; Thomas, R.S.; Pike, J.W.; McDonnell, D.P. Regulation of aryl hydrocarbon receptor function by selective estrogen receptor modulators. *Mol. Endocrinol.* **2010**, *24*, 33–46. [CrossRef]
119. Kim, E.J.; Shin, M.; Park, H.; Hong, J.E.; Shin, H.K.; Kim, J.; Kwon, D.Y.; Park, J.H. Oral administration of 3,3'-diindolylmethane inhibits lung metastasis of 4T1 murine mammary carcinoma cells in BALB/c mice. *J. Nutr.* **2009**, *139*, 2373–2379. [CrossRef]
120. Chang, X.; Tou, J.C.; Hong, C.; Kim, H.A.; Riby, J.E.; Firestone, G.L.; Bjeldanes, L.F. 3,3'-Diindolylmethane inhibits angiogenesis and the growth of transplantable human breast carcinoma in athymic mice. *Carcinogenesis* **2005**, *26*, 771–778. [CrossRef]
121. Hsu, E.L.; Chen, N.; Westbrook, A.; Wang, F.; Zhang, R.; Taylor, R.T.; Hankinson, O. CXCR4 and CXCL12 down-regulation: A novel mechanism for the chemoprotection of 3,3'-diindolylmethane for breast and ovarian cancers. *Cancer Lett.* **2008**, *265*, 113–123. [CrossRef]
122. Yerushalmi, R.; Bargil, S.; Bar, Y.; Ozlavo, R.; Tuval, S.; Rapson, Y.; Pomerantz, A.; Zoref, D.; Sharon, E.; Caspi, O.; et al. 3,3-Diindolylmethane (DIM): A nutritional intervention and its impact on breast density in healthy BRCA carriers. A prospective clinical trial. *Carcinogenesis* **2020**, *41*, 1395–1401. [CrossRef]
123. Bjeldanes, L.F.; Kim, J.Y.; Grose, K.R.; Bartholomew, J.C.; Bradfield, C.A. Aromatic hydrocarbon responsiveness-receptor agonists generated from indole-3-carbinol in vitro and in vivo: Comparisons with 2,3,7,8-tetrachlorodibenzo-p-dioxin. *Proc. Natl. Acad. Sci. USA* **1991**, *88*, 9543–9547. [CrossRef] [PubMed]
124. Moiseeva, E.P.; Heukers, R.; Manson, M.M. EGFR and Src are involved in indole-3-carbinol-induced death and cell cycle arrest of human breast cancer cells. *Carcinogenesis* **2007**, *28*, 435–445. [CrossRef] [PubMed]
125. Ho, J.N.; Jun, W.; Choue, R.; Lee, J. I3C and ICZ inhibit migration by suppressing the EMT process and FAK expression in breast cancer cells. *Mol. Med. Rep.* **2013**, *7*, 384–388. [CrossRef] [PubMed]

126. Hargraves, K.G.; He, L.; Firestone, G.L. Phytochemical regulation of the tumor suppressive microRNA, miR-34a, by p53-dependent and independent responses in human breast cancer cells. *Mol. Carcinog.* **2016**, *55*, 486–498. [CrossRef] [PubMed]
127. Yang, T.; Feng, Y.L.; Chen, L.; Vaziri, N.D.; Zhao, Y.Y. Dietary natural flavonoids treating cancer by targeting aryl hydrocarbon receptor. *Crit. Rev. Toxicol.* **2019**, *49*, 445–460. [CrossRef]
128. Goya-Jorge, E.; Jorge Rodriguez, M.E.; Veitia, M.S.; Giner, R.M. Plant Occurring Flavonoids as Modulators of the Aryl Hydrocarbon Receptor. *Molecules* **2021**, *26*, 2315. [CrossRef]
129. Feng, J.; Zheng, T.; Hou, Z.; Lv, C.; Xue, A.; Han, T.; Han, B.; Sun, X.; Wei, Y. Luteolin, an aryl hydrocarbon receptor ligand, suppresses tumor metastasis in vitro and in vivo. *Oncol. Rep.* **2020**, *44*, 2231–2240. [CrossRef]
130. Tiong, C.T.; Chen, C.; Zhang, S.J.; Li, J.; Soshilov, A.; Denison, M.S.; Lee, L.S.; Tam, V.H.; Wong, S.P.; Xu, H.E.; et al. A novel prenylflavone restricts breast cancer cell growth through AhR-mediated destabilization of ERalpha protein. *Carcinogenesis* **2012**, *33*, 1089–1097. [CrossRef]
131. Hanieh, H.; Mohafez, O.; Hairul-Islam, V.I.; Alzahrani, A.; Bani Ismail, M.; Thirugnanasambantham, K. Novel Aryl Hydrocarbon Receptor Agonist Suppresses Migration and Invasion of Breast Cancer Cells. *PLoS ONE* **2016**, *11*, e0167650. [CrossRef]
132. Pham, T.H.; Lecomte, S.; Le Guevel, R.; Lardenois, A.; Evrard, B.; Chalmel, F.; Ferriere, F.; Balaguer, P.; Efstathiou, T.; Pakdel, F. Characterization of Glyceollins as Novel Aryl Hydrocarbon Receptor Ligands and Their Role in Cell Migration. *Int. J. Mol. Sci.* **2020**, *21*, 1368. [CrossRef]
133. Yamashita, N.; Taga, C.; Ozawa, M.; Kanno, Y.; Sanada, N.; Kizu, R. Camalexin, an indole phytoalexin, inhibits cell proliferation, migration, and mammosphere formation in breast cancer cells via the aryl hydrocarbon receptor. *J. Nat. Med.* **2022**, *76*, 110–118. [CrossRef] [PubMed]
134. Zhou, D.; Jiang, C.; Fu, C.; Chang, P.; Yang, B.; Wu, J.; Zhao, X.; Ma, S. Antiproliferative effect of 2-Hydroxy-6-tridecylbenzoic acid from ginkgo biloba sarcotestas through the aryl hydrocarbon receptor pathway in triple-negative breast cancer cells. *Nat. Prod. Res.* **2020**, *34*, 893–897. [CrossRef] [PubMed]
135. Hanieh, H.; Ibrahim, H.M.; Mohammed, M.; Alwassil, O.I.; Abukhalil, M.H.; Farhan, M. Activation of aryl hydrocarbon receptor signaling by gallic acid suppresses progression of human breast cancer in vitro and in vivo. *Phytomedicine* **2022**, *96*, 153817. [CrossRef] [PubMed]
136. Piwarski, S.A.; Thompson, C.; Chaudhry, A.R.; Denvir, J.; Primerano, D.A.; Fan, J.; Salisbury, T.B. The putative endogenous AHR ligand ITE reduces JAG1 and associated NOTCH1 signaling in triple negative breast cancer cells. *Biochem. Pharmacol.* **2020**, *174*, 113845. [CrossRef] [PubMed]
137. Mobini, K.; Tamaddon, G.; Fardid, R.; Keshavarzi, M.; Mohammadi-Bardbori, A. Aryl hydrocarbon-estrogen alpha receptor-dependent expression of miR-206, miR-27b, and miR-133a suppress cell proliferation and migration in MCF-7 cells. *J. Biochem. Mol. Toxicol.* **2019**, *33*, e22304. [CrossRef] [PubMed]
138. Sari, Z.; Miko, E.; Kovacs, T.; Boratko, A.; Ujlaki, G.; Janko, L.; Kiss, B.; Uray, K.; Bai, P. Indoxylsulfate, a Metabolite of the Microbiome, Has Cytostatic Effects in Breast Cancer via Activation of AHR and PXR Receptors and Induction of Oxidative Stress. *Cancers* **2020**, *12*, 2915. [CrossRef] [PubMed]
139. Sari, Z.; Miko, E.; Kovacs, T.; Janko, L.; Csonka, T.; Lente, G.; Sebo, E.; Toth, J.; Toth, D.; Arkosy, P.; et al. Indolepropionic Acid, a Metabolite of the Microbiome, Has Cytostatic Properties in Breast Cancer by Activating AHR and PXR Receptors and Inducing Oxidative Stress. *Cancers* **2020**, *12*, 2411. [CrossRef] [PubMed]
140. Kim, D.W.; Gazourian, L.; Quadri, S.A.; Romieu-Mourez, R.; Sherr, D.H.; Sonenshein, G.E. The RelA NF-kappaB subunit and the aryl hydrocarbon receptor (AhR) cooperate to transactivate the c-myc promoter in mammary cells. *Oncogene* **2000**, *19*, 5498–5506. [CrossRef] [PubMed]
141. Novikov, O.; Wang, Z.; Stanford, E.A.; Parks, A.J.; Ramirez-Cardenas, A.; Landesman, E.; Laklouk, I.; Sarita-Reyes, C.; Gusenleitner, D.; Li, A.; et al. An Aryl Hydrocarbon Receptor-Mediated Amplification Loop That Enforces Cell Migration in ER-/PR-/Her2- Human Breast Cancer Cells. *Mol. Pharmacol.* **2016**, *90*, 674–688. [CrossRef]
142. Parks, A.J.; Pollastri, M.P.; Hahn, M.E.; Stanford, E.A.; Novikov, O.; Franks, D.G.; Haigh, S.E.; Narasimhan, S.; Ashton, T.D.; Hopper, T.G.; et al. In silico identification of an aryl hydrocarbon receptor antagonist with biological activity in vitro and in vivo. *Mol. Pharmacol.* **2014**, *86*, 593–608. [CrossRef]
143. Murray, T.J.; Yang, X.; Sherr, D.H. Growth of a human mammary tumor cell line is blocked by galangin, a naturally occurring bioflavonoid, and is accompanied by down-regulation of cyclins D3, E, and A. *Breast Cancer Res. BCR* **2006**, *8*, R17. [CrossRef] [PubMed]
144. Stanford, E.A.; Wang, Z.; Novikov, O.; Mulas, F.; Landesman-Bollag, E.; Monti, S.; Smith, B.W.; Seldin, D.C.; Murphy, G.J.; Sherr, D.H. The role of the aryl hydrocarbon receptor in the development of cells with the molecular and functional characteristics of cancer stem-like cells. *BMC Biol.* **2016**, *14*, 1–22. [CrossRef] [PubMed]
145. Degner, S.C.; Papoutsis, A.J.; Selmin, O.; Romagnolo, D.F. Targeting of aryl hydrocarbon receptor-mediated activation of cyclooxygenase-2 expression by the indole-3-carbinol metabolite 3,3'-diindolylmethane in breast cancer cells. *J. Nutr.* **2009**, *139*, 26–32. [CrossRef] [PubMed]
146. D'Amato, N.C.; Rogers, T.J.; Gordon, M.A.; Greene, L.I.; Cochrane, D.R.; Spoelstra, N.S.; Nemkov, T.G.; D'Alessandro, A.; Hansen, K.C.; Richer, J.K. A TDO2-AhR signaling axis facilitates anoikis resistance and metastasis in triple-negative breast cancer. *Cancer Res.* **2015**, *75*, 4651–4664. [CrossRef]

147. Shadboorestan, A.; Tarfiei, G.A.; Montazeri, H.; Sepand, M.R.; Zangooei, M.; Khedri, A.; Ostad, S.N.; Ghahremani, M.H. Invasion and migration of MDA-MB-231 cells are inhibited by block of AhR and NFAT: Role of AhR/NFAT1/β4 integrin signaling. *J. Appl. Toxicol.* **2019**, *39*, 375–384. [CrossRef]
148. Hsieh, T.H.; Tsai, C.F.; Hsu, C.Y.; Kuo, P.L.; Lee, J.N.; Chai, C.Y.; Wang, S.C.; Tsai, E.M. Phthalates induce proliferation and invasiveness of estrogen receptor-negative breast cancer through the AhR/HDAC6/c-Myc signaling pathway. *FASEB J.* **2012**, *26*, 778–787. [CrossRef]
149. Hsieh, T.H.; Hsu, C.Y.; Yang, P.J.; Chiu, C.C.; Liang, S.S.; Ou-Yang, F.; Kan, J.Y.; Hou, M.F.; Wang, T.N.; Tsai, E.M. DEHP mediates drug resistance by directly targeting AhR in human breast cancer. *Biomed. Pharm.* **2022**, *145*, 112400. [CrossRef]
150. Shan, A.; Leng, L.; Li, J.; Luo, X.M.; Fan, Y.J.; Yang, Q.; Xie, Q.H.; Chen, Y.S.; Ni, C.S.; Guo, L.M.; et al. TCDD-induced antagonism of MEHP-mediated migration and invasion partly involves aryl hydrocarbon receptor in MCF7 breast cancer cells. *J. Hazard Mater* **2020**, *398*, 122869. [CrossRef]
151. Bekki, K.; Vogel, H.; Li, W.; Ito, T.; Sweeney, C.; Haarmann-Stemmann, T.; Matsumura, F.; Vogel, C.F. The aryl hydrocarbon receptor (AhR) mediates resistance to apoptosis induced in breast cancer cells. *Pestic. Biochem. Physiol.* **2015**, *120*, 5–13. [CrossRef]
152. Yamashita, N.; Kanno, Y.; Saito, N.; Terai, K.; Sanada, N.; Kizu, R.; Hiruta, N.; Park, Y.; Bujo, H.; Nemoto, K. Aryl hydrocarbon receptor counteracts pharmacological efficacy of doxorubicin via enhanced AKR1C3 expression in triple negative breast cancer cells. *Biochem. Biophys. Res. Commun.* **2019**, *516*, 693–698. [CrossRef]
153. Vogel, C.F.A.; Lazennec, G.; Kado, S.Y.; Dahlem, C.; He, Y.; Castaneda, A.; Ishihara, Y.; Vogeley, C.; Rossi, A.; Haarmann-Stemmann, T.; et al. Targeting the Aryl Hydrocarbon Receptor Signaling Pathway in Breast Cancer Development. *Front. Immunol.* **2021**, *12*, 625346. [CrossRef] [PubMed]
154. Kubli, S.P.; Bassi, C.; Roux, C.; Wakeham, A.; Gobl, C.; Zhou, W.; Jafari, S.M.; Snow, B.; Jones, L.; Palomero, L.; et al. AhR controls redox homeostasis and shapes the tumor microenvironment in BRCA1-associated breast cancer. *Proc. Natl. Acad. Sci. USA* **2019**, *116*, 3604–3613. [CrossRef] [PubMed]
155. Dwyer, A.R.; Kerkvliet, C.P.; Krutilina, R.I.; Playa, H.C.; Parke, D.N.; Thomas, W.A.; Smeester, B.A.; Moriarity, B.S.; Seagroves, T.N.; Lange, C.A. Breast Tumor Kinase (Brk/PTK6) Mediates Advanced Cancer Phenotypes via SH2-Domain Dependent Activation of RhoA and Aryl Hydrocarbon Receptor (AhR) Signaling. *Mol. Cancer Res. MCR* **2021**, *19*, 329–345. [CrossRef] [PubMed]
156. Cirillo, F.; Lappano, R.; Bruno, L.; Rizzuti, B.; Grande, F.; Guzzi, R.; Briguori, S.; Miglietta, A.M.; Nakajima, M.; Di Martino, M.T.; et al. AHR and GPER mediate the stimulatory effects induced by 3-methylcholanthrene in breast cancer cells and cancer-associated fibroblasts (CAFs). *J. Exp. Clin. Cancer Res.* **2019**, *38*, 335. [CrossRef]
157. Hollingshead, B.D.; Beischlag, T.V.; Dinatale, B.C.; Ramadoss, P.; Perdew, G.H. Inflammatory signaling and aryl hydrocarbon receptor mediate synergistic induction of interleukin 6 in MCF-7 cells. *Cancer Res.* **2008**, *68*, 3609–3617. [CrossRef]
158. Yamashita, N.; Saito, N.; Zhao, S.; Terai, K.; Hiruta, N.; Park, Y.; Bujo, H.; Nemoto, K.; Kanno, Y. Heregulin-induced cell migration is promoted by aryl hydrocarbon receptor in HER2-overexpressing breast cancer cells. *Exp. Cell Res.* **2018**, *366*, 34–40. [CrossRef]
159. Liu, Y.; Zhou, N.; Zhou, L.; Wang, J.; Zhou, Y.; Zhang, T.; Fang, Y.; Deng, J.; Gao, Y.; Liang, X.; et al. IL-2 regulates tumor-reactive CD8(+) T cell exhaustion by activating the aryl hydrocarbon receptor. *Nat. Immunol.* **2021**, *22*, 358–369. [CrossRef]

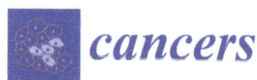 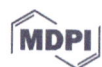

Systematic Review

The Use of Artificial Intelligence (AI) in the Radiology Field: What Is the State of Doctor–Patient Communication in Cancer Diagnosis?

Alexandra Derevianko [1], Silvia Francesca Maria Pizzoli [2,*], Filippo Pesapane [3], Anna Rotili [3], Dario Monzani [4], Roberto Grasso [1,2], Enrico Cassano [3] and Gabriella Pravettoni [1,2]

[1] Applied Research Division for Cognitive and Psychological Science, IEO European Institute of Oncology IRCCS, 20141 Milan, Italy; alexandra.derevianko@ieo.it (A.D.); roberto.grasso@ieo.it (R.G.); gabriella.pravettoni@ieo.it (G.P.)
[2] Department of Oncology and Hemato-Oncology, University of Milan, 20122 Milan, Italy
[3] Breast Imaging Division, IEO European Institute of Oncology IRCCS, 20139 Milan, Italy; filippo.pesapane@ieo.it (F.P.); anna.rotili@ieo.it (A.R.); enrico.cassano@ieo.it (E.C.)
[4] Department of Psychology, Educational Science and Human Movement, University of Palermo, 90128 Palermo, Italy; dario.monzani@unipa.it
* Correspondence: silvia.pizzoli@unimi.it; Tel.: +39-0294372099

Simple Summary: Artificial Intelligence (AI) has been increasingly used in radiology to improve diagnostic procedures over the past decades. The application of AI at the time of cancer diagnosis also creates challenges in the way doctors should communicate the use of AI to patients. The present systematic review deals with the patient's psycho-cognitive perspective on AI and the interpersonal skills between patients and physicians when AI is implemented in cancer diagnosis communication. Evidence from the retrieved studies pointed out that the use of AI in radiology is negatively associated with patient trust in AI and patient-centered communication in cancer disease.

Abstract: Background: In the past decade, interest in applying Artificial Intelligence (AI) in radiology to improve diagnostic procedures increased. AI has potential benefits spanning all steps of the imaging chain, from the prescription of diagnostic tests to the communication of test reports. The use of AI in the field of radiology also poses challenges in doctor–patient communication at the time of the diagnosis. This systematic review focuses on the patient role and the interpersonal skills between patients and physicians when AI is implemented in cancer diagnosis communication. Methods: A systematic search was conducted on PubMed, Embase, Medline, Scopus, and PsycNet from 1990 to 2021. The search terms were: ("artificial intelligence" or "intelligence machine") and "communication" "radiology" and "oncology diagnosis". The PRISMA guidelines were followed. Results: 517 records were identified, and 5 papers met the inclusion criteria and were analyzed. Most of the articles emphasized the success of the technological support of AI in radiology at the expense of patient trust in AI and patient-centered communication in cancer disease. Practical implications and future guidelines were discussed according to the results. Conclusions: AI has proven to be beneficial in helping clinicians with diagnosis. Future research may improve patients' trust through adequate information about the advantageous use of AI and an increase in medical compliance with adequate training on doctor–patient diagnosis communication.

Keywords: artificial intelligence; communication; decision-making; patient empowerment

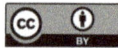

1. Introduction

In the last four decades, medical technology has seen a shift in the development of Artificial Intelligence (AI) which is commonly defined as "a field of computer science that develops systems able to perform tasks commonly associated with intelligent human beings" [1]. AI refers to machines or systems that can act for themselves and make decisions when faced with new situations such as problem-solving or decision-making systems. AI applications include machine learning (ML), natural language processing, automated speech recognition, deep learning (DL), computer vision, and radiomic [2,3]. Particularly, ML, introduced by Arthur Samuel in 1959, defines a field of artificial intelligence where a computer learns automatically from data accumulation, whereas DL emerged as a promising approach for image processing [4], allowing the system to recognize patterns and make predictions [5]. The use of AI demonstrated significant progress in image-recognition tasks [6]. Indeed, AI is one of the fastest-growing areas of informatics and computing with great relevance to healthcare and radiology. Some media headlines claiming doctors' better performances have fueled hype among the public and the press for accelerated implementation of AI techniques. Examples include: "Google says its AI can spot lung cancer a year before doctors" and "AI is better at diagnosing skin cancer than your doctor, study finds" [7,8].

Considering the radiology community, there is a relevant interest in applying AI to improve workflow applications and patient care. AI is considered an optimizing tool to assist the radiologist in detecting suspicious findings in imaging exams, making the diagnosis, choosing a personalized patient protocol, tracking the patient's dose parameters, providing an estimate of the radiation risks [9,10], and also minimizing diagnostic errors. Indeed, despite human intuition on visual perception providing a faithful representation of the world, we often miss salient events in our environment when we are focused on something else. This phenomenon is known as inattentional blindness, i.e., the failure to notice an unexpected but fully visible stimulus when attention is engaged in another task [11]. While enhanced global processing ability generally allows expert radiologists to rapidly detect abnormalities, including unexpected ones [12], inattentional blindness may provide insight into ways to address a growing concern in radiology: missed but clinically significant incidental findings, which are abnormalities in medical images that are unrelated to the patient's main symptomatology and that may even be detected in asymptomatic patients [13]. Furthermore, AI in the medical field might also result in significant support for radiologists' cognitive fatigue, which is often a consequence of their daily demanding medical practice. Medical doctors support the use of AI algorithms as aiding tools for precision medicine. Sarwar and colleagues [14] reported that 75% of 487 interviewed physicians from 54 countries showed positive attitudes toward AI and expressed interest in AI as a diagnostic tool to improve workflow efficiency and quality assurance. A 2018 study pitted dermatologists against a computer that had been trained to differentiate between cancerous skin lesions and benign ones [15]. The results showed dermatologists were only 86.6% accurate at diagnosing skin cancer, while the computer was able to diagnose issues with a 95% accuracy. Another study [16] on AI diagnostic accuracy using endoscopic images for the detection of cancer or neoplastic lesions and the classification of lesions (neoplastic vs. nonneoplastic) in the gastrointestinal tract determined that AI was accurate but had a lower performance compared to the highly accurate endoscopist.

For all these premises, AI holds great promise for the oncology field, and it can be especially useful as a means for mammography screening [17,18]. However, although AI can provide detailed quantifications of tissues on imaging examinations, which can be used for diagnostic, prognostic, and treatment purposes [19], this technology should not be currently used as a standalone medical device, but it should be considered the combination of software and radiologists [20–22]. Furthermore, AI should never outweigh the development of rigorous evidence-based medical practice [15].

Considering the implementation of AI in radiology clinical practice, multiple steps from routine screening based on risk factors to communication reports should be targeted. On one hand, radiologists must play a leading role in developing and validating AI applications for medical imaging; on the other hand, they also must manage the risk that the medical–patient interaction might become more impersonal [23]. To prevent this, patients' points of view should be taken into consideration. The European Union has indeed recognized the problem that algorithm-based medical decision-making poses in this regard and has published a landmark paper highlighting the need for explanations of computerized decision-making in the medical field so that patients can effectively understand the crucial role AI can play in their health [24,25]. The solution is found in the concept of explainable AI (XAI), which is attracting increasing interest in the scientific community [26]. Communication can be seen as a pivotal ingredient in medical care, and XAI might provide a patient-friendly explanation of biomedical decisions based on ML. Particularly, XAI would be highly valuable in the oncology field, where it is essential to consider not only the purely medical aspects but also the patient's psychological and emotional dimensions [27]. Technological aspects of AI systems are largely described by the current literature in different health sectors. However, the patient's standpoint of AI to make decisions on their health is often neglected. Scarce communication between patients and clinicians about the potential benefits of AI is likely to cause to patients' mistrust of such a promising tool. Indeed, most patients perceive an AI-aided diagnosis as not completely reliable [28,29]. One of the reasons behind this mistrust can be identified in the "Third Wheel Effect" [30], whereby the patient considers the AI as an unnecessary intrusion rather than an added value. Specifically, patients may have a perception that their relationship with their doctor will suffer because of the "third wheel", which might then result in "decision paralysis", risk of decision-making delays, "Confusions of the Tongues" and ambiguity.

Overall, current evidence regarding patients' perceptions of AI in radiology and related communication issues is very limited. Since this field is under-explored, this review aims to discuss the use of AI in radiology and the challenges that AI poses in doctor–patient communication. Therefore, the authors propose future research directions to implement doctor–patient communication skills and to support patients' understanding of AI at the time of their cancer diagnosis.

2. Materials and Methods

2.1. Search Strategy

A systematic review of the literature was performed to identify the use of AI in the field of radiology in doctor–patient communication when communicating the diagnosis of cancer. The systematic review was conducted and reported following the Preferred Reporting Items for Systematic Reviews and Meta-Analyses (PRISMA) guidelines [31] (Figure 1). The protocol for this systematic review has not been registered. Digital literature databases, including PubMed, EMBASE, Medline, Scopus, Psycnet, and Medline In-process were searched from 1990 to 2021. Only studies published during the last decade were considered since they are more likely to report current developments in IA in the radiological field and psychological aspects such as the importance of doctor–patient communication. MeSH was used to identify label terms to extract as many articles as possible related to the topic. The keywords and descriptors used in any field were "artificial intelligence" OR "intelligence machine" AND "communication" AND "radiology" AND "oncology diagnosis".

2.2. Inclusion and Exclusion Criteria

All publication types and all study designs were included, with no language or age restriction. The following inclusion criteria were applied: studies that reported the development of AI in radiology in cancer diagnosis; studies with patients' perception of artificial intelligence; studies highlighting the oncological diagnosis communication; studies with patients' point of view on the oncological doctor–patient communication of the AI diagnosis; the use of AI in screening mammography. Medical AI studies without considering doctor–patient communication and papers dealing with the use of AI in other fields were excluded.

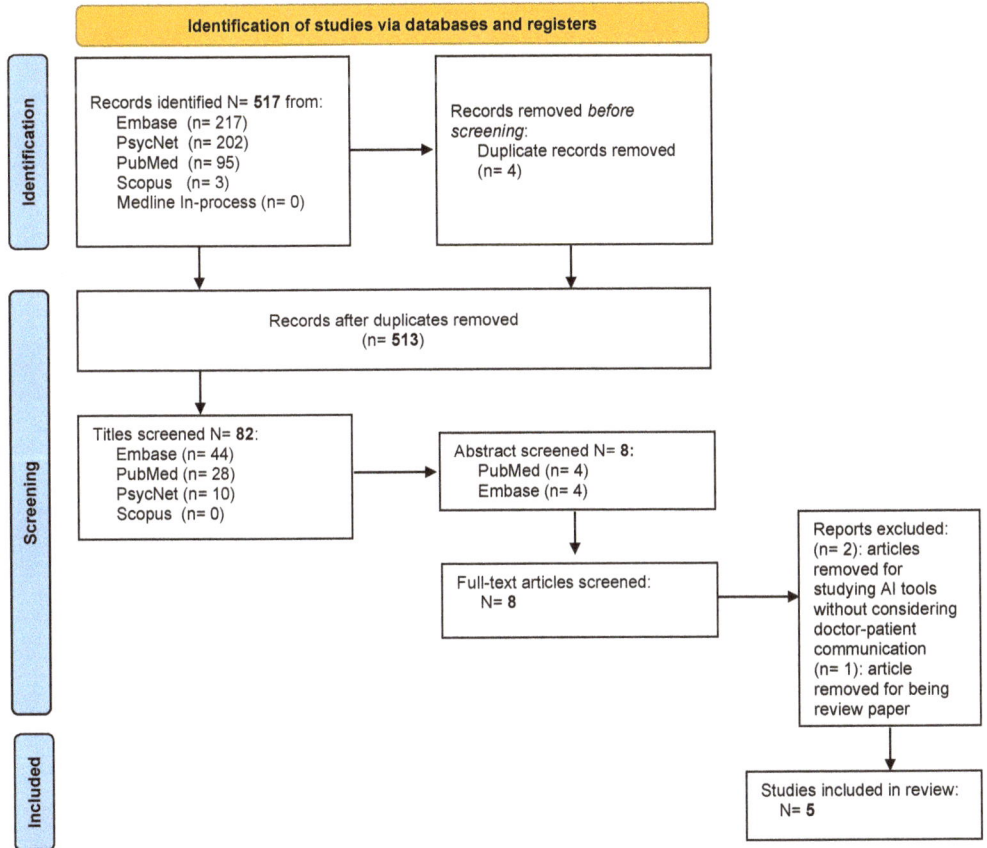

Figure 1. Preferred Reporting Item for Systematic Review (PRISMA) study selection flow diagram.

2.3. Screening and Data Extraction

Two independent reviewers undertook all titles and abstract screening (A.D. and S. F. M. P.) resulting from the literature search for inclusion and exclusion criteria. Disagreements were solved by a discussion with all the members of the research team.

3. Results

In total, 517 publications were identified, and of those, 4 duplicates were removed before the initial screening. Then, 431 articles based on the screening of titles and 74 articles based on the screening of abstracts were excluded. Eight full-text articles were assessed for eligibility. Three articles were excluded, two were removed for studying AI tools without considering doctor–patient communication, and one article removed for being a review paper. Following the full-text screening, five studies met the inclusion criteria.

3.1. Features of the Studies

The study findings are summarized in Table 1. The overall sample size of the studies includes 939 participants. The majority of the participants were over 18 years old and female. Among the retrieved studies, one adopted a longitudinal design, one used a semi-structured interview, and three were qualitative studies regarding the patient's attitude toward AI. Overall, the included studies reported limited data on the characteristics of the patients (diagnosis, cancer stage, etc.). Details of the retrieved studies are reported in Appendix A.

Table 1. Summary of the study sample patients' characteristics, attitudes toward Artificial Intelligence.

References	Patient Characteristics			Attitude toward AI		Patient's Knowledge and Point of View on AI
	Populations	N	Average Age (SD)	Investigated	Language Population	
Ongena et al., 2020 [32]	Breast cancer screening	922	±45	Trust Accountability Personal interaction Efficiency The general attitude toward AI	German	Those who have lower education are less supportive of AI Those who think AI is less efficient had a more negative attitude toward AI
Adams et al., 2020 [33]	/	17	/	Fear of the unknown Trust Human connection Improving communication	English	AI was shaped and viewed as "science fiction"
Carter et al., 2019 [34]	Breast cancer	/	/	Ethical Legal Social implications	English	No deep understanding of the way health technologies work
Mendelson, 2019 [35]	Breast cancer	/	/	Potentials Limitations	English	Education in AI for patients Empowerment skills in doctor–patient communication
Kapoor et al., 2020 [36]	/	/	/	Workflow applications of AI in radiology	English	Closed-loop communication of critical radiology results

3.2. Synthesis of the Results

The most relevant and recurrent variables across studies concerning patients' attitudes toward AI and issues in doctor–patient communication are summarized in Table 2.

Table 2. Main findings on patients' psycho-cognitive attitudes toward Artificial Intelligence and communication issues.

References	Methods	Analysis	Main Variables
Ongena et al., 2020 [32]	Internet Survey with ad hoc 5-point Likert Scale	Quantitative analysis	Patients' education levels shape trust and attitudes toward AI (low education is associated with low trust)
Adams et al., 2020 [33]	Patient engagement Workshop and interviews	Qualitative analysis (thematic analysis)	Trust is linked to the fear of the unknown uses of AI in radiology and the lack of human connections and empathy
Carter et al., 2019 [34]	Narrative review and perspective	Analysis of the ethical issues in doctor–patient communication	Knowledge and understanding of the way AI works are pivotal for the ethical use of AI
Mendelson, 2019 [35]	Narrative review and perspective	Analysis of the pros and cons of using AI in breast cancer imaging	Knowledge and education about AI for patients are as important as the empowerment of skills in communication for physicians
Kapoor et al., 2020 [36]	Overview of the applications of AI in radiology	Qualitative synthesis	Closed-loop communication to provide improved and personalized feedback for patients

Ongena et al. [32] conducted a longitudinal study using an Internet survey for the social science panel on the Dutch population to investigate the general population's view on the use of AI for the diagnostic interpretation of screening mammograms. The study included 922 women from 16 to 75 years old. Five items were measured to investigate the patient's attitude toward AI in mammography: "Necessity of a human check", "AI as a selector for second reading", "AI as a second reader", "Developer is responsible for error", "Radiologist is responsible for error". No standardized questionnaires were used, but a 5-point Likert scale was developed ad hoc to collect patients' agreement or disagreement. The authors analyzed the different items with the variable "education", finding that there were different patients' perceptions between those who have a high level of education and those who do not. Results highlighted that those who find a human check of mammograms necessary tend to prefer a personal interaction in discussion results and consider AI less efficient because of lower education. On the contrary, those who find a human check as neutral tend to view personal interaction in discussing results as less important and consider AI more efficient, keeping a positive attitude towards health technology. Adams et al. [33] hosted a patient engagement workshop and employed qualitative analysis to determine the initial patient perceptions, patient priorities for AI use cases, and patient-identified evaluation metrics. Qualitative interviews were conducted with 17 patients (11 female and 6 male, age and diagnosis were not indicated). The authors identified common themes or patterns from text data. The initial perceptions of AI captured four themes: (1) "Fear of the unknown", (2) "Trust", (3) "Human connection" and (4) "Cultural acceptability". Patients' perceptions of AI were shaped by popular media and science fiction. Some participants expressed fear or described AI as an unknown scary instrument. Trust or lack of trust was the consequence of fear of the unknown AI tool in radiology. For most of the participants, a lack of knowledge also represented a lack of trust in AI, while others displayed a willingness to trust outputs from AI, which might achieve the most accurate information. Furthermore, some participants were concerned about the lack of human connection and that AI might enhance the necessity for "human empathy" and the human "ability to understand with flexibility". Overall, the main result was that all participants underlined the importance of an understandable way to explain the AI results because in some cases medical language emerged as either too difficult or unclear. Indeed, participants emphasized the need to fully understand their imaging results to be engaged in their care and have more productive conversations with their physicians. Carter et al. [34] compiled a narrative review concerning the ethical point of view of doctor–patient communication in radiology using AI. Indeed, patients understand little about health technologies and perhaps do not understand AI systems. Mendelson [35] facets the potential and limitations of AI in breast imaging. The author stressed the importance of the potential of AI in radiology concerning the improvement of the workflow of the algorithms of AI and the outcome analyses that are advancing in the last decades. The main role of the high-tech in AI was the use of imaging data in high quality and quantity, so that AI can support breast imagers in diagnosis and patient management. The importance of physicians' knowledge and expertise was specifically stressed in survival phase decision-making.

Kapoor et al. [36] provided an overview of available tools and developed considerations on the workflow applications of AI. In this work, AI is proposed to optimize patient scheduling, improve worklist management, and help radiologists interpret diagnostic studies. AI applications were described as multiple and complex processes ranging from routine screening to report communication, with several implementation steps. Kapoor et al. [36] highlighted the relevance of the final step in the diagnostic imaging chain that concerns the report communication. The authors described this process as an underrecognized area in which quality of care issues can arise. Moreover, ML algorithms can identify specific disease entities in radiology reports, and can be used to accurately identify tailored follow-up recommendations. The authors concluded that data in feedback reports could be used to ensure appropriate closed-loop communication to monitor radiologist variation in follow-up recommendations [37].

4. Discussion

Our review explored the implications of using AI on doctor–patient communication at the time of cancer diagnosis in the field of radiology. According to our findings, this is still a low-investigated topic in the literature.

The use of AI in healthcare involves not only technical issues but also ethical, psycho-cognitive, and social-demographic considerations of presenting patients with cancer with the presence of AI at the time of the diagnosis. Trust, Accountability, Personal interaction, Efficiency, and General attitude toward AI were identified as five core areas by Ongena et al. [38]. The variables that merge such aspects of patients' attitudes to using and communicating diagnosis with AI are education and knowledge. Accordingly, the authors showed that participants who have lower education are less supportive of AI, and those who have thought AI to be less efficient have a more negative attitude toward AI. Therefore, it is possible to consider that those who do not have a good understanding of the way AI works tend to have a negative attitude toward its effectiveness and less trust in its potential. Moreover, those who mistrust the diagnostic accuracy of AI as well as are not well educated tend to seek interpersonal interaction with doctors much more than those who were neutral about the efficacy of AI. One of the items, the "Necessary of a human check", relates very closely to the importance of doctor–patient communication, focusing on the need to integrate two aspects: the use of high-tech in diagnosis and the need for human–doctor communication about the exam results. This point underlines the pivotal role of the doctor's communication in a circumstance of little knowledge about a new tool in healthcare such as AI. Starting from the premise that the current evidence regarding patients' experiences, perceptions, and priorities for artificial in radiology are limited, Adams et al. [33] investigated a patient's knowledge and perceptions on the use of AI in a care setting. Despite the methodological difference from the previous article, some fundamental and very similar themes emerged. In this case, there are four thematic cores: fear of the unknown, trust, human connection, and improving communication. Therefore, on the patients' side, these aspects are a strong issue of where to place trust. These difficulties in participants' understanding of the use of new technologies, such as AI in radiological diagnosis, imply the need for more human connection, and at least the necessity to improve the quality of communication with the doctors. Indeed, some participants were concerned about the lack of human connection and that AI may emphasize the necessity of "human empathy". The qualitative interviews showed that patients felt the topic of "improving communication" was a priority for AI use cases. This result may reflect again the importance of doctor–patient communication throughout the healthcare process from examination scheduling to diagnosis communication. In addition to the complexity of the different layers of AI involved such as DL and ML, there is a strong debate about the medical decision-making process with such a tool. Carter et al. [34] highlighted that patients are still very hesitant when faced with AI outputs, as the image of the "machine" conveys the idea of something that can make mistakes. On the physician's side, AI has implications for human capacities. Firstly, AI could lead to a change in clinicians' skills. Indeed, they are more likely to lose capabilities they do not regularly use, for example, if they read fewer mammograms. A second point about professional responsibility concerns automation bias which means that humans tend to accept machine decisions, even when they are wrong [39]. To overcome these risks, it is necessary to train clinicians to avoid or lower automation bias. Mendelson [35] focused not only on patients' perceptions and their knowledge about AI, but also on the need for physicians to empower their skills in communication. Although doctors may know very well their medical and scientific language and the functions of their technological tools, they do not systematically train their skills in diagnosis communication, especially when they use AI tools. Recently, a systematic literature review addressed an important gap in cancer care focusing on the impact of Health Information Technology (HIT) on doctor–patient communication. Studies showed that some types of HIT can increase patients' confidence and support their active involvement in the care processes while maintaining a good relationship with the healthcare team (38). Therefore, a patient's knowledge of diagnostic tools is as important as a physician's communication skills. Kapoor et al. [36] shed light on the concept of closed-loop communication. The authors described that sometimes there is variability in radiologists' language and follow-up recommendations and that machines using AI collocated in different hospitals can have different outcomes. The divergence of outcomes requires doctors to understand what is wrong with the machines and discuss the meaning of the discrepant results, while their communication remains in a closed loop, not engaging patients. It is well known that the effectiveness of medical treatment depends on the quality of the patient–clinical relationship [40] and the use of AI in the field of radiology poses challenges in doctor–patient communication at the time of the diagnosis. Therefore, implementing the doctor–patient communication of AI results and issues may change the patient's choice in their health.

4.1. Limitations

Overall, the literature on the topic is scarce. Furthermore, there is high heterogeneity in the methodologies of studies, which range from a longitudinal study to a narrative review, including qualitative analysis. The heterogeneity of studies posed challenges to the systematization of the results. It also shed light on the fact that the main topic, assessed over time and despite different methods, produced similar results. Finally, the heterogeneity of the samples rendered it difficult to define AI attitudes in specific subsamples of patients or specific moments of the cancer care pattern.

4.2. Future Directions

Future research may consider some useful steps in applying AI bearing in mind patients' psycho-cognitive perspectives. We propose the acronym AIR-IUT to highlight the three main steps to be considered in the application of AI in the field of radiology and future studies dealing with the patient's experience of the application of AI. The acronym stands for the fact that in the field of Artificial Intelligence in Radiology, the process is to Inform patients to Understand and Trust the use of AI. Future interventions should consider implementing the use of digital platforms with illustrative videos to inform patients, offering reliable educative means that might be delivered in the waiting rooms. Indeed, involving patients with digital interaction could increase compliance, reduce the fear of the unknown about health technology and psychological feelings, and improve patients' decision-making at the time of treatment, since they are actively involved and informed at the screening time [41]. Concurrently, a training course to enhance doctor–patient communication skills at the time of diagnosis may be developed. Such a course should help clinicians to adopt patient-friendly language (i.e., jargon words must be explained or replaced by simpler words) and an empathetic approach, entailing particular attention to the patient's psychological well-being.

5. Conclusions

In conclusion, doctors should sharpen their communication skills when AI is involved in diagnosis, and patients should be engaged in the process mainly by being informed on the functioning of medical tools used to formulate their diagnosis. One of the most evident elements from the retrieved studies is that patients do not know what AI is and this lack of knowledge affects trust and doctor–patient communication. Since patients should be empowered and tailor informed at all phases of their clinical journey, they should ideally know which diagnostic tools are used by their clinicians and the way they work. Given the outstanding AI's potential, we believe that informing patients about its progress in our field will help them to be more trusting towards it.

Author Contributions: A.D., R.G., S.F.M.P., F.P., A.R. and D.M. conceived and discussed the initial concept of the manuscript; A.D., S.F.M.P. and F.P. wrote the first draft; D.M., R.G. and A.R. revised the draft and the theoretical concepts; G.P. and E.C. supervised the entire process and contributed to it through methodological and theoretical discussion with all the other authors. All authors have read and agreed to the published version of the manuscript.

Funding: This research received no external funding.

Institutional Review Board Statement: The manuscript does not require Institutional Review Board approval.

Informed Consent Statement: No written informed consent has been obtained since no subjects were involved in the study.**Data Availability:** The are no datasets associated with the manuscript.

Acknowledgments: The present work was partially supported by the Italian Ministry of Health with Ricerca Corrente and 5 × 1000 funds for IEO European Institute of Oncology IRCSS.

Conflicts of Interest: The authors declare no conflict of interest.

Appendix A

Table A1. Summary of General Characteristics of Included Studies.

Title	URL	Resource	Type	Identifiers	Db
(1) Workflow Applications of Artificial Intelligence in Radiology and an Overview of Available Tools	doi.org/10.1016/j.jacr.2020.08.016	PubMed	Narrative review	PMID: 33153540	MeSH-PubMed
(2) Artificial Intelligence in Breast Imaging: Potentials and Limitations	doi.org/10.2214/AJR.18.20532	PubMed	Narrative review	PMID: 30422715	MeSH-PubMed
(3) Patient Perspectives and Priorities Regarding Artificial Intelligence in Radiology: Opportunities for Patient-Centered Radiology	doi.org/10.1016/j.jacr.2020.01.007	PubMed	Qualitative	PMID: 32068006	MeSH-PubMed
(4) The ethical, legal and social implications of using artificial intelligence systems in breast cancer care	doi.org/10.1016/j.breast.2019.10.001	PubMed	Narrative review	PMID: 31677530	MeSH-PubMed
(5) Artificial intelligence in screening mammography: A population Survey of Women's Preferences	doi.org/10.1016/j.jacr.2020.09.042	PubMed	Longitudinal study	PMID: 33058789	MeSH-PubMed

References

1. Park, S.H.; Han, K. Methodologic Guide for Evaluating Clinical Performance and Effect of Artificial Intelligence Technology for Medical Diagnosis and Prediction. *Radiology* **2018**, *286*, 800–809. [CrossRef]
2. Martín Noguerol, T.; Paulano-Godino, F.; Martín-Valdivia, M.T.; Menias, C.O.; Luna, A. Strengths, Weaknesses, Opportunities, and Threats Analysis of Artificial Intelligence and Machine Learning Applications in Radiology. *J. Am. Coll. Radiol.* **2019**, *16*, 1239–1247. [CrossRef]
3. Lee, J.G.; Jun, S.; Cho, Y.W.; Lee, H.; Kim, G.B.; Seo, J.B.; Kim, N. Deep Learning in Medical Imaging: General Overview. *Korean J. Radiol.* **2017**, *18*, 570. [CrossRef]
4. King, B.F. Guest Editorial: Discovery and Artificial Intelligence. *Am. J. Roentgenol.* **2017**, *209*, 1189–1190. [CrossRef]
5. King, B.F. Artificial Intelligence and Radiology: What Will the Future Hold? *J. Am. Coll. Radiol.* **2018**, *15*, 501–503. [CrossRef]
6. Hosny, A.; Parmar, C.; Quackenbush, J.; Schwartz, L.H.; Aerts, H.J. Artificial Intelligence in Radiology. *Nat. Rev. Cancer* **2018**, *18*, 500–510. [CrossRef]

7. Google Says Its AI Can Spot Early-Stage Lung Cancer, in Some Cases Better Than Doctors Can—GeekWire. Available online: https://www.geekwire.com/2019/google-says-ai-can-spot-early-stage-lung-cancer-cases-better-doctors-can/ (accessed on 30 November 2022).
8. AI Is Better at Diagnosing Skin Cancer Than Your Doctor, Study Finds. Available online: https://finance.yahoo.com/news/ai-better-diagnosing-skin-cancer-182057234.html?guccounter=1&guce_referrer=aHR0cHM6Ly93d3cuZ29vZ2xlLmNvbS8&guce_referrer_sig=AQAAANisvvSAdl5qYPcgGM6vghzJGoKDCILKb6ZGRYgyzSFEVWdkC4mwZBAxDq42fxoiV3IZEMfLzba8QgjRa2ifcPPF1ln8Lp2GKLxl-pW3muUc2iFRx4jHSPbe9_6AFiy16Ng_oRQlxR-gbT9ShXuKomPU5CN_DzKo7FscfW6YsGNv (accessed on 30 November 2022).
9. Pesapane, F.; Codari, M.; Sardanelli, F. Artificial Intelligence in Medical Imaging: Threat or Opportunity? Radiologists Again at the Forefront of Innovation in Medicine. *Eur. Radiol. Exp.* **2018**, *2*, 35. [CrossRef]
10. Neri, E.; de Souza, N.; Brady, A.; Bayarri, A.A.; Becker, C.D.; Coppola, F.; Visser, J. What the Radiologist Should Know about Artificial Intelligence—An ESR White Paper. *Insights Imaging* **2019**, *10*, 1–8. [CrossRef]
11. Neisser, U.; Becklen, R. Selective Looking: Attending to Visually Specified Events. *Cogn. Psychol.* **1975**, *7*, 480–494. [CrossRef]
12. Carrigan, A.J.; Wardle, S.G.; Rich, A.N. Finding Cancer in Mammograms: If You Know It's There, Do You Know Where? *Cogn. Res. Princ. Implic.* **2018**, *3*, 1–14. [CrossRef] [PubMed]
13. O'Sullivan, J.W.; Muntinga, T.; Grigg, S.; Ioannidis, J.P.A. Prevalence and Outcomes of Incidental Imaging Findings: Umbrella Review. *BMJ* **2018**, *361*, k2387. [CrossRef]
14. Sarwar, S.; Dent, A.; Faust, K.; Richer, M.; Djuric, U.; van Ommeren, R.; Diamandis, P. Physician Perspectives on Integration of Artificial Intelligence into Diagnostic Pathology. *NPJ Digit. Med.* **2019**, *2*, 28. [CrossRef] [PubMed]
15. Haenssle, H.A.; Fink, C.; Schneiderbauer, R.; Toberer, F.; Buhl, T.; Blum, A.; Kalloo, A.; ben Hadj Hassen, A.; Thomas, L.; Enk, A.; et al. Man against Machine: Diagnostic Performance of a Deep Learning Convolutional Neural Network for Dermoscopic Melanoma Recognition in Comparison to 58 Dermatologists. *Ann. Oncol.* **2018**, *29*, 1836–1842. [CrossRef] [PubMed]
16. Cho, B.J.; Bang, C.S.; Park, S.W.; Yang, Y.J.; Seo, S.I.; Lim, H.; Shin, W.G.; Hong, J.T.; Yoo, Y.T.; Hong, S.H.; et al. Automated Classification of Gastric Neoplasms in Endoscopic Images Using a Convolutional Neural Network. *Endoscopy* **2019**, *51*, 1121–1129. [CrossRef]
17. Astley, S.M.; Harkness, E.F.; Sergeant, J.C.; Warwick, J.; Stavrinos, P.; Warren, R.; Wilson, M.; Beetles, U.; Gadde, S.; Lim, Y.; et al. A Comparison of Five Methods of Measuring Mammographic Density: A Case-Control Study. *Breast Cancer Res.* **2018**, *20*, 10. [CrossRef]
18. French, D.P.; Astley, S.; Astley, S.; Brentnall, A.R.; Cuzick, J.; Dobrashian, R.; Duffy, S.W.; Gorman, L.S.; Gorman, L.S.; Harkness, E.F.; et al. What Are the Benefits and Harms of Risk Stratified Screening as Part of the NHS Breast Screening Programme? Study Protocol for a Multi-Site Non-Randomised Comparison of BC-Predict versus Usual Screening (NCT04359420). *BMC Cancer* **2020**, *20*, 570. [CrossRef]
19. Aerts, H.J.W.L. Data Science in Radiology: A Path Forward. *Clin. Cancer Res.* **2018**, *24*, 532. [CrossRef]
20. Alshamrani, K.; Offiah, A.C. Applicability of Two Commonly Used Bone Age Assessment Methods to Twenty-First Century UK Children. *Eur. Radiol.* **2020**, *30*, 504. [CrossRef]
21. Chilamkurthy, S.; Ghosh, R.; Tanamala, S.; Biviji, M.; Campeau, N.G.; Venugopal, V.K.; Mahajan, V.; Rao, P.; Warier, P. Deep Learning Algorithms for Detection of Critical Findings in Head CT Scans: A Retrospective Study. *Lancet* **2018**, *392*, 2388–2396. [CrossRef] [PubMed]
22. Rodriguez-Ruiz, A.; Lång, K.; Gubern-Merida, A.; Broeders, M.; Gennaro, G.; Clauser, P.; Helbich, T.H.; Chevalier, M.; Tan, T.; Mertelmeier, T.; et al. Stand-Alone Artificial Intelligence for Breast Cancer Detection in Mammography: Comparison With 101 Radiologists. *J. Natl. Cancer Inst.* **2019**, *111*, 916–922. [CrossRef]
23. Codari, M.; Melazzini, L.; Morozov, S.P.; van Kuijk, C.C.; Sconfienza, L.M.; Sardanelli, F. Impact of Artificial Intelligence on Radiology: A EuroAIM Survey among Members of the European Society of Radiology. *Insights Imaging* **2019**, *10*, 105. [CrossRef]
24. Hamon, R.; Junklewitz, H.; Sanchez, I.; European Commission. *Joint Research Centre. Robustness and Explainability of Artificial Intelligence*; Publications Office of the European Union: Luxembourg, 2020. [CrossRef]
25. Zanca, F.; Brusasco, C.; Pesapane, F.; Kwade, Z.; Beckers, R.; Avanzo, M. Regulatory Aspects of the Use of Artificial Intelligence Medical Software. *Semin. Radiat. Oncol.* **2022**, *32*, 432–441. [CrossRef] [PubMed]
26. Arrieta, A.; Díaz-Rodríguez, N.; Del Ser, J.; Bennetot, A.; Tabik, S.; Barbado, A.; García, S.; Gil-López, S.; Molina, D.; Benjamins, R.; et al. Explainable Artificial Intelligence (XAI): Concepts, Taxonomies, Opportunities and Challenges toward Responsible AI. *Inf. Fusion* **2020**, *58*, 82–115. [CrossRef]
27. Cortes, C.; Vapnik, V.; Saitta, L. Support-Vector Networks. *Mach. Learn.* **1995**, *20*, 273–297. [CrossRef]
28. Fan, W.; Liu, J.; Zhu, S.; Pardalos, P.M. Investigating the Impacting Factors for the Healthcare Professionals to Adopt Artificial Intelligence-Based Medical Diagnosis Support System (AIMDSS). *Ann. Oper. Res.* **2020**, *294*, 567–592. [CrossRef]
29. Pesapane, F.; Rotili, A.; Valconi, E.; Agazzi, G.M.; Montesano, M.; Penco, S.; Nicosia, L.; Bozzini, A.; Meneghetti, L.; Latronico, A.; et al. Women's Perceptions and Attitudes to the Use of AI in Breast Cancer Screening: A Survey in a Cancer Referral Centre. *Br. J. Radiol.* **2022**, *95*, 20220569. [CrossRef]
30. Triberti, S.; Durosini, I.; Pravettoni, G. A "Third Wheel" Effect in Health Decision Making Involving Artificial Entities: A Psychological Perspective. *Front. Public Health* **2020**, *8*, 117. [CrossRef] [PubMed]

31. McInnes, M.D.F.; Moher, D.; Thombs, B.D.; McGrath, T.A.; Bossuyt, P.M.; Clifford, T.; Cohen, J.F.; Deeks, J.J.; Gatsonis, C.; Hooft, L.; et al. Preferred Reporting Items for a Systematic Review and Meta-Analysis of Diagnostic Test Accuracy Studies: The PRISMA-DTA Statement. *JAMA* **2018**, *319*, 388–396. [CrossRef]
32. Ongena, Y.P.; Yakar, D.; Haan, M.; Kwee, T.C. Artificial Intelligence in Screening Mammography: A Population Survey of Women's Preferences. *J. Am. Coll. Radiol.* **2021**, *18*, 79–86. [CrossRef]
33. Adams, S.J.; Tang, R.; Babyn, P. Patient Perspectives and Priorities Regarding Artificial Intelligence in Radiology: Opportunities for Patient-Centered Radiology. *J. Am. Coll. Radiol.* **2020**, *17*, 1034–1036. [CrossRef] [PubMed]
34. Carter, S.M.; Rogers, W.; Win, K.T.; Frazer, H.; Richards, B.; Houssami, N. The Ethical, Legal and Social Implications of Using Artificial Intelligence Systems in Breast Cancer Care. *Breast* **2020**, *49*, 25–32. [CrossRef]
35. Mendelson, E.B. Artificial Intelligence in Breast Imaging: Potentials and Limitations. *Am. J. Roentgenol.* **2019**, *212*, 293–299. [CrossRef] [PubMed]
36. Kapoor, N.; Lacson, R.; Khorasani, R. Workflow Applications of Artificial Intelligence in Radiology and an Overview of Available Tools. *J. Am. Coll. Radiol.* **2020**, *17*, 1363–1370. [CrossRef] [PubMed]
37. O'Connor, S.D.; Dalal, A.K.; Anik Sahni, V.; Lacson, R.; Khorasani, R. Does Integrating Nonurgent, Clinically Significant Radiology Alerts within the Electronic Health Record Impact Closed-Loop Communication and Follow-Up? *J. Am. Med. Inform. Assoc.* **2016**, *23*, 333. [CrossRef] [PubMed]
38. Haan, M.; Ongena, Y.P.; Hommes, S.; Kwee, T.C.; Yakar, D. A Qualitative Study to Understand Patient Perspective on the Use of Artificial Intelligence in Radiology. *J. Am. Coll. Radiol.* **2019**, *16*, 1416–1419. [CrossRef] [PubMed]
39. Coiera, E. The Fate of Medicine in the Time of AI. *Lancet* **2018**, *392*, 2331–2332. [CrossRef]
40. McCabe, R.; Healey, P.G.T. Miscommunication in Doctor–Patient Communication. *Top. Cogn. Sci.* **2018**, *10*, 409–424. [CrossRef] [PubMed]
41. Ahuja, A.S. The Impact of Artificial Intelligence in Medicine on the Future Role of the Physician. *PeerJ* **2019**, *7*, e7702. [CrossRef]

Disclaimer/Publisher's Note: The statements, opinions and data contained in all publications are solely those of the individual author(s) and contributor(s) and not of MDPI and/or the editor(s). MDPI and/or the editor(s) disclaim responsibility for any injury to people or property resulting from any ideas, methods, instructions or products referred to in the content.

MDPI
St. Alban-Anlage 66
4052 Basel
Switzerland
www.mdpi.com

Cancers Editorial Office
E-mail: cancers@mdpi.com
www.mdpi.com/journal/cancers

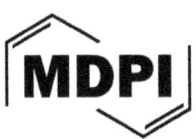

Disclaimer/Publisher's Note: The statements, opinions and data contained in all publications are solely those of the individual author(s) and contributor(s) and not of MDPI and/or the editor(s). MDPI and/or the editor(s) disclaim responsibility for any injury to people or property resulting from any ideas, methods, instructions or products referred to in the content.

www.ingramcontent.com/pod-product-compliance
Lightning Source LLC
LaVergne TN
LVHW070208100526
838202LV00015B/2019